Practical Chronic Pain Management

Tariq Malik
Editor

Practical Chronic Pain Management

A Case-Based Approach

Springer

Editor
Tariq Malik
Department of Anesthesia and Critical Care
University of Chicago
Chicago, IL
USA

ISBN 978-3-030-46674-9 ISBN 978-3-030-46675-6 (eBook)
https://doi.org/10.1007/978-3-030-46675-6

This Springer imprint is published by the registered company Springer Nature Switzerland AG
The registered company address is: Gewerbestrasse 11, 6330 Cham, Switzerland

Foreword

This book is case-based presentation on the management of chronic pain syndromes. The book starts with a nice overview of the evaluation of patients with pain. It is followed by pain syndromes in the head and neck, shoulder and hand, chest, abdomen, pelvis, and inguinal region, then back, buttock, and lower extremity pain. Total body pain, neuropathic and cancer pain, and pain managed by intrathecal medications are also discussed. The chapters follow a similar format. They begin with an introduction, then a case presentation; diagnosis vis-à-vis the patient's history, physical examination, and laboratory and imaging studies; pathophysiology; treatments including pharmacologic, interventional, and other modalities; and finally end with a concluding paragraph. The references, for a case-based manuscript, are more than adequate. They range from 17 to over 70 references.

Books on chronic pain have run the gamut from standard texts, reviews, case presentations, question and answer format, or on specific topics such as complications. The availability of these different formats is to adapt to the preferences and needs of the clinician or researcher. Each format has its own unique style, advantages, and disadvantages. Some clinicians prefer the case-based approach as it provides similarities with patients that they encounter and improved recall of the available tools for management of their patients with difficult pain syndromes. As such, this book has a definite role in a busy clinician's library.

This book by Dr. Tariq Malik provides an opportunity for the reader to gain insights on the signs and symptoms, available therapeutic options, difficulties to be encountered, and possible results of management of the different chronic pain syndromes. The efforts of Dr. Malik and the chapter authors should be recognized and appreciated.

Honorio T. Benzon, MD
Professor Anesthesiology
Northwestern University
Feinberg Medical School
Chicago, IL, USA

Preface

> Divine is the task to relieve pain.
>
> —Hippocrates

Chronic pain is still an enigma. It is poorly understood and poorly managed. The situation is no different than that of general anesthesia, where the physiology and mechanism of general anesthetics is poorly understood but still millions of patients are being administered general anesthesia for various surgical procedures. Same way, millions of people are suffering from chronic pain , they visit primary care clinics, emergency rooms, and pain clinics , and are given various therapies but with little understanding of the underlying disease and even less evidence of support for the various therapies they are being administered. Chronic pain is the most common disease in the world but somehow is quite underappreciated in its burden on humanity and hence poorly taught in medical school, and even during postgraduate medical training. The epidemic nature of the condition is bound to get worse with the inevitable change in demographics that is bound to happen worldwide as the incidence of this condition increases with age. There is a plethora of books on chronic pain management out there. The books range in sizes from being very small to huge. But at the end of the day, a clinician wants a practical way to manage a patient.

This book has been written keeping that aspect in mind. It's not a textbook explaining theory or mechanism of painful conditions. Nor is it a manual of injection techniques. The text is focused on problem-based disease management. The idea is how treat a painful condition in a step-by-step manner and what is the thought process and evidence behind each intervention.

The book covers 45 common painful conditions. Chapters have been written by various physicians who come from various backgrounds. The main focus is to keep the approach evidence based and provide level of evidence for each intervention.

It's a humbling experience to write a book on chronic pain as one gets to know how little is known and how far we have still to go. In the end, I thank everyone who has contributed to this book, as without their effort, nothing would have been possible.

Chicago, IL, USA — Tariq Malik

Contents

Contributors

Alaa Abd-Elsayed, MD, MPH Department of Anesthesiology, University of Wisconsin School of Medicine and Public Health, Madison, WI, USA

Hassan Aboumerhi, MD Department of Anesthesiology, Northwestern University, Chicago, IL, USA

E. B. Braun, MD Department of Anesthesiology, University of Kansas Medical Center, Kansas City, KS, USA

Kenneth D. Candido, MD Department of Anesthesiology, Advocate Illinois Masonic Medical Center, Chicago, IL, USA

Department of Anesthesiology, University of Illinois, Chicago, IL, USA

Department of Surgery, University of Illinois, Chicago, IL, USA

Paul K. Cheng, MD Department of Anesthesiology and Pain Medicine, UC Davis Medical Center, Sacramento, CA, USA

Jonathan Church, MD Department of Anesthesiology, Chicago, IL, USA

University Pain Centers, Chicago, IL, USA

Dalia H. Elmofty, MD Department of Anesthesia, University of Chicago, Chicago, IL, USA

Dan Fischer, MD Department of Anesthesiology and Critical Care, University of Chicago, Chicago, IL, USA

J. M. Foster, MD Department of Anesthesiology, University of Kansas Medical Center, Kansas City, KS, USA

Robert Fuino, MD Department of Neurology, University of Vermont Medical Center, Burlington, VT, USA

Sonia Gill, MD Department of Anesthesiology and Critical Care, University of Chicago, Chicago, IL, USA

Evan Goodman, MD Department of Anesthesiology and Critical Care, University of Chicago, Chicago, IL, USA

Joseph Graham, DO Department of Physical Medicine and Rehabilitation, Schwab Hospital, Chicago, IL, USA

Armen Haroutunian, MD Department of Anesthesiology, Advocate Illinois Masonic Medical Center, Chicago, IL, USA

Sumit Jain, MD Department of Anesthesiology, Northshore University, Evanston, IL, USA

Khyrie Jones, MD Schwab Rehabilitation Hospital & Care Network/ University of Chicago, Chicago, IL, USA

T. W. Khan, MD Department of Anesthesiology, University of Kansas Medical Center, Kansas City, KS, USA

Ahmad Khattab, DO Department of Anesthesiology and Critical Care, University of Chicago, Chicago, IL, USA

David H. Kim, MD, MS Department of Anesthesiology and Pain Medicine, Kansas University Medical Center, Kansas City, KS, USA

Nicholas Kirch, MD Department of Anesthesiology and Critical Care, University of Chicago, Chicago, IL, USA

Nebojsa Nick Knezevic, MD, PhD Department of Anesthesiology, Advocate Illinois Masonic Medical Center, Chicago, IL, USA

Department of Anesthesiology, University of Illinois, Chicago, IL, USA

Department of Surgery, University of Illinois, Chicago, IL, USA

Lynn R. Kohan, MD, MS Department of Anesthesiology, University of Virginia Health System, Charlottesville, VA, USA

Wyatt Kupperman, DO Neurological Institute, Cleveland Clinic, Cleveland, OH, USA

Teresa M. Kusper, DO, MBS Department of Anesthesiology, Advocate Illinois Masonic Medical Center, Chicago, IL, USA

Usman Latif, MD Department of Anesthesiology, University of Kansas Medical Center, Kansas City, KS, USA

Mary Leemputte, MD Department of Anesthesiology, Northwestern University, Chicago, IL, USA

Tariq Malik, MD Department of Physical Medicine and Rehabilitation, Schwab Hospital, Chicago, IL, USA

Naveed Mameghani, MD Department of Anesthesia and Critical Care, University of Chicago, Chicago, IL, USA

Darshan Patel, MD Department of Anesthesiology, St. Francis Medical Center, Evanston, IL, USA

Daneel M. Patoli, MD Department of Anesthesiology and Critical Care, University of Chicago, Chicago, IL, USA

Behnoosh B. Rahavard, MD Department of Anesthesiology, Advocate Illinois Masonic Medical Center, Chicago, IL, USA

Arjun Ramesh, MD Department of Anesthesiology, Rush University, Chicago, IL, USA

Maunak V. Rana, MD Department of Anesthesiology and Critical Care, University of Chicago, Chicago, IL, USA

A. Sack, MD Department of Anesthesiology, University of Kansas Medical Center, Kansas City, KS, USA

Jonathan K. Song, DO Department of Physical Medicine and Rehabilitation, Schwab Rehabilitation Hospital/University of Chicago, Chicago, IL, USA

T. M. Sowder, MD Department of Anesthesiology, University of Kansas Medical Center, Kansas City, KS, USA

Adam S. Sprouse Blum, MD Department of Neurological Sciences, University of Vermont, Burlington, VT, USA

Brady Still, MD Department of Anesthesia and Critical Care, University of Chicago, Chicago, IL, USA

Rup Tandan, MD Department of Neurology, University of Vermont Medical Center, Burlington, VT, USA

Beth VanderWielen, MD Department of Anesthesiology, University of Wisconsin-Madison Hospitals and Clinics, Madison, WI, USA

Waqar Waheed, MD Department of Neurosciences, University of Vermont Medical Center, Burlington, VT, USA

Andrew Wendahl, MD Department of Anesthesiology, University of Wisconsin School of Medicine and Public Health, Madison, WI, USA

Adam C. Young, MD Department of Anesthesiology and Pain Management, Illinois Bone and Joint Institute, Morton Grove, IL, USA

Pain Management Divison, Illinois Bone and Joint Institute, Morton Grove, IL, USA

Sophy C. Zheng, MD Department of Anesthesiology, Northwestern Memorial Hospital, Chicago, IL, USA

Xiaoying Zhu, MD, PhD Department of Anesthesiology, University of Virginia Health System, Charlottesville, VA, USA

Thomas Zouki, MD Department of Anesthesiology, Texas Tech University Health Sciences Center, Lubbock, TX, USA

Muhammad Zubair, MD Department of Anesthesiology, Advocate Illinois Masonic Medical Center, Chicago, IL, USA

ABCs of Chronic Pain Evaluation

1

Tariq Malik

Chronic pain is a debilitating disease. It is the most prevalent chronic disease all over the world. It affects about 20 percent of US adults and 8 percent of them would rate it as high-impact chronic pain—meaning pain limited at least one major life activity per a mail survey conducted in 2016 [1]. It costs US economy roughly 635 billion dollars a year [2]. Chronic pain is quite different from acute pain which is a symptom and is a hallmark of tissue injury, self-limited and quite responsive to medical management invariably. The management of acute pain is directed at the underlying disease causing tissue injury. Chronic pain is not a symptom but a disease itself. It is poorly understood and poorly characterized. Even with all the current treatment options available, less than half of the chronic pain sufferers may have their pain alleviated by about 30–40% on average, rest continue to suffer.

Our understanding of chronic pain as a disease influences how we evaluate a chronic pain patient. Medical schools and medical field in general are traditionally trained to think in terms of mechanical disorder, no different than an auto mechanic who wants to fix a car. Clinicians, and the lay public alike, look for some underlying pathology to account for the chronic pain. Their focus on thorough history and physical examination, followed, by laboratory tests and diagnostic imaging procedures, is an attempt to identify or confirm the presence of any underlying pathology that causes the symptom—the so-called pain generator. This focus on locating an identifiable pathology creates frustration in the mind of chronic pain patients who are looking for answers, which leads to frustration, emotional distress, an illusion of chronic pain being as a psychosomatic illness, financially drain patients, and their loss of faith in the medical system. It is not unusual for the chronic pain patients to doctor shop in desperation. This mechanistic view of diseases in medical practice, dating back at least to Descartes in 1644, who in the era of Kepler and Newton thought human body works like a machine or a clock, just like the solar system, and most likely may follow the same laws as the universe does. It is, however, incomplete and is not supported by available research or the current understanding of chronic pain [3]. The current model of pain has evolved from specificity theory of pain, to gate theory of pain to neuromatrix theory of pain. The poor comprehension of chronic pain disorder is a direct result of the poor understanding of human brain and human mind. So far, we do not have the tools to understand brain physiology. To paraphrase a neuroscientist, "we understand how the action potential happens in a nerve fiber, but how all these action potentials lead to emotions, thoughts or dreams is not

T. Malik (✉)
Department of Anesthesia and Critical Care, University of Chicago, Chicago, IL, USA
e-mail: TMuslim@dacc.uchicago.edu; tmalik@dacc.uchicago.edu

T. Malik (ed.), *Practical Chronic Pain Management*, https://doi.org/10.1007/978-3-030-46675-6_1

understood at all." Brain is more or less a black hole for us so far. This leads to the main problem in chronic pain management—poor pain evaluation. Chronic pain evaluation is purely a clinical affair. There is no lab testing or imaging process that can quantify chronic pain burden. This injects subjectivity in the whole assessment. Chronic pain is a complex, multifaceted disease which affects not only body and mind of the patient, but also has feeds of patient's interaction with his surroundings both at home and at work. Effective treatment can only come from a comprehensive assessment of the biological etiology of the pain in conjunction with the patient's specific psychosocial and behavioral presentation, including their emotional state (e.g., anxiety, depression, and anger), perception and understanding of symptoms, and reactions to those symptoms by people around them [3–5].

Evaluating a Chronic Pain Patient

The evaluation starts with a referral from a primary care physician (PCP). The idea is that the PCP should ensure that there is no medical disease that is responsible for the patient's illness. In short, they should rule out any tumor-related, rheumatological, infectious, or ischemic issues. Pain evaluation is in general no different from any other medical evaluation. The main end point is to arrive at a diagnosis. The process of inquiry or evaluation should continue till a diagnosis is accurate and complete. The key question is what is a complete and accurate diagnosis? One problem that is commonly encountered in chronic pain evaluation is that patients are given presumptive diagnosis without much thought and over times the patient is convinced that he or she has that disease. The author has developed the rule that patient should be given a diagnosis unless it can be backed by evidence acceptable in a court of law, i.e., knowing that it is hard to be sure every time, at least the diagnosis should be backed by evidence that is beyond a reasonable doubt with reasonable degree of medical certainty. The second element deals with completeness of diagnosis. This is important to appreciate as once done, further work is not needed. A complete diagnosis has certain components. (1) It should point out the organ of dysfunction or the pain generator. (2) It should account for the pathophysiology in the organ causing pain. (3) It should account for the extent of dysfunction. (4) It should account for the suffering/loss of function (pain catastrophizing, pain disability, coping skills, and other emotional stresses) [6].

To achieve these endpoints, information is gathered from the patient not only using a standard format of history and physical examination, but also using many standardized assessment instruments/ questionnaires. The idea is to evaluate the "whole person" or the disease and not just the pain or symptom. As there is no "algometer" or a lab test that can quantify suffering or severity of pain experienced by the patient, it can only be assessed by the patient's overt communication, both verbal and nonverbal. Regardless of whether a biological basis for the pain can be ascertained, or whether psychosocial problems were caused by, or resulted from pain, the assessment process can be helpful in identifying how biomedical, psychosocial, and behavioral factors interact to influence the nature, severity, persistence of pain and disability, and response to treatment.

History and Physical Examination

As already mentioned, chronic pain evaluation is completely a clinical process. Just like a psychologist or psychiatrist, it is all between the pain physician and the patient; the physician has to totally rely on his or her clinical skills. Other than gathering data, the aim of this clinical interview is to develop trusting relation with the patient. The general goals of this clinical interaction are as follows: (i) determine the pain generator or pathology; (ii) determine the need for any additional diagnostic testing; (iii) determine extent of loss of quality of life, (iv) examine all previously tied treatments and results of those interventions; (v) determine dosage of medications used and any side effects; and (vi) educate the patient about the plan to manage the problem for which there might not be any cure. Physical examination is more important to develop bond with the patient than to diagnose a chronic pain disorder.

A great number of patients that report chronic pain tend to have no positive finding on plain radiographs, computed axial tomography scans, or on electromyography, making a precise pathological diagnosis difficult or impossible [7].

Standard Questionnaires

In addition to this standard medical evaluation approach, an appropriate patient assessment requires an evaluation of patient's mental condition, coping skills, and disability from pain. A number of questionnaires are available to comprehensively evaluate the patient. These questionnaires are easy and inexpensive to administer, quickly assess a wide range of behaviors, obtain information about behaviors that patients may feel uncomfortable about disclosing (sexual relations) or are unobservable (thoughts, emotional arousal) and, most importantly, their reliability and validity can be assessed. These questionnaires are not a substitute for clinical interview. They complement the clinical interview as the findings may suggest issues that would require greater or more detailed exploration during a subsequent visit or referral to another specialist.

There are a plethora of screening tools available. They vary in which domain of pain they target. They are not only useful as a screening tool but are also very helpful in gauging patient response to any intervention.

Pain intensity scales are limited in their value as in general they do not give the complete picture. The information depends upon the context as some patients would mark the score based on the worst pain score since the last physician visit while others would mark it based on the pain they are experiencing while sitting in the chair at the physician's office. It is important to ask the patient about the pain score if the score reflect resting pain, worst pain during activity, or overall average pain (Table 1.1). It is more important to ask and document pain during various activities and compare the pain score change with interventions. Pain intensity daily diary would be truly helpful if properly filled but many patients forget to follow the instructions and the data is not that useful then.

Table 1.1 Commonly used tools for chronic pain assessment

Pain intensity measurement
(a) Numerical Rating Scale (NRS) 0–10, 0–100
(b) Verbal Rating Scale (VRS) mild, moderate, severe
(c) Visual Analog Scale (VAS) pain intensity using 10 or 100 mm line
(d) Facial Pain Scale (FPS) pain intensity using a range of facial expressions
Pain quality
(a) McGill Pain Questionnaire
(b) Neuropathic Pain Scale (NPS)
(c) Regional Pain Scale (RPS)
(d) Leeds Assessment of Neuropathic Symptoms and Sign Scale (LANSS)
(e) Pain DETECT(PD-Q
(f) Douleur Neuropathique 4 (DN4)
Effect on life
(a) Pain Disability Index
(b) Brief Pain Inventory
(c) Functional Independence Measure
(d) Short-Form Health Survey (SF-36 or SF-12)
Disease-specific pain assessment
(a) Western Ontario McMaster Osteoarthritis Index (WOMAC)
(b) Fibromyalgia Impact Questionnaire
(c) Roland-Morris Disability Questionnaire (for back pain)
Psychosocial measures
(a) Beck Depression Inventory
(b) Pain Catastrophizing Scale
(c) Coping Strategies Questionnaire

Pain Quality

Characterizing pain quality is helpful in some situations (characterizing a neuropathic pain), but in general does not make a huge difference in patient management. Various questionnaires have been developed to diagnose neuropathic pain such as pain DETECT(PD-Q), Leeds Assessment of Neuropathic Symptoms and Sign Scale (LANSS), the Douleur Neuropathique 4 (DN4), and the standardized evaluation of pain (StEP) questionnaire. Screening tools are comprised of an interview component and, in some cases, the addition of a brief bedside clinical assessment. Many of these tools have been translated for application in other languages and populations. There is no recognized objective gold standard for assessing NP. However, the Special Interest Group on Neuropathic Pain (NeuPSIG) of the International Association for the Study of Pain has set out a grading system, which is not often used in routine clinical practice, to guide clinical assessment and diagnosis of neuropathic pain. This approach involves multiple steps including obtaining a clinical history of pain, using any of the standard screening questionnaire, which would be suggestive of neuropathic pain (grade I: neuropathic pain possible), assessing the neuroanatomical plausibility of pain, using sensory assessments during physical examination, loss or diminished sensation to touch, vibration, temperature, or pinprick, to confirm nervous system involvement (grade II:probably neuropathic pain), and running diagnostic tests (skin biopsy to look for reduced intraepidermal nerve fiber density; neurophysiological tests such as nerve conduction velocity, heat and laser evoked potentials, nerve excitability tests, R1 blink reflex demonstrating neural function compromise; microneurography to show aberrant nociceptor activity; and genetic tests confirming a hereditary neuropathic pain disorder such as inherited erythromelalgia) [8]. In general, the screening tools are helpful in pointing toward a direction point but do not make much impact in patient outcome as all neuropathic pain are managed more or less the same.

The McGill Pain Questionnaire (MPQ) [9] assesses three categories of word descriptors of pain qualities (sensory, affective, and evaluative) and includes a body diagram for patients to identify the area of their pain. Patients may take 10–15 minutes to fill the original form, so a revised and version of this scale, Short-Form McGill Pain Questionnaire revised (SF-MPQ-2) was developed and is one of the most frequently used measures to assess pain characteristics [10].

Functional Limitations

This is the most important aspect of evaluation and is the main target of all chronic pain interventions. Chronic pain invariably affects patients' personal physical capacities such as affecting their activities of daily living (ADL), as well as their ability to perform an adult role in the family like keeping a job, supervising, or driving kids to and from school or games. Most patients with chronic pain acknowledge that their overall physical functioning was much below par because of their pain, supporting the recommendation that assessment of functioning should be an integral part of pain assessment [11, 12]. The inability to perform necessary and desired functions and stay involved in family activities significantly impact quality of life. This negative effect cannot be easily picked by physical examination and is the reason that that has led to the development of self-report functional status measures to quantify symptoms, function, and behavior directly, and the severity of pain when performing specific activities (e.g., ability to walk upstairs or lift specific weights, sitting for specific periods of time) associated with different types of painful conditions (e.g., osteoarthritis, low back pain).

Research has shown the importance of assessing overall quality of life in chronic pain patients in addition to function [13]. A number of such questionnaires are available, some are general in application and can be used in any chronic pain condition, namely, Short-Form Health Survey (SF-36) [14] or Pain Disability Index [15]. Disease-specific functional assessment tools are also available, namely, Western Ontario McMaster Osteoarthritis Index (WOMAC) [16] or Roland-Morris Back Pain Disability Questionnaire (RDQ) [17]; these tools are very good measure of assessing disease-related pain burden as well as any improvement after an intervention. The whole purpose of using these questionnaires is to have a more complete picture of chronic pain patient's life which cannot be achieved by a clinical interview solely.

Pain Coping Assessment/Behavioral Assessment

The chronic pain invariably leads to emotional distress, particularly depression, anxiety, anger, and irritability, and sleep disorder [18]. These emotional and psychological issues not only complicate pain evaluation but also complicate how to interpret efficacy of a pain intervention. The presence of fatigue and impairment realted to the cognitive issues can come from medications so assessing them upfront is quite important. Beck Depression Inventory (BDI) or the Profile of Mood States (POMS) can be used to assess mental health of chronic pain patients. Equally important is to screen for anxiety disorder or presence of pain catastrophizing trait using screening tools (Pain Catastrophizing Scale) [19].

Conclusion

The multidimensional nature of chronic pain requires a multidimensional assessment. The proper assessment is crucial in making a proper management plan, and without a proper treatment plan, the treatment is bound to fail. Given the subjective nature of pain, the assessment of pain is always a subjective process and totally relies on optimum communication between the patient and the pain physician. Despite having a good relation, it is quite often that the patient cannot totally express him or herself or cannot convey effectively the loss or suffering in his or her life. In addition to having to express his suffering effectivley, the ability to recall an event or pain experience is flawed or inconsistent and depends on the emotional state of the patient. It is because of all these confounding factors that use self-reported questionnaires are very helpful in developing a complete picture of a patient; they should be used to track progress of the patient during subsequent visits. They add an element of objectivity to a very subjective assessment and can be used to assess an effectiveness of any intervention employed.

At the end of the day, all these questionnaires or screening tools are just what they are—just screening or assessment tools and requires careful clinical interpretation. They are data points and by themselves do not mean anything. They still require a clinician who can put these data points in proper context and make a sense out of them. To interpret these data points and make use of this formation in order to help the patient, one still needs to practice art of medicine for medicine is a still a for a large part a social science and not a pure physical science yet.

References

1. Dahlhamer J, Lucas J, Zelaya C, et al. Prevalence of chronic pain and high-impact chronic pain among adults — United States, 2016. Accessed on 11 Jun 2019 https://www.cdc.gov/mmwr/volumes/67/wr/mm6736a2.htm.
2. Gaskin DJ, Richard P. The economic costs of pain in the United States. J Pain. 2012;13(8):715.
3. Flor H, Turk DC. Chronic pain: an integrated biobehavioral approach. Seattle: IASP Press; 2011.
4. Fordyce WE. Behavioral methods for chronic pain and illness. St. Louis: CV Mosby; 1976.
5. Turk DC, Meichenbaum D, Genest M. Pain and behavior medicine: a cognitive-behavioral perspective. New York: Guilford Press; 1983.
6. Turk DC, Robinson JP. Assessment of patients with chronic pain— a comprehensive approach. In: Turk DC, Melzack R, editors. Handbook of pain assessment. 3rd ed. New York: Guilford Press; 2011. p. 188–210.
7. Turk DC, Melzack R. Handbook of pain assessment. 3rd ed. New York: Guilford Press; 2011.
8. Finnerup NB, Haroutounian S, Kamerman P, et al. Neuropathic pain: an updated grading system for research and clinical practice. Pain. 2016;157(8):1599–606.
9. Melzack R. The McGill pain questionnaire: major properties and scoring methods. Pain. 1975;1:277–99.
10. Melzack R. The short-form McGill pain questionnaire. Pain. 1987;30:191–7.
11. Turk DC, Dworkin RH, Revicki D, et al. Identifying important outcome domains for chronic pain clinical trials: an IMMPACT survey of people with pain. Pain. 2008;137:276–85.
12. Turk DC, Dworkin RH, Allen RR, et al. Core outcome domains for chronic pain clinical trials: IMMPACT recommendations. Pain. 2003;106:337–45.
13. Gladman DD, Mease PJ, Strand V, et al. Consensus on a core set of domains for psoriatic arthritis. J Rheumatol. 2007;34:1167–70.
14. Ware JE Jr, Sherbourne CD. The MOS 36-item short-form health survey (SF-36): I. conceptual framework and item selection. Med Care. 1992;30:473–83.
15. Pollard CA. Preliminary validity study of the pain disability index. Percept Mot Skills. 1984;59:974.
16. Bellamy N, Buchanan WW, Goldsmith CH, Campbell J, Stitt LW. Validation study of WOMAC: a health status instrument for measuring clinically important patient relevant outcomes to antirheumatic drug therapy in patients with osteoarthritis of the hip or knee. J Rheumatol. 1988;15:1833–40.
17. Roland M, Morris R. A study of the natural history of back pain. Part I: development of a reliable and sensitive measure of disability in low-back pain. Spine. 1983;8:141–4.
18. Turk DC, Okifuji A. Psychological factors in chronic pain: evolution and revolution. J Consult Clin Psychol. 2002;70:678–90.
19. Sullivan MJL, Bishop SR, Pivik J. The pain catastrophizing scale: development and validation. Psychol Assess. 1995;7:524–32.

2 A 40-Year-Old Woman with Chronic Recurrent Headache (Migraine)

Adam S. Sprouse Blum

Case Description

Karla M. is a 40-year-old attorney. She was a healthy child, with the exception of asthma which resolved as she got older. She experienced menarche at 11 years old and developed headaches around the same time. Through high school she occasionally missed class because of severe headaches. In college she tended to have attacks around exams, particularly if she stayed up all night studying, and around menses. Changes in weather also seemed to precipitate attacks. At 22 years old, she was diagnosed with irritable bowel syndrome. At 28 and 34 years old, she gave birth to her two children. Headaches improved dramatically during both pregnancies. Her second pregnancy was complicated by pre-eclampsia, which was effectively managed. Within a month of giving birth to her second child, she noticed a change in her headaches. Her headache frequency and severity increased and the location of her head pain shifted from being centered around her left or right temple to involving her entire head as well as her mid face and upper neck. She now experiences some amount of head pain most days, 4–6 days per month they are severe.

Up to 24 hours prior to an attack, her sense of smell is heightened, she feels fatigued, and she has difficulty concentrating. With some, but not all, attacks she experiences tingling numbness affecting her right upper extremity and the right side of her face and tongue. She also reports difficulty expressing herself verbally with these attacks. These symptoms last 5–10 minutes and occur at the onset of headache. Occasionally, she will have these symptoms without headache. When she does experience headaches, they usually involve her entire head and are throbbing in nature, severity achieves 7–8/10, and light and noise bother her for which she seeks a dark quiet room. Associated symptoms frequently include nausea (though she rarely vomits) as well as a sense of disequilibrium. Most attacks last 4–6 hours but lingering non-headache symptoms may persist all day. After an attack, she feels exhausted.

Karla is now trying to become a partner in her law firm, but is finding it increasingly difficult to "just push through." Her headaches are interfering with her career goals which is why she has come to you for help.

What Is Your Preliminary Diagnosis?

Karla's most likely diagnosis is migraine with aura. Migraine is three times more common in women [1] and tends to emerge or shift around a hormonal milestone, as is the case above with onset around menarche. Karla has a history of

A. S. Sprouse Blum (✉)
Department of Neurological Sciences, University of Vermont, Burlington, VT, USA
e-mail: Adam.Sprouse-Blum@uvmhealth.org

T. Malik (ed.), *Practical Chronic Pain Management*, https://doi.org/10.1007/978-3-030-46675-6_2

both asthma and irritable bowel syndrome, both which are more common in people with migraine [2, 3]. Other conditions that are more common in people with migraine include depression, anxiety, Raynaud's phenomenon, obstructive sleep apnea [2], idiopathic gastroparesis [4] and interstitial cystitis [5], among others.

Karla identified specific migraine triggers including stressful life events, lack of sleep, menses, and changes in weather. These are common migraine triggers [6]. During pregnancy, migraine is often variable during the first trimester but improves during the second and third [7]. Preeclampsia is more common in patients with migraine and may share a common pathophysiology [8]. Migraine often shifts after giving birth, as it did for Karla, in terms of frequency, severity, or presentation [9].

Prior to attacks, Karla experiences a heightened sense of smell (osmophobia), fatigue, and difficulty concentrating. These are common components of the migraine premonitory phase which is of variable duration and occurs prior to attacks (Fig. 2.1). Karla also experiences migraine aura in the form of both a sensory disturbance (unilateral tingling numbness) and a speech disturbance. By definition [10], migraine aura must last at least 5 minutes. Migraine aura occurs in about one-third of migraine sufferers [11, 12] and classically presents just prior to the headache phase but may occur during headache or without headache. During an attack, Karla reports pain affecting her entire head including her mid face and upper neck. Mid face pain is common in migraine but often mistaken for sinus disease [13]. Pain at the upper neck is another commonly misdiagnosed and overlooked migraine symptom. It is thought to be due to the connections between the trigeminal nerve and the upper two cervical nerves in the trigeminal nucleus in the pons [14], which may be sensitized in migraine [15]. After an attack, many patients experience a migraine "postdrome" consisting of various symptoms including fatigue, difficulty concentrating, and stiff neck [16].

How Is the Diagnosis Confirmed?

Migraine is a clinical diagnosis made based on the patient's report of their symptoms. The International Classification of Headache Disorders 3rd edition (ICHD-3, available online at: www.ichd-3.org) is a detailed hierarchical classification created as a diagnostic reference for clinicians and researchers.

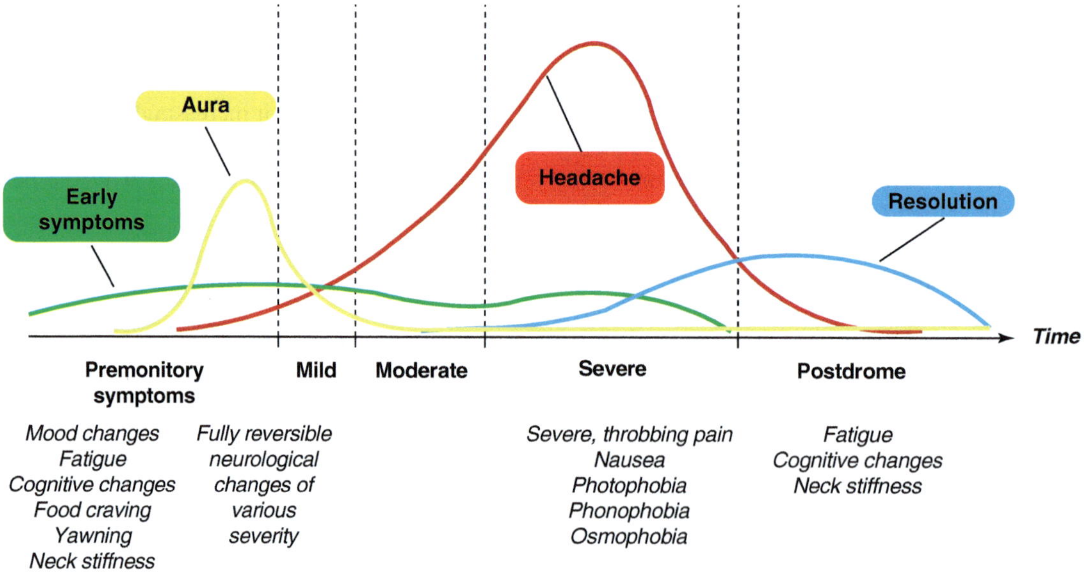

Fig. 2.1 Phases of a migraine attack. (Adapted from Ong et al. [54], with permission)

Keep in mind that both light *and* noise sensitivity are required to fulfill criterion D.2. When a patient is missing one of criteria A through D, they are classified as having "probable" migraine.

Applying the ICHD-3 criteria, Karla's symptoms of repeated attacks of headache lasting at least 4 hours, that are pulsating (throbbing) in nature, with moderate to severe pain intensity, associated with nausea, light and noise sensitivity meet criteria for migraine. When making a migraine diagnosis, it is also important to clarify whether aura is present since aura is associated with increased risk of ischemic stroke and may have important treatment ramifications. Karla's experience of right-sided sensory changes and speech disturbance lasting at least 5 minutes meet criteria for migraine aura.

What Is the Pathophysiology of This Condition?

Our understanding of migraine pathophysiology has evolved over time. For decades, migraine was believed to be a purely vascular condition involving dilation or stretching of cerebral blood vessels. However, as imaging techniques improved we understood that some, but not all subjects experience changes in the caliber of cerebral vessels during attacks [17–19]. This recognition gave rise to the theory that migraine is a primary problem of the nervous system. The nervous system theory of migraine is supported by observations of both anatomical [20] and functional [21] changes in the brain of subjects with migraine. However, the nervous system theory ignores the vascular changes that also occur. We now think of migraine as a neurovascular disorder, appreciating the changes observed in both systems [15]. However, connecting these systems into a unified theory has proven enigmatic.

In an attempt to explain the changes observed in both the vascular and nervous systems in migraine, one prominent theory suggests migraine is due to a cascade of events set off by a process called cortical spreading depression (CSD). CSD is a slow moving (2–5 mm/min) wave of depolarization that spreads through the gray matter of the brain resulting in a decrease in spontaneous cortical activity [22]. CSD has previously been shown to be the cause of migraine visual aura [23]. CSD has also been shown to induce the release of inflammatory mediators [24]. These inflammatory mediators are believed to cause migraine by diffusing toward the surface of the brain to induce a sterile inflammatory reaction of the dura [15]. The dura, unlike the brain, is pain sensitive. Nociceptive information from the dura is transmitted by sensory afferents that travel primarily through the V1 (ophthalmic) branch of the trigeminal nerve to the trigeminal cervical complex then via second order neurons to multiple brainstem structures (e.g., thalamus, hypothalamus, basal ganglia nuclei) which then project to multiple cortical areas (e.g., somatosensory, insula, auditory, visual, olfactory cortices) involved in processing these nociceptive signals and contributing to the varied symptoms of the migraine syndrome [15, 25].

While the current theory successfully connects the neural and vascular systems, some clinical observations still must be reconciled. For example, most subjects with migraine do not experience aura, aura may occur in isolation (without headache), and aura may occur simultaneously with other symptoms of migraine [27], leaving room for modification to the current theory.

How Is This Problem Managed?

The pharmacologic management of migraine can be divided into *acute treatment* and *preventive therapy*.

Acute Treatment

Three groups of medications are commonly used in the acute treatment of migraine: (1) "migraine-specific" treatments (e.g. triptans, gepants, ditans), (2) nonsteroidal anti-inflammatory drugs (NSAIDs), and (3) dopamine antagonists. We often provide patients with one agent from each group, then allow the patient to decide which agent or combination they prefer for a particular attack. Allowing the patient to choose their treatment based on the severity of attack is referred to as stratified care, and is the preferred approach to acute treatment [26]. Many patients prefer to take an NSAID for a low-severity headache and a migraine-specific treatment such as a triptan plus an NSAID and/or dopamine antagonist for a severe attack. There are currently seven triptan medications available. Some triptans are available in more than one mode of delivery (e.g., tablet, oral dissolving tablet, nasal spray, nasal powder, subcutaneous injection). For patients with nausea with vomiting, a non-oral route is preferred. In general, triptans should be taken as early as possible into an attack and may be repeated after 2 hours for incomplete relief. Common side effects include flushing, paresthesia, and chest or jaw discomfort or tightness [28]. Contraindications include ischemic heart disease (e.g., angina, myocardial infarction) and cerebrovascular syndromes (e.g., stroke, transient ischemic attack). Dopamine antagonists are effective for both the nausea and headache of migraine [29]. Common side effects include drowsiness and restlessness. The risk of tardive dyskinesia increases with duration of exposure and cumulative dose [30].

Preventive Therapy

Pharmacologic preventive therapy of migraine can be divided into nutraceuticals and pharmaceuticals.

The currently recommended nutraceuticals are magnesium citrate (400–600 mg/day), riboflavin (400 mg/day), and coenzyme Q10 (300 mg/day) [31].

Pharmaceutical agents which are FDA approved for migraine prevention include topiramate (100 mg/day) [32], divalproex sodium (1000 mg/day) [33], propranolol (80–240 mg/day) [34], timolol (10–30 mg/day) [35], onabotulinumtoxinA (155 units every 12 weeks) [36], erenumab (70–140 mg/month) [37], fremanezumab (225 mg/month or 675 mg/3 months) [38], galcanezumab (240 mg loading dose then 120 mg/month) [39], and eptinezumab (100 mg/month or 300 mg/3 months) [40]. While these are the only currently available FDA-approved options for migraine prevention, many others have demonstrated benefit with variable levels of evidence [41–44] and are used off-label. Agents commonly used for migraine prevention off-label include anti-epileptics (e.g., zonisamide, levetiracetam), beta blockers (e.g., metoprolol, nadolol), tricyclic antidepressants (e.g., amitriptyline, nortriptyline), calcium channel blockers (e.g., verapamil), serotonin-norepinephrine reuptake inhibitors (e.g., venlafaxine, duloxetine), and angiotensin receptor blockers (e.g., candesartan).

Migraine prevention should be offered when a patient has 6 or more days with headache per month and should be considered with fewer headache days when impairment exists and the risk/benefit ratio favors initiation of therapy [1]. When counseling a patient about starting preventive migraine therapy it is important to inform them that prevention typically does not work quickly, often requiring 6–8 weeks at an effective dose to achieve full benefit. Two or more agents may be required to provide sufficient relief. It is important for prescribers to become familiar with the effective dose of common migraine-preventive medications as insufficient doses render patients without relief and higher doses carry an increased risk for side effects without additional benefit. The start low and go slow principle should be followed, titrating to the effective dose over time to limit the development of side effects. Migraine prevention may not be needed indefinitely and attempts to eliminate layers of migraine prevention should be considered periodically. We typically recommend 9–12 months of "good" control before discontinuing an effective migraine preventive. If migraine returns, prevention may be restarted.

What Is the Prognosis of This Condition?

The natural history of migraine is highly variable. For some, migraine presents around puberty then fades over time or presents only occasionally, such as around menses or during times of increased stress. For others, migraine is more pervasive, sometimes becoming a daily debilitating disease. There is some evidence that migraine improves after menopause [45]; though this is certainly not always the case and occasionally migraine first presents during perimenopause.

While the patient is the best gauge of treatment success, a 50% reduction in migraine frequency is a common goal used in studies of migraine-prevention. Objective measures of migraine specific disability, such as the Headache Impact Test (HIT-6™), may be used to track patient progress [46]. We also utilize a simple headache log in which patients indicate, once daily (usually at the end of their day), whether they had a headache that day and the highest severity it achieved. This simple log may be preferable to more complex diaries as it avoids patients feeling the need to constantly log their symptoms, but provides sufficient detail to help guide management.

Discussion

Prevalence

Headache disorders are the most common neurologic disease in the world [47] and the second leading cause of global disability (second only to low back pain) [48]. Migraine affects 1 in 10 people worldwide [49]. The prevalence of migraine is three times greater in women (Fig. 2.2).

Differential Diagnosis

While migraine is exceedingly common, its manifestations are protean. As such, the diagnosis and treatment of migraine are often delayed or missed all together. The "SNOOP" mnemonic

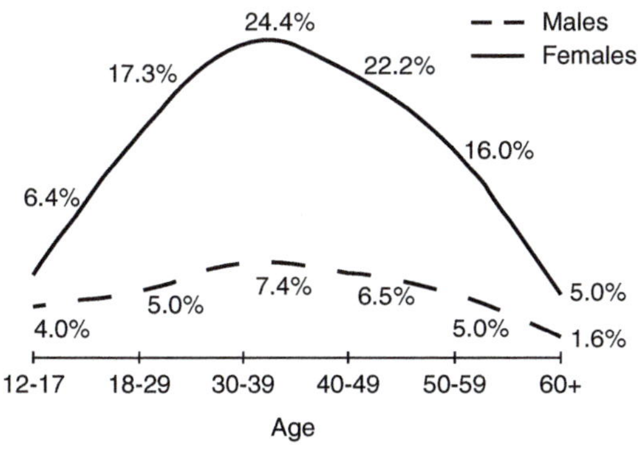

Fig. 2.2 Migraine prevalence in males and females over time. (Adapted from Lipton et al. [1], with permission)

Table 2.1 "SNOOP" mnemonic: red flags associated with secondary headaches

*S*ystemic symptoms (fever, weight loss, myalgias)
*S*econdary risk factors (HIV, cancer, pregnancy)
*N*eurologic exam (focal deficit, confusion, seizures)
*O*nset (sudden/thunderclap)
*O*lder (new or progressive headache, especially over 50 years)
*P*attern change (new symptoms in previously stable pattern)
*P*recipitants (Valsalva maneuver, position change, sexual activity)

Adapted from Dodick [56], with permission

(Table 2.1) is a commonly utilized tool [50] to identify headache red flags, suggesting the possibility of a secondary headache. When a red flag exists, further workup should be considered.

Predictive Value of Different Clinical Features (Both on History and Physical Exam) and Lab Testing/Imaging

History

Migraine is a heritable polygenic disease. Asking about a family history is often helpful in supporting a new migraine diagnosis. Because migraine often emerges or shifts around hormonal milestone (e.g., menarche, birth of a child, or menopause), asking about these milestones in female patients is informative and recommended. Head trauma, even minor head trauma, can lead to chronic headaches. Post-traumatic headaches generally have a phenotype of tension-type, migraine, or a combination of the two. Treatment should be tailored to which ever phenotype the patient's headaches most closely resemble.

Physical Exam

The neurologic exam of a patient with migraine should be normal. An abnormality on neurologic exam should prompt further evaluation for a secondary headache.

Lab Testing

Routine blood work should not be obtained in subjects who meet ICHD-3 criteria for migraine and who do not have a red flag.

Imaging

The American Headache Society "Choosing Wisely" recommendations are clear on this point [51]: "Don't perform neuroimaging studies in patients with stable headaches that meet criteria for migraine" and "Don't perform CT imaging for headache when MRI is available, except in emergency settings." Patients with migraine are four times more likely to have white matter abnormalities on MRI [52]. White matter lesions increase with increasing migraine frequency in some, but not all studies, and have not been associated with cognitive changes. As such, patients with these lesions should be reassured [53].

Strength of Evidence for Different Treatment Modalities

The most recent evidence-based guideline from the American Academy of Neurology and the American Headache Society was published in 2012 and found that "divalproex sodium, sodium valproate, topiramate, metoprolol, propranolol, and timolol are effective for migraine prevention and should be offered to patients with migraine to reduce migraine attack frequency and severity (Level A)." [41] Lamotrigine was established as *not* effective in migraine prevention (Level A) and should *not* be offered. This guideline is currently in the process of being updated.

Future Directions or Clinical Trials in Progress

The future is bright for people suffering with migraine. In 2018, the FDA approved the first new drug class for migraine prevention in over 25 years, the CGRP/CGRP receptor antagonists. These new drugs are the only agents on the market that were created specifically for migraine prevention. All other currently available migraine preventives were created for another purpose and subsequently found to be effective. In 2019 and 2020, the FDA approved two new classes of migraine acute treatments, the gepants (e.g., ubrogepant and rimegepant) and a ditan (lasmiditan). The gepants are oral CGRP receptor antagonists. They are particularly relevant in subjects who do not tolerate or have contraindications to triptans. Lasmiditan is an oral 5-HT_{1F} agonist. The ditans are related to triptans but exhibit minimal effect on vascular tone and may have a particular role in patients with cardiovascular disease, though they carry a warning to avoid driving or operating machinery for at least 8 hours after taking which may be prohibitive [55].

Other novel classes of medication for migraine are also in development including agents that target the pituitary adenylate cyclase activating polypeptide (PACAP) and transient receptor potential cation channel (TRPM8) systems, though much work remains to be done before these drugs end up in the hands of patients suffering with migraine.

Conclusion/Summary

Migraine is a highly prevalent and disabling disease for which clear clinical diagnostic criteria and effective treatments exist. All patients with migraine should be offered an acute treatment regimen for attacks, typically a "migraine-specific" drug (e.g., triptan, gepant, ditan), an NSAID, and/or a dopamine antagonist. These agents can be taken individually or in combination and should be chosen based on the severity of the attack. Prevention should be offered, particularly when patients have headache 6 or more days per month in order to limit the frequency and severity of attacks and related migraine disability. Pharmacologic migraine prevention consists of nutraceuticals and pharmaceuticals. Prescribers should become familiar with the effective dose of commonly prescribed agents, and patients should be reminded that migraine prevention often takes 6–8 weeks to take full effect. More than one layer of migraine prevention may be required to achieve satisfactory migraine control. The SNOOP mnemonic can be used to identify headache red flags. When a red flag exists, secondary headaches should be considered.

The future of migraine care looks bright as our understanding of its pathophysiology is quickly advancing and several new treatment options are on the horizon.

References

1. Lipton RB, Bigal ME, Diamond M, Freitag F, Reed ML, Stewart WF. Migraine prevalence, disease burden, and the need for preventive therapy. Neurology. 2007;68(5):343–9.
2. Bigal ME, Lipton RB. The epidemiology, burden, and comorbidities of migraine. Neurol Clin. 2009;27(2):321–34.
3. Chang FY, Lu CL. Irritable bowel syndrome and migraine: bystanders or partners? J neurogastroenterol mot. 2013;19(3):301–11.
4. Parkman HP, Yates K, Hasler WL, Nguyen L, Pasricha PJ, Snape WJ, et al. Clinical features of idiopathic gastroparesis vary with sex, body mass, symptom onset, delay in gastric emptying, and gastroparesis severity. Gastroenterology. 2011;140(1):101–15.
5. Warren JW, Howard FM, Cross RK, Good JL, Weissman MM, Wesselmann U, et al. Antecedent nonbladder syndromes in case-control study of interstitial cystitis/painful bladder syndrome. Urology. 2009;73(1):52–7.
6. Pavlovic JM, Buse DC, Sollars CM, Haut S, Lipton RB. Trigger factors and premonitory features of migraine attacks: summary of studies. Headache: The Journal of Head and Face Pain. 2014;54(10):1670–9.
7. Sances G, Granella F, Nappi R, Fignon A, Ghiotto N, Polatti F, et al. Course of migraine during pregnancy and postpartum: a prospective study. Cephalalgia : an international journal of headache. 2003;23(3):197–205.
8. Adeney KL, Williams MA. Migraine headaches and preeclampsia: an epidemiologic review. Headache: The Journal of Head and Face Pain. 2006;46(5):794–803.
9. Stein GS. Headaches in the first post partum week and their relationship to migraine. J Head Face Pain. 1981;21(5):201–5.
10. Arnold M. Headache classification committee of the international headache society (IHS) the international classification of headache disorders. Cephalalgia : an international journal of headache. 2018;38(1):1–211.
11. Launer LJ, Terwindt GM, Ferrari MD. The prevalence and characteristics of migraine in a population-based cohort the GEM study. Neurology. 1999;53(3):537.
12. Lipton RB, Stewart WF, Diamond S, Diamond ML, Reed M. Prevalence and burden of migraine in the United States: data from the American migraine study II. Headache. 2001;41(7):646–57.
13. Schreiber CP, Hutchinson S, Webster CJ, Ames M, Richardson MS, Powers C. Prevalence of migraine in patients with a history of self-reported or physician-diagnosed sinus headache. Arch Intern Med. 2004;164(16):1769–72.
14. Johnston MM, Jordan SE, Charles AC. Pain referral patterns of the C1 to C3 nerves: implications for headache disorders. Ann Neurol. 2013;74(1):145–8.
15. Noseda R, Burstein R. Migraine pathophysiology: anatomy of the trigeminovascular pathway and associated neurological symptoms, cortical spreading depression, sensitization, and modulation of pain. Pain. 2013;154:S44–53.
16. Giffin NJ, Lipton RB, Silberstein SD, Olesen J, Goadsby PJ. The migraine postdrome an electronic diary study. Neurology. 2016;87(3):309–13.
17. Gv S, Van der Grond J, Cv K, Van der Geest R, Terwindt G, Ferrari M. Migraine headache is not associated with cerebral or meningeal vasodilatation—a 3T magnetic resonance angiography study. J neurol. 2008;131(8):2192–200.
18. Asghar MS, Hansen AE, Amin FM, Van Der Geest R, Koning P, Larsson HB, et al. Evidence for a vascular factor in migraine. Ann Neurol. 2011;69(4):635–45.
19. Amin FM, Asghar MS, Hougaard A, Hansen AE, Larsen VA, de Koning PJ, et al. Magnetic resonance angiography of intracranial and extracranial arteries in patients with spontaneous migraine without aura: a cross-sectional study. Lancet Neurol. 2013;12(5):454–61.
20. Schwedt TJ, Chong CD, Wu T, Gaw N, Fu Y, Li J. Accurate classification of chronic migraine via brain magnetic resonance imaging. J Head Face Pain. 2015;55(6):762–77.
21. Schwedt TJ, Chiang C-C, Chong CD, Dodick DW. Functional MRI of migraine. The Lancet Neurology. 2015;14(1):81–91.
22. Close LN, Eftekhari S, Wang M, Charles AC, Russo AF. Cortical spreading depression as a site of origin for migraine: role of CGRP. Cephalalgia : An inter J headache. 2019;39(3):428–34.
23. Hadjikhani N, Del Rio MS, Wu O, Schwartz D, Bakker D, Fischl B, et al. Mechanisms of migraine aura revealed by functional MRI in human visual cortex. Proc Natl Acad Sci. 2001;98(8):4687–92.
24. Karatas H, Erdener SE, Gursoy-Ozdemir Y, Lule S, Eren-Koçak E, Sen ZD, et al. Spreading depression triggers headache by activating neuronal Panx1 channels. Science. 2013;339(6123):1092–5.
25. Dodick DW. A phase-by-phase review of migraine pathophysiology. Headache: The Journal of Head and Face Pain. 2018;58:4–16.
26. Lipton RB, Stewart WF, Stone AM, Láinez MJ, Sawyer JP. Stratified care vs step care strategies for migraine: the Disability in Strategies of Care (DISC) Study: a randomized trial. Jama. 2000;284(20):2599–605.
27. Charles A, Hansen JM. Migraine aura: new ideas about cause, classification, and clinical significance. Curr Opin Neurol. 2015;28(3):255–60.
28. Becker WJ. Acute migraine treatment. Cont Lifelong Learning Neurol. 2015;21(4, Headache):953–72.
29. Becker WJ. Acute migraine treatment in adults. Headache. 2015;55(6):778–93.
30. Wijemanne S, Jankovic J, Evans RW. Movement disorders from the use of metoclopramide and other

antiemetics in the treatment of migraine. Headache. 2016;56(1):153–61.
31. Schwedt TJ. Preventive therapy of migraine. Continuum. 2018;24(4):1052–65.
32. Topiramate prescribing information.
33. Divalproex sodium FDA Prescribing Information.
34. Propranolol FDA Prescribing Information.
35. Timolol maleate – Link to FDA Prescribing Information.
36. OnabotulinumtoxinA – FDA Prescribing Information.
37. Erenumab - FDA Prescribing Information.
38. Fremanezumab - FDA Prescribing Information.
39. Galcanezumab - FDA Prescribing Information.
40. Eptinezumab - FDA Prescribing Information. https://www.accessdata.fda.gov/drugsatfda_docs/label/2020/761119s000lbl.pdf.
41. Silberstein S, Holland S, Freitag F, Dodick DW, Argoff C, Ashman E. Evidence-based guideline update: pharmacologic treatment for episodic migraine prevention in adults report of the quality standards Subcommittee of the American Academy of neurology and the American headache society. Neurology. 2012;78(17):1337–45.
42. Linde M, Mulleners WM, Chronicle EP, McCrory DC. Antiepileptics other than gabapentin, pregabalin, topiramate, and valproate for the prophylaxis of episodic migraine in adults. Cochrane Database Syst Rev 2013;(6). https://www.cochranelibrary.com/cdsr/doi/10.1002/14651858.CD010608/epdf/full.
43. Burch R. Antidepressants for preventive treatment of migraine. Curr Treat Options Neurol. 2019;21(4):18.
44. Shamliyan TA, Kane RL, Taylor FR. Migraine in adults: Preventive pharmacologic treatments. 2013.
45. Neri I, Granella F, Nappi R, Manzoni G, Facchinetti F, Genazzani A. Characteristics of headache at menopause: a clinico-epidemiologic study. Maturitas. 1993;17(1):31–7.
46. members: IHSCTS, Tfelt-Hansen P, Pascual J, Ramadan N, Dahlöf C, D'Amico D, et al. Guidelines for controlled trials of drugs in migraine: a guide for investigators. Cephalalgia. 2012;32(1):6–38.
47. Feigin VL, Abajobir AA, Abate KH, Abd-Allah F, Abdulle AM, Abera SF, et al. Global, regional, and national burden of neurological disorders during 1990–2015: a systematic analysis for the global burden of disease study 2015. Lancet Neurol. 2017;16(11):877–97.
48. Global, regional, and national incidence, prevalence, and years lived with disability for 328 diseases and injuries for 195 countries, 1990–2016: a systematic analysis for the Global Burden of Disease Study 2016. Lancet (London, England). 2017;390(10100):1211–1259.
49. Woldeamanuel YW, Cowan RP. Migraine affects 1 in 10 people worldwide featuring recent rise: a systematic review and meta-analysis of community-based studies involving 6 million participants. J Neurol Sci. 2017;372:307–15.
50. Martin VT. The diagnostic evaluation of secondary headache disorders. Headache: The Journal of Head and Face Pain. 2011;51(2):346–52.
51. Loder E, Weizenbaum E, Frishberg B, Silberstein S, Force AHSCWT. Choosing wisely in headache medicine: the a merican headache Society's list of five things physicians and patients should question. Headache: The Journal of Head and Face Pain. 2013;53(10):1651–9.
52. Swartz RH, Kern RZ. Migraine is associated with magnetic resonance imaging white matter abnormalities: a meta-analysis. Arch Neurol. 2004;61(9):1366–8.
53. Bashir A, Lipton RB, Ashina S, Ashina M. Migraine and structural changes in the brain: a systematic review and meta-analysis. Neurology. 2013;81(14):1260–8.
54. Ong JJY, Wei DY, Goadsby PJ. Recent advances in pharmacotherapy for migraine prevention: from pathophysiology to new drugs. Drugs. 2018;78(4):411–37.
55. Lasmiditan - FDA Prescribing Information. https://www.accessdata.fda.gov/drugsatfda_docs/label/2019/211280s000lbl.pdf.
56. Dodick DW. Pearls: headache. Semin Neurol. 2010;30(1):74–81.

3 Cluster Headache

Sonia Gill and Tariq Malik

Case Description

A 41-year-old man presents to clinic with a 3-week history of several "stabbing" right-sided headache with eye pain, conjunctival injection, and tearing of his R eye. Each episode lasts about 20 minutes, and occurs a few times per day, more often at night. "Those are the worst minutes of my life and I've honestly thought about jumping out a window head first, that's how bad they are," he states. His past medical history was unremarkable until 1 year ago, when he has been diagnosed with hypertension, hyperlipidemia, and stable angina for which he sees a cardiologist regularly. His medications include amlodipine, carvedilol, atorvastatin, and an as-needed sublingual nitrate for chest pain. He drinks alcohol occasionally, and denies other drug use. His blood pressure is well controlled in clinic and his exam is unremarkable.

S. Gill
Department of Anesthesiology and Critical Care, University of Chicago, Chicago, IL, USA

T. Malik (✉)
Department of Anesthesia and Critical Care, University of Chicago, Chicago, IL, USA
e-mail: TMuslim@dacc.uchicago.edu; tmalik@dacc.uchicago.edu

What Is Your Preliminary Diagnosis?

Chief complaint of headache carries a long list of possible diagnosis. It is always important to systematically evaluate the patient to ensure that no life-threatening condition or easily treated condition is missed. Using the International Headache Society criteria, the preliminary diagnosis is a cluster headache [1]. The International Classification of Headache Disorders defines cluster headache as a strictly unilateral headache lasting 15–180 minutes, localized within or above the orbit, often accompanied by at least one ipsilateral autonomic symptom or agitation, or both. Autonomic symptoms include conjunctival injection, lacrimation, nasal congestion, rhinorrhea, miosis, ptosis, eyelid edema, and forehead or facial sweating. They occur up between once every other day to as frequently as eight times a day (third international). These frequent, recurrent headaches can be debilitating, affecting quality of life and sometimes, inciting suicidal thoughts [2].

How Is Diagnosis Confirmed?

Diagnosis of CH is based on careful history that elicits the clinical features of attacks with ipsilateral associated symptoms and a cyclic nature. Brain MRI with detailed study of the pituitary area and cavernous sinus is recommended for all

T. Malik (ed.), *Practical Chronic Pain Management*, https://doi.org/10.1007/978-3-030-46675-6_3

trigeminal autonomic cephalgias (TACs) including CH, because even a clinically typical CH can be caused by structural lesions [3].

What Is the Pathophysiology of This Condition?

The exact pathophysiologic mechanism of CH is unknown, but the prior theory of inflammation of the cavernous sinus has been replaced by the theory of a complex neurovascular process that involves a synchronized abnormal activity in the hypothalamus, the trigeminovascular system, and the parasympathetic nervous system [4]. Understanding some of the pathophysiology has guided novel treatment modalities.

Studies of hormone and biomarker levels, as well as neuroimaging studies, suggest the role of the anterior hypothalamus [4–10]. The involvement of the hypothalamus, in particular, the suprachiasmatic nuclei that govern circadian release of hormones, is thought to be involved with gender differences, seasonal variation of headaches, and timing of headaches that is sometimes related to circadian rhythm [11].

A genetic alteration might predispose an individual to cluster headache, as epidemiologic studies show a tendency for cluster headaches to affect families, but the exact mutation and its mode of inheritance has not been identified [4]. *There is preliminary data to suggest that a mutation in the HCRTR2 gene which codes for hypocrein-2 receptor might be involved, but these data have not been confirmed* [4].

Studies in the last decade suggest that anomalies in the metabolism of tyrosine and complex biochemical pathways may play a role in the pathogenesis of CH [12]. *In these patients, the levels of tyramine and other elusive amines are elevated. Their interactions with trace amine-associated receptors, which are expressed in subcortical centers and blood vessels, modulate the release of dopamine and norepinephrine, which may result in the abnormal activation of the autonomic system and hypothalamus* [12].

Higher sympathetic tone has been shown during neurostimulation of the sphenopalatine ganglion preceding cranial autonomic symptoms or cluster pain, while during cluster pain increased parasympathetic activity has been observed [13]. This severe unilateral pain involves activation of the trigeminal-autonomic reflex, via the first (ophthalmic) division of the trigeminal nerve. The associated autonomic symptoms including lacrimation, nasal congestion, and rhinorrhea are due to the activation of the cranial parasympathetic outflow from the seventh cranial nerve [14]. These nerve fibers synapse in the sphenopalatine ganglion, making stimulation of the sphenopalatine ganglion a target for treating CH pain and symptoms.

Activation of the trigeminovascular system leads to neuropeptide release, including calcitonin gene-related peptide (CGRP), vasoactive intestinal peptide (VIP), and pituitary adenylate cyclase-activating peptide (PACAP) [15]. Patients with spontaneous or nitroglycerine-induced CH attacks were found to have increased calcitonin gene-related peptide (CGRP) levels in the external jugular vein that was normalized after O_2 inhalation or treatment with subcutaneous sumatriptan [15]. The release of these peptides leads to a number of downstream effects including arteriolar vasodilation, plasma protein extravasation, and degranulation of mast cells [15].

Cluster headache is associated with psychiatric comorbidities of which depression, anxiety, and aggressive behavior are the most common. The mechanism of the suicidal ideation experienced by some is also unclear, but may be due to the psychological impact of recurrent attacks, a lack of sleep, or possibly, more complex mechanism like an alteration in serotonergic pathways or the production of cytokines.

Attacks occur spontaneously and may be provoked by alcohol, histamine, nitroglycerin, or organic compounds such as perfume and paint. In over half of patients, small quantities of alcohol, particularly red wine, will precipitate an attack, usually within an hour of ingestion [3].

How Is This Problem Managed?

The mainstay of therapy is to abort attacks quickly once they have begun, as there are often a few minutes between onset and peak of symptom intensity, and to prevent future attacks [3].

The 2016 American Headache Society cluster headache treatment guidelines catergorize only 3 Level A recommendations for acute therapy: sumatriptan subcutaneous, zolmitriptan intranasal, and high flow oxygen. High flow oxygen and triptans are the most effective therapies for an acute cluster headache attack. About 60–70% of CH patients respond to inhalation of 100% oxygen via a non-rebreathing face mask. It takes 15 minutes to work and if effective, will completely abort the attack. It is used as first-line treatment when triptans are contraindicated. Unlike triptans, there is no limit as to how often it can used to abort CH attack. Sumatriptan, a 5-HT1B/D agonist, 6 mg injected subcutaneously, is considered the gold standard to abort ongoing CH attacks, and works within 15 minutes. Injected route is more effective than other routes like nasal (zolmitriptan 5–10 mg dose or sumatriptan nasal dose 20 mg) which takes upto 30 minutes to work; oral route is effective but takes longer than 30 minutes to work. There is evidence of tachyphlaxis with escalating doses, and it is contraindicated in those with cardiovascular or cerebrovascular disorders or hypertension [16]. Intranasal lidocaine has been tested in few trials with good response; optimal dose and concentration is not known. It can be used as a spray, drop, or using a cotton swab. It is used if oxygen fails to abort the attack and triptans are contraindicated. Corticosteroids are sometimes prescribed to temporarily improve symptoms while a preventive medication takes effect. One of the older treatments for CH is oral ergotamanine. An intravenous version, dihydroergotamine, can stop attacks in 3 days in about two-thirds of patients [16]. Melatonin might be a useful adjunct as well [17]. Octreotide 100 microgram administered subcutaneously has been found to be effective abortive therapy and is well tolerated. However it is usually considered second line of therapy after triptan and is used when triptans have failed to abort the CH attack.

High-dose oral steroid (prednisolone 1 mg/kg or at least 40 mg orally a day) is quite effective in preventing recurrence of attacks. The oral steroid is given over 1–3 weeks. Single dose of prednisolone (30 mg/kg) given IV can be equally effective. Occipital nerve block done with bupivacaine, and triamcinolone can also provide a longer lasting relief when combined with abortive therapy.

Avoidance of alcohol, napping, and nitrates like nitroglycerine when possible are some of the preventative methods. First-line preventive drugs include verapamil and lithium, but ergot medications, topiramate, and valproic acid may also be used. While corticosteroids are effective in preventing headaches, caution should be used when considering long-term preventive solutions.

Verapamil has Level C recommendation from American Headache Society (AHS) but Level A from the European Federation of Neurological Societies (EFNS) as an effective preventive intervention. Its usual dose is 240–960 mg a day given in divided doses, and median effective dose is 480 mg a day. It takes 2 weeks to work, and usual side effects are constipation, hypotension, peripheral edema, and heart block. Verapamil is usually better tolerated than lithium, and with fewer side effects, though an EKG should be performed because of a risk of heart block. Lithium has Level C recommendation from AHS and Level B from EFNS. Target dose is 600–1500 mg a day. The drug has narrow therapeutic index and requires serum level monitoring. Common side effects are diarrhea, tremors, and polyuria [3]. Melatonin (dose 10–20 mg a day) has Level C recommendation from both societies as though it has better side effect profile than the previous two drugs, but is less effective.

Up to 20% of chronic CH is resistant to pharmacological treatments, in which case interventional procedures that target the various nerves should be considered. The number of different injections or surgcial procedures include block, stimulation of the vagus nerve, occipital nerve, sphenopalatine ganglion, and deep brain stimulation of the hypothalamus) radiofrequency, stereotactic radiosurgery, and vidian neurectomy [18]. These therapies may be considered for episodic CH that is refractory to standard medical therapy [18]. External vagus nerve stimulation (nVNS) is an FDA-approved therapy to abort an acute CH attack as well as to be used an adjunctive therapy for cluster headache prevention. The device is used provide three 2-minute stimulation which are self-administered by the patient by applying the device over the carotid pulsation just below the jaw.

Novel methods like onabotulinum toxin A, neurostimulation including sphenopalatine ganglion stimulation, hypothalamic deep brain stimulation, occipital nerve stimulation, and monoclonal antibodies against calcitonin gene-related peptide, a crucial neurotransmitter of the trigeminal system, are under investigation for the preventive treatment of cluster headache [2].

In 2018, the FDA approved a number of monoclonal antibodies targeted at the CGRP, for migraine treatment. Galcanezumab showed effectiveness in preventing episodic cluster headache, although has not yet been submitted to the FDA for this indication [19]. Clonidine, an $\alpha_1$receptor antagonist, significantly reduces the number of CH attacks [20].

What Is the Prognosis of This Condition?

What is the long-term outcome – complete cure, recurrent, or chronic persistent problem?

The most common presentation is the episodic form, in which attacks occur daily for weeks or months, with complete remission for months or years. Some patients describe one to two episodes a year. Approximately one-fourth of patients will experience only a single episode, and 80% of patients have an episodic pattern of headaches. If the episode does not remit within 1 year, it is characterized as a chronic cluster headache [2]. A study of patients who had cluster headaches for 20 years or longer showed that one-third of patients will experience complete remission, one-third will have a decrease in the severity of headaches and may not require medications, and one-third will remain unchanged [17].

Discussion

Prevalence

Cluster headache is not as common as migraine but is not rare and is often misdiagnosed and hence mismanaged. The prevalence of cluster headache is approximately 0.1% of the general population. One study showed that 85% of patients who suffer from cluster headaches are cigarette smokers, but the link is unclear, as abstinence from nicotine has not been shown to improve symptoms. Men are more frequently affected than women, with a male to female ratio of about 3:1; however, this ratio is decreasing with more women being diagnosed. It is unclear if this reflects a change in diagnostic accuracy. In women, it is often misdiagnosed as migraine, as photophobia and nausea may also occur with cluster headache. Though patients can get CH at any age, attacks typically start in those 20–40 years of age.

There seems to be a hereditary or familial nature in some cases of CH. First-degree relatives of CH patients has an estimated 10- to 50-fold increased risk of developing CH. Several genes have been identified as potential source of problem but none have been validated. A genome-wide analysis study suggested that a variant of the pituitary adenylate cyclase-activating polypeptide (PACAP) receptor gene ADCYAP1R1 could be relevant to cluster headache, which initially was considered a very promising finding, but studies produced conflicting results. The inheritance pattern also seems to vary from autosomal recessive to autosomal dominant. Neuroimaging studies and neuromodulatory therapies are improving our understanding of the disease.

Differential Diagnosis

It is important to have a conclusive diagnosis and other diseases are excluded. The list of diseases include temporal arteritis, migraines, other TACs, sinusitis, glaucoma, and structural lesions in the mid and posterior cranial fossa, including pituitary tumors, aneurysms, AV malformations, carotid dissection, and cavernous sinus pathology [3, 17]. Migraine and trigeminal neuralgia are most often confused with CH. More importantly, some patients may have both conditions.

Predictive Value of Different Clinical Features (Both on History and Physical Exam) and Lab Testing/ Imaging

Eighty percent of patients have lacrimation and conjunctival injection. Nasal stuffiness or rhinorrhea occurs in at least two-thirds of patients. In 3–5% of cases, there is no associated autonomic symptom [21].

Strength of Evidence for Different Treatment Modalities

Sumatriptan to abort ongoing CH attacks has support from both – from data reported in double-blind, placebo-controlled trials and from clinical practice [22, 23]. Few randomized clinical trials have investigated preventive drugs in CH, and much of preventive therapy is based on clinical experience. Surgical procedures should be considered with great caution because there are no reliable long-term observational data and because they can induce trigeminal neuralgia or contralateral cluster headaches.

Future Directions or Clinical Trials in Progress

Phase III clinical trials with CGRP monoclonal antibodies are underway for the preventive treatment of episodic and chronic CH (NCT03107052, NCT02797951).

Conclusion/Summary

Cluster headache is a debilitating condition requiring prompt diagnosis and medical attention. Nicknamed the "suicide headache," patients with CH fear recurrence of attacks and have contemplated taking their own lives, with some actually having committed suicide. It is often an ipsilateral headache in the temporal or orbital region with associated autonomic symptoms. The exact mechanism is not known, but there have been discoveries showing a complex neurovascular pathology, involving the hypothalamus, autonomic pathways, signaling molecules, and resulting tissue and vascular changes. Successful treatment of attacks includes oxygen administration and sumatriptan. There are a number of preventive strategies including pharmacologic ones (verapamil and lithium being the most common) and nonpharmacologic ones (avoidance of triggers). Some patients may require escalating doses, multiple medications and may even be refractory to medications, warranting the use of nerve blocks or nerve stimulation as part of a preventive strategy.

References

1. Diagnostic criteria for episodic and chronic cluster headache. The International Classification of Headache Disorders, 3rd edition, 2018. Headache Classification Committee of the International Headache Society.
2. Hoffmann J, May A. Diagnosis, pathophysiology, and management of cluster headache. Lancet Neurol. 2018;17(1):75–83.
3. Ljubisavljevic S, Zidverc TJ. Cluster headache: pathophysiology, diagnosis and treatment. J Neurol. 2019;266(5):1059–66.
4. Hofman MA, Zhou JN, Swaab DF. Suprachiasmatic nucleus of the human brain: an immunocytochemical and morphometric analysis. J Comp Neurol. 1996;305:552–6.
5. Strittmatter M, Hamann GF, Grauer M, et al. Altered activity of the sympathetic nervous system and changes in the balance of hypophyseal, pituitary and adrenal hormones in patients with cluster headache. Neuroreport. 1996;7:1229–34.

6. May A, Bahra A, Buchel C, et al. Hypothalamic activation in cluster headache attacks. Lancet. 1998;352:275–8.
7. May A, Ashburner J, Buchel C, et al. Correlation between structural and functional changes in brain in an idiopathic headache syndrome. Nat Med. 1999;5:836–8.
8. Lodi R, Pierangeli G, Tonon C, et al. Study of hypothalamic metabolism in cluster headache by proton MR spectroscopy. Neurology. 2006;66:1264–6.
9. Morelli N, Pesaresi I, Cafforio G, et al. Functional magnetic resonance imaging in episodic cluster headache. J Headache Pain. 2009;10:11–4.
10. Yang FC, Chou KH, Kuo CY, et al. The pathophysiology of episodic cluster headache: insights from recent neuroimaging research. Cephalalgia. 2018;38(5):970–83.
11. Lund N, Barloese M, Petersen A, et al. Chronobiology differs between men and women with cluster headache, clinical phenotype does not. Neurology. 2017;88(11):1069–76.
12. D'Andrea G, Gucciardi A, Perini F, Leon A. The role of neurotransmitters and neuromodulators in the pathogenesis of cluster headache: a review. Neurol Sci. 2019;40(1):39–44.
13. Barloese M, Petersen AS, Guo S, et al. Sphenopalatine ganglion stimulation induces changes in cardiac autonomic regulation in cluster headache. Clin Physiol Funct Imaging. 2018;38(5):808–15.
14. Goadsby PJ. Pathophysiology of cluster headache: a trigeminal autonomic cephalgia. Lancet Neurol. 2002;1:251–7.
15. Buture A, Boland JW, Dikomitis L, Ahmed F. Update on the pathophysiology of cluster headache: imaging and neuropeptide studies. J Pain Res. 2019;12:269–81. https://doi.org/10.2147/JPR.S175312. eCollection 2019. Review.
16. Leone M, Giustiniani A, Cecchini AP. Cluster headache: present and future therapy. Neurol Sci. 2017;38(1):45–50. https://doi.org/10.1007/s10072-017-2924-7. Review. PubMed PMID: 28527055.
17. Dodick DW, Rozen TD, Goadsby PJ, Silberstein SD. Cluster headache. Cephalalgia. 2000;20(9):787–803. Review.
18. Rosso C, Felisati G, Bulfamante A, Pipolo C. Cluster headache: crosspoint between otologists and neurologists-treatment of the sphenopalatine ganglion and systematic review. Neurol Sci. 2019;40(1):137–46.
19. Tepper SJ. Anti-calcitonin gene-related peptide (CGRP) therapies: update on a previous review after the American Headache Society 60th Scientific Meeting, San Francisco, June 2018. Headache. 2018;58(3):276–90.
20. D'Andrea G, Perini F, Granella F, Cananzi A, Sergi A. Efficacy of transdermal clonidine in short-term treatment of cluster headache: a pilot study. Cephalalgia. 1995;15(5):430–3.
21. Martins I, Gouveia R, Antunes J. Double dissociation between autonomic symptoms and pain in cluster headache. Cephalalgia. 2005;25:398–400.
22. The Sumatriptan Cluster Headache Study Group. Treatment of acute cluster headache with sumatriptan. N Engl J Med. 1991;325:322–6.
23. Ekbom K, Monstad I, Prusinski A, et al. Subcutaneous sumatriptan in the acute treatment of cluster headache: a dose comparison study. The Sumatriptan Cluster Headache Study Group. Acta Neurol Scand. 1993;88(1):63–9.

4 Atypical Facial Pain/Persistent Idiopathic Facial Pain

Brady Still and Tariq Malik

Case Description

A 35-year-old woman presents to your pain clinic with 6 months of daily left facial pain. She describes the pain as deep, dull, and burning in quality. She indicates it generally begins next to her nose, but often spreads to other parts of her face in a non-dermatomal pattern. She cannot recall anything that may have triggered the pain, though she has had facial botulinum toxin injections in the past. She denies pain on the right. The pain is not changed with chewing or talking, and she experiences no difficulties with facial movement or sensation. She denies current or prior rashes or blisters on her face. She saw her regular dentist last month, who told her there were no issues with her teeth or gums. She takes no medications. Her only other medical problems are anxiety and depression, for which she sees a therapist.

What Is Your Preliminary Diagnosis?

Facial pain or headache is a very common complaint. Common conditions causing pain in this location are migraine, trigeminal neuralgia, sinusitis, or dental related. The patient in the case presented would need a thorough evaluation by a medical doctor including an ENT or dental consultation if needed. After such complete evaluation including imaging of the head or face, should she be referred to a pain clinic. The preliminary diagnosis is atypical facial pain (AFP), also called persistent idiopathic facial pain (PIFP). As defined by the International Headache Society (IHS), PIFP is "[p]ersistent facial and/or oral pain, with varying presentations but recurring daily for more than 2 hours per day over more than 3 months, in the absence of clinical neurological deficit" [1]. This pain is typically ill-defined, both in character and in location, but is often dull and unilateral. It notably does not follow a dermatomal distribution. Though the disease is persistent in nature, patients often describe exacerbations during periods of stress. Motor function is preserved, and there are no sensory deficits. Patients often endorse minor maxillofacial trauma or procedures preceding the onset of pain, though many patients are unable to definitively establish an inciting event. Psychiatric comorbidities, particularly anxiety and depression, are common [2–5]. The IHS further notes a proposed variant of PIFP, atypical odontalgia, referring to "continuous pain in one or more teeth or in a tooth socket after extraction," but does not provide formal diagnostic criteria due to a dearth of research [1].

B. Still · T. Malik (✉)
Department of Anesthesia and Critical Care, University of Chicago, Chicago, IL, USA
e-mail: TMuslim@dacc.uchicago.edu; tmalik@dacc.uchicago.edu

T. Malik (ed.), *Practical Chronic Pain Management*, https://doi.org/10.1007/978-3-030-46675-6_4

The formal IHS diagnostic criteria for PIFP are as follows [1]:

A. Facial and/or oral pain fulfilling criteria B and C.
B. Recurring daily for >2 h per day for >3 months.
C. Pain has both of the following characteristics:
    1. Poorly localized, and not following the distribution of a peripheral nerve.
    2. Dull, aching, or nagging quality.
D. Clinical neurological examination is normal.
E. A dental cause has been excluded by appropriate investigations.

There are no other diagnostic criteria in common clinical use.

How Is the Diagnosis Confirmed?

As PIFP is a diagnosis of exclusion, there is no confirmatory testing. Other common causes of facial pain, including temporomandibular dysfunction, regional myofascial pain, trigeminal neuralgia, and the common headache disorders, must be excluded via a thorough history and physical and appropriate imaging. Particular care should be given to establishing a lack of sensory changes, which would suggest the more common entities of trigeminal neuralgia and trigeminal neuropathy [3, 5]. Magnetic resonance imaging (MRI) may be useful in ruling out central nervous system or trigeminal pathology.

What Is the Pathophysiology of This Condition?

The pathophysiology of PIFP, like many idiopathic chronic pain conditions, is poorly understood, and is thought to result from a combination of biological and psychological factors [5–7]. PET imaging of patients with PIFP exposed to a thermally noxious stimulus reveals differences in activity suggestive of globally altered processing of noxious stimuli [8]. More specifically, derangements in striatal dopaminergic signaling are thought to play a key role [9]. Habituation of the blink reflex (BR), a process under dopaminergic control, is often deficient in patients with PIFP; in addition, D1- and D2-labeled PET imaging of patients with PIFP demonstrates abnormalities in dopaminergic signaling [6, 9, 10]. Quantitative sensory testing (QST) additionally reveals that many patients with PIFP have abnormalities in small-fiber function [10]. Though the exact small-fiber abnormality seen in QST is highly variable, the most common finding is thermal hypoesthesia [10]. These findings are similar to those in patients with overt trigeminal neuropathy, leading some to hypothesize that PIFP and trigeminal neuropathy may represent a continuum of pain pathology [10]. Unlike the trigeminal neuralgias and neuropathies, there is limited to no evidence of neurovascular compression of the trigeminal nerve in patients with PIFP [11].

How Is This Problem Managed?

As PIFP is a chronic, persistent pain syndrome with both biological and psychological components, a multidisciplinary pain management strategy incorporating both pharmacologic agents and cognitive behavioral therapy is recommended [2, 3, 5, 7]. Medical management includes the following agents:

A. *Amitriptyline:* Dose: 25 mg once per day, titrated to symptom relief and side-effect tolerance to a maximum of 100 mg once per day [5, 12]. Side effects include sedation, headache, gastrointestinal upset.
B. *Fluoxetine:* Dose: 20 mg once per day, with no consensus as to titration strategy [7]. Side effects include sexual dysfunction, headache, gastrointestinal upset, and discontinuation syndrome.
C. *Venlafaxine: D*ose: 75 mg once per day, with no consensus as to titration strategy [13]. Side effects include sexual dysfunction, headache, gastrointestinal upset, and insomnia.

Anticonvulsant agents such as gabapentin and pregabalin have been trialed in individual patients; however, no compelling evidence exists for their use in PIFP [5].

Cognitive-behavioral therapy is recommended in conjunction with medical management as outlined above [5, 7].

Invasive strategies, including trigeminal vascular decompression surgery and deep brain stimulator placement, are generally ineffective. Despite this, many patients with PIFP have undergone invasive procedures in an attempt to treat their facial pain by the time they present to a pain specialist [3].

The most commonly used interventional pain strategy is pulsed radiofrequency (PRF) treatment of the sphenopalatine ganglion (SPG). In this interventional strategy, the SPG is ablated under fluoroscopic guidance following a diagnostic local anesthetic block [14].

No clear treatment guidelines have been promulgated by the IHS or other professional societies. Reviews of PIFP emphasize the primacy of combined medical/psychological intervention, with a role for PRF of the SPG in patients whose pain is refractory to these interventions [2, 3, 5, 7]. There are case reports of percutaneous peripheral neuromodulation having some success in treating atypical facial pain in refractory patients, but the level of evidence is poor and effectiveness not well documented.

What Is the Prognosis of This Condition?

As with many idiopathic chronic pain syndromes, cure is not possible and prognosis is poor. Few patients achieve complete remission, though many do attain partial response to the treatment modalities outlined previously.

Discussion

Prevalence

As with many chronic pain conditions, especially those that are diagnoses of exclusion, the exact epidemiology of PIFP remains difficult to determine. A population-based study of 3336 German citizens found a prevalence of 0.03% (1 of 3336) [15]. A prospective, clinic-based study of 307 patients with side-locked headache found a prevalence of 3%, with no statistically significant difference between male and female patients [16]. A large retrospective examination of the Integrated Primary Care Information Database of approximately 800,000 Dutch patients found 362 patients with chronic facial pain, of which 11.3% (41 of 362) were diagnosed as having PIFP. 75.6% of these patients were female, suggesting a female predominance. The same study found an incidence rate of 4.4 per 100,000 person-years (PY), with a peak incidence between age 30 and 39 [17]. A cohort-based study of 53 patients diagnosed with PIFP at the Danish Headache Centre found that 75% (40 of 53) were female, with a mean age of 49.8 [4]

Differential Diagnosis

As PIFP is a diagnosis of exclusion with often nonspecific features, the differential diagnosis is broad, including but not limited to [1, 3]:

A. Headache disorders
   (a) Migraine with or without aura
   (b) Cluster headache
   (c) Cervicogenic headache
B. Trigeminal neuropathies/neuralgias
   (a) Posttraumatic trigeminal neuropathy (PTTN)
   (b) Trigeminal neuralgia
C. Temporomandibular disorders
D. Dental and gingival pathologies
E. Ocular disorders
   (a) Glaucoma
F. Infectious etiologies
   (a) Herpes zoster
   (b) Sinusitis
G. Regional myofascial pain (RMP)
H. Central facial pain

Predictive Value of Clinical Features

The clinical features of PIFP are relatively nonspecific, and individual features lack predictive value. The literature is limited with regard to the test characteristics of clinical features of PIFP.

Strength of Evidence for Treatment Modalities

Studies evaluating the treatment modalities for PIFP are limited. The primary evidence for each of the three primary pharmacologic treatments and the one interventional management are outlined in the following:

A. *Amitriptyline:* Single crossover RCT, $n = 32$. Patients randomized to amitriptyline 30 mg once per day ("low dose") versus placebo, amitriptyline 150 mg once per day ("high dose") versus placebo, or amitriptyline 150 mg versus amitriptyline 30 mg. Statistically significant decrease in pain relative to placebo occurred for both the low dose and high dose group, with no difference in the direct comparison group [12].
B. *Fluoxetine:* Single RCT, $n = 178$. Patients randomized to fluoxetine 20 mg once per day, CBT alone, CBT plus fluoxetine 20 mg once per day, or placebo. Fluoxetine reduced pain intensity; CBT in addition to fluoxetine reduced patient distress and functional interference [7].
C. *Venlafaxine:* Single crossover RCT, $n = 30$. Patients randomized to venlafaxine 37.5–75 mg once per day (titrated as patient tolerated) followed by placebo, or placebo followed by venlafaxine 37.5–75 mg once per day. Modest relief of pain on one rating scale was achieved, though no statistically significant difference was observed on the pain scale used as the primary outcome [13].
D. *Radiofrequency ablation of the sphenopalatine ganglion.* Single retrospective analysis of patients with chronic head and face pain who underwent RFA, $n = 46$. 21% reported complete pain relief; 65% reported mild to moderate pain relief [14].

Future Directions

Given that PIFP remains a poorly understood entity, much of the literature emphasizes the need for further neuroimaging to better elucidate the pathophysiology of the condition. The paucity of high-quality randomized controlled trials additionally limits effective treatment of the condition; further trials are needed to determine both the ideal agents and ideal doses. An area of active research with regard to interventional pain management is the application of peripheral nerve field stimulation (PNFS) in patients with PIFP. In one retrospective study of PNFS of patients with facial pain, the single patient with PIFP demonstrated an improvement in VAS pain score from 7 to 3 following implantation of an infraorbital nerve stimulator [18].

Conclusion/Summary

Atypical facial pain (AFP) or persistent idiopathic facial pain (PIFP) is a chronic pain syndrome characterized by persistent facial and/or oral pain not clearly attributable to other facial or dental pathology. It appears to have a female predominance, with onset in middle age. There are no pathognomonic or highly suggestive clinical features or imaging findings associated with the condition, and it remains a diagnosis of exclusion. Prognosis is generally poor, though positive results have been achieved with amitriptyline, fluoxetine, and venlafaxine. RFA of the sphenopalatine ganglion remains the interventional strategy of choice in patients who fail medical management. Further work will aim to better determine the pathophysiology of the condition, as well as determine effective treatments.

References

1. Headache Classification Committee of the International Headache Society (IHS). The international classification of headache disorders, 3rd edition (beta version). Cephalalgia. 2013;33(9):629–808.
2. Benoliel R, Gaul C. Persistent idiopathic facial pain. Cephalalgia. 2017;37(7):680–91.
3. Cornelissen P, van Kleef M, Mekhail N, Day M, van Zundert J. 3. Persistent idiopathic facial pain. Pain Pract. 2009;9(6):443–8.
4. Maarbjerg S, Wolfram F, Heinskou TB, Rochat P, Gozalov A, Brennum J, et al. Persistent idiopathic facial pain – a prospective systematic study of clinical

characteristics and neuroanatomical findings at 3.0 T MRI. Cephalalgia. 2017;37(13):1231–40.
5. Weiss AL, Ehrhardt KP, Tolba R. Atypical Facial Pain: a Comprehensive, Evidence-Based Review. Curr Pain Headache Rep. 2017;21(2). Available from: http://link.springer.com/10.1007/s11916-017-0609-9.
6. Forssell H, Jääskeläinen S, List T, Svensson P, Baad-Hansen L. An update on pathophysiological mechanisms related to idiopathic oro-facial pain conditions with implications for management. J Oral Rehabil. 2015;42(4):300–22.
7. Zakrzewska JM. Chronic/persistent idiopathic facial pain. Neurosurg Clin N Am. 2016;27(3):345–51.
8. Derbyshire SW, Jones AK, Devani P, Friston KJ, Feinmann C, Harris M, et al. Cerebral responses to pain in patients with atypical facial pain measured by positron emission tomography. J Neurol Neurosurg Psychiatry. 1994;57(10):1166–72.
9. Hagelberg N, Forssell H, Aalto S, Rinne JO, Scheinin H, Taiminen T, et al. Altered dopamine D2 receptor binding in atypical facial pain. Pain. 2003;106(1):43–8.
10. Forssell H, Tenovuo O, Silvoniemi P, Jääskeläinen SK. Differences and similarities between atypical facial pain and trigeminal neuropathic pain. Neurology. 2007;69(14):1451–9.
11. Kuncz A, Vörös E, Barzó P, Tajti J, Milassin P, Mucsi Z, et al. Comparison of clinical symptoms and magnetic resonance angiographic (MRA) results in patients with trigeminal neuralgia and persistent idiopathic facial pain. Medium-term outcome after microvascular decompression of cases with positive MRA findings. Cephalalgia. 2006;26(3):266–76.
12. Sharav Y, Singer E, Schmidt E, Dionne RA, Dubner R. The analgesic effect of amitriptyline on chronic facial pain. Pain. 1987;31(2):199–209.
13. Forssell H, Tasmuth T, Tenovuo O, Hampf G, Kalso E. Venlafaxine in the treatment of atypical facial pain: a randomized controlled trial. J Orofac Pain. 2004;18(2):131–7.
14. Bayer E, Racz GB, Miles D, Heavner J. Sphenopalatine ganglion pulsed radiofrequency treatment in 30 patients suffering from chronic face and head pain. Pain Pract. 2005;5(3):223–7.
15. Mueller D, Obermann M, Yoon M-S, Poitz F, Hansen N, Slomke M-A, et al. Prevalence of trigeminal neuralgia and persistent idiopathic facial pain: a population-based study. Cephalalgia. 2011;31(15):1542–8.
16. Prakash S, Rathore C, Makwana P, Dave A. A cross-sectional clinic-based study in patients with side-locked unilateral headache and facial pain. Headache J Head Face Pain. 2016;56(7):1183–93.
17. Koopman JSHA, Dieleman JP, Huygen FJ, de Mos M, Martin CGM, MCJM S. Incidence of facial pain in the general population. Pain. 2009;147(1):122–7.
18. Klein J, Sandi-Gahun S, Schackert G, Juratli TA. Peripheral nerve field stimulation for trigeminal neuralgia, trigeminal neuropathic pain, and persistent idiopathic facial pain. Cephalalgia. 2016;36(5):445–53.

A 75-Year-Old Woman with Frequent Fleeting Face Pain (Trigeminal Neuralgia)

5

Armen Haroutunian, Kenneth D. Candido, and Nebojsa Nick Knezevic

Case Description

This is a case report of a 75-year-old female presenting to the pain management department with the description of a 10-year history of intermittent, sharp, stabbing left-sided facial pain radiating along the cheekbone and her jawbone all the way to her chin. The patient described that on most days she had mild pain and denied any baseline pain between the episodes of pain exacerbation. Aggravating factors included eating, swallowing, brushing her teeth, washing her face, clenching her teeth, light touch, and cold/windy weather. She denied any pain while sleeping, or waking up from the pain. She described trigger points including touching her left cheek and a few intra-oral points. Her dental history revealed a diagnosis of trigeminal neuralgia controlled with carbamazepine 100 mg twice daily, which relieved her pain temporarily. The patient stated that she often forgot to take her medication and had started to experience similar pain over the course of the last 6 months, gradually increasing in intensity. Her past medical history was only significant for hypertension, and occasional migraines, controlled with oral pharmacologic therapy. She denied any past surgical history. Review of systems is negative.

The patient's vitals were within normal limits. Physical examination demonstrated a patient in visible distress. Cranial nerves were intact, as well as the remainder of the neurologic examination. On oral examination, pain was present on palpitation of the mandibular and maxillary alveolar ridge and on the left side of the tongue. Review of her brain magnetic resonance imaging did not demonstrate any abnormalities. The decision was made to proceed with a Gasserian ganglion nerve block under computed tomography (CT) guidance (Fig. 5.1). She tolerated the procedure well and reported an excellent response with complete resolution of symptoms.

A. Haroutunian
Department of Anesthesiology, Advocate Illinois Masonic Medical Center, Chicago, IL, USA

K. D. Candido · N. N. Knezevic (✉)
Department of Anesthesiology, Advocate Illinois Masonic Medical Center, Chicago, IL, USA

Department of Anesthesiology, University of Illinois, Chicago, IL, USA

Department of Surgery, University of Illinois, Chicago, IL, USA

What Is Your Preliminary Diagnosis?

The preliminary diagnosis, exacerbation of trigeminal neuralgia, was based primarily on the history of the patient. Patients often described the pain as stabbing, momentary, and electric-like, often coming in clusters with periods of remission that may lasted a few months to a few years [1].

T. Malik (ed.), *Practical Chronic Pain Management*, https://doi.org/10.1007/978-3-030-46675-6_5

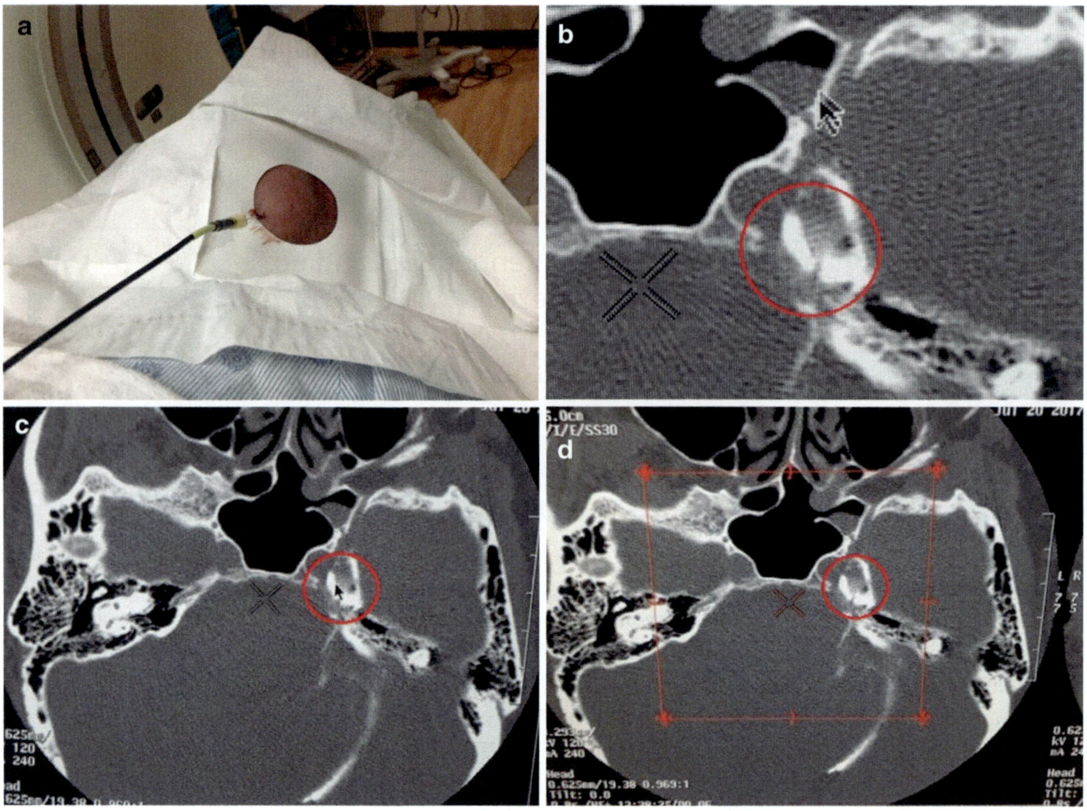

Fig. 5.1 (a–d) Gasserian ganglion block for trigeminal neuralgia under CT guidance

How is the Diagnosis Confirmed?

The pain is unilateral and upon examination the provider should confirm that the pain is in the distribution of the trigeminal nerve. Laboratory, radiologic, or electrophysiologic testing was not needed to confirm the diagnosis of TN, since patients with the characteristic signs and symptoms with a negative neurologic examination could commence treatment [2]. Preoperative MRI should be ordered to rule out other etiologies such as tumor or demyelinating disease. In most cases, no specific laboratory tests are needed, unless therapy with carbamazepine is started at which point blood count and liver function tests are required [2].

What Is the Pathophysiology of This Condition?

The trigeminal nerve is the sensory supply to the face as well as sensory and motor supply to the muscles of mastication. The three major divisions of the trigeminal nerve are the ophthalmic (V1), maxillary (V2), and mandibular (V3) nerves (Fig. 5.2). In 35% of patients, the pain typically radiates only to the maxillary or mandibular divisions accompanied by a brief spasm or tic [2]. The nerve exits at the level of the mid-lateral pons with its ganglion (the Gasserian ganglion) located at the trigeminal fossa (also known as Meckel's cave) (Fig. 5.3). These first-order

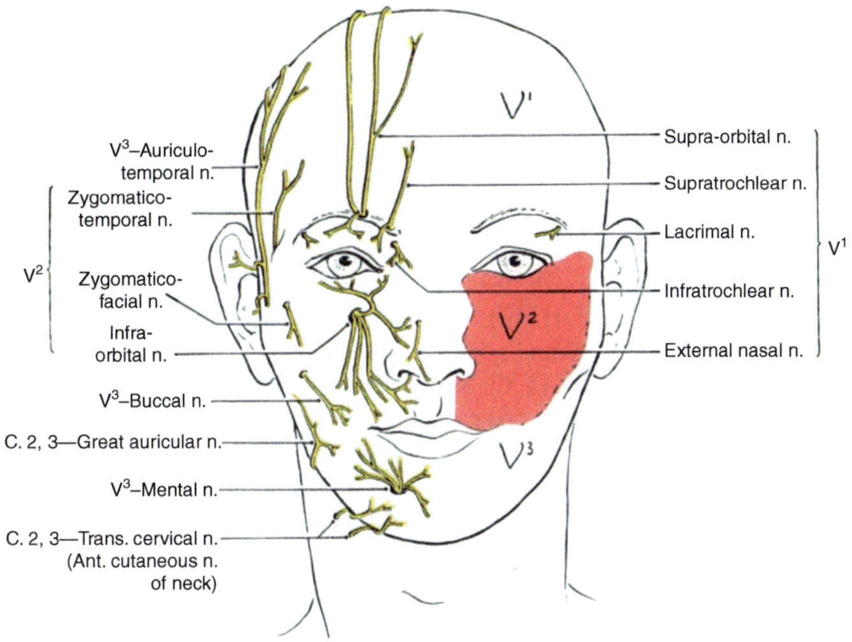

Fig. 5.2 Sensory Innervation of the branches of the trigeminal nerve

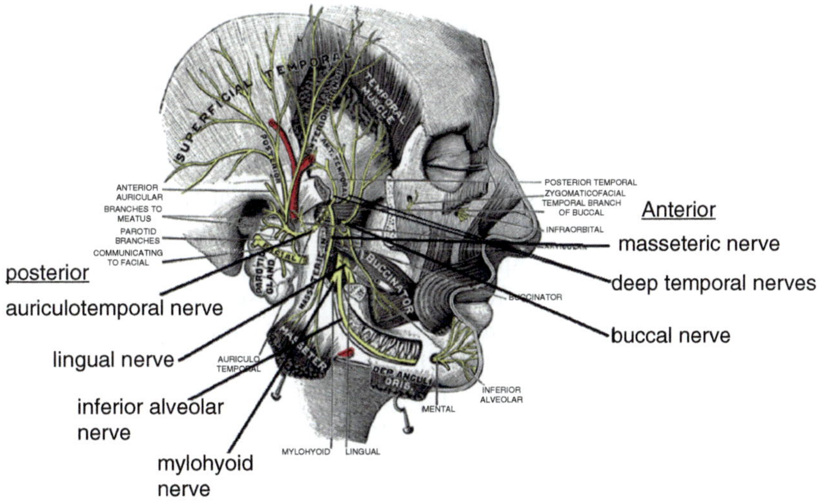

Fig. 5.3 The Gasserian ganglion and branches of the trigeminal nerve. (From Carter HV, Gray H, Anatomy of the Human Body, 1918)

neurons carry pain, temperature, and touch [2]. The majority of TN is caused by vascular compression of the nerve root, known as classic TN. Other causes of TN are schwannoma, meningioma, epidermoid cyst, aneurysm, and AV malformation [3]. The pathogenesis of neuropathy seems to be related to demyelination secondary to the area compressed and resultant ectopic impulse generation; however, the exact mechanism remains unclear [4]. Higher order complex pain mechanisms and central sensitization are also believed to play a role [5, 6]. Knowledge of the pathogenesis is important and can help direct treatment; structural compression can be addressed with surgical decompression while abnormal neuronal firing can be treated with anticonvulsant medications, and hypersensitivity can be treated with ablative techniques [7].

How Is the Problem Managed?

Management of TN is multimodal and includes pharmacologic therapy, percutaneous procedures, surgery, and radiation therapy. Medical management is often the initial treatment in patients with classic or vascular compressive TN. The first drug of choice is carbamazepine, an anticonvulsant that stabilizes neurons by blocking sodium channels. Studies demonstrate complete or near complete control of the pain in 60–100% of patients as compared to placebo [8]. Doses of 100–200 mg are started for two or three times daily, and are increased in increments of 200 mg until pain relief is achieved. The maximum recommended daily dose is 1200 mg daily. Side effects include dizziness, nausea, and vomiting. Laboratory analysis and blood count can reveal leukopenia, and rarely, aplastic anemia. Screening in the Asian population is recommended as the HLA-B 15:02 haplotype is associated with development of Stevens-Johnson syndrome or life-threatening toxic epidermal necrolysis [4]. Oxcarbazepine, an anticonvulsant that also blocks sodium channels, is as equally effective as carbamazepine [4]. The starting dose is 600 mg daily, increased in 300 mg increments to a total dose of 1200–1800 mg daily. A secondary medication, baclofen, binds the gaba-B receptor and blocks mono-and-polysynaptic reflexes by acting as an inhibitory neurotransmitter, hyperpolarizing the terminal, thus relieving muscle spasticity [4]. The starting dose is typically 15 mg daily in three divided doses, titrated up to 60 mg daily. Side effects include dizziness, sedation, and dyspepsia. The drug should be discontinued slowly since abrupt stoppage can cause seizures and hallucinations. If symptoms fail to subside, then tertiary medications such as lamotrigine, phenytoin, valproic acid, gabapentin, pregabalin, and clonazepam should be considered. Lamotrigine has been recommended as the drug of choice in patients with secondary TN caused by multiple sclerosis [9]. Opioids such as morphine, hydromorphone, and oxycodone are sometimes required to help treat the acute exacerbation of pain lasting days to weeks. When used in combination with neuropathic medications, opioids are more effective at lower doses [4].

When medical management does not provide adequate relief and the pain becomes refractory, surgery may be indicated. The two main surgical categories include microvascular decompression or ablative procedures (rhizotomy, radiosurgery, peripheral neurectomy, and nerve blocks) [4]. Ablative techniques are less invasive; however, recurrence may be more common. Microvascular decompression is achieved with a craniotomy and most frequently requires mobilization of the superior cerebellar artery loop, which is often the culprit responsible for the compression of the TN nerve [10]. A study in 1996 in the New England Journal of Medicine demonstrated that microvascular decompression is safe and effective, with a high rate of long-term success [11]. The most common complication is aseptic meningitis (11%), followed by hearing loss (10%) and sensory loss (7%) [4].

Ablative procedures include rhizotomy, radiosurgery, peripheral neurectomy, and nerve block. Rhizotomy can be achieved with radiofrequency thermocoagulation, mechanical balloon compression (Fogarty catheter), or chemical (glycerol) injection. With these procedures, a cannula is passed through the foramen ovale, and the sensory division of the trigeminal nerve is destroyed by one of the aforementioned methods. Initial pain relief can be as high as 90%, declining to 68–85% by 2 years, and by 54–64% in 3 years [8]. A major complication is meningitis, occurring in 0.2% of patients. Paresthesias can occur in up to 12% [4]. Radiosurgery describes the use of Gamma Knife to deploy high-dose radiation to the cisternal portion of the trigeminal nerve. Placement of a head frame and use of stereotactic MRI allow for specific nerve identification. These beams cause degeneration and death of the nerve axon. Pain relief can sometimes take up to 1 month to evolve [12]. Pain relief at 1 year was 69%, and 52% at 3 years. Worsening sensory impairment can occur in 9–37% of patients [4]. Peripheral neurectomy describes ablation of the branches of the trigeminal nerve (supraorbital, infraorbital, alveolar, and lingual nerves) via alcohol injection, cryotherapy, incision, or radiofrequency lesioning [4]. The evidence for each of these respective techniques is inconclusive.

Patients who do not respond well to medication or patients who are not suited for surgical decompression are often good candidates for trigeminal nerve block [13]. The peripheral nerve block can also be diagnostic as well as therapeutic for other conditions as well, such as recalcitrant herpes zoster ophthalmicus and postherpetic neuralgia [14]. Contraindications to the block include patient refusal, active anti-coagulation therapy, antiplatelet medications, or in pregnant women. Complications include hematoma, intravascular injection, or total spinal anesthesia. For these reasons, performing the block under image guidance is crucial [15]. Instead of blocking the trigeminal ganglion, the branches of the TN corresponding to the distribution of pain are blocked (typically V2 and V3 branches).

Trigeminal Nerve Block Technique

Ophthalmic Branch (V1) Nerve Block

In clinical practice, the branches of the ophthalmic nerve are blocked to treat pain around the eyes and nose. The nerve splits into lacrimal, frontal, and nasociliary branches. The frontal nerve further divides into the supraorbital and supratrochlear nerves. The supraorbital nerve supplies sensation to the forehead, scalp, and upper eyelid. The supratrochlear nerve supplies sensation to the upper nose, as well as the upper eyelid and conjunctivae. These two divisions of the frontal nerve are the main treatment targets in upper facial pain [1]. With the patient prepped and draped in the supine position, the supraorbital notch is palpated or identified using ultrasound guidance, and a short (1/2 in. or 3/4 in.; 22- or 25-gauge) needle is placed and advanced until contact with the bone is made, then withdrawn 1 mm. After negative aspiration, 1.5 mL of a combination of local anesthetic and steroid are injected (typically 0.25% bupivacaine with 20 mg of triamcinolone) [1]. Either a particulate steroid such as triamcinolone or nonparticulate such as dexamethasone can be used without any difference in outcomes or neurologic sequelae [16]. By needle redirection to the upper medial aspect of the superior orbital bone, the supratrochlear nerve is encountered, which sits just lateral to the base of the nose. With the same entry point used for the supraorbital nerve injection, injecting 1.5 mL of the local anesthetic and steroid mixture is undertaken [1].

Maxillary (V2) and Mandibular (V3) Nerve Block

With the patient in the supine position on the fluoroscopic table (alternative is to use ultrasound guidance), palpitation of the groove under the zygomatic arch will allow for identification of the coronoid notch. After 2–3 mL skin infiltration of local anesthetic, a 22-gauge 2.5-inch blunt (Whitacre, or equivalent) spinal needle is advanced under fluoroscopy at a perpendicular plane until contact with the pterygoid plate is made. The needle should be slightly withdrawn, and 1–2 mm and 3 mL of contrast is injected with confirmation of appropriate spread on imaging. Then, a mixture of local anesthetic and steroid (2 mL 0.25% bupivacaine with 20 mg triamcinolone) should be administered [1]. This will target the mandibular division (V3) of the trigeminal nerve. Redirection of the needle anterior and superior (approximately 1 cm past the pterygoid plate) will target the maxillary division (V2). Repeat the same injection technique with the mixture of local anesthetic with steroid. Again, proper needle placement prior to injection is critical, as advancement into the orbit can result in catastrophic outcomes [1].

What Is the Prognosis of This Condition?

The prognosis of disease is variable and episodes may last weeks to months. Recurrence of symptoms characterized as "waxing and waning" is common in the setting of background facial pain [4]. Lack of response to treatment therapy or pain in the V1 distribution are poor predictors of outcome. However, up to 90% of patients are pain-free soon after any of the operations, and the pain relief lasts longer with surgical decompression [17]. The chronic pain associated with the disease can cause depression or affect daily functioning, sometimes leading to death or suicide [2].

Discussion

Prevalence

Trigeminal neuralgia was first described by Dr. Johannes Laurentis Bausch in the mid-seventeenth century, who, in the midst of suffering from the disease himself, managed to detail the course of illness. Coined as "tic douloureux" by Nicolaus Andre in 1704, the condition is characterized by brief episodes of electric shock-like pain in one or more of the divisions of the trigeminal nerve, occurring in paroxysms, sometimes associated with facial spasms. The pain is typically unilateral and is often along the distribution of V2 and V3 branches of the TN, rarely affecting V1. Touching of certain trigger zones can lead to attacks, as can simple tasks such as chewing, talking, and grimacing. Seasonal changes, resulting in temperature changes and wind exposure, can precipitate attacks. The condition is rare (4–13 per 100,000 people) and affects women more than men in a 1:1.5–1:1.7 ratio [4]. It is more common after the age of 50, but can start as early as the second decade. There is weak evidence linking hypertension and migraine headaches as risk factors [18–20]. Patients who develop the disease during the second to fourth decade are more likely to be suffering from multiple sclerosis [2].

Differential Diagnosis

Based on the International Headache Society's (IHS) 3rd Edition of Classification of Headache Disorders, TN is divided into classic TN (or primary) and painful trigeminal neuropathy (secondary). Classic TN entails idiopathic TN as well as vascular compression as the causes of TN. Painful trigeminal neuropathy, however, is caused by lesions other than vascular compression, such as postherpetic trigeminal neuropathy, acute herpes zoster, post-traumatic trigeminal neuropathy, multiple sclerosis, and space-occupying lesions [4]. Diagnostic criteria (as defined by the IHS third edition) are as follows [4]:

1. Three attacks of unilateral face pain that must fulfill criteria 2 and 3.
2. Pain occurs along the distribution of the trigeminal nerve.
3. The pain has at least three of these following features:
   (a) Recurrent attacks lasting from a second to two minutes.
   (b) Severe in intensity (VAS $\geq$ 8/10).
   (c) Shock-like or stabbing in nature.
   (d) At least three attacks precipitated by stimulus that is not noxious in nature.
4. No neurologic deficit.
5. Not accounted for by another ICHD-3 diagnosis.

Predictive Value of Different Clinical Features and Lab Testing/Imaging

MRI with and without contrast is recommended for patients who meet the clinical criteria in order to differentiate classic TN from painful trigeminal neuropathy. Imaging can help identify or rule out multiple sclerosis, mass effect, vascular compression at the nerve root, and ultimately aid in preoperative planning.

Strength of Evidence for Different Treatment Modalities

The decision to pursue a certain therapy is multifaceted and depends on clinical findings and the underlying pathology, at which point an individualized treatment plan can be instituted. First-line therapy is medical management with carbamazepine; however, 15% of patients do not derive any benefits from this medication. Younger patients with classic TN refractory to medication treatment are good candidates for surgical decompression and can sometimes achieve complete cure. For elderly patients with active comorbidities, ablative therapies carry low risk and can produce quick relief.

Future Directions or Clinical Trials in Progress

There is much hope for future therapy. A 2014 literature review identified injection of botulinum toxin type A as an effective treatment therapy for patients refractory to medical management [17]. Already used to treat headaches and a number of other pain conditions, botulinum toxin type A inhibits the release of acetylcholine at the neuromuscular junction and decreases substance P, calcitonin gene-related peptide (CGRP), and glutamate. Although more studies are needed to substantiate its use, it does show much promise in the future treatment of TN [17]. Another emerging novel pharmacologic option currently under investigation is a sodium channel blocker (CNV1014802), shown to decrease paroxysmal attacks by 60% and pain scores by 55% [21]. Future nonpharmacological options include transcranial direct current stimulation or repetitive transcranial magnetic stimulation [22].

The sphenopalatine ganglion (SPG) block has recently re-emerged as a treatment option for patients with headache and face pain [23]. Described in 1908 by Dr. Sluder at Washington University and first used for treatment of trigeminal neuralgia by Dr. Ruskin in 1925, the SPG is the parasympathetic ganglia found in the pterygopalatine fossa, located posterior to the middle nasal turbinate [24, 25]. Although the mechanism is not exactly understood, interference with the parasympathetic outflow as well as modulation of the trigeminal nucleus caudalis via the afferent sensory fibers (believed to play a role in central sensitization) are two supported theories behind how the SPG block works [26]. The most common methods for SPG blockade include the transnasal, transoral, and lateral infratemporal approaches. The injectate is a local anesthetic, either alone or in combination with a depot steroid. Although the transnasal approach is the simplest and is typically devoid of major complications while being well tolerated, anatomic variability in patients creates uncertainty in the efficacy of the procedure and includes rare complications such as epistaxis and even rarer possible infection [27]. However, a new transnasal applicator, the Tx360, allows for a more precise delivery of analgesics and has popularized the technique due to its inexpensive, fast, and easy-to-use interface [28]. Further investigations comparing the new application to traditional techniques are still warranted.

Conclusion

Facial pain affects many people worldwide with costs of many billions of dollars per year. The pain causes an extensive burden on the individual, families, society, healthcare, and healthcare providers. In addition, trigeminal neuralgia causes debilitating disease, depression, and suicide if left untreated. The diagnosis is made based upon clinical judgment and imaging helps identify underlying disease and helps guide therapy. Treatment options include pharmacologic and nonpharmacologic therapies. First-line medication is with carbamazepine. Surgery is reserved for patients refractory to medical management. Emerging new pharmacologic and interventional therapies provide much promise in the treatment of trigeminal neuralgia.

References

1. Hoppenfeld JD. Fundamentals of pain medicine: how to diagnose and treat your patients. Philadelphia: Wolters Kluwer Health; 2014.
2. Singh MK. Trigeminal Neuralgia. In: Egan RA, Editor. 2016. Retrieved 06 July 2018, from https://emedicine.medscape.com/article/1145144-overview.
3. Love S, Coakham HB. Trigeminal neuralgia: pathology and pathogenesis. Brain. 2001;124:2347–60.
4. Bajwa ZH, Ho CC, Khan SA. Trigeminal neuralgia. In: Dashe JF, Editor. 2018. Retrieved 6 July 2018, from https://www.uptodate.com/contents/trigeminal-neuralgia/print.
5. Fromm GH, Terrence CF, Maroon JC. Trigeminal neuralgia: current concepts regarding etiology and pathogenesis. Arch Neurol. 1984;41:1204–7.
6. Obermann M, Yoon MS, Ese D. Impaired trigeminal nociceptive processing in patients with trigeminal neuralgia. Neurology. 2007;69:835–41.
7. Zussman BM, Moshel YA. Trigeminal Neuralgia: case report and review. JHN J. 2012;7(2).:Article 3.
8. Gronseth G, Cruccu G, Alksne J, Argoff C, Brainin M, Burchiel K, Nurmikko T, Zakrzewska JM. Practice parameter: the diagnostic evaluation and treatment of trigeminal neuralgia (an evidence-based review): report of the Quality Standards Subcommittee of the American Academy of Neurology and the European Federation of Neurological Societies. Neurology. 2008;71(15):1183–90.
9. Swathi T. Trigeminal neuralgia - a case report with review of literature. SAJ Case Report. 2017;4:102.
10. Jannetta PJ. Microsurgical management of trigeminal neuralgia. Arch Neurol. 1985;42(8):800–1.
11. Barker FG, Janetta PJ, Bissonette DJ, Larkins MV, Jho HD. The long-term outcome of microvascular decompression for trigeminal neuralgia. N Engl J Med. 1996;334:1077–83.
12. Young RF, Vermeulen SS, Grimm P, Blasko J, Posewitz A. Gamma Knife radiosurgery for treatment of trigeminal neuralgia, idiopathic and tumor related. Neurology. 1997;48:608–14.
13. Scrivani SJ, Mathews ES, Maciewicz RJ. Trigeminal neuralgia. Oral Surg Oral Med Oral Pathol Oral Radiol Endod. 2005;100(5):527–38.
14. Greenberg C, Papper EM. The indications for Gasserian ganglion block for trigeminal neuralgia. Anesthesiology. 1969;31:566–73.
15. Cherian A. Trigeminal Nerve Block Technique. In: Raghavendra MR, editor. 2016. Retrieved 6 July 2018, from https://emedicine.medscape.com/article/2040595-technique.
16. Nader A, Kendall MC. Dexamethasone versus triamcinolone side effects for ultrasound-guided trigeminal nerve block for the treatment of refractory typical or atypical facial pain. J Pain. 2016;17(4):S72.
17. Guardiani E, Sadoughi B, Blitzer A, Sirois D. A new treatment paradigm for trigeminal neuralgia using Botulinum toxin type A. Laryngoscope. 2014;124:413–7.
18. Maarbjerg S, Gozalov A, Olesen J, Bendtsen L. Trigeminal neuralgia—a prospective systematic study of clinical characteristics in 158 patients. Headache. 2014;54:1574–82.
19. Teruel A, Ram S, Kumar SK, Hariri S, Clark GT. Prevalence of hypertension in patients with trigeminal neuralgia. J Headache Pain. 2009;10(3):199–201.
20. Lin KH, Chen YT, Fuh JL, Wang SJ. Increased risk of trigeminal neuralgia in patients with migraine: a nationwide population-based study. Cephalalgia. 2015.
21. Versavel M. Efficacy and safety of the novel sodium channel Blocker CNV1014802 in Trigeminal Neuralgia and Lumbosacral Radiculopathy Scientific Tracks Abstracts. J Pain Relief. https://doi.org/10.4172/2167-0846.S1.002.
22. Obermann M, Katsarava Z, Holle D. An update on emerging therapeutic options for the treatment of trigeminal neuralgia. Expert Opin Orphan Drugs. 2017;5(11):859–63. https://doi.org/10.1080/21678707.2017.1394183.
23. Spector S, Srivastava SS. A new look at sphenopalatine ganglion blocks for chronic migraine. Practical Pain Management. 2017;16:1.
24. Sluder G. The role of the sphenopalatine ganglion in nasal headaches. AR Elliott Publishing Company. N Y State J Med. 1908;27:8–13.
25. Ruskin SL. Techniques of sphenopalatine therapy for chorioretinitis. Eye Ear Nose Throat Mon. 1951;30(1):28–31.
26. Yarnitsky D, Goor-Aryeh I, Bajwa ZH, Ransil BI, Cutrer FM, Sottile A, Burstein R. Possible parasympathetic contributions to peripheral and central sensitization during migraine. Headache. 2003;43(7):704–14.
27. Bonica JJ. The management of pain with special emphasis on the use of analgesic block in diagnosis, prognosis, and therapy. Philadelphia: Lea & Febinger; 1953.
28. Candido KD, Massey ST, Sauer R, Darabad RR, Knezevic NN. A novel revision to the classical transnasal topical sphenopalatine ganglion block for the treatment of headache and facial pain. Pain Physician. 2013;16(6):E769–78.

A Patient with Chronic Pain in the Back of the Head

6

Usman Latif

Case Description

A 43-year-old woman presents to chronic pain clinic with complaint of chronic headache. She has a history of diabetes mellitus, hypertension, gastroesophageal reflux disease, seasonal allergies, and childhood asthma. She denies any drug allergies. She takes metformin, lisinopril, pantoprazole, and cetirizine on a daily basis. She also takes Aspirin 81 mg on most days. She does not smoke. She drinks a few glasses of wine per month. She works a software developer and spends a lot of time seated at a workstation. She has several family members with a history of breast cancer.

She reports pain from the occiput extending over the scalp towards her forehead. The pain is over the entire scalp, but is worst on the left side. On the left side, it feels as the pain is shooting forward towards the eye. The pain is described as shooting, electric, and tingling. She states that her scalp feels very sensitive to touch at times. Pressure over the back of the head can be painful. Brushing her hair and lying on a pillow can also be uncomfortable at times.

Sometimes, she feels that the pain triggers generalized headaches. She denies any photophobia, phonophobia, nausea, or vomiting. Her headaches are not preceded by an aura. There is no clear trigger for the headaches. She does not believe there is any correlation with food, drink, or alcohol intake. She denies any other associated neurologic symptom. She cannot recall any specific injury to her head or neck.

U. Latif (✉)
Department of Anesthesiology, University of Kansas Medical Center, Kansas City, KS, USA
e-mail: ulatif@KUMC.edu

What Is Your Preliminary Diagnosis?

Every headache complaint should be thoroughly evaluated to rule out concerning pathology. Symptoms that might increase need for further workup include headache onset after the age of 50, loss of consciousness or collapse, description as first or worst headache patient has experienced, thunderclap nature of headache, focal neurologic deficit, papilledema, neck stiffness, an immunocompromised state, personality changes, headache after trauma, new onset of severe headache in pregnancy or postpartum, and headache that is worse with exercise, cough, or sexual intercourse [1, 2]. Patients with sudden onset of the first or worst headache of their life should be evaluated with computed tomography of the head without contrast. Immunocompromised patients with severe headache should be evaluated with magnetic resonance imaging with and without contrast.

The differential diagnosis should initially include migraine, cluster headache, tension-type headache, temporal arteritis, and hemicrania

T. Malik (ed.), *Practical Chronic Pain Management*, https://doi.org/10.1007/978-3-030-46675-6_6

continua. Following exclusion of these and other possibilities, occipital neuralgia can be considered. C2 neuralgia can also have a very similar presentation with occipital pain, but is more likely to have associated ciliary injection and ipsilateral lacrimation [3]. Postherpetic neuralgia involving the C2 root can be investigated by examining the scalp for lesions and eliciting a history to evaluate for prior shingles in the distribution. The upper cervical facets, particularly C2–3, can potentially be the cause of a dull, aching occipital head and neck pain. Medial branch blocks could be employed to differentiate facetogenic pain.

How Is Diagnosis Confirmed?

The International Headache Society diagnostic criteria for occipital neuralgia provide some guidance for making a diagnosis of occipital neuralgia [4]. Criteria include unilateral or bilateral pain located in the distribution of the greater, lesser, and/or third occipital nerves, associated with dysesthesia and/or allodynia during innocuous stimulation of the scalp and/or hair and either tenderness over the affected nerve branches or trigger points at the emergence of the greater occipital nerve or in the area of distribution of C2. The pain must have at least two of the following three characteristics: recurring paroxysmal attacks of a few seconds to minutes, severe intensity, and a shooting, stabbing, or sharp quality of the pain. Pain should be eased temporarily with local anesthetic block of the affected nerve.

There is some overlap with migraine and other headache syndromes. Therefore, the headache symptoms should not be better accounted for by another diagnosis. Additionally, in some patients, lying on a pillow and hyperextending the neck may result in pain [5]. This is termed the pillow sign. The use of ultrasound to aid in diagnosis has been reported in the literature [6]. Sonographic visualization of the GON or LON at the origination or anywhere along the course to the occiput may reveal neural edema, entrapment, or adjacent muscle spasm. This could potentially be of utility in the hands of a practitioner experienced in ultrasound of the posterior head and neck.

What Is the Pathophysiology of This Condition?

The greater occipital nerve (GON) originates from the medial branch of the dorsal ramus of C2 [3]. It then runs between the inferior oblique capitis muscle and the semispinalis capitis. It then travels lateral and deep to the trapezius before piercing it just inferior to the superior nuchal ridge. The GON is medial to the occipital artery. Sensory innervation is provided by the GON from the occipital protuberance to the vertex.

Branches of C2 and C3 in the cervical plexus come together to form the lesser occipital nerve (LON) [3]. The nerve runs along the posterior border of the sternocleidomastoid muscle. The lateral scalp superior and posterior to the ear is innervated by the LON. The third occipital nerve arises as a branch from C3 and provides sensation over the upper neck and lower occipital scalp.

Occipital neuralgia results with irritation of the nerve and can be primary or secondary. Some possible causes of occipital neuralgia may include trauma to the greater or lesser occipital nerves, upper cervical facet arthritis, tumors affecting the C2 and C3 nerve roots, history of radiation to the neck, diabetes, gout, vasculitis, irritation of the C1/2 nerve roots by an aberrant branch of the inferior cerebellar artery, dural AV fistula at the cervical level, bleeding from a bulbocervical cavernoma, fenestrated vertebral artery pressing on the C1/2 nerve roots, aberrant course of the vertebral artery, schwannoma in the craniocervical junction or of the occipital nerve, C2 myelitis, multiple sclerosis, cervical osteochondroma, osteolytic lesion of the cranium, and muscle tension at the occiput [5, 7]. Prolonged and frequent periods of keeping the head in a forward and downward position can also be associated with occipital neuralgia.

Occipital neuralgia typically involves a pain from the base of the head, or occiput, across the scalp towards the front of the head. It can approach near the forehead. It is also possible to have pain which shoots forward from the posterior scalp towards the eye. Pain may be unilateral or bilateral. The pain may be described as electric, tinging, aching, burning, throbbing, and shooting. Patients may have continuous aching, throbbing, or burning along with intermittent shooting or shock-like pains. Alternately, there may be intermittent pain episodes with no pain in the intervening periods.

Sensitivity to light, scalp tenderness, and pain with movement of the neck can be associated with the condition. Headaches associated with occipital neuralgia can occasionally be confused with other headache syndromes and are most commonly misdiagnosed as migraines or tension headaches. In particular, this can be possible when a practitioner does not recognize that pain behind the eye can potentially be attributed to occipital neuralgia in the appropriate setting.

Associated symptoms can be broad due to connections with the VIII, IX, and X cranial nerve and can include vision impairment/ocular pain (67%), tinnitus (33%), dizziness (50%), nausea (50%), and congested nose (17%) [5].

Imaging is generally not helpful in making the diagnosis of occipital neuralgia, but may be of utility in evaluating associated concerning neurologic symptoms or excluding other pathologies. There should be a low threshold to order magnetic resonance imaging of the brain in the presence of headache with any concerning or severe symptoms. Plain radiographs of the cervical spine can also be helpful in ruling out other abnormalities of the spine and cranium, such as Arnold-Chiari malformations [7]. Occipital neuralgia is generally a clinic diagnosis and may require exclusion of other headache pathologies.

How Is This Problem Managed?

Initial management is conservative and includes heat, rest, physical therapy, NSAIDs, and muscle relaxants [8]. In some cases, massage might be helpful, but sensitivity in the area may limit utility or exacerbate the condition in some patients. Pharmacologic treatment can include serotonin reuptake inhibitors, tricyclic antidepressants, and anticonvulsants such as gabapentin, pregabalin, and carbamazepine [5]. Because many cases respond to interventional treatment, it is not unreasonable to defer pharmacologic trial until after initial injection therapy as it might spare the patient from chronic medication. Ultimately, the order and prioritization of the various treatments should be customized to the patient and their preferences.

Occipital nerve diagnostic and therapeutic blocks can be employed for diagnosis and treatment of this condition. Loukas et al. determine the ideal injection site with a large study of 100 cadavers [9]. The ideal injection site was found to be 2 cm lateral and 2 cm inferior to the occipital protuberance. At this location, the occipital artery should be palpable laterally. To identify the LON, a line can be envisioned running from the mastoid to the occipital protuberance [3]. The LON should lie at the one-third mark closest to the mastoid [10]. There is great variability of the course of the nerves described in the literature [5]. One study performed dissection on embalmed cadavers and then employed a 3D digitizer [11]. The authors found that the most medial branch of the GON was 33.5 mm from the external occipital protuberance (EOP). The mean distance between the occipital artery and the EOP was 37.4 mm. This indicated that the GON was generally about 4 mm medial to the occipital artery. This study also concluded that on the EOP-mastoid process line, the medial third mark corresponded to the GON and the lateral third mark to the LON. Because of variation in anatomy, these injections should be considered field blocks to maximize coverage.

Diagnostic blocks can be performed with the clinician's choice of local anesthetic, and this author prefers bupivacaine 0.5% with 0.75 mL at each site. Published accounts advocate for a wide range of volumes of injection as high as 3–4 mL per side, but low-volume injections are also supported in the literature [7]. For therapeutic blocks, a solution of local anesthetic combined with steroids can be utilized. This author prefers a solution of 1 mL lidocaine 2%, 1 mL bupivacaine 0.5%, and 1 mL dexamethasone (10 mg), with 0.75 mL injected at each of the bilateral greater and lesser occipital nerves. For strictly unilateral pain, the procedure is performed only on the affected side.

The risk of adverse reactions is increased with steroid injection and can include alopecia and cutaneous atrophy [3]. Because of the proximity to the occipital artery, aspiration should be performed prior to injection. Common side effects can include dizziness, lightheadedness, soreness at the injection site, and as with most injection procedures, the possibility of vasovagal syncope.

A small study evaluated efficacy and found 80% or greater pain relief acutely with duration lasting from 1 week to 4 months [3]. Another study, retrospectively analyzed 184 patients and demonstrated a mean duration of benefit of 31 days [3]. There are published reports of pain resolving with diagnostic blocks only. Injections with local anesthetic only can be repeated every 2–4 weeks, and some published protocols advocate for a frequency as often as every week for initial treatment [12]. Injections with corticosteroids should be limited to once every 3 months.

Ultrasound-guided technique is also possible, but rarely employed due to the relative ease and success of the anatomic-guided approach, the minimal depth of insertion, the field block nature of the block, and patient aversion to having ultrasound gel in their hair. The occipital artery is palpated at the superior nuchal ridge. A linear high-frequency transducer is placed in transverse orientation to the ridge and overlying the occipital artery. The greater occipital nerve should be proximal to the occipital artery on the medial aspect. The artery should appear as pulsatile and may be partly compressible due to its small size. The nerve will appear hypoechoic and noncompressible [7].

A needle can be inserted in plane once the nerve is optimally visualized. A 2-inch 25-gauge needle can be used, but the author prefers a 1.75-inch 27- or 25-gauge needle on a 3 mL syringe. The needle should then be advanced to the periosteum in close proximity to the nerve. The needle is then retracted slightly and after aspiration, 0.25 mL of injectate can be injected in the area with visualized perineural spread. The remaining 0.5 mL of injectate can be injected in a fan-like distribution in the area as the greater occipital nerve branches extensively as it moves superiorly over the skull.

The probe can then be moved laterally and inferiorly in relation to the occipital artery. The lesser occipital nerve should be apparent overlying the semispinalis capitis muscle. Following negative aspiration, 0.25 mL of inject can be injected in the area with visualized perineural spread. The remaining 0.5 mL of injectate can be injected in a fan-like distribution in the area.

Contraindications to injection include infection, malformations such as hemangioma at the injection site, allergy to the medications to be administered, and patients on anticoagulants or with medical conditions which significantly increase the risk of bleeding. Consideration should be taken with patients who are pregnant or breastfeeding, and, generally, it is best to coordinate any interventional and pharmacological plans with the obstetrician. Additionally, patients with certain conditions such as ulcerative colitis, active infection, hypertension, congestive heart failure, renal disease, and psychiatric illness are more likely to have side effects [10].

Complications are rare but can include those which are common to most nerve blocks such as infection, bleeding, and allergic reaction to injectate. Since the scalp is well vascularized and the block is performed in the vicinity of the occipital artery, local anesthetic toxicity is a possibility, particularly when performed with larger volume injectate. Post-injection pressure in the punctured areas will help reduce bleeding and ecchymosis incidence [7].

While there has long been ample evidence that occipital nerve injection can be beneficial for occipital neuralgia, the 2016 American Headache Society Guidelines now also recommend suboccipital steroid injections as prophylactic treatment for cluster headaches [13, 14]. It is the only prophylactic treatment with Level A evidence for that indication.

Pulsed radiofrequency (PRF) has also been employed in the treatment of occipital neuralgia. Conventional radiofrequency (CRF) is typically not an option due to the superficial nature of the occipital nerves. PRF can be considered in cases where patients respond to anesthetic blocks of the GON and/or LON but have insufficient or no long-term relief with corticosteroid injection.

Unlike CRF, PRF is hypothesized to act through a temperature-independent, neuromodulatory process which alters synaptic transmission and pain signaling via the emission of electric fields with little or no tissue destruction [15]. Case reports and small trials have shown anywhere from 50% to 70% improvement in pain for durations of 4–6 months [16]. Reviews of PRF as a treatment for occipital neuralgia are promising, but further research is needed to support its use [15, 16]. In particular, high-quality randomized, controlled trials are lacking [16]. At this time, the Congress of Neurological Surgeons Guidelines recommend occipital nerve stimulation as a Level III recommendation for patients with medically refractory occipital neuralgia [17].

Two studies have evaluated the efficacy of botulinum toxin type A for the treatment of ON. One retrospective study of 6 patients demonstrated a reduction of 6 points on the VAS for a mean duration of greater than 16 weeks [3]. A prospective pilot study of 6 patients with a 12-week follow-up found some improvement in sharp, shooting pain and quality-of-life measures, but no improvement in dull pain or pain medication usage. Given the small sample sizes and variable results, botulinum toxin A injection is not routinely utilized in the occipital neuralgia treatment algorithm, but it is may be of utility in select patients, and future research will hopefully provide further insight into efficacy. Ultrasound-guided techniques have been described in the literature to facilitate targeted botox injection of muscles in presumed areas of occipital nerve entrapment [6].

Surgical management might include microvascular decompression if mechanical vascular compression of the nerve is felt to be the underlying pathology. In this case, displacement of the vessel away from the nerve may be of benefit. Neuromodulation with stimulator leads placed in the posterior scalp superficial to the cervical muscular fascia in the suboccipital area in proximity to the greater and lesser occipital nerves can be considered in limited cases [18]. This procedure carries the benefit of being less invasive than other surgical options, but risks include bleeding, infection, lead migration, difficulties with insurance coverage, and possibility of poor efficacy. Use of neurostimulation is FDA approved, but not for headache and craniofacial pain [12]. Therefore, occipital nerve stimulation is an off-label use.

There are also some nontraditional treatments which are not well supported in the literature due to a lack of studies in the subject areas, but there are case studies, series, and small studies support other alternate treatments. One report advocates for transcutaneous electrical nerve stimulation with three sessions per week [14]. Maintenance treatment consisted of physical therapy, deep tissue massage, and muscle relaxants. In this case, there was resolution of pain at the 12-month follow-up.

What Is the Prognosis of This Condition?

A study in the Dutch population reported an incidence of 3.2 per 100,000 people [5]. There was some increased female representation, but it was not significant. Eighty-five percent of patients have unilateral involvement. The GON is involved in 90% of cases, the LON in 10%, and both nerves in 9% [3].

Prognosis and cure rate varies widely and is not well elucidated in the literature. There are varying descriptions of the course of the condition including resolution with a single or series of injections, a recurring condition with intermittent periods of resolution, and a chronic, recalcitrant pain [10].

Conclusion/Summary

Occipital neuralgia is a relatively uncommon condition in the general population but more prevalent among the subset of patients with cephalgia. While there are many characteristic features, it is also a diagnosis of exclusion. Multiple treatment modalities exist including pharmacologic, physical therapy, and interventional treatment. Occipital nerve blocks are the most common and prevalent treatment with reasonable evidence supporting efficacy. Other interventional treatments include pulsed radiofrequency, neuromodulation, and surgical procedures.

References

1. Lynch KM, Brett F. Headaches that kill: a retrospective study of incidence, etiology and clinical features in cases of sudden death. Cephalalgia. 2012;32(13):972–8.
2. Hainer BL, Matheson EM. Approach to acute headache in adults. Am Fam Physician. 2013;87(10):682–7.
3. Dougherty C. Occipital neuralgia. Curr Pain Headache Rep. 2014;18(5):411.
4. Headache Classification Committee of the International Headache S. The international classification of headache disorders, 3rd edition (beta version). Cephalalgia. 2013;33(9):629–808.
5. Choi I, Jeon SR. Neuralgias of the head: occipital neuralgia. J Korean Med Sci. 2016;31(4):479–88.
6. Narouze S. Occipital neuralgia diagnosis and treatment: the role of ultrasound. Headache. 2016;56(4):801–7.
7. Waldman SD. Ultrasound-guided greater and lesser occipital nerve block. Comprehensive atlas of ultrasound-guided pain management injection techniques. Philadelphia: Lippincott Williams and Wilkins; 2014.
8. NIH. Occipital Neuralgia National Institute of Neurologic Disorders and Stroke 2018. Available from: https://www.ninds.nih.gov/Disorders/All-Disorders/Occipital-Neuralgia-Information-Page.
9. Loukas M, El-Sedfy A, Tubbs RS, Louis RG Jr, Wartmann CH, Curry B, et al. Identification of greater occipital nerve landmarks for the treatment of occipital neuralgia. Folia Morphol (Warsz). 2006;65(4):337–42.
10. Dach F, Eckeli AL, Ferreira Kdos S, Speciali JG. Nerve block for the treatment of headaches and cranial neuralgias – a practical approach. Headache. 2015;55 Suppl 1:59–71.
11. Shin KJ, Kim HS, Jehoon O, Kwon HJ, Yang HM. Anatomical consideration of the occipital cutaneous nerves and artery for the safe treatment of occipital neuralgia. Clin Anat. 2018;31(7):1058–64.
12. Mammis A, Gupta G. Occipital nerve stimulation: medscape. 2015. Available from: https://emedicine.medscape.com/article/2094731-overview.
13. Robbins MS, Starling AJ, Pringsheim TM, Becker WJ, Schwedt TJ. Treatment of cluster headache: the American headache society evidence-based guidelines. Headache. 2016;56(7):1093–106.
14. Ghaly RF, Plesca A, Candido KD, Knezevic NN. Transcutaneous electrical nerve stimulation in treatment of occipital neuralgia: a case report. A A Pract. 2018;11(1):4–7.
15. Manolitsis N, Elahi F. Pulsed radiofrequency for occipital neuralgia. Pain Physician. 2014;17(6):E709–17.
16. Vanneste T, Van Lantschoot A, Van Boxem K, Van Zundert J. Pulsed radiofrequency in chronic pain. Curr Opin Anaesthesiol. 2017;30(5):577–82.
17. Sweet JA, Mitchell LS, Narouze S, Sharan AD, Falowski SM, Schwalb JM, et al. Occipital nerve stimulation for the treatment of patients with medically refractory occipital neuralgia: Congress of Neurological Surgeons systematic review and evidence-based guideline. Neurosurgery. 2015;77(3):332–41.
18. Viswanath O, Rasekhi R, Suthar R, Jones MR, Peck J, Kaye AD. Novel interventional nonopioid therapies in headache management. Curr Pain Headache Rep. 2018;22(4):29.

7 A 35-Year-Old Man with Neck Pain Since a Car Accident (Whiplash Injury)

David H. Kim, Jonathan Church, and Adam C. Young

Case Presentation

A 35-year-old male presents to your clinic with new onset neck pain and headaches. His symptoms began 3 week prior when he was involved in a motor vehicle collision. He was a restrained driver, stopped at a stop sign when a vehicle going 20 miles per hour struck his vehicle from behind. He did not lose consciousness, his airbags did not deploy, and he was ambulatory at the scene. He noted neck pain that required emergency room evaluation at that time. He received an X-ray (Fig. 7.1) and was diagnosed with cervical myofascial strain. The emergency room physician prescribed cyclobenzaprine 5 mg three times daily as needed for muscle spasms and suggested he apply heat as well. He was instructed to follow up with his primary care provider should his symptoms worsen or continue. Over the next few weeks, he experienced worsening neck stiffness, which is worse in the morning and with moving his head in any direction. He complains of headaches that radiate from the occiput to the vertex and throb continuously. Lastly, he reports that his sleep has been interrupted because of the pain.

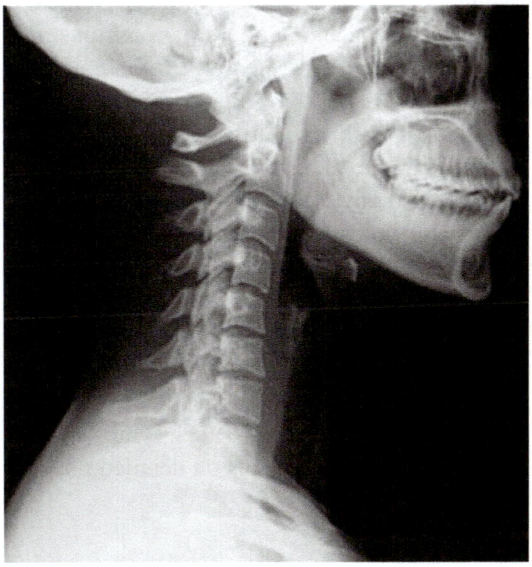

Fig. 7.1 Lateral view radiograph in a 35-year-old man with neck pain

His past medical history is significant for well-controlled gastroesophageal reflux disease. His surgical history is significant for a right knee meniscectomy at age 31. Current medications include ranitidine 75 mg BID prn for dyspepsia, cyclobenzaprine 5 mg TID prn for muscle spasms, and acetaminophen 500 mg TID prn for

D. H. Kim
Department of Anesthesiology and Pain Medicine, Kansas University Medical Center, Kansas City, KS, USA

J. Church
University Pain Centers, Chicago, IL, USA

A. C. Young (✉)
Department of Anesthesiology and Pain Management, Illinois Bone & Joint Institute, Morton Grove, IL, USA
e-mail: Adam_Young@Rush.Edu

T. Malik (ed.), *Practical Chronic Pain Management*, https://doi.org/10.1007/978-3-030-46675-6_7

pain. He is allergic to penicillin. Social history is significant for alcohol use 6 drinks per week, no tobacco or illicit drug use; he works as a financial advisor. Review of systems is positive for neck pain, muscle stiffness, and headaches. He specifically denies and numbness, tingling, or weakness of the upper extremities.

How Do You Evaluate the Patient?

Detailed history and physical examination is always important. History should include elucidating mechanism of injury, speed of vehicle at the time of accident, any loss of conscious, outcome of evaluation by the first ER visit, and any imaging done and its result. Idea is to look for any sign of neck instability or any other major injury. How the patients are managed since the accident and any other follow-up recommended and its outcome is important to know to avoid any duplication of effort.

This patient noticed new onset pain in the head and neck after being rear-ended. Negative X-ray of the spine and absence of neuro-deficit is quite reassuring. In presence of negative spine X-ray and absence of any other symptoms, the next step would be to focus on detailed physical examination.

What Do You Expect on His Physical Examination?

Physical examination findings of patients with suspected whiplash injury are variable. These findings are often used to classify severity of whiplash-related disorders and to follow improvement in the condition with treatment. It can range from a completely normal physical examination to limited range of motion, weak muscles, presence of trigger points, delayed or absence reflexes, and altered pain or touch threshold.

After neck and neuro stability has been established during initial evaluation, i.e., by an ER visit, focus should be on evaluation range of motion of neck in all directions, looking for any trigger points, evaluating muscle strength, and any other neurodeficits (reflexes/sensory loss/weakness) in the upper extremities.

How Do You Establish Diagnosis?

Whiplash-associated disorder is a clinical diagnosis. There are no pathognomonic signs or symptoms. It is a diagnosis of exclusion and is established using history of acceleration-deceleration as mechanism of injury in the absence of any other disorder. There is imaging or any other test that establishes the diagnosis except they are done to rule out other pathologies.

When Would You Order Additional Tests?

Additional tests are ordered to elicit information that can alter treatment plan. Patients with normal physical examination do not need additional imaging or any nerve conduction studies. About half the patients with whiplash pain after car accident may have cervical facet joint pain. This pain can only be diagnosed with diagnostic injections, which should be done if the conservative therapy fails to improve patients.

What Is the Natural Prognosis of This Condition?

A majority of people (>75%) complain of neck pain after a car accident. Roughly 80% of them are asymptomatic within 3 months. It becomes a chronic problem in 10–15% of patients. Intense initial pain is a strong predictor of poor outcome. Other factors predicting chronicity or poor outcome include older age, female gender, intense psychological response to initial pain, litigation, multiple pain complaints, and unprepared at the time of impact.

What Is the Underlying Pathophysiology of This Condition?

The underlying pathology is unclear. The imaging studies reveal no obvious damage. Cervical facet joints are source of nociception in certain patients and can be easily diagnosed using diagnostic injection techniques, but in others source of pain is not clear. Imbalance of muscle movements or abnormal muscle recruitment has been proposed. This includes less contribution from deeper cervical muscles putting more strain on superficial cervical muscles, excessive activation of trapezius muscle, and switch to fast-twitch muscle fibers from slow-twitch fibers resulting in easy fatigability. Sensorimotor symptoms of paresthesia, allodynia, and hyperalgesia may be due to central sensitization of both nociceptive and non-nociceptive sensory pathways. Psychological factors may contribute to the above physiological abnormalities. Whiplash-related pain condition is often associated with depression, anxiety disorder, and fear of pain with work.

How Is the Condition Managed?

Whiplash-associated pain is poorly understood. The first step is comprehensive medical evaluation of patient including psychological aspects. Mainstay of treatment is to restore range of motion, strength, and endurance of the muscles. In acute phase, within 3 weeks of injury, nonsteroidal and muscle relaxer agents help, but these agents have no proven role in chronic phase. Manual manipulation, chiropractor therapy, acupuncture, and trigger point injections all are equally effective in short term. Best long-term relief comes from RF ablation of medial nerve branches resulting in denervation of cervical facet joints when done in patients in whom diagnostic blocks provide complete relief. Early mobilization is encouraged and results in better long-term outcome. Cognitive behavior therapy should be employed along with physical therapy whenever indicated. Active physical therapy is the focus of treatment.

Background

Whiplash or whiplash-associated disorder (WAD) is a relatively prevalent condition with an estimated 3.8/1000 people are affected [1]. The incidence of the condition is high with close to a million people per year evaluated and treated for neck strain injury in US emergency departments [2]. Many patients experience symptoms that can be protracted, some being severe enough to lead to disability [3]. Economic impact and litigation involved with this condition is also remarkably high with motor vehicle accidents as one of the leading causes of personal injury and 29 billion dollars per year spent on whiplash injuries and litigation alone in the United States [4]. Whiplash-associated disorder (WAD) is defined as by the Quebec Task Force in 1995 as an acceleration-deceleration mechanism of energy transfer to the neck resulting in bony or soft tissue injuries, which may in turn result in a variety of clinical manifestations [5]. The disorder encompasses the cervical spine and nervous system injuries that arise from inertial forces being applied to the head in from the rapid back and forth motion of the head and neck. The force of this whiplash motion can result in damage to bony or soft tissue structures, which include the intervertebral discs, face joints, muscle, ligaments, and dorsal root ganglia; common sources of pain include cervical spine ligaments, cervical spine muscles, or facet joints. The clinical manifestations of whiplash include principally neck pain, headache, and decreased neck range of motion. In addition, other symptoms include tenderness and pain in the shoulders and upper extremities, paresthesias in the upper extremities, visual symptoms, tinnitus, dizziness, fatigue, cognitive impairment, and mood disorders. WAD is classified according to the Quebec classification based on both signs and symptoms (Table 7.1). Of note, the pain associated with WAD may not develop immediately with one study reporting that complete reporting of neck pain after neck injury can take up to 72 hours. [6] This is similarly reflected in the clinical spectrum of whiplash-associated disorders per the Quebec Task Force, which has timing

Table 7.1 Quebec classification of whiplash injuries

Grade	Clinical presentation
0	No complaint of neck pain. No physical signs.
I	Neck pain, stiffness, tenderness. No physical signs.
II	Neck complaints. Musculoskeletal signs including decreased range of motion or point tenderness.
III	Neck complaints. Neurological signs including decreased deep tendon reflexes, weakness, sensory deficits
IV	Neck complaints. Fracture or dislocation.

From Spitzer et al. [5], with permission

of presentation correlated with severity of pathology and symptoms [5].

The etiology of chronic pain in WAD is inconclusive. It has been theorized that the delayed but sometimes persistent pain in whiplash is secondary to cervical facet joint synovitis [7, 8]. This theory is supported by clinical response to cervical zygapophyseal injections [9]. Other potential etiologies include persistent posterior branch irritation of cervical nerve roots or muscle spasm causing impingement of the nerve roots. It has also been shown that pre-existing disc degeneration on MRI is not correlated with clinical presentation or prognosis for WAD [10]. However, it appears that there may be a central nervous system component to the development of pain. An MRI study comparing healthy controls with WAD patients demonstrated regional decreases of gray matter volume in several cortical regions and was also correlated with behavior and physiologic measures such as cognitive performance, maladaptive pain response, central sensitization, hyperalgesia [11]. This is also supported by a study demonstrating altered regional cerebral blood flow PET scans in WAD patients [12].

Besides the aforementioned theories of cervical facet joint synovitis and muscular dysfunction, another theory of the etiology of neck pain is neck musculature contraction and subsequent chronic compression of the cervical nerve roots. The symptom of neck pain can also be attributed to neck muscle dysfunction and degeneration. One study has demonstrated correlation of muscle fatty infiltrates in the cervical multifidi muscles after whiplash with degree of symptoms [13]. Functional measures of control of head movements is also altered in whiplash patients with average time to peak force significantly longer for flexion and extension movements of the neck. This has also been followed up in the rehabilitation literature with reduction in neck strength and extensor endurance [14].

The numerous associated symptoms of WAD may be attributed to cranial nerve dysfunction, central nervous system, cervical radiculopathy, and/or plexopathy. Headaches are one of the more common symptoms, occurring in up to 70% of these patients. The etiology of occipital headaches associated with WAD can be attributed to zones of reference from the cervical facet joints. Evidence of this is response to anesthetic blockade of the C2/C3 facet in cervicogenic headache [15]. Furthermore, surgical decompression of the occipital nerve has alleviated chronic headaches in WAD patients [16]. In addition, the C2 nerve root has a known anatomic connection through the spinal trigeminal nucleus that may mediate headache in the trigeminal nerve distributions [17, 18]. This may similarly lead to numbness of loss of sensation in the face in whiplash with one study demonstrating altered thermal sensitivity in facial distributions in whiplash patients [19]. For cervicogenic headache, neural blockade of the C2/C3 nerve roots and greater occipital nerve has also been shown to be effective in treating headache symptoms [20].

Visual symptoms may also occur with whiplash and are typically self-limited but may be relatively common. One prospective case series of 39 patients with whiplash injury tested for ophthalmic and oculomotor function demonstrated that 10 of the 39 patients had ocular symptoms and signs, which fully resolved in all but 2 patients by 9 months [21]. The most common complaint was blurry vision. This may be due to eye coordination, gaze stability, or convergence insufficiency. In one study of 20 WAD patients and 20 asymptomatic controls, significant deficits in gaze stability and eye coordination were noted in the WAD patients during head rotation and sequential head and eye movements [22]. However, other studies have demonstrated no differences between WAD patients and controls for examinations of smooth pursuit eye movements or convergence [23, 24]. One study has linked restricted cervical movements and differences in proprioceptive information from the cervical spine with oculomotor dysfunction, which may explain why significant results were seen in the aforementioned study with head rotation and movements, while stationary oculomotor testing in the latter two studies had non-significant differences [25]. Similarly, limited neck movement has been correlated with reduction of the cervico-ocular reflex in these patients.

Complaints of dizziness and vertigo may be attributed to neck dysfunction with altered cervical proprioception. Significant differences in postural stability have been quantified in whiplash patients compared to controls [26]. Additionally, head extension has been linked with postural instability in whiplash patients [27]. Given the possible cervical etiology of dizziness and vertigo in WAD patients, it has also been demonstrated that cervical medial branch blockade can alleviate presumed cases of cervicogenic vertigo [28]. The etiology of dizziness and vertigo may also be due to cervicocranial junction compression secondary to ligament laxity, which has also been noted in other cervicocranial disorders such as Chiari malformation.

In the absence of imaging or neurophysiologic findings consistent with a radiculopathy, central stenosis, cervical myelopathy, or plexopathy, complaints of arm pain or numbness may be attributed to referred pain from cervical facet joints. One study examined upper extremity reaction time, movement speed, accuracy, coordination, and tapping speed and found no difference in WAD patients aside from reaction time [29].

Differential Diagnosis

The differential diagnosis for whiplash injury includes those that affect the cervical spine, skull, and central nervous system. They can be related to the muscular, ligamentous, neurological, or bony structures. Diagnosis is often based on physical exam and history, and supported by radiologic findings. These include the following:

- Whiplash injury
- Cervical spondylosis
- Cervical herniated nucleus pulposus
- Cervical facet syndrome
- Cervical myofascial strain
- Cervical radiculopathy
- Cervical central canal stenosis
- Cervical myelopathy
- Fracture
- Thoracic outlet syndrome
- Vascular injury (vertebral or carotid dissection)
- Referred shoulder or acromioclavicular joint pain
- Referred pain from myocardial infarction
- Inflammatory rheumatologic diseases
- Malignancy of cervical spine
- Infection (e.g., meningitis, herpes zoster)
- Traumatic brain injury
- Malingering, factitious disorder, psychogenic pain

Confirming the Diagnosis

The diagnosis of WAD is clinical. No single radiologic, electrophysiologic, or physical test is sensitive and specific for the condition. Per the Quebec task force, whiplash is defined as "bony or soft tissue injury from an acceleration-deceleration mechanism of energy transfer to the neck" [5]. The clinical history should elicit factors such as mechanism of injury and symptoms such as neck pain, limited neck mobility, headaches, upper extremity pain and paresthesia, visual disturbances, dizziness and vertigo, temporomandibular joint dysfunction, cognitive impairment, and mood disorders. No physical examination finding is specific to WAD. The physical examination should focus on range of motion and exclusion of other diagnoses such as signs of cervical myelopathy, radiculopathy, plexopathy, facet arthropathy, and occipital neuralgia. Radiologic findings are often not present in the acute phase. Certain findings such as loss of cervical spine lordosis may be correlated with WAD.

X-ray, CT, and MRI may be used to identify structural injuries associated with WAD. The lack of correlation with radiologic evidence is shown by the Quebec classification of whiplash injuries, which relies on radiologic findings in only Grade IV (Table 7.1). X-ray of the cervical spine is the first line of assessment and can be used to rule out significant bony injury as seen in WAD IV. CT may be a better option for patients with more acute trauma with high probability of injury or fractures requiring rapid evaluation. MRI can be used to better evaluate soft tissue and neurologic structures of the cervical spine, which may reveal ligamentous injuries or the cause for a neurologic deficit [30]. Radiologic testing should be guided by clinical necessity at time of acute injury and clinical suspicion for other etiologies at the subacute and chronic phases. Imaging may help rule out other etiologies such as malignancy, infection, or vascular injuries in addition to relatively common cervical spine pathology. Prolonged peripheral motor latency on electrophysiologic testing may be present but is not specific.

Treatment

The treatment of whiplash includes several different modalities with varying degrees of evidence, clinical indications, and efficacy. A comprehensive five-part review is provided by Teasell et al. in 2010 [31]. To summarize, current evidence supports exercise, physiotherapy, and mobility training programs. Other therapies have equivocal or conflicting studies or are limited by low number of studies with small sample sizes. For patients presenting within 3 months of Grade I-III WAD, initial recommendations to patients should include advice, reassurance, encouragement to resume normal activity, and cervical spine exercises. For those with persistent symptoms for greater than 3 months, supervised exercises with advice are recommended.

In the acute setting, within 2 weeks of injury, there are several treatments that have been tested. Educational interventions have had conflicting results. Physical therapy and active exercise treatment have been shown to have significant effects on reducing pain and disability scores post-acute phase [32]. In one study of 200 patients with acute WAD, patients who received physiotherapy for 2 weeks, as opposed to cervical immobilization with a soft collar, experienced a 50% reduction in pain and disability at 6-month follow-up [33]. One well-designed randomized controlled trial with 200 acute WAD patients compared soft collar immobilization for 1 week versus physiotherapist instruction for mobilization for 1 week. Patients with early mobilization significantly lowered mean pain intensity, disability, neck pain, headache, and shoulder pain [34]. In terms of pharmacologic treatment, one study has examined steroid use in a series of 40 acute WAD patients and demonstrated significant reduction of symptoms, sick days, and sick leave with methylprednisolone infusion for the first 23 hours after initial presentation [35]. Other interventions such as pulsed electromagnetic field therapy and laser acupuncture lack evidence to support their use.

For management of chronic whiplash, exercise remains the standard non-interventional treatment. Multiple randomized controlled trials have examined the use of guided exercise programs for chronic WAD. In one randomized controlled trial with a treatment regimen of 12 exercise sessions over 6 weeks, significant improvements were made in pain, disability, and functional disability. However, in this particular study, these improvements were not maintained at 1-year follow-up [36]. This may imply that exercise must be sustained to have a sustained effect on pain control. A review of chiropractic manipulation has found that although there are a number of articles and studies that support chiropractic manipulation in whiplash associated disorder, the quality of evidence is low [37]. Although a number of cognitive behavioral, counseling, and psychologic interventions have been trialed, the varying interventions make it difficult to formulate conclusions. In general, psychologic intervention is associated with improvement in pain, disability, return to work, and coping. Biofeedback training has promising evidence for its use. One case series of 11 patients demonstrated clear improvements in pain in the neck and upper back region and a non-significant trend towards decreased disability [38].

Interventional therapies for whiplash span injection-based therapies, radiofrequency neurotomy, to surgical options such as cervical spine fusion and occipital nerve decompression. For injection-based therapies, various agents have been attempted including water, saline, and botulinum toxin A injections into trigger points and steroid and local anesthetic injections into zygopophyseal joints and selective nerve blocks. Botulinum toxin A has had several randomized controlled trials with two demonstrating no significant difference between botulinum toxin A and placebo injections and one demonstrating improvement in pain scores and cervical range of motion [39, 40]. The cumulative evidence is inconclusive regarding the efficacy of botulinum toxin A for whiplash-associated disorder. A meta-analysis of trigger point injections including botulinum toxin A studies and local anesthetic studies similarly was inconclusive regarding the benefit of trigger point injections [41].

Facet joint injections have a modicum of evidence in favor of their usage. One study by Slipman et al. demonstrated that intra-articular injections of corticosteroids were able to reduce headache frequency in 61% of patients [42]. However, this study was limited by its retrospective structure and small sample size of 18 patients. In addition, one study has attempted to stimulate regeneration of the zygapophyseal joints via intra-articular dextrose-lidocaine injections, which had significant improvements in pain and function that persisted through 12 months of follow-up [43]. It has been hypothesized that the injection of local anesthetic alone is equally efficacious as when steroid is added; a prior study with whiplash patients and intra-articular injection of betamethasone did not demonstrate any significant improvement in pain relief compared with local anesthetic [44].

Occipital nerve or C2/C3 nerve root blocks have been used successfully to treat the cervicogenic headache associated with whiplash. In contrast to injections or blockade of the facet joints or medial branches, radiofrequency neurotomy of the cervical medial branches has had robust data demonstrating pain relief that persists for several months to years [45–47]. Improvements in several studies also included reduction in disability measures, cervical range of motion, and muscle strength.

Surgical interventions are highly variable in terms of treatment offered with oftentimes a single supporting study regarding any given technique. Occipital nerve decompression has been successfully utilized for whiplash-related headache. Another study has examined surgical fasciectomy of the trapezius muscle with neurolysis of the spinal accessory nerve with improvements in pain, headaches, insomnia, weakness, and stiffness [48]. Cervical fusion has a select few studies that demonstrate improvement in pain [49]. These studies had relatively few patients but also had subjects who had been refractory to other forms of treatment and were screened and selected based on symptoms and signs demonstrating a potential affected segment in the cervical spine.

All interventions are meant to improve range of motion and strength of muscles which is ultimately achieved through an active exercise program. The aim of the program is to prevent development of chronic pain behavior and improve functionality. The program usually focuses on improving mobility, muscle coordination and proprioception, and endurance.

References

1. Overmeer T, Peterson G, Landén Ludvigsson M, Peolsson A. The effect of neck specific exercises with or without a behavioral approach on psychological factors in chronic whiplash associated disorders. A randomized controlled trial with a 2 year follow up. Medicine (Baltimore). 2016;95(34):e4430.
2. Quinlan KP, Annest JL, Myers B, et al. Neck strains and sprains among motor vehicle occupants – United States, 2000. Accid Anal Prev. 2004;36:21–7.

3. Carroll LJ, Holm LW, Hogg-Johnson S, et al. Bone and joint decade 2000-2010 task force on neck pain and its associated disorders. Course and prognostic factors for neck pain in whiplash-associated disorders (WAD): results of the bone and joint decade 2000–2010 task force on neck pain and its associated disorders. Spine. 2008;33:S83–92.
4. Freeman MD, Croft AC, Rossignol AM, et al. A review and methodologic critique of the literature refuting whiplash syndrome. Spine. 1999;24:86–98.
5. Spitzer WO, Skovron ML, Salmi LR, et al. Scientific monograph of the Quebec task force on whiplash-associated disorders: redefining 'whiplash' and its management. Spine. 1995;20:2S–73S.
6. Deans GT, Magalliard JN, Kerr M, Rutherford WH. Neck sprain-a major cause of disability following car accidents. Injury. 1987;18(1):10–2.
7. Tanaka N, Atesok K, Nakanishi K, et al. Pathology and treatment of traumatic cervical spine syndrome: whiplash injury. Adv Orthop. 2018;28:1–6.
8. Endo K. Whiplash injury handbook. Tokyo: Springer-Japan; 2006.
9. Persson M, Sörensen J, Gerdle B. Chronic whiplash associated disorders (WAD): responses to nerve blocks of cervical zygapophyseal joints. Pain Med. 2016;17(12):2162–75.
10. Chung NS, Jeon CH, Lee YS, et al. Is preexisting cervical disk degeneration a prognostic factor in whiplash-associated disorders? Clin Spine Surg. 2017;30(9):E1251–5.
11. Coppieters I, De Pauw R, Caeyenberghs K, et al. Decreased regional grey matter volume in women with chronic whiplash-associated disorders: relationships with cognitive deficits and disturbed pain processing. Pain Physician. 2017;20(7):E1025–51.
12. Vállez García D, Doorduin J, Willemsen AT, et al. Altered regional cerebral blood flow in chronic whiplash associated disorders. EBioMedicine. 2016;10:249–57.
13. Elliott JM, Courtney DM, Rademaker A, Pinto D, Sterling MM, Parrish TB. The rapid and progressive degeneration of the cervical multifidus in whiplash: an MRI study of fatty infiltration. Spine. 2015;40(12):E694–700.
14. Krogh S, Kasch H. Whiplash injury results in sustained impairments of cervical muscle function: a one-year prospective, controlled study. J Rehabil Med. 2018;50(6):548–55.
15. Bovim G, Berg R, Dale LG. Cervicogenic headache: anesthetic blockades of cervical nerves (C2-C5) and facet joint (C2/C3). Pain. 1992;49(3):315–20.
16. Magnússon T, Ragnarsson T, Björnsson A. Occipital nerve release in patients with whiplash trauma and occipital neuralgia. Headache. 1996;36(1):32–6.
17. Kerr FW. Structural relation of the trigeminal spinal tract to upper cervical roots and the solitary nucleus in the cat. Exp Neurol. 1961;4:134–48.
18. Piovesan EJ, Kowacs PA, Oshinsky ML. Convergence of cervical and trigeminal sensory afferents. Curr Pain Headache Rep. 2003;7(5):377–83.
19. Häggman-Henrikson B, Lampa E, Nordh E. Altered thermal sensitivity in facial skin in chronic whiplash-associated disorders. Int J Oral Sci. 2013;5(3):150–4.
20. Inan N, Ceyhan A, Inan L, et al. C2/C3 nerve blocks and greater occipital nerve block in cervicogenic headache treatment. Funct Neurol. 2001;16(3):239–43.
21. Burke JP, Orton HP, West J, et al. Whiplash and its effect on the visual system. Graefes Arch Clin Exp Ophthalmol. 1992;230(4):335–9.
22. Treleaven J, Jull G, Grip H. Head eye coordination and gaze stability in subjects with persistent whiplash associated disorders. Man Ther. 2011;16(3):252–7.
23. Kongsted A, Jørgensen LV, Bendix T, et al. Are smooth pursuit eye movements altered in chronic whiplash-associated disorders? A cross-sectional study. Clin Rehabil. 2007;21(11):1038–49.
24. Stiebel-Kalish H, Amitai A, Mimouni M, et al. The discrepancy between subjective and objective measures of convergence insufficiency in whiplash-associated disorder versus control participants. Ophthalmology. 2018;125(6):924–8.
25. Heikkilä HV, Wenngren BI. Cervicocephalic kinesthetic sensibility, active range of cervical motion, and oculomotor function in patients with whiplash injury. Arch Phys Med Rehabil. 1998;79(9):1089–94.
26. Bianco A, Pomara F, Petrucci M, et al. Postural stability in subjects with whiplash injury symptoms: results of a pilot study. Acta Otolaryngol. 2014;134(9):947–51.
27. Kogler A, Lindfors J, Odkvist LM, Ledin T. Postural stability using different neck positions in normal subjects and patients with neck trauma. Acta Otolaryngol. 2000;120(2):151–5.
28. Hahn T, Halatsch ME, Wirtz C, Klessinger S. Response to cervical medial branch blocks in patients with cervicogenic vertigo. Pain Physician. 2018;21(3):285–94.
29. See KS, Treleaven J. Identifying upper limb disability in patients with persistent whiplash. Man Ther. 2015;20(3):487–93.
30. Strudwick K, McPhee M, Bell A, et al. Review article: best practice management of neck pain in the emergency department (part 6 of the musculoskeletal injuries rapid review series). Emerg Med Australas. 2018;30(6):754–72.
31. Teasell RW, McClure JA, Walton D, et al. A research synthesis of therapeutic interventions for whiplash-associated disorder: part 1 - overview and summary. Pain Res Manag. 2010;15(5):287–94.
32. Teasell RW, McClure JA, Walton D, et al. A research synthesis of therapeutic interventions for whiplash-associated disorder: part 2 - interventions for acute WAD. Pain Res Manag. 2010;15(5):295–304.
33. Vassiliou T, Kaluza G, Putzke C, et al. Physical therapy and active exercises – an adequate treatment for prevention of late whiplash syndrome? Randomized controlled trial in 200 patients. Pain. 2006;124(1–2):69–76.
34. Schnabel M, Ferrari R, Vassiliou T, Kaluza G. Randomised, controlled outcome study of active

mobilisation compared with collar therapy for whiplash injury. Emerg Med J. 2004;21(3):306–10.
35. Pettersson K, Toolanen G. High-dose methylprednisolone prevents extensive sick leave after whiplash injury. A prospective, randomized, double-blind study. Spine. 1998;23(9):984–9.
36. Stewart MJ, Maher CG, Refshauge KM, et al. Randomized controlled trial of exercise for chronic whiplash-associated disorders. Pain. 2007;128(1–2):59–68.
37. Shaw L, Descarreaux M, Bryans R, et al. A systematic review of chiropractic management of adults with Whiplash-Associated Disorders: recommendations for advancing evidence-based practice and research. Work. 2010;35(3):369–94.
38. Voerman GE, Vollenbroek-Hutten MM, Hermens HJ. Changes in pain, disability, and muscle activation patterns in chronic whiplash patients after ambulant myofeedback training. Clin J Pain. 2006;22(7):656–63.
39. Braker C, Yariv S, Adler R, et al. The analgesic effect of botulinum-toxin a on post-whiplash neck pain. Clin J Pain. 2008;24(1):5–10.
40. Padberg M, de Bruijn SF, Tavy DL. Neck pain in chronic whiplash syndrome treated with botulinum toxin. A double-blind, placebo-controlled clinical trial. J Neurol. 2007;254(3):290–5.
41. Scott NA, Guo B, Barton PM, Gerwin RD. Trigger point injections for chronic non-malignant musculoskeletal pain: a systematic review. Pain Med. 2009;10(1):54–69.
42. Slipman CW, Lipetz JS, Plastaras CT, et al. Therapeutic zygapophyseal joint injections for headaches emanating from the C2-3 joint. Am J Phys Med Rehabil. 2001;80(3):182–8.
43. Hooper RA, Frizzell JB, Faris P. Case series on chronic whiplash related neck pain treated with intraarticular zygapophysial joint regeneration injection therapy. Pain Physician. 2007;10(2):313–8.
44. Barnsley L, Lord SM, Wallis BJ, Bogduk N. Lack of effect of intraarticular corticosteroids for chronic pain in the cervical zygapophysealjoints. N Engl J Med. 1994;330(15):1047–50.
45. Smith AD, Jull G, Schneider G, et al. Cervical radiofrequency neurotomy reduces psychological features in individuals with chronic whiplash symptoms. Pain Physician. 2014;17(3):265–74.
46. Prushansky T, Pevzner E, Gordon C, Dvir Z. Cervical radiofrequency neurotomy in patients with chronic whiplash: a study of multiple outcome measures. J Neurosurg Spine. 2006;4(5):365–73.
47. Teasell RW, McClure JA, Walton D, et al. A research synthesis of therapeutic interventions for whiplash-associated disorder: part 5 - surgical and injection-based interventions for chronic WAD. Pain Res Manag. 2010;15(5):287–94.
48. Nystrom NA, Champagne LP, Freeman M, Blix E. Surgical fasciectomy of the trapezius muscle combined with neurolysis of the spinal accessory nerve; results and long-term follow-up in 30 consecutive cases of refractory chronic whiplash syndrome. J Brachial Plex Peripher Nerve Inj. 2010;5:7.
49. Nyström B, Svensson E, Larsson S, et al. A small group whiplash-associated disorders (WAD) patients with central neck pain and movement induced stabbing pain, the painful segment determined by mechanical provocation: fusion surgery was superior to multimodal rehabilitation in a randomized trial. Scand J Pain. 2016;12:33–42.

8 A 45-Year-Old Man with Chronic Neck Pain of Insidious Onset

Joseph Graham and Tariq Malik

Case Description

A 45-year-old male is referred to the pain clinic with complaints of bilateral neck and upper back pain of slow onset over the last 6 months by his primary care physician. There is no precipitating factor. He denies any trauma. He played football in high school and college and never had few neck pain episodes back then, but they were self-limited and resolved with no intervention. He recently has changed desk jobs, and has been working longer hours at the office but nothing unusual. His PCP first prescribed him a short course of NSAIDs and recommended he complete comprehensive physical therapy for his neck pain. The pateint states that he gets only short-lived pain relief from the medications, but his pain always returns later that day. He feels physical therapy helped his strength and flexibility, but his pain was worse after each session. He tried massage which helped for a few days, but again, the pain returned. He describes the pain as fluctuating between dull and achy to intermittent stabbing sensation in his neck, and surrounding his shoulder blades bilaterally. His pain is worse with prolonged sitting, especially at his desk, sleeping on his side with his arms relaxed, and most all arm movements, including over-head activities. On examination, he displays slightly asymmetry in shoulder height and exaggerated cervical lordosis. Palpation of his neck and back reveal multiple discreet tender bands of muscle tissue located in his trapezius, rhomboids, and latissimus dorsi muscles. He has good range of motion but feels some pain at the end of neck flexion, extension, and rotation.

What Is Your Preliminary Diagnosis?

In any patient presenting with pain, it is important to rule out serious pathology from CNS abnormality or malignancy. In the absence of red flag symptoms such as new onset objective weakness, radicular pain, bowel/ bladder incontinence, weight loss, skin changes, or fever, pain with palpation of soft tissues and active range of motion is likely musculoskeletal in origin. MSK pain carries a wide differential. Underlying bony pathology including trauma, facet arthropathy, other arthritic conditions, and alignment issues can all lead to musculoskeletal pain [1–5]. Specific to myofascial pain, confounding diagnoses such as muscle spasm, and fibromyalgia carry similar presentations and can make diagnosis

J. Graham · T. Malik (✉)
Department of Physical Medicine and Rehabilitation, Schwab Hospital, Chicago, IL, USA
e-mail: joseph.graham@sinai.org; TMuslim@dacc.uchicago.edu; tmalik@dacc.uchicago.edu

T. Malik (ed.), *Practical Chronic Pain Management*, https://doi.org/10.1007/978-3-030-46675-6_8

more challenging. Myofascial pain typically is associated with underlying structural or postural abnormalities which must be considered during the diagnostic and treatment process. Patients may have a history of traumatic incident (acute sprain or strain), general overuse, whiplash, or chronic underlying postural issues which can predispose them to developing myofascial pain. It is important to look for medical conditions that predispose patients to musculoskeletal injury. Any rheumatological disease, hypermobility disorders, metabolic disorders (parathyroid disease, Vita-D deficiency), or mechanical issues (scoliosis, leg length discrepancy, joint disease). In the case above, the patient has been working at his desk, likely with poor posture and poor ergonomics which have placed strain on his cervical paraspinals, scapular stabilizers, and trapezius muscles. This patient's history and physical examination are highly suggestive of myofascial pain syndrome resulting from chronic postural changes.

How Is Diagnosis Confirmed?

The hallmark feature of myofascial pain syndromes is the presence of myofascial trigger points (MTrPs) in conjunction with a supporting history. Trigger points are defined as hyperirri nodules which can cause local or referred pain spontaneously or when palpated with manual compression [6]. Another defining feature of trigger points is the presence of fasciculation when dry needled or stimulated with snapping palpation [7, 8]. Patients will complain of pain with postural changes, stretching, and compression/massage of the area. Myofascial pain is often described as dull, achy, or deep. Often times, a supporting history includes insidious onset of worsening axial pain with areas of tenderness located over soft tissues.

Physical examination is used to rule in/out axial and joint pathology that could be contributing to a patient's pain, and is also used to confirm the presence of trigger points, if myofascial pain syndrome is suspected. The original diagnostic approach and criteria by Simons and Travell were recently revised in 2018. This revision proposed that myofascial pain is present when two of the following are found on physical exam: taut band of tissue, hypersensitivity, and/or referred pain [9]. Palpation of tissues is done with the examiner's fingers perpendicular to the muscle fibers. Slow dragging over the deep muscular structures around the area of pain may reproduce the pain, or cause a radiation of pain in a consistent distribution. Through this palpation, the examiner can ask questions to fulfill the diagnostic criteria for trigger points. Asking if the pain produced is similar to their typical complaints, and if the pain radiates, allows the examiner to determine how many of the diagnostic factors are present. Diagnosis of myofascial pain syndrome is heavily dependent on the examiner's ability to obtain a comprehensive history, as well as execute manual palpation accurately enough to identify trigger points.

Imaging is useful in the workup of myofascial pain to help rule in or out underlying structural conditions that may be contributing to the etiology of the myofascial syndrome. Imaging usually begins with plain film X-ray of surrounding structures to evaluate for occult fracture, degenerative changes, or congenital structural abnormalities. Patients with any of these conditions can present with subsequent myofascial pain stemming from muscular compensation. Because myofascial pain is a soft tissue disorder, X-ray, CT, and MRI are of little utility in actual diagnosis of the condition. MRI may show soft tissue edema, but this is not specific enough to myofascial pain syndrome to make the diagnosis. Ultrasound evaluation of the tender areas may show changes in the muscle body, but is less diagnostic and more commonly used for anatomy-directed treatment. One low-powered study showed evidence of soft tissue changes in MTrPs. Trigger points appeared as focal, hypoechoic regions on ultrasound, and displayed reduced vibration amplitude indicating localized stiff nodules [10].

Clinical Features of Myofascial Pain

1. Palpable taut band
2. Tenderness on palpation (trigger point)
3. Referred pain – partial or full on palpation
4. Local twitch on palpation or injection
5. Weakness in the muscle group
6. Restricted range of motion both passive and active

What Is the Pathophysiology of This Condition?

The exact pathophysiology of trigger point generation is unknown. The accepted explanation is that it develops after a muscle is supramaximally loaded or exposed to repeated low-level stress. Taut bands develop within the muscle that later on develop trigger points. Trigger points are called active if pain is present without putting any pressure on the muscle, or latent trigger point, if pain is present only on palpation. Taut muscle bands develop from local micro-injury to the muscle that result in capillary leak, inflammation, ischemia, and hypoxia causing a sustained local contraction. Excess activity by the acetylcholine at the NM junction and or abnormal calcium channel modulation leading to excess calcium influx is also claimed – all leading to sustained contraction. The local inflammation or release of inflammatory chemicals may even precipitate sensitization of afferent peripheral nerve fibers as well as central sensitization as demonstrated by lower pain perception threshold and pain referred to distant part of the limb, across the body, or from dorsal to ventral side of the body. Biochemistry of the trigger point studied using micro-dialysis probe reveals elevation of substance P, CGRP, bradykinin, serotonin, and cytokines. The disturbed concentration is confined to within 1 cm of the trigger point area. The trigger point region pH is found to be low [4–5]. This is said to be due to poor blood flow leading to ischemia and hypoxia in the area. Biopsy of the muscle from the trigger point in animal shows contracted sarcomeres, torn muscle fibers, and longitudinal stripes – but these have been replicated in humans. This is attributed to excess activity of acetylcholine. In one human study, biopsy of muscle showed nonspecific myopathic changes: fiber size variation, cell death, and moth-eaten fibers. Mitochondrial changes were also seen in some.

In short, acitivities that cause sudden or sustained muscle use lead to muscle damage by creating areas of energy supply vs demand mismatch within the muscle tisssue, triggering series of event from release of number of biochemical which create swelling, worsening capillary flow and ischemia, to sustained muscle contraction from abnormal calcium ion influx, poor activity of acetylcholinesterase from low pH, activation of nociception that eventually leads to peripheral sensitization causing pain in the muscle and twitch response and central sensitization that cause referred pain and even pain in other muscle from affecting synaptic transmission at the dorsal horn of spinal cord most likely via glutamate receptor over activity.

As stated above, myofascial trigger points are the hallmark feature of myofascial pain syndromes. They are postulated to exist in two clinical stages, active and latent. Their active form is the main cause for patient presentation to a healthcare practitioner; however, latent trigger points have been shown to affect patients function as well. Active trigger points cause local pain and radiating pain to surrounding tissues when palpated. Active trigger points may also display overlying autonomic skin changes such as redness, sweating, and goose bumps. Trigger points in their latent stage do not cause spontaneous pain, but will be painful locally or with radiation when deeply palpated [9]. Latent trigger points display mechanical hyperesthesia, pressure/pain hyperalgesia, and vibration hypoesthesia [11]. Latent trigger points do not cause spontaneous pain, and therefore are not typically the reason someone will present to a healthcare provider. They do however alter the activation patterns of muscles and can cause weakness and restricted range of motion [12]. Active trigger points can also limit range of motion. It is thought that muscles with active MTrPs exhibit limited extensibility, and this has a negative effect on involved joints, resulting in functional limitation [13].

Current research supports local sensitization of low-threshold mechanosensitive afferents in the motor endplates of the trigger points. These travel to the centrally sensitized dorsal horn neurons in the spinal cord [9, 14].

How Is This Problem Managed?

Management of most all pain conditions consists of a step-wise escalation of care. Conservative treatments can be tailored to the condition and often times can address patient's complaints sufficiently. Conservative approaches for myofascial pain and general musculoskeletal pain alike include a comprehensive routine of stretching, massage, ice/heat, and gradual range of motion exercises. If these simple approaches fail, moving to pharmacologic therapies and formal physical therapy would be an appropriate next step. Physical therapy is useful and effective in the treatment of myofascial pain syndromes if the patient can tolerate the treatment. Physical therapy should be targeted toward mobility, stretching of affected areas, and strengthening of core and extremities. Attention to correcting aggravating postural and biomechanical factors is also important. Use of deep tissue massage, as well as ultrasound massage, can improve blood flow and help relax tight muscles and taut muscle bands associated with myofascial pain syndrome. Modalities include phonphoresis, EMG biofeedback, electrical muscle stimulation, and transcutaneous electrical nerve stimulation (TENS) [3].

If patients are unable to tolerate physical activity due to pain, a combination of therapy and oral agents together can produce pain relief sufficient to participate in formal physical therapy. Oral analgesics such as Acetaminophen can improve pain related to general musculoskeletal pain, arthritis, and other ligament/tendon issues, including myofascial pain. NSAIDs can be used more specifically to target pain generated from muscle pathology such as trigger points, sprains, and spasms. Ibuprofen 600 mg TID or Naproxen 250 mg TID for a short 5–7-day course is appropriate, with careful consideration for side effects of nephrotoxicity and gastrointestinal irritation. Addition of gentle muscle relaxants such as Tizanidine or Baclofen can be employed next. Tizanidine has less sedating side effects, but a trial of both is warranted prior to more invasive treatments.

When patients fail the conservative treatments listed above, they are appropriate for evaluation by a pain physician. Interventional treatments for myofascial pain syndromes are targeted at trigger points in the muscle tissue as well as addressing any underlying structural or psychological contributing factors. After collecting a thorough history and physical, and making the diagnosis of myofascial pain syndrome, the pain physician must determine location of trigger points in the muscle tissue. As addressed above, discrete bands of hypersensitive tissue are located and marked. Trigger points may be addressed with dry needling or wet needling. Wet needling involves an injectate of local anesthetic, corticosteroid, or a combination of both [15]. Ultrasound guidance can aid in the localization of the muscle targeted, and help to avoid vasculature and underlying lung tissue. Botulinum toxin is also used if initial needling only gives short-term relief. The randomized controlled studies on the effectiveness of botulinum use were variable in quality, used different doses, small in size, and had mixed results. In open non-randomized trials, the results were positive. In general, there is no difference in outcome irrespective of what is injected – local anesthetic with or without steroids, botulinum toxins, or just dry needling.

When injecting trigger points, certain precautions must be taken. Avoiding non-targeted tissues such as vasculature, lungs, and nerves is paramount to reduce patient's discomfort and adverse outcomes. Diabetic patients benefit from reduced corticosteroid dose, due to hyperglycemic side effects of systemic absorption. Patients with diabetes should be counseled to monitor blood glucose levels closely over the days following any injection with corticosteroid.

What Is the Prognosis of This Condition?

When addressed properly, myofascial pain syndrome can be cured. Because of the multifaceted nature of the disease, myofascial pain requires a multifaceted approach. The patient may have chronic complaints of pain, underlying structural and postural abnormalities, and psychological factors contributing to their overall state. Myofascial pain is a cyclical issue that compounds, as more pain causes more muscular/postural compensation and guarding, which ultimately worsens the condition. Myofascial interventions are aimed to break this cycle, and allow for a reset of the tissue. Once trigger points are treated and underlying causes are addressed, the patient can make a full recovery to a pain-free life. When patients present to a pain clinic, the problem is often chronic, and therefore difficult to resolve quickly. The underlying pathogenesis of chronic myofascial pain is unknown, hence hard to cure. There is significant similarity with fibromyalgia syndrome at that time, and it is hard to know if myofascial pain is a version of fibromyalgia or is coexisting with it. Careful consideration in diagnosis with a stepwise holistic approach to the patient's treatment plan can produce satisfactory results.

Discussion

Prevalence

Due to the wide differential diagnosis of musculoskeletal pain that can present similarly to myofascial pain, and the wide range of etiologies that can be associated with or cause myofascial pain, prevalence is difficult to determine. In primary care clinic setup, the prevalence was noticed to be around 9%, while in a rehab clinic setup, it was reported at 85%. The presence of trigger points were found in 61% of patients with CRPS, in 67% of patients with post stroke central pain, and high incidence was also found after many upper limb or chest surgeries. No gender difference in trigger point prevalence has been noticed. A cross-sectional population study of patients with presenting complaints of pain found a prevalence of around 30% fulfilling diagnostic criteria for myofascial pain syndrome [16].

Very likely a number of cases of myofascial pain go undiagnosed for a number of reasons. A patient's symptoms may not be severe enough to present to a healthcare provider who is able to make the diagnosis, or the patient may self manage the condition with over-the-counter remedies. Additionally, if a patient's myofascial pain syndrome is chronic and trigger points are in the latent stage, the patient may continue living life with modified function to compensate for any decreased range of motion and minor weakness the MTrPs cause.

Differential Diagnosis

The differential diagnosis of myofascial pain syndrome includes a number of conditions that present similarly to MPS. Fibromyalgia, muscle overuse, and muscle spasm can mimic myofascial pain syndrome. Fibromyalgia typically presents with chronic widespread musculoskeletal pain, fatigue, psychiatric symptoms, and multiple somatic symptoms. Etiology and pathophysiology of this condition are unknown, but it is postulated that fibromyalgia is a disorder of pain regulation, and is a form of central sensitization. Muscle overuse and muscle spasm tend to have a more clear etiology, and tend to be isolated to specific muscle groups with clearer inciting events or activities [17].

Additionally, patients with myofascial pain often have other underlying conditions that are contributing to their myofascial pain that can cloud the diagnosis. Often, the underlying abnormalities are more readily diagnosed and may garner more focus of treatment initially. These conditions include, but are not limited to, facet arthopathy, peripheral osteoarthritis, spondylolisthesis, disc bulge, scoliosis, and poor posture. While these carry their own diagnostic workup and treatment, if present, they must be addressed in the treatment of myofascial pain syndrome.

Predictive Value of Different Clinical Features (Both on History and Physical Exam) and Lab Testing/Imaging

Predictive factors for diagnosing myofascial pain syndrome lie mostly in the thorough history and physical. Factors include age, gender, previous trauma (whiplash, falls, and fractures), and occupation with prolonged positioning, hobbies with repetitive motions, posture, and time course of symptoms. Physical exam findings of regional tenderness which is responsive to position changes and palpation, discreet taut bands of muscle, as well as pain limited range of motion are predictive. Imaging findings showing underlying abnormalities that contribute to the syndrome are predictive, but not diagnostic to myofascial pain syndrome.

Strength of Evidence for Different Treatment Modalities

A systematic review of literature comparing needling techniques was conducted in 2000, which showed efficacy of dry needling for treatment of active trigger points. This review included 23 papers which all included dry needling with varying injected substances. Different combinations of local anesthetic, saline, and corticosteroids were included. Effects of dry needling were independent of injected substance, but showed dry needling to be an effective treatment [15].

Without clear guidelines, selection of injected substance remains largely provider preference, and is typically based on training, experience, and other anecdotal evidence.

In a randomized, double-blind prospective study of botulinum toxin type A versus injection of normal saline was conducted in 1998. The study was low power, with only 33 total subjects, and no statistically significant benefit of botulinum toxin injection was found over placebo [18]. However, this study did note a high incidence of patients who were asymptomatic after a second botulinum injection into previously symptomatic trigger points.

Future Directions or Clinical Trials in Progress

Current literature on myofascial pain suffers from lack of objective criteria to diagnose the condition. The key diagnostic feature is physical examination and suffers from great inter-observer variability. There is no pathognomic laboratory or microscopic findings, exact mechanism is unknown. There is need for basic and clinical research to better characterize the disease.

There is an urgent need for clinical research to develop evidence-based guidelines for treatments. Currently there are small-power studies providing some guidance, as well as anecdotal evidence of treatment efficacy. There is a need for larger, higher power studies looking into the efficacy of treatment modalities of myofascial trigger points in myofascial pain syndrome.

Additionally there is a need for studies focusing on better detection and diagnosis of myofascial pain in patients with other pathological conditions, both structurally and psychologically to determine comorbidities and predisposing conditions that may lead to or contribute to myofascial pain syndrome.

Conclusion/Summary

Myofascial pain syndrome is a painful disorder that is a common reason for pain clinic visits. It can affect all skeletal muscles in the body, but is most commonly located in the back. It is involved in many cases of chronic pain, but the diagnosis is often missed. Pain is typically regional and has associated tightness in muscle tissue with tenderness to palpation, decreased range of motion, and muscle weakness without atrophy. Myofascial trigger points are at the center of the pathology and exist in two forms, active and latent. Active trigger points account for the vast majority of presenting complaints of patients. These points are discreet areas of taut muscle tissue which can exhibit hypersensitivity and referred pain. The pathophysiology of myofascial pain syndrome is not well understood, but current research supports sensitization of motor endplates, and the dorsal horn in the spinal cord. The diagnosis of the syndrome relies heavily on the ability of the healthcare provider to take an accurate history and physical. Radiographic imaging is of little utility in the diagnosis of the syndrome, but can be helpful in identifying underlying conditions that coexist with or contributing to the myofascial pain. First steps in management include conservative measures such as physical therapy, oral analgesics, and lifestyle/postural modifications. Once conservative measures are failed, patients may benefit from interventional procedures. Current research is limited and consensus guidelines do not exist for interventional treatment; however, there are small studies and anecdotal evidence which support dry needling and wet needling with a range of injected substances. These interventions have been shown to provide symptomatic relief and improve function temporarily. As stated above, careful consideration must be made to underlying structural, postural, or psychological factors that may be contributing to the syndrome. Further investigative efforts are needed to establish consensus guidelines outlining which injected substances provide the most relief, and overall efficacy of treatments in this condition.

References

1. Salaffi F, De Angelis R, Stancati A, et al. Health-related quality of life on multiple musculoskeletal conditions: a cross-sectional population based epidemiological study. II. The MAPPING study. Clin Exp Rheumatol. 2005;23:829–39.
2. Travell JG, Simons DG. Myofascial pain and dysfunction: the trigger point manual. Baltimore: Williams & Wilkins; 1983.
3. Fleckenstein J, Zaps D, Ruger LJ, et al. Discrepancy between prevalence and perceived effectiveness of treatment methods in myofascial pain syndrome: results of a cross sectional, nationwide survey. BMC Musculoskelet Disord. 2010;11:32.
4. Bogduk N. On the definitions and physiology of back pain, referred pain, and radicular pain. Pain. 2009;147(1–3):17–9.
5. Langford CA, Mandell BF. Arthritis Associated with Systemic Disease, and Other Arthritides. In: Jameson J, Fauci AS, Kasper DL, Hauser SL, Longo DL, Loscalzo J. eds. Harrison's Principle of Internal Medicine, 20e New York, NY: McGraw-Hill; 2020. http://accessmedicine.mhmedcial.com.proxy.uchicago.edu/content.aspx?bookid=2129§ionid=192286220. Accessed April 30.
6. Alonso Bianco C, Femandez de Las Peñas C, de la Uave Rincón AI, et al. Characteristics of referred muscle pain to the head from active trigger points in women with myofascial temporomandibular pain and fibromyalgia syndrome. J Headache Pain. 2012;13:625–37.
7. Rha OW, Shin JC, Kim YK, et al. Detecting local twitch responses of myolascial trigger points in the low back muscles using ultrasonography. Arch Phys Med Rehabil. 2011;92:1576–80.
8. Koppenhaver SL, Walker MJ, Rettig C, et al. The assocration between dry needling induced twitch response and change in pain and muscle function in patients with low back pain: a quasi-experimental study. Physiotherapy. 2017;103:131–7.
9. Fernandez-de-Las-Penas C, Dommerholt J. International consensus on diagnostic criteria and clinical considerations of myofascial trigger points: a Delphi Study. Pain Med. 2018;19(1):142–50.
10. Sikdar S, Shah J, et al. Novel applications of ultrasound technology to visualize and characterize myofascial trigger points and surrounding soft tissue. Arch Phys Med Rehabil. 2009;90(11):1829–38.
11. Ambite Ouesada S, Arias Buria JL, Courtney CA, et al. Exploration of quantitative sensory testing in latent trigger points and referred pain areas. Clin J Pain. 2018;34:409–14.
12. Cellk O, Yeldan I. The relationship between latent trigger point and muscle strength in healthy subjects: a double-blind study. J Back Musculoskelet Rehabil. 2011;24:251–6.
13. Fernandez Perez AM, Villaverde-Gutierrez C, Mora-Sanchez A, et al. Muscle trigger points, pressure pam threshold, and cervical range of motion m patients with high level of disability related to acute whiplash injury. J Orthop Sports Phys Ther. 2012;42:634–41.
14. Hong CZ, Simons DG. Pathophysiologic and electrophysiologic mechanisms of myofascial trigger points. Arch Phys Med Rehabil. 1998;79(7):863–72.
15. Cummings M, White AR. Needling therapies in the management of myofascial trigger point pain: a systematic review. Arch Phys Med Rehabil. 2001;82(7):986–92.
16. Skootsky SA, Jaeger B, Oye RK. Prevalence of myofascial pain in general internal medicine practice. West J Med. 1989;151(2):157–60.
17. Pomares FB, Funck T, et al. Histological underpiinnings of grey matter changes in fibromyalgia infestigated using multimodal brain imaging. J Neurosci. 2017;37(5):1090–101.
18. Wheeler AH, Goolkasian P, Gretz S. A randomized, double-blind, prospective pilot study of botulinum toxin injection for refractory, unilateral, cervicothoracic, paraspinal, myofascial pain syndrome. Spine. 1998;23(15):1662–6.

Cervical Spondylosis

9

Andrew Wendahl and Alaa Abd-Elsayed

Case Description

A 75-year-old man presents to your clinic complaining of neck pain. Past medical history includes hypertension, hyperlipidemia, hypothyroidism, and a 50 pack-year smoking history. He is on appropriate medications for his conditions but has been on the same doses for years. This patient has had a total knee surgery in the past year but has not otherwise had regular medical follow-up. He reports that he has had dull aching pain for as long as he can remember with no precipitating event. He denies any recent eliciting event. He does endorse a motor vehicle accident 25 years ago in which he believes he did suffer a whiplash injury. The patient denies weakness to his extremities or loss of bowel or bladder function. He does endorse inability to sit still for long because of the nagging neck pain that gets worse. The neck pain is often associated with headache radiating up the back of his head, bilateral shoulder pain, and achiness between his shoulder blades.

What Is Your Preliminary Diagnosis?

An elderly patient with neck pain with no injury most likely has a degenerative process causing neck pain. However other pathologies such as infection, tumor, and any other neurological disorder should be ruled out. It is important to inquire about weight loss, fever, or any history of tumor. A careful history includes symptom and severity, mechanism of injury and was there trauma or loss of consciousness, number of episodes, sites and boundaries of the pain, radiation, frequency of pain, aggravating factors, alleviating factors, and specific characterization of the symptoms. Does the patient exhibit or complain of any sympathetic symptoms? Severe acceleration/whiplash-type injury can lead to hypertonia of the sympathetic nervous system [1, 2]. The top of your differential should include cervical spondylosis, cervical spinal stenosis, and cervical disc herniation [2]. Spondylosis (also called spondylosis deformans) is present in 60% of those older than 45 years and 85% of those older than 65 years old [3]. Symptoms of this osteoarthritis usually do not manifest until 60 years of age or older. Examination begins with careful observation of the patient's motion and posture, specifically head and neck. Do they have the normal lordotic curvature (~30–40 degrees) and is the head in the midline? [4] Physical examination should actively rule out or rule in any evidence of neurological compression or injury. Look for any sign any muscle spasticity, atrophy, or asymmetry in the upper limb muscles. Evaluate passive and active neck range of motion. Look for differences in range of motion and willingness to do

A. Wendahl · A. Abd-Elsayed (✉)
Department of Anesthesiology, University of Wisconsin School of Medicine and Public Health, Madison, WI, USA

T. Malik (ed.), *Practical Chronic Pain Management*, https://doi.org/10.1007/978-3-030-46675-6_9

the movement. Range of motion decreases with age, except for at C1 to C2, and females tend to have greater active range of motion [5]. The examiner may apply passive overpressure to test the end feel of the movement while remaining vigilant of vertebral artery compression which can lead to a decrease in blood supply to the brain.

Key tests can be performed on the cervical spine depending on suspected pathology. Foraminal compression (Spurling's) test is a popular test that has been reported as 28% sensitive and 100% specific for radicular symptoms. The brachial plexus compression test is useful in ruling in more distal compression causing upper extremity symptoms. Pain at the site is not diagnostic; the test is positive only if pain radiates into the shoulder or upper extremity [6]. Shoulder abduction test, relieve of pain when painful arm is placed on head is suggestive of foraminal stenosis. Neck distraction test, relieve of pain when distraction is applied to the cervical spine with patient lying supine favors foraminal stenosis pathology. The shoulder pathology can mimic or exacerbate neck pain. Detailed shoulder evaluation is important whenever neck pain is being evaluated. Shoulder evaluation is covered in another chapter in the book. Presence of hypo- or hyperreflexia should be ruled out. Patient with any radiation down the arm should have their sensory dermatome carefully evaluated. Palpation is an important part of the examination in order to rule in or out point tenderness. It is done to look for the presence of trigger points or facet joint tenderness. Primary purpose of history and physical examination is to diagnose the site and pathology of the pain generator as this will lead to organized ordering of tests to confirm the diagnosis.

How Is the Diagnosis Confirmed?

A diagnosis for cervical spondylosis is suggested by the history and physical examination. This diagnosis should be considered in patients with chronic age-related cervical pain. Cervical facet is the other chronic pain condition most prevalent in this age group. Cervical spondylosis is diagnosed by ruling out cervical facet disease using diagnostic injection. This is further discussed in the book in another chapter. The following recommendations are based off of the North American Spine Society's Evidence-Based Clinical Guidelines for Multidisciplinary Spine Care. To begin, the question you need to answer is, "What are the most appropriate diagnostic tests and when are these tests indicated?" Provocative tests including the shoulder abduction and Spurling's tests may be considered in evaluating patients with clinical signs and symptoms consistent with spondylosis. MRI is suggested for the confirmation of correlative compressive lesions (disc herniation and spondylosis) in cervical spine patients who have failed a course of conservative therapy. In the absence of reliable evidence, it is the work group's opinion that CT may be considered as the initial study to confirm a correlative compressive lesion if MRI is contraindicated. The evidence is insufficient to make a recommendation for or against the use of EMG for patients in whom the diagnosis of cervical radiculopathy is unclear after clinical exam and MRI [7].

What Is the Pathophysiology of This Condition?

The pathophysiology of spondylosis is not completely understood. A widely cited theory states that the sequence of degenerative changes seen in spondylosis begins with desiccation of the vertebral disc, estimated to be 90 percent water in early adult life, but an estimated 69 percent water by the eighth decade. As this disc loses water, the annulus fibrosis weakens and disc height depression occurs. This leads to increased stress at the zygapophyseal joints, vertebral end plates, and the uncovertebral joints (joints of Luschka). The increased stress is hypothesized to lead to osseous and ligamentous hypertrophy and osteopathy formation. Osteophyte formation is most commonly found in mobile cervical and lumbar regions, supporting this theory [8].

Pain centered in the neck with radiation into the upper thoracic region could be from any source so it is imperative to think through the associated anatomy. The cervical spine is divided into two areas, the cervicoencephalic for the upper cervical spine and the cervicobrachial for the lower cervical spine. Cervicoencephalic injuries have the potential of involving the brain, brainstem, and spinal cord presenting with symptoms of headache, fatigue, vertigo, poor concentration, hypertonia, and irritability. This presentation is expected to be acutely related to some injury and should be emergently referred to neurosurgery. The lower cervical spine is called the cervicobrachial area, often referring pain into the upper extremity [4]. This is more likely the source of our patients pain as pathology in this region often leads to neck pain alone, arm pain alone, or both. Associated symptoms commonly include neck and/or arm pain, headaches, restricted range of motion (ROM), paresthesia, altered myotomes and dermatomes, and radicular signs. Cognitive and cranial nerve dysfunction are alarm signs and should not be associated with this region. There are seven vertebrae in the cervical spine with the body of each vertebra (except C1) supporting the weight of those above it. The facet joints bear some weight of the vertebrae above, although the weight is minimal if the normal lordotic posture is maintained. However, even a slight amount of weight bearing can lead to spondylitic changes at these joints.

How Is This Problem Managed?

Cervical spondylosis is a broad diagnosis used to include soft tissue, disc degeneration, and degenerative bony lesions (osteophytes). Degenerative changes are widespread, often apparent on radiographs of adults over the age of 30. There is a broad continuum from normal aging to the overtly pathologic state. There is poor correlation between the degree of radiographic change and severity [9]. After ruling out neurologic compromise, it is a multimodal approach to pain management that is best for treating general chronic osteoarthritic pain. Conservative management (nonsurgical) is the initial approach following a thorough evaluation and can be broken down into two components: conservative therapy and epidural glucocorticoid injections. Conservative therapy generally includes a combination of the following modalities: physical therapy with exercise and gradual mobilization, avoidance of provocative activities, and a short course of oral prednisone and oral analgesics. There is not a consensus regarding the proper sequence of conservative modalities. There is no proper order or combination of modalities that has been established with society guidelines. Following is an example of how a treatment regimen could be instituted. Treatment can begin with oral analgesics and avoidance of provocative activities. Some providers will add in a short course of oral prednisone at this time if pain is severe at this time. Analgesics may include NSAIDs as first-line therapy. Neuropathic medications including gabapentin and pregabalin may be used in treating cervical pain if there seems to be a component of radiculopathy, although evidence is weak for this indication. Based on your examination and history, if the patient has a component of spasticity there may be benefit to adding in a muscle relaxant such as cyclobenzaprine. Dosing typically starts at 5 mg two to three times per day in order to reduce drowsiness. Depending on the nature of the patient's spasticity, the dose may be doubled if adequate relief is not achieved. Once a point of relief is met, the patient should begin physical therapy with strengthening and mobilization. Prolonged inactivity is widely believed to delay recovery. This conservative regimen may be prescribed for 6–8 weeks, and if there is no improvement, the patient should be reexamined. At this time and if not done already, neuroimaging and electrodiagnostic studies should be performed. Careful assessment of weakness and myelopathic findings are prudent if refractory or progressive symptoms are apparent at this time. Progressive neurologic deficit could be an indication for surgery and the patient should be referred for surgical evaluation. Other symptoms on reevaluation that warrant surgical evaluation include progressive motor weakness or signs of myelopathy (in the presence of imaging studies showing a surgically anatomical spinal cord compression) [10]. Persistent cervical radicular pain, with or without radiculopathy, may benefit from epidural glucocorticoid injections, despite mixed data [11]. Treatment begins with a single injection followed by assessment of response. Clinical practice is variable; however, one approach is to repeat one or two times if needed separated by 3 weeks between each injection [12]. Fluoroscopic guidance is mandatory during these interventions due to the rare but serious complications with cervical epidural glucocorticoid injections. Well-documented reports exist of death or severe neurologic sequelae from hemorrhage or infarction involving the brain, brainstem, cerebellum, or spinal cord [13, 14].

Cervical spondylosis is a prevalent age-degenerative process that may reach nearly 95% by the age 65. This process is driven by the formation of osteophytes and compression of the spinal cord. These changes are associated with disc protrusion, neuroforaminal narrowing, and spinal cord counter changes in up to 78% of asymptomatic individuals [15]. The treatment guidelines should follow those of the specific disorders spondylosis causes including radiculopathy, facet joint pain, disc herniation, and spondylitic myelopathy.

What Is the Prognosis of This Condition?

There are not an abundance of randomized controlled studies. One trial of 205 adults with acute cervical radiculopathy found physical therapy and home exercises for 6 weeks or a cervical collar and rest for 3–6 weeks was superior to no treatment (control) for reduction in neck and arm pain [16]. Small prospective and retrospective observational studies suggest that transforaminal or interlaminar epidural glucocorticoid injections are associated with relief 6 months or longer in 40–60% of patients [17, 18]. These studies do not distinguish between treatment improvement versus the natural history of cervical radiculopathy complicating the picture. This is a point of further investigation.

What Is the Long-Term Outcome: Complete Cure, Recurrent or Chronic Persistent Problem?

Degenerative changes leading to spondylosis and facet pain are chronic anatomical changes. These changes of the cervical spine are seen in approximately 10% of individuals by age 25 and in 95% by the age of 65. The levels most commonly affected by both disc herniation and chronic spondylosis are C6/C7 followed by C5/C6 as these are the cervical segments where the most extension and flexion occurs [19]. Relief is often obtained over time. Although data are limited, many patients struggling with compressive radiculopathy improve without specific treatment [20]. Nondegenerative radiculopathy can be related to diabetes mellitus, tumor infiltration, demyelination, and other causes that are influenced by the natural history and dependent on the response to treatment of the condition.

Discussion

Prevalence

The lifetime prevalence of spinal pain has been reported as 54% to 80%, with as many as 60% of patients continuing to have chronic pain 5 years or longer after the initial episode [21]. Myelopathy occurs in 5 to 10 percent of patients with symptomatic cervical spondylosis [22].

Differential Diagnosis

The differential diagnosis is broad for neck/arm pain and must be narrowed down based on a thorough history and physical examination. One can begin to narrow this down by first thinking through the broader categories including degenerative spinal disorders, soft tissue disorders, inflammatory disorders, infections, tumors, intraspinal disorders, systemic disorders with referred pain, shoulder and elbow pathology, peripheral nerve entrapment syndromes, thoracic outlet syndrome, and psychogenic pain. For the purpose of this chapter, one should narrow our differential down to those in the degenerative versus soft tissue disorders. The degenerative spinal disorders differential should include discogenic pain, radiculopathy, myeloradiculopathy, and myelopathy. The differential within the soft tissue disorders category should include sprains, myofascial pain syndromes, fibromyalgia, and whiplash syndrome [23]. Cervical spondylotic myelopathy (also called radiculomyelopathy) must remain on the differential as it can damage spinal nerve roots as well as the cord itself. The C5-7 regions are most commonly affected, so the lower motor neuron or segmental signs would generally be observed in these myotomes.

Predictive Value of Different Clinical Features (Both on History and Physical Exam) and Lab Testing/Imaging

Provocative tests including the shoulder abduction and Spurling's tests may be considered in evaluating patients with clinical signs and symptoms consistent with the diagnosis of cervical radiculopathy. This is a Grade C recommendation from the North American Spine Society (NASS) guidelines published in 2010. NASS also published Grade B recommendations in their 2010 guidelines promoting CT, CT myelography, or MRI in the face of dermatomal arm pain because the predictive value is not specific for identifying pathologic level in patients with cervical radiculopathy. MRI is suggested for the confirmation of correlative compressive lesions (disc herniation and spondylosis) in cervical spine patients who have failed a course of conservative therapy and who may be candidates for interventional or surgical treatment. CT myelography is suggested for the evaluation of patients with clinical symptoms or signs discordant with MRI findings. CT myelography is also suggested in patients with contraindication to MRI. The evidence is insufficient to make a recommendation for or against the use of EMG for patients in whom the diagnosis of cervical radiculopathy is unclear after clinical exam or MRI [24].

Strength of Evidence for Different Treatment Modalities

Selective nerve root block with specific dosing and technique protocols may be considered in the evaluation of patients with cervical radiculopathy and compressive lesions identified at multiple levels on MRI or CT myelography to discern the symptomatic level(s) or differentiate in the face of discordant symptoms or imaging findings [22].

Future Directions or Clinical Trials in Progress

Future progress should be directed toward focused diagnosis and treatment with the goal of improving upon success rates. The field of pain medicine continues to need studies to improve upon strength in recommendations for treatment.

Conclusion/Summary

Cervical spondylosis refers to a progressive degenerative process affecting the vertebral bodies and intervertebral discs which can lead to stenosis of the central spinal canal. Progression of this disease can result in compression of the cervical spinal cord leading to a syndrome of spinal cord dysfunction known as cervical spondylitis myelopathy. Cervical spondylotic myelopathy is the most common cause of myelopathy in adults over 55, leading to disability and impaired quality of life [22]. Once this difficult diagnosis is made, the patient should be immediately referred to surgery. Other less emergent sequelae of cervical spondylosis lead to osteophyte formation leading to neck pain, cervical radiculopathy, and degeneration of intervertebral discs resulting in disc herniation. Additionally, ossification and hypertrophy of the posterior longitudinal ligament and ligaments flava occur. Society guidelines recommend 6–8 weeks of conservative management before referral for surgical evaluation or interventional pain procedures. Imaging should be pursued in the case of refractory or progressive symptoms. MRI is recommended by the North America Spine Society, unless contraindicated or non-diagnostic at which time they recommend going to CT myelography. There is no cure for the condition. Cervical epidural steroid injection helps for term only. Surgery is only indicated in the presence of instability or signs of nerve compression. In the absence of nerve injury, the role of surgery is inconclusive.

References

1. Teresi LM, Lufkin RB, Reicher MA, Moffit BJ, Vinuela FV, Wilson GM, Bentsen JR, Hanafee WN. Asymptomatic degenerative disk disease and spondylosis of the cervical spine: MR imaging. Radiology. 1987;164(1):83.
2. Boswell MV, Shah RV. Interventional techniques in the management of chronic spinal pain: evidence-based practice guidelines. Pain Physician. 2005;8:1–47, ISSN 1533-3159.
3. Rao RD, Currier BL, Albert TJ, et al. Degenerative cervical spondylosis: cervical syndromes, pathogenesis and management. J Bone Joint Surg Am. 2007;89:1360–78.
4. Porterfield JA, DeRosa C. Mechanical neck pain—perspective in functional anatomy. Philadelphia: WB Saunders; 1995.
5. Youdas JW, Garrett TR, Suman VJ, et al. Normal range of motion of the cervical spine: an initial goniometric study. Phys Ther. 1992;72:770–80.
6. Uchihara T, Furukawa T, Tsukagoshi H. Compression of brachial plexus as a diagnostic test of a cervical cord lesion. Spine. 1994;19:2170–3.
7. Bono CM, Ghiselli G. Diagnosis and treatment of cervical radiculopathy from degenerative disorders: USA: North American Spine Society; 2010.
8. Lestini WF, Wiesel SW. The pathogenesis of cervical spondylosis. Can Orthop Relat Res. 1989;(239):69–93.
9. Resnick D. Degenerative diseases of the vertebral column. Radiology. 1985;156(1):3.
10. Ellenberg MR, Honet JC, Treanor WJ. Cervical radiculopathy. Arch Phys Med Rehabil. 1994;75(3):342.
11. Engel A, Wade K, MacVicar J, Standards Division of the International Spine Intervention Society. The effectiveness and risks of fluoroscopically guided cervical transforaminal injections of steroids: a systematic review with comprehensive analysis of the published data. Pain Med. 2014;15(3):386.
12. Persson L, Anderberg L. Repetitive transforaminal steroid injections in cervical radiculopathy: a prospective outcome study including 140 patients. Evid Based Spine Care J. 2012;3(3):13.
13. Engel A, King W. The effectiveness and risks of fluoroscopically guided cervical transforaminal injections of steroids: a systematic review with comprehensive analysis of the published data. Pain Med. 2014;15(3):386.
14. Scanlon GC, Moeller-Bertram T, Romanowsky SM, Wallace MS. Cervical transforaminal epidural steroid injections: more dangerous than we think? Spine (Phila Pa 1976). 2007;32(11):1249.
15. Siivola SM, Levoska S, Tervonen O, Ilkko E, Vanharanta H, Keinanen-Kiukaanniemi S. MRI changes of cervical spine in asymptomatic and symptomatic young adults. Eur Spine J. 2002;11:358–63. 1609.
16. Kuijper B, Tans JT, Beelan A. Cervical collar or physiotherapy versus wait and see policy for recent onset cervical radiculopathy: randomized trial. BMJ. 2009;339:b3883. Pub 2009 Oct 7.
17. Slipman CW, Lipetz JS. Therapeutic selective nerve root block in the nonsurgical treatment of atraumatic cervical spondylitis radicular pain: a retrospective analysis with independent clinical review. Arch Phys Med Rehabil. 2000;81(6):741.
18. Vallee JN, Feydy A. Chronic cervical radiculopathy: lateral-approach periradicular corticosteroid injection. Radiology. 2001;218(3):886.
19. Manchikanti L, et al. An update of comprehensive evidence-based guidelines for interventional techniques in chronic spinal pain. Part I: introduction and general considerations. Pain Physician. 2013;16:S1–S48.
20. Radhakrishnan K, Litchy WJ, O'Fallon WM, Kurland LT. Epidemiology of cervical radiculopathy. A population-based study from Rochester, Minnesota, 1976 through 1990. Brain. 1994;117(Pt 2):325.
21. American Society of Anesthesiologists Task Force on Chronic Pain Management; American Society of Regional Anesthesia and Pain Medicine. Practice guidelines for chronic pain management: an updated report by the American Society of Anesthesiologists Task Force on Chronic Pain Management and the American Society of Regional Anesthesia and Pain Medicine. Anesthesiology. 2010;112(4):810–33.
22. McCormick WE, Steinmetz MP, Benzel EC. Cervical spondylotic myelopathy: make the difficult diagnosis, then refer for surgery. Cleve Clin J Med. 2003;70(10):899.
23. Fong W, McGovern SC, Wang JC. Evaluation of cervical spine disorders. Chapter 4: Spine Secrets Plus. USA. p. 33–9.
24. Bono CM, et al. Evidence-based clinical guidelines for multidisciplinary spine care. USA: North American Spine Society (NASS); 2010.

A 65-Year-Old Man with Chronic Neck Pain (Cervical Facet Disease)

10

Andrew Wendahl and Alaa Abd-Elsayed

Case Description

A 65-year-old man walks into your clinic complaining of a headache with dull posterior neck pain radiating to the mid back region and limited range of motion. The patient has had limited improvement with conservative management over the past year including physical therapy, chiropractic treatment, massage, acupuncture, and NSAID use. He endorses a constant 7/10 on the visual analog scale and reports it is limiting to his daily activities. The patient denies any recent trauma including whiplash, motor vehicle accident, or any other isolated event. On exam, the patient had positive facet loading test of the cervical spine with tenderness on palpating the cervical vertebrae just lateral to the spinous process. The patient had a cervical spine series prior to chiropractic treatment to rule out any fracture or tumor. No other imaging has been done up until this point.

What Is Your Preliminary Diagnosis?

My preliminary diagnosis would include facet joint pain while keeping in mind other pain generators in the anatomical region [1–4]. These include intervertebral disks, ligaments, muscles, and nerve roots. Other syndromes overlapping with signs and symptoms include cervicodynia, cervical myofascial pain syndrome, cervical degenerative disk disease, ligamentous laxity, neck strain, compression fracture, cervical radiculopathy, and cervical stenosis [1].

How Is the Diagnosis Confirmed?

Diagnosis is confirmed by putting many elements together including the clinical exam, imaging techniques, and the use of diagnostic blocks. Before performing any tests on a patient with chronic spinal pain, the clinician should decide whether testing for facet pain is the priority, or if other sources should be investigated.

Diagnosis is made including a thorough history and physical exam, imaging techniques, and the use of diagnostic blocks. The pain distribution and quality produces a "pain map" as well as joint provocation on physical exam. The pain maps of the specific joints and nerve distributions overlap considerably, so although they provide clues to origin they do not specify exact location [4]. The first diagnostic study should include radiographs in the neutral, flexed, and extended positions with a documented range of motion exam. Although cervical spine MRI may reveal degenerative changes consistent with cervical facet arthropathy, imaging alone cannot reveal

A. Wendahl · A. Abd-Elsayed (✉)
Department of Anesthesiology, University of Wisconsin School of Medicine and Public Health, Madison, WI, USA

T. Malik (ed.), *Practical Chronic Pain Management*, https://doi.org/10.1007/978-3-030-46675-6_10

the facet joints [1]. Cervical facet joint injections are often performed to test the hypothesis that the target joint is the source of pain. The cervical facet joints can be anesthetized with local anesthetic injected directly into the intraarticular joint space or with anesthetizing the medial branches of the dorsal rami innervating the corresponding joint [5, 6].

What Is the Pathophysiology of This Condition?

The facet joint is also referred to as a zygaphophysial joint (ZJ) which are paired synovial joints that link the posterior elements of the spine from the C2-3 level down to the lowest spinal motion segment, L5-S1. The ZJ is made up of two bony processes or apophyses, a superior and an inferior articular process, each of which has an articular surface (or facet) lined with hyaline cartilage about 1–2 mm thick. The nerve supply of the ZJ is via the medial branches of the dorsal rami of the spinal nerves. The joint capsules are richly innervated by sensory afferent fibers (first order neurons) which transmit neural impulses from each joint via the medial branch nerves to their cell bodies in the dorsal root ganglia and then on to synapse with second-order neurons in the dorsal horn of the spinal cord; from there impulses transmit via central pathways to the sensory cortex [4]. Facet pain is typically dull and aching in quality indicating local somatic pain although can also be referred to more distant regions.

How Is This Problem Managed?

A rehabilitation program is pertinent to the treatment of a patient with cervical facet disease. One should begin with a conservative approach. Conservative management includes reducing pain and inflammation while increasing pain-free range of motion and functionality. Pertinent to this phase of recovery is strength and flexibility training. Application of ice during the acute phase can decrease blood flow, hemorrhage into local tissues, and therefore reduces local edema. Therapeutic modalities, such as ultrasound scan and electrical stimulation, manual therapy, joint mobilization, soft tissue massage, and muscle stretching are often helpful. Medication management should be instituted in certain circumstances. Non-steroidal anti-inflammatory medications may be started at the lowest possible doses to decrease inflammation and pain in the acute setting. The American Geriatric Society (AGS) suggests that NSAIDs should be avoided when possible to decrease the risk of gastropathy, nephrotoxicity, and increased cardiac risk in chronic use [7]. Acetaminophen, Para-acetylaminophenol, can be helpful as part of a multimodal analgesic regimen but is not an anti-inflammatory in contrast to NSAIDs. Gabapentin and pregabalin have proven efficacy versus placebo in several neuropathic conditions. Gabapentin has been primarily studied and found effective in post-herpetic neuralgia and painful diabetic neuropathy. Treatment with gabapentin should be initiated at a low dose with gradual increases until pain relief, dose limiting adverse effects, or 3600 mg per day in three divided doses. An adequate trial of gabapentin can require 2 months or more [8].

If a conservative approach does not suffice, then more invasive procedures should be considered and used. These options include therapeutic facet joint injections, with intraarticular facet joint injections, medial branch blocks, or medial branch neurotomy. The duration of pain relief from intraarticular facet joint injection varies among investigators. Medial branch blocks have also been used therapeutically in the cervical spine. If positive response is seen, a series of three medial branch blocks should be performed over 12–18 weeks to document length of time with good response. If a patient has significant relief lasting 2–3 months, they may need a maintenance program. A positive response with quick dissolution may be an indication for radio frequency ablation in hopes for longer term relief usually maxing at 4 treatments per year.

Medial branch neurotomy has been described with many trials with inconclusive results reported. Many investigators in the field have found radio frequency thermocoagulation of medial branches to be safe and efficacious. This lesioning is performed with continuous or pulsed mode radio frequency. Radio frequency neurotomy denervates the facet joint by coagulating the medial branch of the dorsal ramus, thus denaturing the nerve proteins. The dorsal root ganglion is preserved, not destroyed, so the cell bodies remain intact and the nerve may grow back in 6–9 months. This could reproduce facet joint pain and repeating neurotomy could be a viable option [9]. Cervical fusion should only be considered after failed aggressive nonsurgical care. This treatment is less successful in treating cervical facet disease than for radicular pain.

Complications are associated with facet joint injections, as with all invasive procedures including headache, syncope, hypotension, nausea, sweating, flushing, and lightheadedness. Bleeding is a rare complication but if a patient has a bleeding disorder, is anticoagulated, or vascular proximity to injection location can increase risk. Infection is rare with <1–2% of injections resulting in minor infection and 0.1–0.01% resulting in severe infection with the most serious being epidural abscess and bacterial meningitis. Worsening of pain symptoms may occur, and this may include pain at the injection site. The most feared complication includes nerve or spinal cord damage or paralysis from direct needle trauma. Complications of radio frequency thermoneurolysis are rare and include the above risks as well as deafferentation pain, sensory or motor deficits, and allodynia [10].

The facet or zygapophysial joints are paired diarthrodial articulations between posterior elements of adjacent vertebrae. These joints are well innervated by the medial branches of the dorsal rami, contain free and encapsulated nerve endings, and nociceptors and mechanoreceptors. Based on controlled diagnostic blocks of facet joints, in accordance with the criteria established by the International Association for the Study of Pain (IASP), facet joints have been implicated as responsible for spinal pain in 54–67% of patients with neck pain [11].

Society treatment guidelines were discussed in the aforementioned management section. The highlights included first beginning with conservative management. In case of continued refractory or progressive symptoms, it is important to acquire imaging and pursue more serious pathology including ruling out surgical indications before attempting invasive interventional pain procedures.

What Is the Prognosis of This Condition?

Prognosis referring to the whiplash-induced facet pain has been studied. In a study in the United Kingdom, the most important predictors of pain at 1 year were severity at the time of rear-end collision [12]. In addition to pain symptoms, neck mobility is another important risk factor that predicts disability 1 year after whiplash injury [13].

Abstracted from the 2013 ASIPP guidelines and recommendations, the current evidence shows the prevalence utilization criteria of 75–100% pain relief to range from 36 to 67% in cervical facet joint pain based on diagnostic blocks [14].

Discussion

Prevalence

Facet or zygapophysial joints have been implicated as the source of chronic spinal pain in 54–67% of heterogeneous groups of patients with chronic neck pain.

Differential Diagnosis

Pain generators in the cervical spine include intervertebral disks, facet joints, ligaments, muscles, and nerve roots. Other painful conditions can overlap in symptoms including cervicodynia, cervical myofascial pain syndrome, cervical degenerative disk disease, ligamentous laxity, neck strain, compression fracture, cervical radiculopathy, and cervical stenosis [1]. Manchikanti et al. evaluated a sample of 56 patients from a previous study population with neck pain undergoing cervical diskography and facet joint nerve blocks at the same level for diagnostic purposes. The findings were that 64% of disk disease identified with diskography had a positive cervical medial branch block. Further results concluded the 41% of patients had a symptomatic disk and a symptomatic facet joint at the same segment, and an additional 23% had a painful facet joint without associated same level disk pain [15].

Predictive Value of Different Clinical Features (Both on History and Physical Exam) and Lab Testing/Imaging

Predictive factors for persistent neck pain including greater age, accompanying low back pain, neck trauma, headache, radiation of pain, being employed, and prior episodes of neck pain are described by Schellingerhout [16]. Psychosocial and neurophysiological factors including having a depressed mood, weak cervical muscle endurance, and impaired pain inhibition were positive factors for developing chronic neck pain. Also, poor sleep is a complicating comorbidity found in 70% of patients with chronic neck pain [17, 18].

Strength of Evidence for Different Treatment Modalities

Diagnostic cervical facet joint nerve blocks are recommended in patients with somatic or nonradicular neck pain or headache and upper extremity pain, with duration of pain of at least 3 months. This is without preponderance of evidence of discogenic pain, disc herniation, or radiculitis [19]. Controlled diagnostic blocks with two local anesthetics (or placebo-controlled) are the only means of confirming the diagnosis of facet joint pain. The hypothesis that testing a patient first with lidocaine and subsequently with bupivacaine provides a means of identifying the placebo response has been tested and proven. The specificity of the effect of cervical and lumbar facet joint blocks was demonstrated in controlled trials [11]. Based on the updated guidelines for interventional techniques in the *Pain Physician* journal, indicated evidence for radio frequency neurotomy and cervical medial branch blocks is fair. This is based upon one randomized, double-blind, active-controlled trial, and one prospective evaluation. Based on two RCTs, the evidence for cervical intraarticular injections is limited [19]. Consequently, the recommendation is that therapeutic facet joint nerve blocks or conventional radio frequency neurotomy may be provided based on the response from controlled diagnostic blocks.

Future Directions or Clinical Trials in Progress

Future clinical trials are warranted in order to improve accuracy of diagnosis and treatment while decreasing complication rates.

Conclusion/Summary

Cervical facet disease, otherwise referred to as the zygapophyseal joint disease, can cause axial pain and some experts say the most common cause of headaches and whiplash-related neck pain [20–22]. Patients will often present with a history of trauma with an abrupt flexion-extension type injury or an occupation requiring persistent neck extension. Pain symptoms often refer to the occiput, shoulders, periscapular region, or proximal limbs. Axial symptoms are greater than extremity symptoms, as is the case with cervical discogenic pain. There is no specific examination or imaging finding to provide confirmatory diagnostic information. Diagnosis is difficult and requires putting all aspects together including a thorough history and physical exam, imaging techniques, and diagnostic blocks. Fluoroscopically guided intraarticular injection with local anesthetic or ablation of the innervation to the joint are the definitive diagnostic tests. This is done by injecting local anesthetic either directly into the joint space or anesthetizing the medial branches of the dorsal rami of a corresponding joint. However, there is limited evidence for intraarticular injection. Therapeutic nerve blocks should be provided based on response from controlled diagnostic blocks. Potential risks and complications can be disastrous related to needle placement and administration of various drugs. For this reason, meticulous safety guidelines and proper use of fluoroscopic imaging are indispensable for effective injection of cervical anatomy.

References

1. Sial KA, Simopoulos TT, Bajwa ZH, Warfield CA. Cervical facet syndrome. In: Waldman pain management. Netherlands: Elsevier; 2011. Chapter 57. p. 516–21.
2. Johnson RM, Hart DL, Simmons EF, et al. Cervical orthoses. A study comparing their effectiveness in restricting cervical motion in normal subjects. J Bone Joint Surg Am. 1977;59A:332–9.
3. Alund M, Larsson SE. Three-dimensional analysis of neck motion: a clinical method. Spine. 1990;15:87–91.
4. King W, Borowczyk JMI. Zygapophysial joint pain: procedures for diagnosis and treatment. In: Pain procedures in clinical practice, vol. 36. 3rd ed. Netherlands: Elsevier; 2011. p. 357–89.
5. Fukui S, Ohseto K, Saiotam M, et al. Referred pain distribution of the cervical zygapophyseal joints and cervical dorsal rami. Pain. 1996;68:79.
6. Cole A, Farrell J, Stratton S. Functional rehabilitation of cervical spine athletic injuries. In: Kibler B, Herring S, Press J, editors. Functional rehabilitation of sports and musculoskeletal injuries. Gaithersburg: Aspen Publication; 1998. p. 127.
7. National Collaborating Centre for Chronic Conditions (NCCCC). Osteoarthritis: the care and management of osteoarthritis in adults. London: Royal College of Physicians; 2008.
8. Moore RA, Wiffen PJ, Derry S. McQuay HJ. Cochrane Database Syst Rev: Gabapentin for chronic neuropathic pain and fibromyalgia in adults; 2011.
9. Manchikanti L, Falco FJE. An update of comprehensive evidence-based guidelines for interventional techniques in chronic spinal pain. Part I: introduction and general considerations. Pain Physician. 2013;16:S1–S48. ISSN 1533-3159.
10. Bogduk N. International Spinal Injection Society guidelines for the performance of spinal injection procedures: part 1: zygapophyseal joint blocks. Clin J Pain. 1997;13:285.
11. Boswell MV, Shah RV. Interventional techniques in the management of chronic spinal pain: evidence-based practice guidelines. Pain Physician. 2005;8:1–47, ISSN 1533-3159.
12. Pobereskin LH. Whiplash following rear end collisions: a prospective cohort study. J Neurol Neurosurg Psychiatry. 2005;76(8):1146.
13. Kasch H. The risk assessment score in acute whiplash injury predicts outcome and reflects biopsychosocial factors. Spine (Phila Pa 1976). 2011;36(25 Suppl):S263.
14. Falco FJE, et al. An updated review of diagnostic utility of cervical facet joint injections. Pain Physician. 2012;15:E807–38.
15. Bono CM, Ghiselli G. Diagnosis and treatment of cervical radiculopathy from degenerative disorders: USA: North American Spine Society; 2010.
16. Schellingerhout JM. Prognosis of patients with nonspecific neck pain: development and external validation of a prediction rule for persistence of complaints. Spine (Phila Pa 1976). 2010;35(17):E827.
17. Shahidi B, Curran-Everett D, Maluf KS. Psychosocial, physical, and neurophysiological risk factors for chronic neck pain: a prospective inception cohort study. J Pain. 2015;16(12):1288. Epub 2015 Sep 21.
18. Valenza MC, Valenza G. Alteration in sleep quality in patients with mechanical insidious neck pain and whiplash-associated neck pain. Am J Phys Med Rehabil. 2012;91(7):584.
19. Manchikanti L, et al. An update of comprehensive evidence-based guidelines for interventional techniques in chronic spinal pain. Part I: introduction and general considerations. Pain Physician. 2013;16:S1–S48.
20. Lord SM, Barnsley L, Wallis BJ, Bogduk N. Chronic cervical zygapophysial joint pain after whiplash. A placebo-controlled prevalence study. Spine (Phila Pa 1976). 1996;21(15):1737.
21. Bogduk N, Lord S. Cervical zygapophysial joint pain. Neurosurgery. 1998;8:107.
22. Manchikanti L, Siugh V, Rivera J, et al. Prevalence of cervical facet joint pain in chronic neck pain. Pain Physician. 2002;5:243.

Cervical Radicular Pain

11

Andrew Wendahl and Alaa Abd-Elsayed

Case Description

A 35-year-old woman walks into your clinic complaining of neck and right arm pain since a recent fall on ice from a standing position. Besides pain, the patient also complains of weakness with using a screwdriver in her right hand. This is important to her job description involving furniture restoration. Since the fall, she reports difficulty sleeping due to neck stiffness. Pain between the shoulder blades has become commonplace. She has trialed conservative management with nonsteroidal anti-inflammatories and acetaminophen. She has undergone 4 weeks of physical therapy exercises as prescribed with minimal improvement. She reported temporary improvement with heating pad therapy.

What Is Your Preliminary Diagnosis?

The diagnosis begins with the history and physical exam. Clinical features should guide the exam. The acute onset following an antecedent event leads me down the path of a herniated nucleus pulposus versus spondylosis which is often more indolent. However, most cases have no readily identifiable precipitant. The first aim is to find evidence of weakness and sensory disturbance in myotomal and dermatomal patterns as well as to catch any signs of myelopathy from cord compression. Assess passive and active range of motion if any shoulder weakness or wasting is apparent. Spurling's maneuver (neck compression) is performed by extending and rotating the neck to the side of pain with a downward pressure [2]. This test is positive if limb pain or paresthesias are reproduced. Neck pain alone is nonspecific and constitutes a negative test. The Spurling's test is highly specific but sensitivity is low to moderate. Another test, with low to moderate sensitivity and moderate to high specificity is the shoulder abduction relief test based on a 2006 systematic review [3].

How Is Diagnosis Confirmed?

Cervical radiculopathy is a clinical diagnosis and made on the basis of history and physical findings. Neuroimaging and electrodiagnostic testing are indicated for most patients if myotomal weakness or myelopathy, increased risk of or suspicion for an atypical underlying nondegenerative cause (i.e., neoplastic, infectious, or inflammatory), or when symptoms persist beyond 4–6 weeks of conservative therapy. In the proper setting of radiculopathy symptoms, imaging studies of the cervical spine can confirm the diagnosis. MRI is currently the study of choice for

A. Wendahl · A. Abd-Elsayed (✉)
Department of Anesthesiology, University of Wisconsin School of Medicine and Public Health, Madison, WI, USA

T. Malik (ed.), *Practical Chronic Pain Management*, https://doi.org/10.1007/978-3-030-46675-6_11

initial neuroimaging evaluation of the cervical spine, unless contraindicated. CT myelography is the superior study for diagnosing foramina compression for its distinction of osteophyte from soft tissue material [4]. Plain radiographs are rarely diagnostic because soft tissue is not well visualized. Radiculopathy is nondiagnostic, but usually confirmed by electromyography. This study usually consists of nerve conduction studies (NCS) and a needle EMG of the upper arm and neck [5].

What Is the Pathophysiology of This Condition?

A radiculopathy is a pathologic process affecting the nerve root. The causes of radiculopathy can be divided into nondegenerative and compressive etiologies. The two main causes of compressive radiculopathy are cervical spondylosis and disk herniation. Compressive radiculopathy is by far the most common pathophysiology, but nondegenerative disorders should always be considered.

Cervical spondylosis is a general term for nonspecific, degenerative changes of the spine. Degenerative changes occur in the vertebral disks, the zygapophysial (facet) and uncovertebral joints, and the vertebral bodies. Bone formation occurs in these areas as osteophytes [5]. Spondylosis is theorized to be from increased stress from the aging process leading to osseous and ligamentous hypertrophy and osteophyte formation. Disk herniation is another common cause of compressive radiculopathy as prolapsed material presses on a nerve root. This root compression with radicular symptoms is most likely to occur if herniation occurs laterally. In a large epidemiological survey of patients with cervical radiculopathy, disk protrusion was found to be the case in 21.9% of patients [6]. Nondegenerative radiculopathy can be from causes including infectious processes (i.e., herpes zoster and Lyme disease), nerve root infarction, root avulsion, infiltration by tumor, granulomatous tissue infiltration, and demyelination. Deficits associated with nondegenerative radiculopathy often spans multiple myotomes and dermatomes. This is more complete than a typical compressive radiculopathy due to the more diffuse ventral and dorsal affect [5].

How Is This Problem Managed?

Recommendations for diagnosis and treatment of cervical radiculopathy from degenerative disorders have been described by the North American Spine Society (NASS) Clinical Guidelines, 2010. It is recommended that diagnosis be considered in patients with arm pain, neck pain, scapular or periscapular pain, paresthesias, numbness and sensory changes, and weakness or abnormal deep tendon reflexes in the arm. This grade B recommendation was based off of the findings presented by Henderson et al. following a retrospective observational study reporting results in the treatment of 736 patients with cervical radiculopathy. Of these patients, the reported symptoms were as follows: arm pain (99.4%), neck pain (79.7%), scapular pain (52.5%), anterior chest pain (17.8%), and headache (9.7%). Dermatomal arm pain alone is not specific in identifying the pathologic level in patients with cervical radiculopathy. For this reason, CT, CT myelography (CTM), or MRI is suggested prior to any surgical decompression. This suggestion is of course after a failed course of conservative therapy in most cases. Modic et al. conducted a prospective study comparing the accuracy of MRI, CTM, and myelography in the evaluation of cervical radiculopathy. This study included 52 patients who underwent MRI, myelography, and CTM; 28 went on to surgery. Findings confirmed in surgery identified diagnostic accuracy rates of 74% for MRI, 85% for CTM, and 67% for myelography. The author concluded that MR with CTM used jointly was a viable alternative to myelography with 90% of patients having diagnostic agreement with surgical findings [7]. CT alone is recommended by work group consensus if MRI is contraindicated. Evidence is insufficient to make a recommendation for or against the use of EMG for patients in whom the diagnosis of cervical radiculopathy is unclear after clinical exam and MRI [8].

Selective nerve root block with specific dosing and technique protocols may be considered in the evaluation of patients with cervical radiculopathy and compressive lesions identified at multiple levels on MRI or CT myelography to discern the symptomatic level(s). Selective nerve root block may also be considered to confirm a symptomatic level in patients with discordant clinical symptoms and MRI or CTM findings [9, 10]. There are no studies to adequately address the role of physical therapy, exercise, chiropractic manipulation, or massage therapy in the management of cervical radiculopathy from degenerative disorders. The aforementioned treatment modalities should be considered carefully given case reports of adverse outcomes including radiculopathy, myelopathy, disk herniation, and vertebral artery compression with manipulative therapy. Transforaminal epidural steroid injections using fluoroscopic or CT guidance may be considered when developing a medical/interventional treatment plan for patients with cervical radiculopathy from degenerative disorders. There are many studies reporting up to 65% of patients reporting good or excellent results with regard to pain relief and many opting out of surgery. For instance, Lin et al. described a retrospective case series of 70 patients considered potential surgical candidates for cervical radiculopathy, underwent cervical transforaminal epidural steroid injections, of which the 65% with good or excellent results was abstracted [11]. Ancillary treatments such as bracing, traction, electrical stimulation, acupuncture, and transcutaneous electrical stimulation have been associated with improvements in uncontrolled case series. These modalities may be considered recognizing that no improvement relative to natural history of cervical radiculopathy has been demonstrated. Overall, surgical intervention is suggested for the rapid relief of symptoms of cervical radiculopathy from degenerative disorders when compared to medical/interventional treatment.

There is good evidence for cervical epidural steroid injections for radiculitis secondary to disk herniation with local anesthetics and steroids. Manchikanti et al., in a large randomized trial with 120 participants receiving cervical interlaminar epidural steroid injections under fluoroscopy with long-term follow-up yielded positive results. Outcome measures showed significant improvement in pain relief and functional status >50% at 3, 6, and 12 months out [12].

What Is the Prognosis of This Condition?

The North American Spine Society work group found no validated outcome measures to be utilized in prognostication of the subset of patients with cervical radiculopathy from degenerative disorders. The Neck Disability Index (NDI), SF-36, SF-12, and VAS are recommended outcome measures for assessing treatment of cervical radiculopathy from degenerative disorders, with a grade A recommendation [11].

The majority of radiculopathies arise from nerve root compression; the two predominant mechanisms are cervical spondylosis and disk herniation. Although data are limited, some, if not most, patients with compressive cervical radiculopathy improve without specific treatment [13–15]. Evidence that improvement is not treatment specific comes from a population-based study of 561 patients with cervical radiculopathy from Rochester, Minnesota. This was not a natural history study, since most patients received some treatment and 26 percent had surgery for cervical radiculopathy. Nevertheless, at last follow-up, 90 percent of patients were asymptomatic or only mildly incapacitated.

What Is the Long-Term Outcome: Complete Cure, Recurrent or Chronic Persistent Problem?

Symptoms of cervical radiculopathy recur in up to one-third of patients after initial improvement [14]. Conservative management should be reemployed when symptoms recur, unless a significant motor deficit or myelopathy is present. Abstracted from the 2013 ASIPP guidelines, most evidence indicates that between 50 and 75% of people who have neck pain initially also report pain 1 to 5 years later [16].

Discussion

Prevalence

One of the largest epidemiological studies of cervical radiculopathy was a retrospective population-based review of 561 patients (332 men and 229 women) with cervical radiculopathy seen from 1976 to 1990 in Rochester, Minnesota [14]. All patients with complaints of neck pain were screened, and clinical criteria using symptoms, signs, and diagnostic testing were used to retrospectively make the diagnosis of definite, probable, or possible cervical radiculopathy. A total of 561 cases (332 men and 229 women) with cervical radiculopathy were identified.

The following observations were reported in an epidemiological review [14]:

- The mean age at diagnosis was 47.9 years (range 13–91 years).
- Average annual incidence rates per 100,000 people for men and women were 107.3 and 63.5, respectively; the male to female ratio was 1.7:1.
- Age-specific incidence rates per 100,000 people were highest for the 50–54 year age group, 245.1 in males and 164.5 in females, and declined steeply after the age of 60 years.
- Lower cervical roots, particularly C7, are more frequently affected by compression than higher cervical roots. In a series of cases that came to surgery, the following observations were made [15]:
  - C7 was the most frequently affected nerve root, accounting for approximately 70 percent of patients with cervical radiculopathy.
  - C6 root involvement was found in approximately 20%.
  - Involvement of the C5, C8, and T1 levels together accounted for the remaining 10 percent.

Differential Diagnosis

As mentioned, cervical radiculopathy is a clinical, and to some extent subjective, diagnosis made on the basis of history and clinical findings. Typical findings of solitary root lesions may include pain, numbness, weakness, reflex changes, as well as overlapping dermatomes. Neuroimaging and electrodiagnostic studies are indicated for most especially in the setting of significant neurologic deficit, suspicion for an atypical underlying (nondegenerative) cause, or when persistent symptoms do not resolve with 4–6 weeks of conservative therapy. The differential should include entrapment neuropathy, zygapophyseal (facet) joint pain, brachial plexus syndromes, nondegenerative etiologies (neoplastic, infectious, or inflammatory), myalgia, nerve root infarction, root avulsion, demyelination, and traumatic causes to name a few other possible etiologies.

Predictive Value of Different Clinical Features (Both on History and Physical Exam) and Lab Testing/Imaging

- MRI is currently the study of choice in most patients for the initial neuroimaging evaluation of the cervical spine. CT myelography is superior to MRI in the distinction of osteophyte from soft tissue and remains superior to MRI.
- The diagnosis of radiculopathy is usually confirmed by needle electromyography, frequently involving a myotomal pattern of denervation. Nerve conduction studies alone are not sensitive for radiculopathy and should be done beyond 3 weeks of symptoms to improve sensitivity.
- Due to a high prevalence of asymptomatic degenerative changes in the cervical spine, an imaging evaluation revealing evidence of degenerative changes or disk herniation can only support the diagnosis of cervical radiculopathy and cannot by itself establish a diagnosis [17].

Strength of Evidence for Different Treatment Modalities

In summary, the evidence for cervical epidural injections is good for radiculitis secondary to disk herniation with local anesthetics and steroids, fair with local anesthetic only; whereas it is fair for local anesthetics with or without steroids for axial or discogenic pain, pain of central spinal stenosis, and pain of post-surgery syndrome [12].

Future Directions or Clinical Trials in Progress

Future clinical trials are needed to describe improved and effective nonsurgical means of treating radicular pain. While serious complications of cervical interlaminar epidural procedures are rare, future research should be directed at improved complication rates. A cervical spinal cord injection of corticosteroids is a devastating complication, and multiple cases of intramedullary injection have been described after interlaminar approach [12].

Conclusion/Summary

Cervical radiculopathy is a term applied when a nerve root is inflamed, irritated, and has produced a clinically significant motor or sensory neurologic deficit in that nerves distribution. The most common cause for this includes disk protrusion and cervical spondylosis. The common view is that this compressive force on the affected nerve is what leads to common symptoms being numbness, paresthesia, weakness, and hyporeflexia by blocking conduction and causing ischemia. There is another theory that inflammatory markers are irritants of the spinal nerves leading to pain. History and physical exam are critical to the diagnosis although dermatomal patterns are often overlapping. Many specialized tests exist including the Spurling's compression test, Lhermitte's sign, neck distraction test, shoulder abduction test, Adson's test, and Hoffmann's sign [17]. Imaging is the most useful in diagnosis, and MRI is the society-supported gold standard. The prevalence of abnormalities on MRI in asymptomatic individuals is of concern, however [18]. Multimodal conservative therapy is always the first recommendation. Interventional pain management has been described with substantial differences in technique and outcomes. Thus, characteristics applicable to each technique including interlaminar and transforaminal approaches are considered as separate entities. Response has also been found quite variable to epidural injections depending on pathologic condition (i.e., disk herniation, radiculitis, discogenic pain without herniation, spinal stenosis, and post-surgery syndrome) [1]. One must be attentive to the severity of complications when considering invasive techniques [19]. Surgery is typically indicated when all of the following criteria are met: MRI or CT myelography indicating compressive etiology, pain persistence after 6–12 weeks of conservative treatment; a progressive motor deficit; or cervical spinal cord compression on imaging and/or clinically significant myelopathy. There is no good consensus on proper timing of surgery, however [12, 20].

References

1. Boswell MV, Trescot AM, Datta S, et al. American Society of Interventional Pain Physicians. Interventional techniques: evidence-based practice guidelines in the management of chronic spinal pain. Pain Physician. 2007;10(1):7–111.
2. Rubinstein SM, Pool JJ, van Tulder MW, Riphagen II, de Vet HC. A systematic review of the diagnostic accuracy of provocative tests of the neck for diagnosing cervical radiculopathy. Eur Spine J. 2007;16(3):307. Pub 2006 Sep 30.
3. Bartlett RJ, Hill CR, Gardiner E. A comparison of T2 and gadolinium enhanced MRI with CT pyelography in cervical radiculopathy. Br J Radiol. 1998;71(841):11.
4. Bono CM, Ghiselli G. Diagnosis and treatment of cervical radiculopathy from degenerative disorders: USA: North American Spine Society; 2010.

5. Radhakrishnan K, Litchy WJ, O'Fallon WM, Kurland LT. Epidemiology of cervical radiculopathy. A population-based study from Rochester, Minnesota, 1976 through 1990. Brain. 1994;117(Pt 2):325.
6. Semmes R, Murphey M. A report of four cases with symptoms simulating coronary disease. JAMA. 1943;121:1209.
7. Alrawi MF, Khalil NM, Mitchell P, Hughes SP. The value of neurophysiological and imaging studies in predicting outcomein the surgical treatment of cervical radiculopathy. Eur Spine J. 2007;16(4):495–500.
8. Anderberg L, Annertz M, Rydholm U, Brandt L, Saveland H. Selective diagnostic nerve root block for the evaluation of radicular pain in the multilevel degenerated cervical spine. Eur Spine J. 2006;15(6):794–801.
9. Modic MT, Masaryk TJ, Mulopulos GP. Cervical radiculopathy:prospective evaluation with surface coil MR imaging, CT with metrizamide, and metrizamide myelography. Radiology. 1986;161(3):753–9.
10. Lin EL, Lieu V, Halevi L, Shamie AN, Wang JC. Cervical epidural steroid injections for symptomatic disc herniations. Agri. 2012;24:130–4.
11. Lees F, Turner JW. Natural history and prognosis of cervical spondylosis. Br Med J. 1963;2(5373):1607.
12. Diwan SA, et al. Effectiveness of cervical epidural injections in the management of chronic neck and upper extremity pain. Pain Physician. 2012;15:E405–34.
13. Radhakrishnan K, Litchy WJ, O'Fallon WM, Kurland LT. Epidemiology of cervical radiculopathy. A population-based study from Rochester, MN, 1976 through 1990. Brain. 1994;117(Pt 2):325.
14. Kujjper B, Tans JT, Schimsheimer RJ, van der Kallen BF, Beelen A, Nollet F, de Visser M. Degenerative cervical radiculopathy: diagnosis and conservative treatment. A review. Our J Neurol. 2009;16(1):15–20.
15. Loss RE, Corbin KB, Maccarty CS, Love JG. Significance of symptoms and signs in localization of involved root in cervical disk protrusion. Neurology. 1957;7(10):673.
16. Manchikanti L, et al. An update of comprehensive evidence-based guidelines for interventional techniques in chronic spinal pain. Part I: introduction and general considerations. Pain Physician. 2013;16:S1–S48.
17. Bogduk N. Differential diagnosis. In: Medical management of acute cervical radicular pain: an evidence-based approach. Newcastle: University of Newcastle, Australia, Newcastle Bone and Joint Institute; 1999. p. 51.
18. Bush K, Hillier S. Outcome of cervical radiculopathy treated with periradicular/epidural corticosteroid injections: a prospective study with independent clinical review. Eur Spine J. 1996;5:319.
19. Heckmann JG, Lang CJG, Zöbelien I, et al. Herniated cervical intervertebral discs with radiculopathy: an outcome study of conservatively or surgically treated patients. J Spinal Disord. 1999;12:396.
20. Carette S, Fehlings MG. Clinical practice: cervical radiculopathy. N Engl J Med. 2005;353:392.

12 Temporomandibular Joint Dysfunction

Ahmad Khattab and Tariq Malik

Case Description

A 50-year-old female patient presents to your pain management clinic with 3 months of pain over her left jaw, just anterior to the ear. Pain started insidiously, with no known precipitating factors. She has been to her primary care physician who then referred her to an ENT specialist, but all the work-up is negative. She reports the pain is an intermittent, dull ache that occasionally radiates to her left ear and chin. The pain is made worse with chewing food and when she clenches her teeth in stressful situations. She also has noticed that her left jaw sometimes "pops" when she opens her mouth. Pain is affecting her appetite and mood now. She has tried over-the-counter medications such as acetaminophen and ibuprofen but has not had adequate relief.

What Is Your Preliminary Diagnosis?

In the absence of negative medical work-up, the most likely preliminary diagnosis is temporomandibular joint (TMJ) dysfunction. This is a chronic dysfunction of TMJ joints. Exact etiology of pain is unknown and is multifactorial encompassing biological and psychological factors. Quite often there is a myofascial pain dysfunction of the muscles of mastication. Patients with TMJ dysfunction commonly present with pain in the joint area that may radiate into the mandible, the ear, the neck, and the tonsillar pillars [1]. The pain is usually described as a dull ache and can be triggered by chewing and teeth clenching. Palpation over the TMJ itself or the surrounding muscles of mastication may reproduce the pain. The American Association for Dental Research has recommended that the diagnosis of TMJ dysfunction should be primarily based on the presenting patient's history and physical exam findings, but imaging modalities may also be helpful in confirming the suspected diagnosis. Furthermore, TMJ dysfunction should be distinguished from other common facial pain syndromes that may present similarly clinically [2].

How Is Diagnosis Confirmed?

Diagnostic Criteria

The first diagnostic criteria for TMJ disorders were established by a panel of TMD experts and published in the *Journal of Craniomandibular Disorders* in 1992 and they were termed the

A. Khattab
Department of Anesthesiology and Critical Care, University of Chicago, Chicago, IL, USA

T. Malik (✉)
Department of Anesthesia and Critical Care, University of Chicago, Chicago, IL, USA
e-mail: TMuslim@dacc.uchicago.edu; tmalik@dacc.uchicago.edu

T. Malik (ed.), *Practical Chronic Pain Management*, https://doi.org/10.1007/978-3-030-46675-6_12

Research Diagnostic Criteria for Temporomandibular Disorders (RDC/TMD) [3]. The RDC/TMD criteria were built upon a dual axis assessment. Axis I described standard diagnostic criteria for TMD based on clinical presentation of the patient. Axis II described using psychosocial and behavioral patient factors to help further identify patients with TMD. The RDC/TMD Axis I criteria group temporomandibular disorders into three subcategories as described below [3]:

A. Group 1: Muscle Disorders
   (a) Myofascial pain
      - Pain reported by the patient in masticatory muscles, including jaw, temples, face, preauricular area, or inside the ear
      - Pain with palpation in at least three sites, with at least one site being on the side that the patient is reporting the pain
         1. There are 20 sites total, 10 sites on each side: posterior, middle, and anterior temporalis; origin, body, and insertion of masseter; posterior mandibular region; submandibular region; lateral pterygoid; tendon of temporalis.
   (b) Myofascial pain with limited opening
      - Myofascial pain
      - Pain-free unassisted opening <40 mm and passive stretch >5 mm where the examiner uses their index finger and thumb to passively stretch the patient's mouth to open wider than unassisted opening. The patient uses a hand signal to indicate discomfort.
B. Group 2: Disc Displacements
   (a) Disc displacements with reduction
      - Lack of pain in the joint
      - Reproducible click on excursion with opening or closing
      - With click on opening or closing (unless excursive click confirmed):
         1. Click on opening happens at greater than or equal to 5 mm interincisal distance than on closing
         2. Clicks eliminated by protrusive opening
   (b) Disc displacements without reduction with limited opening
      - History of locking or catching that interferes with eating
      - No TMJ clicking
      - Unassisted opening less than or equal to 35 mm and passive stretch less than or equal to 4 mm
      - Contralateral excursion <7 mm *OR* uncorrected ipsilateral deviation on opening
   (c) Disc displacements without reduction without limited opening
      - History of locking or catching that interferes with eating
      - Presence of TMJ sounds excluding DDR clicking
      - Unassisted opening >35 mm and passive stretch >4 mm
      - Contralateral excursion greater than or equal to 7 mm
      - Optional imaging (arthrography or MRI) to confirm disc displacement
C. Group 3: Other Common Joint Disorders
   (a) Arthralgia
      - Pain with TMJ palpation either laterally or intra auricular
      - Self-reported joint pain with or without jaw movement
      - Absence of crepitus and possibility of clicking
   (b) Osteoarthritis
      - Pain as described for arthralgia
      - Crepitus on any movement OR radiologic evidence of joint changes, which include erosion of cortical delineation, sclerosis of parts or all the condyle and articular eminence, flattening of joint surfaces, and osteophyte formation.
   (c) Osteoarthrosis
      - Crepitus on any movement OR radiologic evidence of joint changes, which include erosion of cortical delineation, sclerosis of parts or all the condyle and articular eminence, flattening of

joint surfaces, and osteophyte formation.
- No reported joint pain
- No pain on any movement

These criteria were used for a number of years until around the mid-2000s. A multi-site Validation Project was initiated in an attempt to assess the validity of the RDC/TMD criteria as compared to the gold standard criteria. The gold standard diagnoses for pain-related TMD were established by consensus between two TMD and orofacial pain experts at three different sites using patient history, physical exam findings, and panoramic radiograph. They concluded that the Axis I criteria needed improvement [4]. Listed in Tables 12.1 and 12.2 are the revised criteria, which are now referred to as the Diagnostic Criteria for Temporomandibular Disorders [5].

Table 12.1 Validated Axis I Pain-Related TMD Diagnoses

Disorder	History	Exam findings
Myalgia[a]		
Sensitivity: 90% Specificity: 99%	Pain in a masticatory structure modified by jaw movement, function, or parafunction	Report of familiar pain[b] in temporalis or masseter muscle(s) with: (1) palpation of these muscles, or (2) maximum unassisted or assisted opening movements(s). Note: Assessment of other masticatory muscles may be indicated in some clinical situations.
Myofascial pain with referral		
Sensitivity: 86% Specificity: 98%	Same as for myalgia	(1) Report of familiar pain[b] with palpation of the temporalis or masseter muscle(s) and (2) Report of pain at a site beyond the boundary of the muscle being palpated (e.g., referral to a tooth)
Arthralgia		
Sensitivity: 89% Specificity: 98%	Same as for myalgia	Report of familiar pain[b] in TMJ with (1) Palpation of the TMJ or (2) Maximum unassisted or assisted opening, right or left lateral, or protrusive movements.
Headache attributed to TMD		
Sensitivity: 89% Specificity: 87%	Headache in temporal area modified by jaw movement, function, or parafunction	Report of familiar headache[c] in temple area with (1) Palpation of temporalis muscle(s) or (2) Maximum unassisted or assisted opening, right or left lateral, or protrusive movement(s). Note: A diagnosis of pain-related TMD must also be present (e.g., myalgia, arthralgia)

From Schiffman and Ohrbach [5], with permission

[a]Myalgia can be subclassified into three disorders: local myalgia, myofascial pain, and myofascial pain with referral; only myofascial pain with referral has been validated. See Schiffman et al., 2014, for diagnostic criteria for local myalgia and myofascial pain

[b]Familiar pain is similar to the pain the patient has been experiencing. The intent is to replicate the patient's pain complaint

[c]Familiar headache is similar to the headache the patient has been experiencing. The intent is to replicate the patient's headache complaint

What Is the Pathophysiology of This Condition?

The pathophysiology of TMD is not well understood. Due to the complex nature of the joint itself and the multifactorial causes of symptoms, there is no known single etiology that is found commonly among all TMD. However, there are many factors that have been studied that potentially could contribute to the development of TMD.

Direct trauma to the joint, such as that experienced in mandibular fractures causing disc displacement, intubation, and prolonged yawning or significant mouth opening, have all been reported in patients with TMD [6]. Some forms of microtrauma, such as teeth grinding, teeth clenching, and other forms of abnormal posturing of the mandible have also been thought to contribute to TMD [6]. Malocclusion of the structures surrounding the TMJ were historically thought to lead to dysfunction of the joint but recent data suggests that occlusive disorders such as overbite, crossbite, and occlusal sliding may develop as a result of joint disease progression rather than being the cause [6].

Table 12.2 Validated Axis I TMJ Diagnoses

Disorder	History	Exam Findings
Disc displacement with reduction		
Sensitivity: 34% Specificity: 92%	TMJ noise(s) present	Clicking, popping, or snapping noise present with: (1) Opening and closing, or (2) Opening or closing and lateral or protrusive movements
Disc displacement with reduction with intermittent locking		
Sensitivity: 38% Specificity: 98%	(1) TMJ noise(s) present, and (2) Jaw locks with limited opening and then unlocks	Same as disc displacement with reduction. Note: When the jaw gets lock in the clinic, maneuver is required to open the mouth.
Disc displacement without reduction with limited opening		
Sensitivity: 80% Specificity: 97%	(1) TMJ locking with limited opening, and (2) Limitation severe enough to interfere with the ability to eat	Maximum assisted opening (passive stretch) <40 mm. Note: Maximum opening includes inter-incisal opening plus vertical overlap of incisors
Disc displacement without reduction without limited opening		
Sensitivity: 54% Specificity: 79%	(1) TMJ locking with limited opening, and (2) Limitation severe enough to interfere with the ability to eat	Maximum assisted opening (passive stretch) >40 mm. Note: Maximum opening includes inter-incisal opening plus vertical overlap of incisors
Degenerative joint disease		
Sensitivity: 55% Specificity: 61%	TMJ noise(s) present	Crepitus * present during maximum active opening, passive opening, right lateral, left lateral, or protrusive movement(s). Note: Crepitus is defined as crunching, grinding, or grating noise(s)
Subluxation		
Sensitivity: 98% Specificity: 100%	TMJ locking or catching in a wide open position that resolves with a specific maneuver (e.g., moving the jaw)	Note: When the jaw gets stuck in a locked position in the clinic, maneuver is required to close mouth

From Schiffman and Ohrbach [5], with permission

TMJ extracellular matrix (ECM) is a form of fibrocartilage tissue that serves as a lubricant for the joint. The ECM may become compromised and become inflamed due to factors such as direct mechanical injury, hypoxia-reperfusion injury, and neurogenic inflammation [7]. Furthermore, some studies have shown that patient with degeneration of the TMJ had increased levels of Interleukin 1β (IL–1β), IL-6, TNF-α, IL-8, and Endothelin-1 in the TMJ synovial fluid [6, 7]. These cytokines contribute to the degradation of cartilage and bone within the joint by facilitating release of proteinases and inflammatory mediators [6, 7].

How Is This Problem Managed?

Treatment for TMJ disorders can be divided into three general categories – non-medication management, pharmacologic therapies, and interventional modalities.

Non-medication Management

Patients with TMJ disorders should be educated about the disease process and the non-invasive treatment options should be targeted to the suspected underlying cause of each patient's pain process. Every patient should be given techniques to deal with behavioral issues (such as teeth clenching, teeth grinding, stress-related habits, and diet) that may be contributing to the symptoms [8]. Any underlying anxiety disorders should also be addressed. Physical therapy techniques involving range of motion exercises and manual therapies targeting the TMJ and muscles of mastication and cervical spine muscles can be helpful in reducing pain by strengthening and improving mobility in the muscles [9, 10]. If a patient has known issues with malocclusion, then they may benefit from occlusal splints and occlusal adjustments by promoting stability of the joint and minimizing joint-traumatizing factors [8].

Pharmacologic Therapies

Multiple options for oral medications exist for the treatment of TMJ disorders. NSAIDs such as Ibuprofen and Naproxen are commonly used to address the inflammatory aspect of pain with TMJ disorders. The benefit of using NSAIDs should be weighed against the potential risks associated with long-term NSAID use, and using NSAIDs should only be considered if the benefits outweigh those risks. Muscle relaxants such as Cyclobenzaprine may also play a role in reducing pain and symptoms in patients with primarily a myofascial component to their TMJ disorders [11]. Antidepressant and anticonvulsant medications such as Amitriptyline and Gabapentin may also be beneficial in offering a multimodal approach to treating the neuropathic aspect of TMJ pain [11]. Benzodiazepines such as Diazepam and Clonazepam may also provide benefit in treatment, although the data is not conclusive and the risk of sedation, misuse, and drug interactions likely outweighs the potential benefit from long-term use [11].

Interventional Modalities

If more-conservative therapies fail to improve pain and quality of life in patients with TMJ disorders, advanced-level injections/procedures can be considered. Risks associated with injections should always be discussed with patients and include bleeding, infection, damage to the intra-articular disc, and failure to relieve the pain. There are various injection techniques that can be used to inject the joint to help improve pain in the TMJ disorder. Injections can be performed with the aid of fluoroscopy, CT guidance, or ultrasound guidance. Figure 12.1 depicts the approach to performing an intra-articular TMJ injection [1].

Intra-articular injections with either local anesthetic plus steroid mixture or hyaluronate can be used to relieve symptoms of TMJ disorders, specifically those with internal derangements [12]. A literature review looking at nine randomized control trials of patients receiving intra-articular injections with corticosteroids and/or hyaluronate showed that patients had improved pain levels after the injections, but some studies did not reflect statistically significant results [12]. Another systematic review looking at multiple studies involving hyaluronate

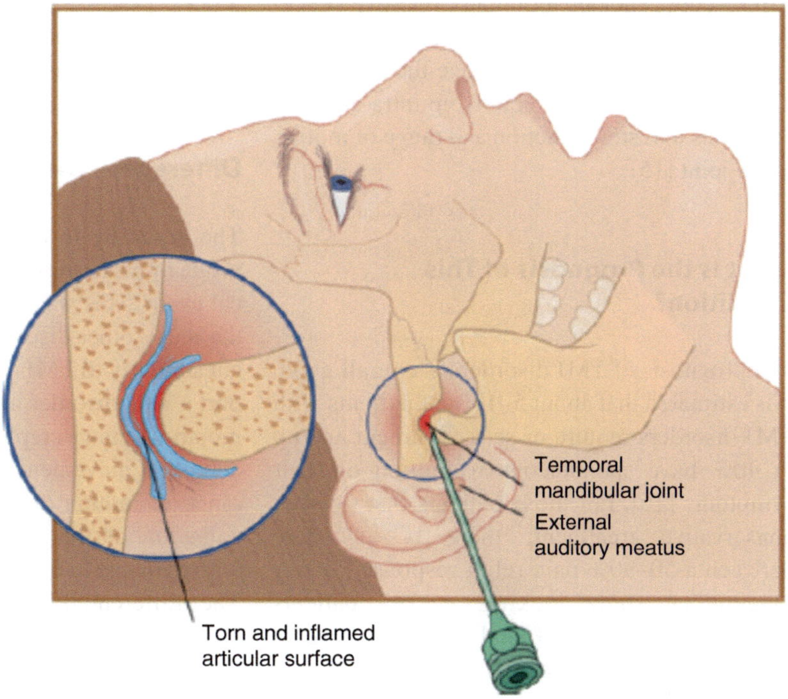

Fig. 12.1 The approach to performing an intra-articular TMJ injection. (From Waldman [1], with permission)

injections in patients with TMJ disc displacements and inflammatory-degenerative disorders found that all groups of patients had a decrease in their pain levels for anywhere between 15 days to 24 months [13].

If the patient's underlying TMJ disorder is primarily attributed to spasms of muscles of mastication, one may consider performing botulinum toxin A injections. These injections are primarily performed in the lateral pterygoid muscle but can also be targeted toward surrounding muscles of mastication that may be contributing to TMJ dysfunction. A review article looked at lateral pterygoid botulinum toxin A injections in 24 studies and found that, regardless of the number of injections or dosages used, patients had a decreased amount of clicking sounds, pain, hyperactivity, and dysfunction [14].

If patients fail to have relief of symptoms with injections, then surgical procedures addressing deformity of the TMJ and its contents may be considered. Arthrocentesis is a minimally invasive procedure that involves a sterile needle being advanced into the joint and draining the fluid, followed by flushing the joint with sterile solution to evacuate debris and inflammatory cytokines. Arthroscopy, another minimally invasive procedure, can also be performed to evaluate the damage within the joint, to help stage the severity of TMJ disease, and also to break up intra-articular adhesions to restore function and range of motion to the joint [15].

What Is the Prognosis of This Condition?

The prognosis of TMJ disorders is overall good. It is estimated that about 5–10% of patients with TMJ disorders require or seek treatment and up to 40% have spontaneous resolution of their symptoms [16]. For those patients that do seek conservative treatment, there is anywhere between a 50–90% pain relief response [16]. A longitudinal study looking at 195 patients treated conservatively found that after 2 years about two-third of the patients had complete resolution of symptoms, about one-fourth had slight symptoms that persisted, and 3% of patients had intermittently recurring symptoms [17]. Ultimately, the prognosis of this complex, multifactorial disease process is dependent on the patient's underlying cause of symptoms, the patient's risk factors, and the chronicity of the condition.

Discussion

Prevalence

It is estimated that anywhere from 5% to 25% of adults experience symptoms of TMJ disorders, with peak incidence at 20 to 40 years of age and sometimes as late as 50 years of age [8, 16]. There is a much higher incidence in females as compared to males with reported ratios of anywhere between 2:1 to 8:1 [8, 16]. It is difficult to establish an accurate prevalence of TMJ disorders because, although many people may have symptoms, only a small proportion of those people will actually seek treatment for the symptoms they are experiencing [8]. Furthermore, this complex disease process may be confused with other disease processes that may present in a similar fashion, leading to underestimation of the prevalence of the disease.

Differential Diagnosis

The best way to diagnose TMJ disorders is by virtue of performing a detailed history and physical exam. This will help the practitioner rule out the many other disease processes that may present similarly to TMJ disorders. Findings that support a TMJ disorder include clicking sounds with mouth opening, crepitus or locking of the TMJ, abnormal movement of the mandible, decreased range of motion of the mandible, tenderness to palpation of the muscles of mastication, pain with dynamic loading, and signs of bruxism [16]. The differential diagnosis for TMJ disorder should include the following: dental conditions (infections, cavities, dry socket), giant cell arteritis, mandibular malignancies/tumors, migraine headache, glossopharyngeal neuralgia, postherpetic neuralgia, trigeminal neuralgia, otitis, complex regional pain syndrome, salivary stone, and sinusitis [1, 16]. Many of these differential diagnoses may be ruled out with history/exam findings as well as obtaining imaging of the head and neck structures surrounding the TMJ with modalities such as CT scan or MRI.

Predictive Value of Different Clinical Features and Lab Testing/Imaging

Listed earlier in Tables 12.1 and 12.2 are the diagnostic criteria for the spectrum of TMJ disorders with their respective specificities and sensitivities for each TMJ sub-classification. A review article looked at seven main articles to determine sensitivity, specificity, and negative/positive likelihood ratios for findings such as joint sounds, pain in the TMJ, and movements of the TMJ [18]. They found that each of these findings had a wide range of predictability and that most of the articles they looked at compared findings within the TMJ disorder spectrum (osteoarthritis vs. joint effusion vs. disc displacement). Unfortunately, there are no major studies comparing these findings with patients who have TMJ disorders compared to patients with non-TMJ disorders.

Many different imaging modalities can be used as part of the diagnosis and treatment of TMJ disorders. These modalities include but are not limited to conventional radiography, CT scan, MRI, and ultrasonography. In general, starting with a plain radiograph is recommended and will help identify most acute fractures, dislocations, or severe degenerative changes within the joint [16]. CT scans are more sensitive for detecting fractures or bony abnormalities when compared to the other imaging modalities. MRI is overall the best imaging modality for comprehensive joint evaluation, with up to a 95% correlation between MRI findings and structural joint issues in symptomatic patients [16]. However, false positive findings can be found in up to 34% of asymptomatic patients. Ultrasonography can be considered when MRI or CT are not available, and offers the benefit of examining the TMJ in a dynamic setting, which may reveal issues that may not be evident on a static image performed with the other imaging modalities [16].

Strength of Evidence for Different Treatment Modalities

There are currently no publications by any professional societies regarding the strength of evidence for the treatment modalities for TMJ disorders. The recommendations are to start with conservative treatments and attempt more invasive treatments if conservative modalities are unsuccessful [16].

Future Directions or Clinical Trials in Progress

The most recent interesting development in addressing TMJ disorders involves tissue-engineering strategies that involve the TMJ disc. The biggest challenge in addressing TMJ disorders where disc thinning and degeneration has occurred is that the treatments are palliative but not curative. There have been animal studies conducted with tissue-engineered implants derived from allogenic costal chondrocytes that have shown promising results [19]. At 8 weeks post implantation, the implants showed complete stability and no evidence of breakdown or fragmentation. There was also minimal immune response to the tissue-engineered implants and no acute implant rejection was noted [19]. This strategy could prove to be promising in addressing TMJ disorders involving disc thinning in the early phases to help prevent advancement of joint degeneration.

Conclusion/Summary

TMJ disorders are chronic pain syndromes with complex etiologies that primarily affect the TMJ and surrounding musculoskeletal structures and in severe cases can significantly affect quality of life. The diagnosis of TMJ disorders has historically been challenging due to the wide spectrum of presenting signs and symptoms, as well as the differential diagnoses that present similarly. Treatment consists of a variety of conservative treatment modalities such as behavior modification, oral occlusal splints, and physical therapy. There are a number of pharmacologic drug classes such as NSAIDs, muscle relaxants, and neuropathic agents that have been shown to help relieve symptoms as well. If symptoms are not relieved with conservative therapies, there are different injections into or around the TMJ that may offer benefit. Surgery should only be considered when addressing severe internal derangements and significant symptoms not relieved with other modalities. Further research is needed to develop additional pharmacotherapies and interventions to help treat TMJ disorders.

References

1. Waldman SD. Temporomandibular joint dysfunction. In: Atlas of common pain syndromes: Philadelphia, PA: Elsevier; 2019. p. 42–6.
2. The TMJ Association, Ltd. http://www.tmj.org/Page/37/19.
3. Dworkin SF, LeResche L. Research diagnostic criteria for temporomandibular disorders: review, criteria, examinations and specifications, critique. J Craniomandib Disord. 1992;6(4):301–55.
4. Truelove E, Pan W, Look JO, et al. The research diagnostic criteria for temporomandibular disorders. III: validity of axis I diagnoses. J Orofac Pain. 2010;24(1):35–47.
5. Schiffman E, Ohrbach R. Executive summary of the diagnostic criteria for temporomandibular disorders (DC/TMD) for clinical and research applications. J Am Dent Assoc. 2016;147(6):438–45. Epub 2016 Feb 26.
6. Chang CL, Wang DH, Yang MC, Hsu WE, Hsu ML. Functional disorders of the temporomandibular joints: internal derangement of the temporomandibular joint. Kaohsiung J Med Sci. 2018;34(4):223–30.
7. Milam SB, Schmitz JP. Molecular biology of temporomandibular joint disorders: proposed mechanisms of disease. J Oral Maxillofac Surg. 1995;53(12):1448–54.
8. Meghan MK, MacBarb RF, Wong ME, Athanasiou KA. Temporomandibular joint disorders: a review of etiology, clinical management, and tissue engineering strategies. Int J Oral Maxillofac Implants. 2013;28(6):e393–414.
9. McNeely ML, Armijo Olivo S, Magee DJ. A systematic review of the effectiveness of physical therapy interventions for temporomandibular disorders. Phys Ther. 2006;86:710–25.
10. Rocabado M. The importance of soft tissue mechanics in stability and instability of the cervical spine: a functional diagnosis for treatment planning. Cranio. 1987;5:130–8.
11. Ouanounou A, Goldberg M, Haas DA. Pharmacotherapy in temporomandibular disorders: a review. J Can Dent Assoic. 2017 Jul;83:h7.
12. Machado E, Bonotto D, Cunali PA. Intra-articular injections with corticosteroids and sodium hyaluronate for treating temporomandibular joint disorders: a systematic review. Dental Press J Orthod. 2013;18(5):128–33.
13. Manfredini D, Piccotti F, Guarda-Nardini L. Hyaluronic acid in the treatment of TMJ disorders: a systematic review of the literature. Cranio. 2010;28(3):166–76.
14. Ataran R, et al. The role of botulinum toxin A in treatment of temporomandibular joint disorders: a review. J Dent (Shiraz). 2017;18(3):157–64.
15. Tanaka E, Detamore MS, Mercuri LG. Degenerative disorders of the temporomandibular joint: etiology, diagnosis, and treatment. J Dent Res. 2008;87(4):296–307.
16. Gauer RL, Semidey MJ, Womack Army Medical Center, Fort Bragg, North Carolina. Diagnosis and treatment of temporomandibular disorders. Am Fam Physician. 2015;91(6):378–86.
17. Garefis P, Grigoriadou E, Zarifi A, et al. Effectiveness of conservative treatment for craniomandibular disorders: a 2-year longitudinal study. J Orofac Pain. 1994;8(3):309–14.
18. Reneker J, Paz J, Petrosino C, Cook C. Diagnostic accuracy of clinical tests and signs of temporomandibular joint disorders: a systematic review of the literature. J Orthop Sports Phys Ther. 2011;41(6):408–16. Epub 2011 Feb 18.
19. Vapniarsky N, et al. Tissue engineering toward temporomandibular joint disc regeneration. Sci Transl Med. 2018;10(446) https://doi.org/10.1126/scitranslmed.aaq1802.

A 45-Year-Old Patient with Persistent Shoulder Pain (Rotator Cuff Injury)

13

Teresa M. Kusper, Nebojsa Nick Knezevic, and Kenneth D. Candido

Case Description

A 45-year-old previously healthy construction worker presented to the clinic with a complaint of severe pain and weakness in his right shoulder for 1 month's duration. He reported dragging a heavy piece of equipment across the construction site when he felt a sudden "pop" followed by an intense pain in his shoulder. Since the injury, he was unable to use his arm at work, especially raising his arm overhead. He had been treating his pain with hot packs and over-the-counter acetaminophen and ibuprofen, but his pain continued especially at nighttime and during work. On visual inspection, the shoulders appeared symmetrical, and there were no signs of swelling, ecchymosis, muscle atrophy, or deformity noted. Physical exam was significant for mild tenderness to palpation over the anterior aspect of the glenohumeral joint, positive Jobe's, Hornblower's and Shrug signs, positive drop arm test, and weakness in external rotation of the arm at the right shoulder. Spurling's test, cross arm test, sulcus sign, apprehension sign, Neer's and Hawkins tests were all negative. Neurologic exam demonstrated intact and symmetric sensation along all dermatomes and normal strength of the biceps, triceps, and intrinsic hand muscles.

What Is Your Preliminary Diagnosis?

Given the history of injury, clinical presentation, and pertinent findings noted on the physical exam, a provisional diagnosis of rotator cuff tear was made. The provocative tests were employed to help elucidate the diagnosis and the extent of the tear. A positive Jobe's, Hornblower's, and drop arm tests along with weak external rotation are consistent with a complete rotator cuff tear possibly involving all four muscle tendons.

How Is the Diagnosis Confirmed?

The clinical diagnosis of rotator cuff tear can be confirmed with the use of plain radiography, ultrasound, magnetic resonance imaging (MRI), and computed tomography (CT) imaging. Plain radiography is considered the initial imaging test of choice, as it may support the diagnosis of the rotator cuff tear but also offer important information about other structures, which may be used to guide medical management. Ultrasound is a

T. M. Kusper
Department of Anesthesiology, Advocate Illinois Masonic Medical Center, Chicago, IL, USA

N. N. Knezevic (✉) · K. D. Candido
Department of Anesthesiology, Advocate Illinois Masonic Medical Center, Chicago, IL, USA

Department of Anesthesiology, University of Illinois, Chicago, IL, USA

Department of Surgery, University of Illinois, Chicago, IL, USA

T. Malik (ed.), *Practical Chronic Pain Management*, https://doi.org/10.1007/978-3-030-46675-6_13

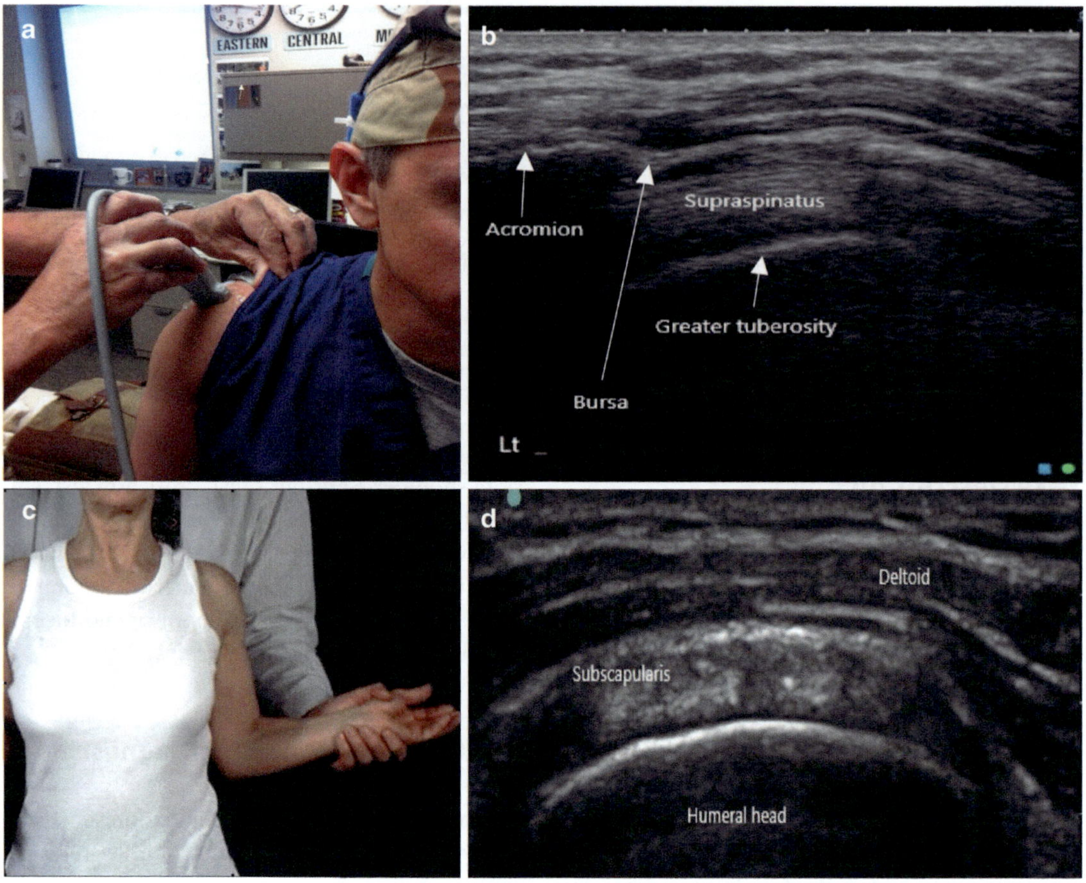

Fig. 13.1 (**a–d**) Ultrasonographic evaluation of the rotator cuff complex. Superior (**a**, **b**) and anterior (**c**, **d**) placement of the transducer and corresponding ultrasound view delineating main muscles of the rotator cuff complex. (Photo courtesy of Ian M. Fowler, MD)

quick and inexpensive diagnostic tool, which can be used at the bedside to visualize the rotator cuff components, (Fig. 13.1a–d) and to diagnose rotator cuff injuries, specifically full- and partial-thickness rotator cuff tears [1].

What Is the Pathophysiology of This Condition?

The exact mechanisms leading to rotator cuff injuries are most likely multifactorial and encompass both intrinsic and extrinsic factors, although the former ones appear to play a greater role [2]. Extrinsic factors include traumatic events causing tear(s) in one or more tendons. The most common inciting event is a fall onto an outstretched arm and it most frequently occurs in younger males (average age 54.7) [3]. Among the traumatic rotator cuff tears, supraspinatus tendon is the most commonly implicated (84%), followed by subscapularis (78%), and infraspinatus (38%) [3]. Other extrinsic factors include postural abnormalities, anatomical variants of the acromion, altered humeral or scapular kinematics, rotator cuff and scapular performance deficits, decreased extensibility of the pectoralis minor or posterior shoulder, and internal impingement of the tendons between the humeral head and glenoid [4]. Intrinsic mechanisms leading to rotator cuff tendinopathy include alterations in biology, morphology, vascularity, and mechanics

[4]. Rotator cuff (RC) degeneration is a well-described intrinsic factor, which may arise due to the irritation or inflammation of the rotator cuff tendons or subacromial bursa leading to diminished tensile strength of the RC fibers, and ultimately resulting in RC tears [5]. In his landmark publications, Neer hypothesized that most rotator cuff injuries (95%) arise due to the irritation of the rotator cuff tendons and subacromial bursa from the overlying acromion, hence the name subacromial impingement syndrome (SIS) [6, 7]. Stage I SIS involves the inflammation of the subacromial bursa (acute bursitis) associated with rotator cuff tendinopathy. Stage II SIS characterizes fibrosis and partial tear of the rotator cuff tendons, whereas Stage III SIS denotes a full-thickness tear of the rotator cuff [8].

How Is the Problem Managed?

Decision-making in the management of rotator cuff tears hinges upon a detailed assessment and robust physical evaluation to exclude the common etiologies of shoulder pain. The key elements of the history include information about the location of the pain and radiation pattern, duration of the pain, the course of pain progression, and response to prior therapy and interventions. It is important to ask questions about hand dominance, occupation, level of physical activity, participation in any athletic activities, and history of trauma or injuries. A complete physical exam should be conducted in a systematic fashion and consist of inspection, palpation, range of motion evaluation, neurologic exam, and provocative testing [9]. Radiographic imaging can be used to exclude other causes of shoulder pain, whereas both ultrasound and magnetic resonance imaging are useful in confirming the diagnosis and quantifying the extent of the tear, since the management might be different for small partial and large full rotator cuff tears [10].

The management of RCTs includes nonsurgical conservative therapy and surgical measures (partial repair and/or debridement, open or arthroscopic repair, reconstruction, and arthroplasty) [11]. Nonsurgical conservative treatment generally is employed for small partial RCTs and seldom for large RCTs, whereas the surgical approach is reserved for cases involving large full-thickness tears (citation). Activity modification (avoidance of overhead activity, heavy loading of the shoulder, bench pressing, overhead throwing, and kayaking), anti-inflammatory medications, corticosteroid injections with or without local anesthetics, and physical therapy are the main pillars of the conservative approach to RCT management [12]. Adequate pain control is imperative to allow the participation in physical therapy and successful progression of the treatment. *Non-steroidal anti-inflammatory drugs (NSAIDs)* are the first-line option, which reduces pain in 3–4 weeks but does not improve function [10]. Main adverse effects of the NSAIDs therapy include gastrointestinal (ulcers, bleeding, perforations, and colitis), [13] renal (acute and chronic renal failure, renal papillary necrosis, nephrotic syndrome with interstitial nephritis, electrolyte and fluid retention leading to increased blood pressure), and cardiovascular side effects (risk of hypertension, atrial fibrillation, myocardial infarction, stroke, and thromboembolic event) [14]. Although these effects are influenced by the dosage and type of the NSAID (Cox-1 vs. Cox-2 or combined selectivity), it is recommended to limit the duration of the therapy to a short period of time (<1 month). Possible complications of joint and tendon injections include septic arthritis, post-injection flare/synovitis, pain or swelling at the side of injection, tendon weakening/rupture, muscle wasting, fat atrophy, nerve/blood vessel injury, steroid arthropathy, and skin pigment changes [15, 16]. Systemic effects of corticosteroid injections include, among others, elevated blood pressure, increase in blood glucose, Cushing's syndrome, insomnia, and steroid psychosis [17–19].

Patients should be regularly assessed to determine their response to the conservative therapy and the need for referral to an orthopedic specialist. Based on the clinical assessment, the following recommendations have been made regarding the reasonable waiting period before referral for an orthopedic evaluation: (a) intact rotator cuffs should be treated conservatively for 3–6 months; (b) small tears should be treated conservatively for 12 weeks; and (c) patients with large tears, history of trauma or dislocation, young healthy active individuals without history of tears, and those with tears >50% should receive a prompt referral and undergo surgical treatment [12, 20].

What Is the Prognosis of This Condition?

The literature shows improved structural and functional recovery after operative treatment compared to the nonoperative approaches. The natural course of unoperated rotator cuff tears involves progressive tear extension, muscle atrophy, fatty infiltration, and degeneration of the long head of the biceps tendon, which correlate with poorer functional outcome [21, 22]. In certain instances, the tears might advance with time from operable to inoperable [23]. Moosmayer et al. examined 89 patients with nonsurgical management of rotator cuff tears (mean follow-up of 8.8 years), and reported a mean increase in tear size of 5.0–9.9 mm in 33 patients, 10.0–19.9 mm in 8 patients, and >20.0 mm in 8 patients [21]. Twenty-three patients initially treated with physiotherapy required surgical intervention at a later date. The same author investigated the course of asymptomatic full-thickness tears in 50 patients and described a development of symptoms in 18 cases [22]. Intuitively, symptomatic patients demonstrated larger cuff tears, and higher rates of muscle atrophy, fatty degeneration, and biceps tendon pathology than the asymptomatic counterparts. Mall et al. followed a cohort of 195 subjects with asymptomatic rotator cuff tears over a period of several years, and reported a development of pain and progression of the disease in 44 patients [24]. In the newly symptomatic group, 18% of full-thickness tears increased by >5.0 mm, and in 40% of subjects the pathology progressed from a partial to full-size tears. Moreover, significant changes were noted in the glenohumeral kinematics, such as decrease in all shoulder motions except external rotation at 90 degrees of abduction, and pain-related increase in compensatory scapulothoracic movement during early shoulder abduction. These findings raise a question about the utility of prophylactic surgical repair of asymptomatic rotator cuff tears in preventing the development of pain, progressive anatomic deterioration, and impairment of function.

Several prognostic factors have been identified, which influence the outcome and recovery after the surgical repair (Table 13.1) [25–31]. The main factors are larger size of the rotator cuff tears [25, 32] and older age of the patients [25]. Park et al. gave the following predictive cut-off values for the increased failure rate after the operative treatment of rotator cuff tears: age >69 years and tear size >2 cm (90% specificity) [33, 34]. A prospective analysis of 105 patients with chronic rotator cuff tears (11 massive, 38 large, 40 medium, and 16 small-size) who underwent open surgical repair and acromioplasty demonstrated substantial pain relief and improvement in active abduction and external rotation in 96 cases [32]. Sixty-eight patients rated the results as excellent, 16 as satisfactory, and 21 as unsatisfactory. A systematic review by Mall et al. shows good post-surgical outcomes in patients with traumatic rotator cuff tears, with the improvement in active forward elevation from 81 to 150 degrees [3].

Table 13.1 Prognostic factors influencing recovery after surgical repair of rotator cuff tears

Demographic	Clinical
Patient age Gender Duration of symptoms Length of the follow-up	Bone mineral density Body mass index Diabetes mellitus Hypercholesterolemia Smoking Level of physical activity Pre-op range of motion NSAIDs
Structural	**Surgical**
Size of the rotator cuff lesion Retraction of the cuff (acromiohumeral distance) Fatty infiltration of the muscles Multiple tendon involvement	Timing of the intervention Concomitant biceps or AC joint procedure Platelet-rich plasma injection

Data from [26, 28–34]

Discussion

Prevalence

Rotator cuff injuries are one of the leading causes of shoulder pain and disability accounting for 4.5 million physician visits in the United States each year [35]. Several epidemiological studies show increasing prevalence of rotator cuff repairs in different regions of the world. For example, an increase of 204% was noted in Finland between 1998 and 2011, [36] and 141% increase was recorded in the United States between 1996 and 2006 [37]. It is challenging to establish the exact prevalence of the condition, which is attributed to the fact that only a portion of the rotator cuff tears is symptomatic. The reported prevalence of rotator cuff tears in the general population ranges between 7.6–36%, [38–40] and it is higher for the asymptomatic versus symptomatic tears [41–43]. The prevalence increases with age for both genders, albeit it is higher for males in the fifth and sixth decades [42]. A systematic review of 6112 shoulders by Teunis et al. showed the overall prevalence of RC abnormalities in individuals <20 years of age compared to 62% in those above the age of 80 [39]. Additionally, the size of the tears varies based on the age of the subjects as well. Small-sized tears are more common in patients in the 50s, while large-sized tears are more prominent in the subsequent decades. The supraspinatus tendon tear is most frequently affected (13.8% of patients), with whole tendon tear in 7.4% of subjects, anterior half tear in 3.6%, and posterior half tear in 2.8% shoulders [42]. Rotator cuff tears are associated with older age, males, smoking, hypercholesterolemia, arm dominance, posture, occupational dispositions, history of trauma, contralateral arm tears, positive impingement sign, diminished active forward elevation, and weakness in abduction and external rotation of the affected limb [11, 41]. Patients over the age of 60 presenting with two out of three of the following findings: weak external rotators or supraspinatus muscles, or signs of impingement (difficulty elevating the arm, inflamed subdeltoid bursa, or positive provocative tests) have 98% chance of having a rotator cuff tear [44]. Large tears are associated with older age, diminished preoperative active motion and weakness, distal clavicular excision, and transposition repair techniques [25].

Differential Diagnosis

Rotator cuff tendinopathy typically manifests as shoulder pain with movement or at rest, painful overhead reaching, shoulder dyskinesis and stiffness, weakness (usually secondary to pain), and nighttime pain while lying on the affected shoulder or with the arm positioned overhead. The pain might radiate to the lateral mid-humerus or anterolateral acromion [45]. Shoulder pain, weakness, and loss of motion are shared with many pathologies involving structures other than the rotator cuff complex. Therefore, the differential diagnosis includes any condition related to the shoulder and other nearby structures: glenohumeral joint instability, glenohumeral joint arthritis, and adhesive capsulitis (frozen shoulder), coracoacromial injury, acromioclavicular injury, suprascapular impingement syndrome, subacromial/subdeltoid tendinitis/bursitis, bicipital tendinopathy, and cervical radiculopathy. A detailed, structured physical exam can help elucidate a potential etiology of the shoulder pain. For example, active and passive range of motion testing differentiates between the two separate etiologies: glenohumeral instability and rotator cuff injury. In the former, both active and passive ROMs are impaired, whereas rotator cuff injuries result in reduction or loss of active ROM. Each rotator cuff muscle plays distinct functional role in the rotator cuff complex: abduction (supraspinatus m.), external rotation (subscapularis m. and teres minor m.), and internal rotation (infraspinatus m.). Therefore, strength and motion testing in abduction and external and internal rotation will allow for isolation of a specific muscle of the rotator cuff complex that is contributing to the pathology.

Predictive Value of Different Clinical Features and Lab Testing/Imaging

Distinct provocative maneuvers have been developed that, when positive, aid the physician in developing an accurate clinical diagnosis. Van Kampen et al. conducted a prospective cohort study of 169 patients with shoulder complaints to examine the diagnostic value of clinical tests in evaluating for rotator cuff tear [46]. Twenty-five different tests were performed by an orthopedist and final diagnosis was confirmed with magnetic resonance arthrography (MRA). The study revealed that advanced age and a positive Neer's test are the most important independent predictors of rotator cuff tear. The overall accuracy of the clinical tests in picking up RCTs ranges between 61% and75%, and the "empty can test" (Jobe's test) is the most sensitive (68.4%), whereas the lift-off and the drop arm tests are most specific in diagnosing RCTs. Select tests and their sensitivity and specificity are presented in Table 13.2.

Imaging studies are an invaluable tool allowing one to confirm a suspected diagnosis, and guide surgical and non-surgical treatment by detailed visualization of the changes indicative of impingement or rotator cuff tendon tears. Conventional radiography is the initial study of the radiological assessment before other, more detailed exams are utilized [47]. X-ray of the shoulder may be preceded or supplanted by the sonographic study, which is a convenient, quick, non-irradiating, inexpensive, and reliable way of assessing rotator cuff pathologies in an office setting. Smith et al. assessed the diagnostic accuracy of ultrasonography (USG) in a meta-analysis of 6066 shoulders and found a sensitivity of 84% and specificity of 89% for partial and full tendon tears [48]. Another meta-analysis by De Jesus et al. (n = 140) showed a similar sensitivity of 85.1 and specificity of 86.1 for partial and full tendon tears [49]. Superior accuracy of USG has been reported in detecting large tendon tears compared to small partial tears [49–52].

Magnetic resonance imaging (MRI), especially when combined with arthrography, offers more detail and clarity than USG and enables to visualize morphology not readily evident on the USG pictures. MRI has higher positive predictive

Table 13.2 Characteristics of the main clinical tests used for the diagnosis of rotator cuff tears

Provocative clinical tests				
Test name	Purpose of the test	Maneuvers	Positive finding	Diagnostic value
Drop arm test	Supraspinatus and infraspinatus tendons; rotator cuff tear	Passive abduction of the shoulder to 180 degrees.	Arm drop	Sensitivity: 10–73% Specificity: 77–100%
Empty can test (Jobe's)	Supraspinatus and infraspinatus tendons; rotator cuff tear	Shoulder abduction to 90° scapular plane and full internal rotation. Thumbs pointing downward.	Pain or weakness during applied resistance by the examiner	Sensitivity: 53–89% Specificity: 65–82%
Hornblower's sign	Teres minor tendon; rotator cuff tear	Arm supported at 90° of abduction with elbow flexed at 90°. Patient externally rotates against the resistance.	Wrist drops when released while elbow supported	Sensitivity: 100% Specificity: 93%
Hawkin's sign	Impingement syndrome	Forward flexion of the humerus of 90° with forced internal rotation of the shoulder	Pain	Sensitivity: 72–92% Specificity: 44–78%
Neer's sign	Impingement syndrome	Forced forward elevation while scapular rotation prevented.	Pain	Sensitivity: 68–89% Specificity: 49–98%

Data from [46, 54–59]

value (PPV) in detecting rotator cuff tears compared to USG (92% versus 88%); [53] however, many studies revealed a comparable diagnostic accuracy in detecting full tears for the two modalities, although USG is more accurate and cost-effective technique in evaluating partial tendon tears [49, 52, 53]. MR arthrography is the most sensitive and specific among the three modalities, but the utility is limited by the invasiveness and discomfort of the study [49, 54–59].

Strength of Evidence for Different Treatment Modalities

Nonsteroidal anti-inflammatory drugs (NSAIDs) and corticosteroid injections are considered the first-line options for rotator cuff disease. A recommendation is made for the use of both NSAIDs (Strength of recommendation (SOR) (B) and steroid injections (SOR A) for the acute treatment of SIS Stage I [60–63]. Good evidence has been presented supporting the benefits of nonsurgical management of Stage II and Stage III SIS [64, 65]. A short-term benefit of NSAIDs has been demonstrated after 1–2 weeks of therapy (Level of evidence II) [60, 61]. The effectiveness of glucocorticoid injections has been extensively studied and is supported by clinical trials and systematic reviews [63, 66–68]. Injections using steroids and local anesthetics are efficacious in relieving pain and improving function in rotator cuff injuries (Level of recommendation B) [10]. Studies reveal similar short-term effectiveness between corticosteroid injections and NSAIDs (Level of evidence IA) [69, 70]. Corticosteroid injections are superior to physical therapy for the treatment of painful rotator cuff conditions (Level of evidence II) [66, 67].

In regard to physical therapy, a systematic review and meta-analysis of 21 studies reported possible pain relief, but unclear improvement in function, for rotator cuff tendinopathy (Level of evidence IA) [71]. No statistical difference has been noted between physical therapy and surgical repair in patients with rotator cuff tendinitis/tendinopathy (Level of evidence IIA) [8]. For full-thickness RC tears, physical therapy provides a long-term pain relief and improved functional abilities (Strength of recommendation B) [8].

Future Directions or Clinical Trials in Progress

As with many other pain syndromes, a growing interest and application of regenerative therapies can be observed for the non-surgical management of rotator cuff tears. The number of studies and reports describing potential benefits of platelet-rich plasma and stem cell engineering continue to increase. As illustrated by several publications, these treatment options show a great deal of promise in the successful recovery of rotator cuff injuries by promoting regeneration of the rotator cuff tendons. The utility of mesenchymal stem cells (MSCs) was examined in a trial involving 20 patients, who received an intratendinous injection of the autologous adipose-derived mesenchymal stem cells for symptomatic rotator cuff disease [72]. The results demonstrated a 71% reduction in pain in the high-dose group, and 80% and 77% decrease in the Shoulder Pain And Disability Index (SPADI) in the mid- and high-dose groups, respectively as well as and 83% and 90% decrease in the articular and bursal defects in the mid- and high-dose groups, respectively. Structural improvements were investigated by Kim et al. in 35 patients treated with arthroscopic rotator cuff repair alone compared to 35 patients treated with the arthroscopic repair with an injection of MSCs, but no clinically significant differences in outcomes were noted [73]. The value of platelet-rich plasma in the treatment of chronic tendinopathy was evaluated by a meta-analysis of RCTs (18 studies; $n = 1066$) [74], and a systematic review of 389 articles [75]. The former publication noted strong evidence supporting the administration of platelet-rich plasma under ultrasound guidance for the management of tendinopathy, whereas the latter work revealed benefits for patellar and lateral epicondylar but not for Achilles and rotator cuff tendinopathy.

Conclusion

Rotator cuff disease is a common cause of shoulder pain, functional loss, and disability affecting a large percentage of population. Rotator cuff injuries, also known as subacromial impingement syndrome, encompass several abnormalities including subacromial bursitis, RC tendinopathy, RC tendinitis, and various degrees of RC tears. Although these pathologies have been a focus of extensive and active research, more work needs to be completed to fully elucidate the mechanisms governing the pathophysiology of the RT injuries, understand the progression of the disease, and gain knowledge of the most optimal therapeutic options available.

References

1. Singh JP. Shoulder ultrasound: what you need to know. Indian J Radiol Imaging. 2012;22(4):284–92.
2. Factor D, Dale B. Current concepts of rotator cuff tendinopathy. Int J Sports Phys Ther. 2014;9(2):274–88.
3. Mall NA, Lee AS, Chahal J, Sherman SL, Romeo AA, Verma NN, et al. An evidenced-based examination of the epidemiology and outcomes of traumatic rotator cuff tears. Arthroscopy. 2013;29(2):366–76.
4. Seitz AL, McClure PW, Finucane S, Boardman ND 3rd, Michener LA. Mechanisms of rotator cuff tendinopathy: intrinsic, extrinsic, or both? Clin Biomech (Bristol, Avon). 2011;26(1):1–12.
5. Lewis J. Rotator cuff related shoulder pain: assessment, management and uncertainties. Man Ther. 2016;23:57–68.
6. Neer CS 2nd. Anterior acromioplasty for the chronic impingement syndrome in the shoulder: a preliminary report. J Bone Joint Surg Am. 1972;54(1):41–50.
7. Neer CS 2nd. Impingement lesions. Clin Orthop Relat Res. 1983;(173):70–7.
8. Trojian T, Stevenson JH, Agrawal N. What can we expect from nonoperative treatment options for shoulder pain? J Fam Pract. 2005;54(3):216–23.
9. Woodward TW, Best TM. The painful shoulder: part I. Clinical evaluation. Am Fam Physician. 2000;61(10):3079–88.
10. Oliva F, Piccirilli E, Bossa M, Via AG, Colombo A, Chillemi C, et al. I.S.Mu.L.T – rotator cuff tears guidelines. Muscles Ligaments Tendons J. 2015;5(4):227–63.
11. Sambandam SN, Khanna V, Gul A, Mounasamy V. Rotator cuff tears: an evidence based approach. World J Orthop. 2015;6(11):902–18.
12. Burbank KM, Stevenson JH, Czarnecki GR, Dorfman J. Chronic shoulder pain: part II. Treatment. Am Fam Physician. 2008;77(4):493–7.
13. Bjarnason I, Hayllar J, MacPherson AJ, Russell AS. Side effects of nonsteroidal anti-inflammatory drugs on the small and large intestine in humans. Gastroenterology. 1993;104(6):1832–47.
14. Harirforoosh S, Asghar W, Jamali F. Adverse effects of nonsteroidal antiinflammatory drugs: an update of gastrointestinal, cardiovascular and renal complications. J Pharm Pharm Sci. 2013;16(5):821–47.
15. Cheng J, Abdi S. Complications of joint, tendon, and muscle injections. Tech Reg Anesth Pain Manag. 2007;11(3):141–7.
16. Brinks A, Koes BW, Volkers AC, Verhaar JA, Bierma-Zeinstra SM. Adverse effects of extra-articular corticosteroid injections: a systematic review. BMC Musculoskelet Disord. 2010;11:206.
17. Habib GS. Systemic effects of intra-articular corticosteroids. Clin Rheumatol. 2009;28(7):749–56.
18. Goldzweig O, Carrasco R, Hashkes PJ. Systemic adverse events following intraarticular corticosteroid injections for the treatment of juvenile idiopathic arthritis: two patients with dermatologic adverse events and review of the literature. Semin Arthritis Rheum. 2013;43(1):71–6.
19. Robinson DE, Harrison-Hansley E, Spencer RF. Steroid psychosis after an intra-articular injection. Ann Rheum Dis. 2000;59(11):927.
20. Shin KM. Partial-thickness rotator cuff tears. Korean J Pain. 2011;24(2):69–73.
21. Moosmayer S, Gartner AV, Tariq R. The natural course of nonoperatively treated rotator cuff tears: an 8.8-year follow-up of tear anatomy and clinical outcome in 49 patients. J Shoulder Elb Surg. 2017;26(4):627–34.
22. Moosmayer S, Tariq R, Stiris M, Smith HJ. The natural history of asymptomatic rotator cuff tears: a three-year follow-up of fifty cases. J Bone Joint Surg Am. 2013;95(14):1249–55.
23. Zingg PO, Jost B, Sukthankar A, Buhler M, Pfirrmann CW, Gerber C. Clinical and structural outcomes of nonoperative management of massive rotator cuff tears. J Bone Joint Surg Am. 2007;89(9):1928–34.
24. Mall NA, Kim HM, Keener JD, Steger-May K, Teefey SA, Middleton WD, et al. Symptomatic progression of asymptomatic rotator cuff tears: a prospective study of clinical and sonographic variables. J Bone Joint Surg Am. 2010;92(16):2623–33.
25. Saccomanno MF, Sircana G, Cazzato G, Donati F, Randelli P, Milano G. Prognostic factors influencing the outcome of rotator cuff repair: a systematic review. Knee Surg Sports Traumatol Arthrosc. 2016;24(12):3809–19.
26. Fermont AJ, Wolterbeek N, Wessel RN, Baeyens JP, de Bie RA. Prognostic factors for successful recovery after arthroscopic rotator cuff repair: a systematic literature review. J Orthop Sports Phys Ther. 2014;44(3):153–63.

27. Lambers Heerspink FO, Dorrestijn O, van Raay JJ, Diercks RL. Specific patient-related prognostic factors for rotator cuff repair: a systematic review. J Shoulder Elb Surg. 2014;23(7):1073–80.
28. Chung SW, Oh JH, Gong HS, Kim JY, Kim SH. Factors affecting rotator cuff healing after arthroscopic repair: osteoporosis as one of the independent risk factors. Am J Sports Med. 2011;39(10):2099–107.
29. Nho SJ, Brown BS, Lyman S, Adler RS, Altchek DW, MacGillivray JD. Prospective analysis of arthroscopic rotator cuff repair: prognostic factors affecting clinical and ultrasound outcome. J Shoulder Elb Surg. 2009;18(1):13–20.
30. Tashjian RZ, Hollins AM, Kim HM, Teefey SA, Middleton WD, Steger-May K, et al. Factors affecting healing rates after arthroscopic double-row rotator cuff repair. Am J Sports Med. 2010;38(12):2435–42.
31. Lundgreen K, Lian OB, Scott A, Nassab P, Fearon A, Engebretsen L. Rotator cuff tear degeneration and cell apoptosis in smokers versus nonsmokers. Arthroscopy. 2014;30(8):936–41.
32. Meyer DC, Wieser K, Farshad M, Gerber C. Retraction of supraspinatus muscle and tendon as predictors of success of rotator cuff repair. Am J Sports Med. 2012;40(10):2242–7.
33. Cofield RH, Parvizi J, Hoffmeyer PJ, Lanzer WL, Ilstrup DM, Rowland CM. Surgical repair of chronic rotator cuff tears. A prospective long-term study. J Bone Joint Surg Am. 2001;83-A(1):71–7.
34. Park JS, Park HJ, Kim SH, Oh JH. Prognostic factors affecting rotator cuff healing after arthroscopic repair in small to medium-sized tears. Am J Sports Med. 2015;43(10):2386–92.
35. Oh LS, Wolf BR, Hall MP, Levy BA, Marx RG. Indications for rotator cuff repair: a systematic review. Clin Orthop Relat Res. 2007;455:52–63.
36. Paloneva J, Lepola V, Aarimaa V, Joukainen A, Ylinen J, Mattila VM. Increasing incidence of rotator cuff repairs – a nationwide registry study in Finland. BMC Musculoskelet Disord. 2015;16:189.
37. Colvin AC, Egorova N, Harrison AK, Moskowitz A, Flatow EL. National trends in rotator cuff repair. J Bone Joint Surg Am. 2012;94(3):227–33.
38. Yamaguchi K, Ditsios K, Middleton WD, Hildebolt CF, Galatz LM, Teefey SA. The demographic and morphological features of rotator cuff disease. A comparison of asymptomatic and symptomatic shoulders. J Bone Joint Surg Am. 2006;88(8):1699–704.
39. Teunis T, Lubberts B, Reilly BT, Ring D. A systematic review and pooled analysis of the prevalence of rotator cuff disease with increasing age. J Shoulder Elb Surg. 2014;23(12):1913–21.
40. Moosmayer S, Smith HJ, Tariq R, Larmo A. Prevalence and characteristics of asymptomatic tears of the rotator cuff: an ultrasonographic and clinical study. J Bone Joint Surg Br. 2009;91(2):196–200.
41. Yamamoto A, Takagishi K, Osawa T, Yanagawa T, Nakajima D, Shitara H, et al. Prevalence and risk factors of a rotator cuff tear in the general population. J Shoulder Elb Surg. 2010;19(1):116–20.
42. Minagawa H, Yamamoto N, Abe H, Fukuda M, Seki N, Kikuchi K, et al. Prevalence of symptomatic and asymptomatic rotator cuff tears in the general population: from mass-screening in one village. J Orthop. 2013;10(1):8–12.
43. Reilly P, Macleod I, Macfarlane R, Windley J, Emery RJ. Dead men and radiologists don't lie: a review of cadaveric and radiological studies of rotator cuff tear prevalence. Ann R Coll Surg Engl. 2006;88(2):116–21.
44. Murrell GA, Walton JR. Diagnosis of rotator cuff tears. Lancet. 2001;357(9258):769–70.
45. Umer M, Qadir I, Azam M. Subacromial impingement syndrome. Orthop Rev (Pavia). 2012;4(2):e18.
46. van Kampen DA, van den Berg T, van der Woude HJ, Castelein RM, Scholtes VA, Terwee CB, et al. The diagnostic value of the combination of patient characteristics, history, and clinical shoulder tests for the diagnosis of rotator cuff tear. J Orthop Surg Res. 2014;9:70.
47. Expert Panel on Musculoskeletal Imaging, Amini B, Beckmann NM, Beaman FD, Wessell DE, Bernard SA, et al. ACR appropriateness criteria((R)) shoulder pain-traumatic. J Am Coll Radiol. 2018;15(5S):S171–S88.
48. Smith TO, Back T, Toms AP, Hing CB. Diagnostic accuracy of ultrasound for rotator cuff tears in adults: a systematic review and meta-analysis. Clin Radiol. 2011;66(11):1036–48.
49. de Jesus JO, Parker L, Frangos AJ, Nazarian LN. Accuracy of MRI, MR arthrography, and ultrasound in the diagnosis of rotator cuff tears: a meta-analysis. AJR Am J Roentgenol. 2009;192(6):1701–7.
50. Lenza M, Buchbinder R, Takwoingi Y, Johnston RV, Hanchard NC, Faloppa F. Magnetic resonance imaging, magnetic resonance arthrography and ultrasonography for assessing rotator cuff tears in people with shoulder pain for whom surgery is being considered. Cochrane Database Syst Rev. 2013;9:CD009020.
51. Al-Shawi A, Badge R, Bunker T. The detection of full thickness rotator cuff tears using ultrasound. J Bone Joint Surg Br. 2008;90(7):889–92.
52. Dinnes J, Loveman E, McIntyre L, Waugh N. The effectiveness of diagnostic tests for the assessment of shoulder pain due to soft tissue disorders: a systematic review. Health Technol Assess. 2003;7(29):iii, 1–166.
53. Naqvi GA, Jadaan M, Harrington P. Accuracy of ultrasonography and magnetic resonance imaging for detection of full thickness rotator cuff tears. Int J Shoulder Surg. 2009;3(4):94–7.
54. Jain NB, Wilcox RB 3rd, Katz JN, Higgins LD. Clinical examination of the rotator cuff. PM R. 2013;5(1):45–56.
55. MacDonald PB, Clark P, Sutherland K. An analysis of the diagnostic accuracy of the Hawkins and Neer subacromial impingement signs. J Shoulder Elb Surg. 2000;9(4):299–301.
56. Miller CA, Forrester GA, Lewis JS. The validity of the lag signs in diagnosing full-thickness tears of the rotator cuff: a preliminary investigation. Arch Phys Med Rehabil. 2008;89(6):1162–8.

57. Park HB, Yokota A, Gill HS, El Rassi G, McFarland EG. Diagnostic accuracy of clinical tests for the different degrees of subacromial impingement syndrome. J Bone Joint Surg Am. 2005;87(7):1446–55.
58. Yuen CK, Mok KL, Kan PG. The validity of 9 physical tests for full-thickness rotator cuff tears after primary anterior shoulder dislocation in ED patients. Am J Emerg Med. 2012;30(8):1522–9.
59. Walch G, Boulahia A, Calderone S, Robinson AH. The 'dropping' and 'hornblower's' signs in evaluation of rotator-cuff tears. J Bone Joint Surg Br. 1998;80(4):624–8.
60. Ginsberg F, Famaey JP. A double-blind comparison of slow-release and standard tablet formulations of fentiazac in the treatment of patients with tendinitis and bursitis. Curr Med Res Opin. 1985;9(7):442–8.
61. Lopez JM. Treatment of acute tendinitis and bursitis with fentiazac--a double-blind comparison with placebo. Clin Ther. 1982;5(1):79–84.
62. Blair B, Rokito AS, Cuomo F, Jarolem K, Zuckerman JD. Efficacy of injections of corticosteroids for subacromial impingement syndrome. J Bone Joint Surg Am. 1996;78(11):1685–9.
63. Withrington RH, Girgis FL, Seifert MH. A placebo-controlled trial of steroid injections in the treatment of supraspinatus tendonitis. Scand J Rheumatol. 1985;14(1):76–8.
64. Bokor DJ, Hawkins RJ, Huckell GH, Angelo RL, Schickendantz MS. Results of nonoperative management of full-thickness tears of the rotator cuff. Clin Orthop Relat Res. 1993;294:103–10.
65. Itoi E, Tabata S. Conservative treatment of rotator cuff tears. Clin Orthop Relat Res. 1992;275:165–73.
66. Winters JC, Sobel JS, Groenier KH, Arendzen HJ, Meyboom-de Jong B. Comparison of physiotherapy, manipulation, and corticosteroid injection for treating shoulder complaints in general practice: randomised, single blind study. BMJ. 1997;314(7090):1320–5.
67. van der Windt DA, Koes BW, Deville W, Boeke AJ, de Jong BA, Bouter LM. Effectiveness of corticosteroid injections versus physiotherapy for treatment of painful stiff shoulder in primary care: randomised trial. BMJ. 1998;317(7168):1292–6.
68. Vecchio PC, Hazleman BL, King RH. A double-blind trial comparing subacromial methylprednisolone and lignocaine in acute rotator cuff tendinitis. Br J Rheumatol. 1993;32(8):743–5.
69. White RH, Paull DM, Fleming KW. Rotator cuff tendinitis: comparison of subacromial injection of a long acting corticosteroid versus oral indomethacin therapy. J Rheumatol. 1986;13(3):608–13.
70. Adebajo AO, Nash P, Hazleman BL. A prospective double blind dummy placebo controlled study comparing triamcinolone hexacetonide injection with oral diclofenac 50 mg TDS in patients with rotator cuff tendinitis. J Rheumatol. 1990;17(9):1207–10.
71. Desjardins-Charbonneau A, Roy JS, Dionne CE, Fremont P, MacDermid JC, Desmeules F. The efficacy of manual therapy for rotator cuff tendinopathy: a systematic review and meta-analysis. J Orthop Sports Phys Ther. 2015;45(5):330–50.
72. Jo CH, Chai JW, Jeong EC, Oh S, Kim PS, Yoon JY, et al. Intratendinous injection of autologous adipose tissue derived mesenchymal stem cells for the treatment of rotator cuff disease: a first-in-human trial. Stem Cells. 2018;36(9):1441–50.
73. Kim YS, Sung CH, Chung SH, Kwak SJ, Koh YG. Does an injection of adipose-derived mesenchymal stem cells loaded in fibrin glue influence rotator cuff repair outcomes? A clinical and magnetic resonance imaging study. Am J Sports Med. 2017;45(9):2010–8.
74. Fitzpatrick J, Bulsara MK, O'Donnell J, McCrory PR, Zheng MH. The effectiveness of platelet-rich plasma injections in gluteal tendinopathy: a randomized, double-blind controlled trial comparing a single platelet-rich plasma injection with a single corticosteroid injection. Am J Sports Med. 2018;46(4):933–9.
75. Balasubramaniam U, Dissanayake R, Annabell L. Efficacy of platelet-rich plasma injections in pain associated with chronic tendinopathy: a systematic review. Phys Sportsmed. 2015;43(3):253–61.

A 75-Year-Old Man with Chronic Shoulder Pain (Shoulder Arthritis)

14

Behnoosh B. Rahavard, Nebojsa Nick Knezevic, and Kenneth D. Candido

Case Description

The patient is a 75-year-old male with chronic progressive right shoulder pain. He mentioned that pain is aggravated by physical activity especially following the period of resting and he experienced morning stiffness, which lasted less than 30 minutes. The patient has pain on palpation and decreased range of motion (ROM), especially external rotation due to pain, and crepitus was felt on ROM examination of his shoulder.

What is the Your Preliminary Diagnosis?

Clinical diagnosis of osteoarthritis had been made based on patient's history and physical exam findings.

B. B. Rahavard
Department of Anesthesiology, Advocate Illinois Masonic Medical Center, Chicago, IL, USA

N. N. Knezevic (✉) · K. D. Candido
Department of Anesthesiology, Advocate Illinois Masonic Medical Center, Chicago, IL, USA

Department of Anesthesiology, University of Illinois, Chicago, IL, USA

Department of Surgery, University of Illinois, Chicago, IL, USA

How Is Diagnosis Confirmed?

Although a clinical diagnosis of osteoarthritis had been made based on the patient's history and physical examination, shoulder X-ray was done in order to rule out other differential diagnosis.

What Is the Pathophysiology of This Condition?

The common contributing factors for OA have been identified including systemic factors such as genetics, estrogen therapy, and bone density as well as biomechanical factors such as obesity, joint laxity, and muscle weakness [1, 2]. Furthermore, it has been shown that cytokines [3, 4] and chondrocytes [5] play the primary role in the pathogenesis of OA.

In one study, the OA following trauma and shoulder instability was studied [6]. Older age and time from injury to surgery were identified as independent predictors for shoulder OA in patients with shoulder instability. However, no association was found between the direction of instability and the presence of osteoarthritis. In summary, the most common risk factors for shoulder OA discussed in the literature include genetics, female sex, past trauma, advancing age, and obesity.

T. Malik (ed.), *Practical Chronic Pain Management*, https://doi.org/10.1007/978-3-030-46675-6_14

How Is the Problem Managed?

After the diagnosis of shoulder OA had been confirmed, the patient was consulted for lifestyle modifications including weight loss and regular exercise. Non-pharmacologic therapies were started for the patient, beginning first with exercise with the main focus on muscle strengthening and improving range of motion. Oral acetaminophen was started later using a dose of 650 mg, four times per day. Patient's liver function had been tested every 6 months since acetaminophen had been initiated for him. Considering the patient's age and borderline glomerular filtration rate, NSAIDs were not prescribed. Due to inadequate pain relief, the patient was referred to a physical therapist and a shoulder joint intra-articular corticosteroid injection was tried (Fig. 14.1). The patient experienced immediate pain relief following the injection, which lasted 9–10 weeks. Intra-articular corticosteroid was repeated every 3 months, and the patient was satisfied with the results.

What Is the Prognosis of This Condition?

Continuing the multimodal pain management including lifestyle modifications, physical therapy, oral acetaminophen therapy, and intra-articular corticosteroids injection, the more invasive methods, including surgical treatments, had been reserved for the more progressive stages of shoulder OA, when other less invasive modalities did not improve the patient's OA symptoms sufficiently.

Discussion

Prevalence

Chronic shoulder pain is a very prevalent condition and is usually associated with a multifactorial pathology and can lead to high costs and patient burden. OA has become a very prevalent

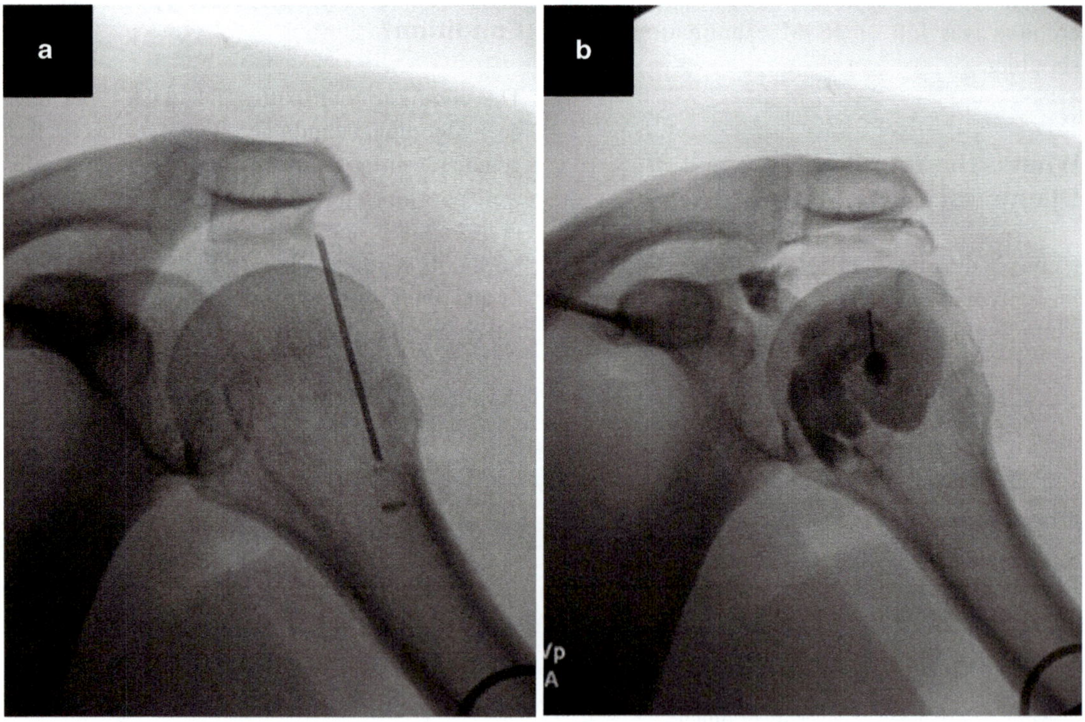

Fig. 14.1 (**a** and **b**) Fluoroscopic images of left shoulder corticosteroid injections

pathology in the United States as the population ages and becomes more obese.

An estimated 15% (40 million) of Americans had some form or arthritis in 1995. By the year 2020, an estimated 18.2% (59.4 million) will have been affected [7]. The prevalence and incidence of shoulder pain were studied in a systematic review study [8], and the incidence of 0.9–2.5% and prevalence of 6.9–26% had been reported. In another study, the higher prevalence of shoulder OA was reported in elderly patients and patients with OA in other joins (e.g., knee OA) [9].

The total costs for the management of chronic shoulder pain in 2000 was reportedly approximately $7 billion in the United States [10]. Approximately 16% of all musculoskeletal complaints of patients are due to shoulder pain [11], and the yearly incidence of 1.5% for patients is seen in primary care settings [12].

Differential Diagnosis

The common manifestation of shoulder OA, in addition to shoulder stiffness, is chronic pain with insidious onset. Pain is aggravated in the morning, with weather changes and increased physical activity, especially following a period of rest that has been termed the "gelling phenomenon." OA can cause morning stiffness, which usually lasts less than half an hour as compared to morning stiffness in rheumatoid arthritis that lasts for 45 minutes or longer [13]. Shoulder OA is often asymmetric.

Patients with shoulder OA may complain of shoulder joint locking or instability. Pain and stiffness of the shoulder can lead to loss of function of the joint and limit the physical activity of patients with shoulder OA.

The most common pathologies that can lead to persistent shoulder pain either in combination or as a separate entity are bursitis, tendinitis, rotator cuff tear, adhesive capsulitis, impingement syndrome, avascular necrosis, glenohumeral osteoarthritis (OA), and other causes of degenerative joint disease or from a traumatic injury. Among all these pathologies, rotator cuff injuries (10%), adhesive capsulitis (6%), and glenohumeral OA (2–5%) are more prevalent and associated with more complex etiologies. A focused medical history and physical examination combined with imaging studies can be utilized to differentiate these pathologies [14].

OA is a common degenerative disorder of the articular cartilage with multifactorial pathology that is caused by a heterogeneous group of conditions associated with the loss of integrity of articular cartilage and defective changes at the joint margins and underlying bone that leads to hypertrophic changes in the bone [15].

Predictive Value of Different Clinical Features and Lab Testing/Imaging

Considerations for physical examination start with a thorough inspection of the entire shoulder girdle for visualizing any deformity or posture changes that may be affecting the biomechanics of the shoulder, as well as investigations for scars from previous trauma, surgery, or atrophy of supraspinatus and infraspinatus as the potential indicators of rotator cuff pathology. Pain on range of motion and limitation of range of motion, especially external rotation as well as crepitus on range of motion, are common findings on the physical exam in patients with shoulder OA [16].

Shoulder OA can be complicated by secondary adhesive capsulitis due to incongruous joint surfaces, osteophytes, and capsular scarring. Both active and passive range of motion should be checked and compared to the contralateral side.

Acromioclavicular (AC) joint should be palpated for swelling, deformity, and instability as the signs for AC joint arthritis, and the positive "cross body adduction test" would be an indicator of this pathology. "Compression rotation test" could be another indicator of shoulder OA and can be performed as a part of physical examination by positioning the patient in the lateral decubitus with the affected side up. The shoulder is internally and externally rotated as the humeral head is compressed into the glenoid. The test would be positive if pain is elicited by the compression of the arthritic glenohumeral surfaces [17]. The results of this test will be more specific following subacromial injection of lidocaine to minimize the contributing effect of subacromial bursitis [18].

The rotator cuff should also be examined properly as subacromial bursitis can be a contributing factor for the patient's pain. Therefore, active external rotation, internal rotation, abduction, and forward flexion strength should be examined.

The anterior and posterior apprehension and relocation tests should be performed in the case of shoulder instability.

Shoulder OA is primarily a clinical diagnosis; however, plain radiography can aid in confirming the diagnosis and to rule out other pathologies. Advanced imaging studies including computed tomography (CT) or magnetic resonance imaging (MRI) are not usually required unless there is a suspicion for another pathology. For instance, MRI is more practical for diagnosing the conditions that cause a rapid change in bone, such as avascular necrosis or subchondral insufficiency fracture, in addition to being able to evaluate the soft tissue such as the rotator cuff, biceps tendon, and glenoid labrum. Despite the high sensitivity of MRI, the specificity of this imaging modality has been shown to be low for the determination of articular cartilage lesions in the shoulder [19]. Ultrasound can be utilized for rapid assessment of joints and inflammatory arthritis. CT is faster than MRI and can provide an assessment of the extent of arthritic deformity, osteophyte formation, and subchondral bone; however, it involves the use of ionizing radiation [20].

Laboratory studies are not needed to confirm the shoulder OA diagnosis, and inflammatory markers including erythrocyte sedimentation rate (ESR) and C-reactive protein (CRP) levels are usually normal. Immunologic tests, including antinuclear antibodies (ANA) and rheumatoid factor (RF) are not recommended to be ordered unless there is evidence for autoimmune arthritis such as shoulder joint inflammation or synovitis. Uric acid levels should be tested only if there is a suspicion for gout. Due to the false positive results of these laboratory tests in the low pretest probability of shoulder gout or autoimmune arthritis, ordering unnecessary tests can lead to misunderstanding and confusion. Furthermore, it would be against the American College of Rheumatology guidelines to order an arthritis panel routinely for patients with joint problem [21].

True glenohumeral AP, scapular "Y", and axillary X-rays should be shown in the plain radiographs [18]. The radiographic classification of shoulder OA has been described as follows [22]. In stage I, the radiographs are normal; however, some arthroscopic evidence of articular cartilage changes exists. Minimal narrowing of the joint space associated with concentricity of the humeral head and glenoid would be seen in stage II. Moderate joint space narrowing with early inferior osteophyte formation can be shown by plain radiographs in stage III. Stage IV is associated with severe loss of joint space with osteophyte formation and loss of concentricity of the humeral head and glenoid.

The classification of shoulder OA, according to arthroscopic evidence, is based on the Outerbridge classification.

Grade I is defined as the softening or blistering of the articular cartilage, while fissuring and fibrillation of the articular surface is classified as grade II. Grade III is associated with deep ulceration of articular cartilage without exposed bone. Loss of full thickness of cartilage with exposed subchondral bone can be seen in grade IV [23].

Shoulder OA treatment falls into four main categories including nonpharmacological, pharmacological, complementary and alternative, and surgical strategies [21].

Treatment should begin with less invasive and safer therapies. Therefore, nonsurgical management should be attempted as the first step for the treatment of patients with shoulder OA.

Strength of Evidence for Different Treatment Modalities

The most common noninvasive strategies recommended are anti-inflammatory medication therapy, physical therapy, and steroid injection. Early studies are assessing and encouraging viscosupplementation injections [24]. Surgical strategies should be utilized as the last resort for patients who do not improve with behavioral and pharmacological therapies and have intractable pain and loss of function.

American and British specialty societies have recommended clinical practice guidelines for a stepped care approach for treating OA starting with nonpharmacologic therapies [25, 26].

Nonpharmacologic therapies for patients with shoulder OA often begin with exercise with the main focus on muscle strengthening and range of motion improving. Swimming, elliptical training, and upper body exercise may be helpful. Other nonpharmacologic therapies, including bracing and splinting of the shoulder in order to support the painful or unstable joint, have been offered in some studies.

Acetaminophen is the mainstay of pharmacologic treatment for mild shoulder OA. It is an effective, inexpensive, and relatively safe medicine. In a review, it was shown that Acetaminophen was more effective than placebo for treating mild OA and was equal to non-steroidal anti-inflammatory drugs (NSIADs) with less gastrointestinal side effects [27].

NSAID therapy is recommended if shoulder OA is moderate to severe and Acetaminophen fails. Caution should be undertaken for the adverse effects of NSAIDs. Opioids, due to the potential for abuse, should be used only if Acetaminophen and NSAIDs fail or if patients cannot tolerate these medications because of adverse side effects. Low doses of opioids should be started first and monitored closely to assess for potential dependence. Corticosteroid and hyaluronic intra-articular injections are other modalities used to treat shoulder OA. Corticosteroid intra-articular injection can cause short-term pain relief lasting 4–8 weeks. The efficacy of this treatment has been proven for the treatment of knee OA, but may not be as effective for shoulder OA. The local anesthetics (mostly Lidocaine) can be utilized in combination with corticosteroids for intra-articular injections, which can lead to immediate pain relief. However, patients should be warned for a potential initial flare-up of symptoms in the first 24 hours, followed by improvement after 48 hours. Intra-articular injections can be repeated at the same joint, although in the usual practice, the number of annual injection is limited to four [28].

Intra-articular hyaluronic acid injections have been shown to be more effective than corticosteroids injection for knee OA [29], but may not be as effective for osteoarthritis of the shoulder [30]. Repeat injections can be done in the same joint; however, it is usually limited to four injections over a year [28]. It has been shown that intra-articular corticosteroid injection has better short-term outcome (1–4 weeks), while intra-articular hyaluronic acid injection has superior results in the long-term (8 weeks or longer) [29]. Thus, in patients with stable OA who develop acute flare-ups of OA, intra-articular corticosteroids injection may be a better choice, and intra-articular hyaluronic acid can be used in patients with chronic OA.

No promising results for long-term efficacy of acupuncture for the treatment of OA have been shown in different studies [31].

In a review, the effects of balneotherapy, defined as a heterogeneous group of treatments known as spa therapy or mineral baths, were demonstrated for the treatment of OA. However, due to methodologic flaws in the reviewed studies, the results may not be reliable [32].

Capsaicin cream has been shown to be superior to placebo when combined with standard treatment of OA [33].

Surgery should be reserved for patients with chronic pain and disability despite conservative therapies. Total joint replacement is considered as the most effective surgical intervention for patients with OA [13, 34, 35]. The average expected length of joint prostheses to function well is 15–20 years [36].

Other surgical options have not been shown to be as effective as total joint arthroplasty for the treatment of OA [37].

Shoulder arthroscopy, as one of the less invasive surgical strategies, should be considered in patients with severe shoulder OA, who are willing to avoid major surgeries or who are not good candidates for arthroplasty due to activity level or young age. Patients who undergo shoulder arthroscopy experience faster recovery [38, 39].

All the loose bodies, chondral flaps, and degenerative tissues are removed during the arthroscopic surgery of the arthritic glenohumeral joint [18]. Pain improvement due to the diluting effect of arthroscopic lavage and removal of debris on degenerative enzymes in OA is a hypothesis that has been discussed recently [22].

Subacromial bursitis frequently exists concurrently with glenohumeral OA; therefore, subacromial decompression surgery can be utilized as another strategy for the management of shoulder OA [22].

Future Directions or Clinical Trials in Progress

Biologic resurfacing has been offered and discussed recently for the management of shoulder OA. Interposing a synthetic or biologic scaffold of sufficiently high tensile strength and repopulation by the host cells have been discussed as the main goals of this new treatment [40].

Furthermore, utilizing the regenerative tissue matrix for arthroscopic resurfacing has been recently studied and postoperative arthroscopic results showed fibrocartilage ingrowth after 3 months [40].

In another article, a bovine patch had been utilized for arthroscopic resurfacing, which led to 50 degrees increase in abduction and 60 degrees increase in forward flexion of the shoulder in patients with shoulder OA [41].

In another study, the arthroscopic lateral meniscal allograft resurfacing was studied for patients with OA; the results showed a promising short-term outcome [42].

Conclusion

OA has become a very prevalent pathology in the United States as the population ages and becomes more obese. Shoulder OA is primarily a clinical diagnosis; however, plain radiography can aid confirming the diagnosis and to rule out other pathologies.

Treatment should begin with less invasive and safer therapies. Therefore, nonsurgical managements should be attempted as the first step in the treatment of patients with shoulder OA. Surgery should be the reserved for patients with chronic pain and disability that persists despite conservative therapies.

References

1. Sharma L, Song J, Felson DT, et al. The role of knee alignment in disease progression and functional decline in knee osteoarthritis. JAMA. 2001;286:188–95.
2. Felson DT, Lawrence RC, Dieppe PA, Hirsch R, Helmick CG, Jordan JM, et al. Osteoarthritis: new insights. Part 1: the disease and its risk factors. Ann Intern Med. 2000;133:635–46.
3. Ruddy S, Harris ED Jr, Sledge CB. Kelley's textbook of rheumatology. 6th ed. WB Saunders Co: Philadelphia; 2001.
4. Cotran RS, Kumar V, Collins T, editors. Robbins pathologic basis of disease. 6th ed. Philadelphia: WB Saunders Company; 1999.
5. Kraus VB. Pathogenesis and treatment of osteoarthritis. Med Clin North Am. 1997;81:85–112.
6. Cameron ML, Kocher MS, Briggs KK, Horan MP, Hawkins RJ. The prevalence of glenohumeral osteoarthrosis in unstable shoulders. Am J Sports Med. 2003;31:53–5.
7. Lawrence RC, Helmick CG, Arnett FC, Deyo RA, Felson DT, Giannini EH, et al. Estimates of the prevalence of arthritis and selected musculoskeletal disorders in the United States. Arthritis Rheum. 1998;41:778–99.
8. Luime JJ, Koes BW, Hendriksen IJ, et al. Prevalence and incidence of shoulder pain in the general population; a systematic review. Scand J Rheumatol. 2004;33:73–81.

9. Oh JH, Chung SW, Oh CH, Kim SH, Park SJ, Kim KW, et al. The prevalence of shoulder osteoarthritis in the elderly Korean population: association with risk factors and function. J Shoulder Elb Surg. 2011;20(5):756–63.
10. Meislin RJ, Sperling JW, Stitik TP. Persistent shoulder pain: epidemiology, pathophysiology, and diagnosis. Am J Orthop. 2005;34:5–9.
11. Urwin M, Symmons D, Allison T, Brammah T, Busby H, Roxby M, et al. Estimating the burden of musculoskeletal disorders in the community: the comparative prevalence of symptoms at different anatomical sites, and the relation to social deprivation. Ann Rheum Dis. 1998;57:649–55.
12. van der Windt DA, Koes BW, de Jong BA, Bouter LM. Shoulder disorders in general practice: incidence, patient characteristics, and management. Ann Rheum Dis. 1995;54(12):959–64.
13. Manek NJ, Lane NE. Osteoarthritis: current concepts in diagnosis and management. Am Fam Physician. 2000;61(6):1795–804.
14. Burbank KM, Stevenson JH, Czarnecki GR, Dorfman J. Chronic shoulder pain: part I. Evaluation and diagnosis. Am Fam Physician. 2008;77(4):453–60.
15. Altman R, Asch E, Bloch D, Bole G, Borenstein D, Brandt K, et al. Development of criteria for the classification and reporting of osteoarthritis. Classification of osteoarthritis of the knee. Diagnostic and Therapeutic Criteria Committee of the American Rheumatism Association. Arthritis and Rheum. 1986;29:1039–49.
16. Sinusas K. Osteoarthritis: diagnosis and treatment. Am Fam Physician. 2012;85(1):49–56.
17. Ellman H, Harris E, Kay SP. Early degenerative joint disease simulating impingement syndrome: arthroscopic findings. Arthroscopy. 1992;8(4):482–7.
18. McCarty LP 3rd, Cole BJ. Nonarthroplasty treatment of glenohumeral cartilage lesions. Arthroscopy. 2005;21(9):1131–42.
19. Yoshioka H, Stevens K, Hargreaves BA, et al. Magnetic resonance imaging of articular cartilage of the knee: comparison between fat-suppressed three-dimensional SPGR imaging, fat-suppressed FSE imaging, and fat-suppressed three-dimensional DEFT imaging, and correlation with arthroscopy. J Magn Reson Imaging. 2004;20(5):857–64.
20. Wenham C, Grainger A, Conaghan P. The role of imaging modalities in the diagnosis, differential diagnosis and clinical assessment of peripheral joint osteoarthritis. Osteoarthr Cartil. 2014;22:1692–702.
21. Guidelines for the initial evaluation of the adult patient with acute musculoskeletal symptoms. American College of Rheumatology Ad Hoc Committee on Clinical Guidelines. Arthritis Rheum. 1996;39(1):1–8.
22. Weinstein DM, Bucchieri JS, Pollock RG, Flatow EL, Bigliani LU. Arthroscopic debridement of the shoulder for osteoarthritis. Arthroscopy. 2000;16(5):471–6.
23. Outerbridge RE, Dunlop JA. The problem of chondromalacia patellae. Clin Orthop Relat Res. 1975;110:177–96.
24. Valiveti M, Reginato AJ, Falasca GF. Viscosupplementation for degenerative joint disease of the shoulder and ankle. J Clin Rheumatol. 2006;12(3):162–3.
25. American College of Rheumatology. Practice guidelines. Recommendations for the medical management of osteoarthritis of the hip and knee. http://www.rheumatology.org/practice/clinical/guidelines/oa-mgmt.asp. Accessed 9 Aug 2011.
26. Scott DL, Shipley M, Dawson A, Edwards S, Symmons DP, Woolf AD. The clinical management of rheumatoid arthritis and osteoarthritis: strategies for improving clinical effectiveness. Br J Rheumatol. 1998;37(5):546–54.
27. Towheed TE, Maxwell L, Judd MG, Catton M, Hochberg MC, Wells G. Acetaminophen for osteoarthritis. Cochrane Database Syst Rev. 2006;1:CD004257.
28. Bettencourt RB, Linder MM. Arthrocentesis and therapeutic joint injection: an overview for the primary care physician. Prim Care. 2010;37(4):691–702.
29. Bannuru RR, Natov NS, Obadan IE, Price LL, Schmid CH, McAlindon TE. Therapeutic trajectory of hyaluronic acid versus corticosteroids in the treatment of knee osteoarthritis: a systematic review and meta-analysis. Arthritis Rheum. 2009;61(12):1704–11.
30. American Academy of Orthopaedic Surgeons. The treatment of glenohumeral joint osteoarthritis: guideline and evidence report. Rosemont: American Academy of Orthopaedic Surgeons; 2009. http://www.aaos.org/research/guidelines/gloguideline.pdf. Accessed 9 Aug 2011.
31. Manheimer E, Linde K, Lao L, Bouter LM, Berman BM. Meta-analysis: acupuncture for osteoarthritis of the knee. Ann Intern Med. 2007;146(12):868–77.
32. Verhagen AP, Bierma-Zeinstra SM, Boers M, et al. Balneotherapy for osteoarthritis. Cochrane Database Syst Rev. 2007;(4):CD006864.
33. Ernst E. Complementary treatments in rheumatic diseases. Rheum Dis Clin N Am. 2008;34(2):455–67.
34. Goodman S. Osteoarthritis. In: Yee A, Paget S, editors. Expert guide to rheumatology. Philadelphia: American College of Physicians; 2005. p. 269–83.
35. Lichtenstein MJ, Pincus T. How useful are combinations of blood tests in "rheumatic panels" in diagnosis of rheumatic diseases? J Gen Intern Med. 1988;3(5):435–42.
36. St Clair SF, Higuera C, Krebs V, Tadross NA, Dumpe J, Barsoum WK. Hip and knee arthroplasty in the geriatric population. Clin Geriatr Med. 2006;22(3):515–33.
37. Kirkley A, Birmingham TB, Litcheld RB, et al. A randomized trial of arthroscopic surgery for osteoarthritis of the knee. N Engl J Med. 2008;359(11):1097–107.
38. Bishop JY, Flatow EL. Management of glenohumeral arthritis: a role for arthroscopy? Orthop Clin North Am. 2003;34(4):559–66.

39. Sperling JW, Steinmann SP, Cordasco FA, Henshaw DR, Coons DA, Burkhead WZ. Shoulder arthritis in the young adult: arthroscopy to arthroplasty. Instr Course Lect. 2006;55:67–74.
40. Bhatia DN, van Rooyen KS, du Toit DF, de Beer JF. Arthroscopic technique of interposition arthroplasty of the glenohumeral joint. Arthroscopy. 2006;22(5):570.e1–5.
41. Brislin KJ, Savoie FH, Field LD, Ramsey JR. Surgical treatment for glenohumeral arthritis in the young patient. Tech Shoulder Elbow Surg. 2004;5:165–9.
42. Pennington WT, Bartz BA. Arthroscopic glenoid resurfacing with meniscal allograft: a minimally invasive alternative for treating glenohumeral arthritis. Arthroscopy. 2005;21(12):1517–20.

A 35-Year-Old Man with Persistent Pain After Hand Injury (Complex Regional Pain Syndrome)

15

Xiaoying Zhu and Lynn R. Kohan

Case Description

A 35-year-old man with no significant past medical history presented to a tertiary medical center pain clinic with right wrist and hand pain following a right wrist fracture and subsequent internal fixation surgery. A few weeks after surgery, the patient's pain still persisted even though the surgical wound healed well. His pain was described as sharp, burning, throbbing, and constant. It was located in the entire right hand and wrist, and sometimes in the forearm. He rated his pain as a constant 7 out of 10 on the Visual Analog Scale (VAS), going up to a 9 out of 10 with movement and cold air. It was worse at night, and he got little sleep due to his pain. In addition to pain, the patient also noticed his right hand felt freezing cold, turned dark purple, and swelled without any triggers. He stated that his hand had limited range of motion, felt weak, and had muscle twitches. He reported the area was extremely sensitive to touch even with clothing or wind. He could barely use his right hand due to pain and weakness. He was on lidocaine patch and oxycodone/acetaminophen with mild relief. He followed up with his surgeon who prescribed him Meloxicam and ordered an X-ray and ultrasound of his wrist. The X-ray showed osteopenia, and his ultrasound was unremarkable for vascular problems. He was referred to the pain clinic for management of his pain. Physical exam showed a well-healed scar at the palmar aspect of the right wrist, mottled purple color and edema at right wrist and hand, and no obvious hair or nail changes between his two hands. His right hand was colder to touch than the left and he had 2+ pulses. Other pertinent findings included positive allodynia to light touch, limited extension and flexion of right wrist and fingers, and weak hand grip. Temperature: Right hand dorsum 28.9 °C, Left Hand dorsum 26.7 °C.

X. Zhu · L. R. Kohan (✉)
Department of Anesthesiology, University of Virginia Health System, Charlottesville, VA, USA
e-mail: xz6b@virginia.edu; xz6b@hscmail.mcc.virginia.edu; lrk9g@virginia.edu

What Is Your Preliminary Diagnosis?

The preliminary diagnosis was complex regional pain syndrome (CRPS) based on his reported symptoms and clinical findings. He had pain out of proportion to the inciting event as well as sensory, motor, vasomotor, and sudomotor changes.

How Is Diagnosis Confirmed?

He was diagnosed with right upper extremity CRPS type I based on the Budapest Criteria for diagnosis of CRPS [1] (Table 15.1). CRPS is a clinical diagnosis based on a person's medical history, symptoms, and signs. Currently there is

T. Malik (ed.), *Practical Chronic Pain Management*, https://doi.org/10.1007/978-3-030-46675-6_15

Table 15.1 Budapest clinical diagnostic criteria for CRPS

1. Continuing pain, which is disproportionate to any inciting event
2. Must report at least one symptom in *three of the four* following categories: *Sensory:* Reports of hyperesthesia and/or allodynia *Vasomotor:* Reports of temperature asymmetry and/or skin color changes and/or skin color asymmetry *Sudomotor/edema:* Reports of edema and/or sweating changes and/or sweating asymmetry *Motor/trophic:* Reports of decreased range of motion and/or motor dysfunction (weakness, tremor, dystonia) and/or trophic changes (hair, nail, skin)
3. Must display at least one sign at the time of evaluation in *two or more* of the following categories: *Sensory:* Evidence of hyperalgesia (to pinprick) and/or allodynia (to light touch and/or deep somatic pressure and/or joint movement) *Vasomotor:* Evidence of temperature asymmetry and/or skin color changes and/or asymmetry *Sudomotor/edema:* Evidence of edema and/or sweating changes and/or sweating asymmetry *Motor/trophic:* Evidence of decreased range of motion and/or motor dysfunction (weakness, tremor, dystonia) and/or trophic changes (hair, nail, skin)
4. There is no other diagnosis that better explains the signs and symptoms.

From Harden et al. [1], with permission

no specific test that can confirm CRPS. Since other conditions can cause similar symptoms, careful examination is important, and testing may be used to help rule out other conditions, such as vascular disease, muscle disease, or nerve injury. This patient had an unremarkable ultrasound exam and normal nerve conduction study/electromyography.

What Is the Pathophysiology of This Condition?

CRPS is a systemic disease involving both the central and peripheral nervous systems. The pathophysiology underlying CRPS remains unclear and controversial despite many advances in the understanding of CRPS in recent years. CRPS appears to be multifactorial with evidence pointing to components of inflammation, peripheral and central sensitization, autoimmune factors, altered cutaneous innervation, autonomic dysregulation, and neuronal plasticity [2, 3]. Symptoms change through the course of CRPS as a result of the varying pathophysiology.

Clinically, there appear to be two subtypes of CRPS, warm CRPS and cold CRPS. And warm CRPS can "transition" into cold CRPS. Inflammatory mechanisms seem to contribute prominently to warm CRPS [4].

Inflammation Exaggerated inflammation is likely involved in CRPS. Tissue injury with or without nerve injury in CRPS seems to lead to the release of pro-inflammatory cytokines and neuropeptides. These substances act on blood vessels, local immune cells, and neural structures, subsequently increasing plasma extravasation and vasodilation, producing inflammatory signs of CRPS – erythema, elevated temperature (warm CRPS), edema, pain, and impaired function [5]. At the same time, these substances also activate local nociceptors, resulting in enhanced sensitivity of peripheral tissue to non-noxious and noxious stimuli (allodynia and hyperalgesia) (peripheral sensitization) [6, 7]. However, it is not clear whether inflammation is a state of chronic pain or a primary mediator of CRPS. Moreover, there is no evidence to show a higher level of inflammatory mediators in the affected limb than the unaffected limb [7].

Central Sensitization The persistent and intense noxious stimulation of peripheral nociceptors results in sensitization of the central nervous system. This is mediated by the release of neuropeptides such as substance P, bradykinin, and glutamate by peripheral nerves, which sensitize and increase the excitability of peripheral and secondary central nociceptive neurons, resulting in allodynia and hyperalgesia [8]. Studies have shown that CRPS patients demonstrate a significantly greater windup to repeated stimulation of the affected limb compared to the contralateral limb [9].

Autoimmunity Autoantibodies against surface antigens on autonomic neurons have been shown to be present in the serum of patients with CRPS suggesting that autoimmunity may play a role in the development of CRPS [10]. Goebel et al. postulated that, in CRPS patients, pathogenic autoimmune features likely develop in the preexisting circulating antibodies after exposure to certain antigens following trauma [11].

Altered Cutaneous Innervation Studies [12, 13] have demonstrated a reduction in cutaneous nociceptive (C-type and Aδ-type) nerve fiber density and altered innervation of hair follicles, sweat glands, and vasculature in the CRPS-affected limb compared to the unaffected limb. And the decrease in C-type and Aδ-type fibers is associated with an increase in aberrant fibers of unknown origin. It has been hypothesized that the amplified pain sensation may be due to altered function of these fibers [12]. It is not clear whether the reduction in nociceptive fiber density is an epiphenomenon or directly related to the condition.

Autonomic Dysregulation Transition of clinical features from warm CRPS to cold CRPS may be related to alterations in catecholamine and the sympathetic system [14]. In warm CRPS, there is a reduction in the circulating plasma norepinephrine level in the CRPS-affected limb compared to the unaffected limb [15]. This results in compensatory upregulation of peripheral adrenergic receptors, causing exaggerated sensitivity to circulating catecholamines [16]. Consequently, excessive vasoconstriction and sweating occur following exposure to catecholamines, giving rise to the characteristic cyanosed and clammy extremity seen during cold CRPS. Studies have also demonstrated impaired endothelial function and vascular reflexes causing exaggerated vasoconstriction in CRPS-affected limbs [12, 17, 18]. Vasoconstriction may further contribute to tissue hypoxia and trophic changes [19]. Animal studies have shown that adrenergic receptors are expressed on nociceptive fibers following nerve trauma, which may contribute to sympathetic-nociceptive coupling, a possible mechanism for the sympathetically mediated pain in CRPS [14]. This has been demonstrated in patients with sympathetically mediated CRPS pain where high sympathetic nervous system activity increases spontaneous pain and hyperalgesia [20].

Neuronal Plasticity In addition to peripheral mechanisms, the central nervous system seems to be implicated in the pathogenesis of CRPS. The progressively worsening signs of impaired recognition, neglect, and motor dysfunction in patients with CRPS point to an important role of the CNS [21]. For example, people with long-standing CRPS tend to perceive their affected limb to be larger than it really is [22]. They also report distortions of the mental image of their limb, like missing parts, alterations in shape, posture, and temperature of the whole limb, or of discrete parts of the limb [23]. The motor dysfunctions associated with CRPS commonly mimic those of movement disorders: tremors, dystonia, and sometimes myoclonus, suggesting the basal ganglia is implicated in the development of CRPS symptoms [24]. In line with these clinical findings, neuroimaging studies of patients with CRPS have demonstrated a decrease in area representing the CRPS-affected limb in the somatosensory cortex compared to the unaffected limb [25, 26]. The sensory representation of the affected limb, as part of the Penfield's homunculus, is distorted, with shrinkage and shifting of the area [26]. The extent of reorganization significantly correlates with the intensity of pain and hyperalgesia experienced by the patient, and these alterations return to normal following successful CRPS treatment [26, 27]. Furthermore, despite its unilateral clinical manifestation, it has been shown that, in CRPS, alterations in cortical excitability occur bilaterally, both in sensory and motor regions. Therefore, a more widespread and bilateral pattern of CNS reorganization appears to characterize CRPS, which may be related to dysfunctions in the basal ganglia or in thalamo-cortical structures [21].

How Is This Problem Managed?

At the patient's first visit, he was started on gabapentin and slowly increased to 600 mg three times a day (TID) (Table 15.2) as tolerated. Diclofenac gel was prescribed in place of Meloxicam because of stomach upset (Table 15.3). Lidocaine patches were discontin-

Table 15.2 Typical doses and titration schedule for medications

Medication	Starting dose	Titration	Medium dose	Maximum dose
Gabapentin	300 mg QHS	Increase by 300 mg/day every 3–5 days	600 mg TID	1200 mg TID
Topiramate	25 mg QHS	Increase by 25 mg/day every week	100 mg BID	200 mg BID
Amitriptyline	25 mg QHS	Increase by 25 mg/day every week	50 mg QHS	100 mg QHS
Duloxetine	30 mg QHS	Increase by 30 mg/day every week	60 mg QHS	120 mg QHS[a]
Baclofen	10 mg QHS	Increase by 10 mg/day every 3–5 days	10 mg TID	10 mg TID
Meloxicam	7.5 mg BID	Not needed		
Ketamine infusion	0.1 mg/kg/h	Increase by 0.1 mg/kg/h every 2 h		0.5–0.7 mg/kg/h

Increase medication dose as tolerated. For patients who are sensitive to medications, lower starting and goal doses, and slower increases are recommended

[a]Some studies suggest no difference in pain relief between 60 and 120 mg

Table 15.3 Common side effects of medications

Medications	Common side effects
Gabapentin	Fatigue, ataxia, nystagmus, peripheral edema, nausea, vomiting
Topiramate	Fatigue, somnolence, dizziness, impaired cognition, paresthesia, mood disorder, loss of appetite, weight loss
Amitriptyline	Somnolence, dizziness, headache, blurred vision, constipation, xerostomia, weight gain
Duloxetine	Fatigue, somnolence, insomnia, dizziness, headache, diaphoresis, xerostomia, nausea, vomiting, diarrhea, constipation, hypertension
Meloxicam	Dizziness, headache, abdominal pain, indigestion, nausea, vomiting, constipation, diarrhea
Baclofen	Fatigue, dizziness, somnolence, headache, weakness, hypotension, nausea, vomiting, constipation
Ketamine infusion	Hallucination, vivid dreams, nightmare, confusion, agitation, anxiety, flashback, dysphoria, insomnia, disorientation, psychotic episodes, hypertension, tachycardia, nystagmus, diplopia, nausea, vomiting, constipation, anorexia, salivary hypersecretion, elevated liver enzymes, cystitis

ued due to lack of effect. He was sent for more physical therapy and scheduled for right stellate ganglion block (SGB) under Fluoroscopy (Fig. 15.1), three in a row, about 2 weeks apart.

Four weeks later, the patient presented for the first SGB. He reported that the Diclofenac gel helped some with his pain, and he had been on the goal dose of gabapentin and noticed minimal benefits, but no side effects. He was instructed to increase his gabapentin dose to 1200 mg TID (Table 15.2) in a similar manner. His first SGB with 10 ml of 1% lidocaine was technically successful and provided about 60–70% relief for 5 days. During that time, his right hand felt warmer and stronger. He was able to use his hand more and tolerated gentle rubbing. Then the effect abated and his pain returned to baseline.

When he presented for the second SGB, he stated that he did not get much pain relief from Gabapentin at 1200 mg TID. At this point, he was instructed to stay on it for longer and amitriptyline was added to his regimen. He was to increase the amitriptyline to 50 mg once a day at bedtime (QHS) (Table 15.2). For this second block, clonidine 50 mcg was added to 10 ml of 1% lidocaine to hopefully achieve better and longer-lasting relief.

Two weeks later, the patient presented for the third SGB. He reported he was taking Amitriptyline 50 mg QHS, which helped with his pain and sleep, but caused intolerable dry mouth (Table 15.3). Instructions were given for him to wean off of Amitriptyline, then start Duloxetine and increase to 60 mg QHS (Table 15.2). He stated the second SGB provided 70% pain relief and functional improvement for 1.5 weeks without side effects. For the third block, 100 mcg of clonidine was added. Following the block, there was significant rise in temperature in his right upper extremity, just like his previous blocks. He had good immediate pain relief too. The plan was for him to follow up in the clinic in 4 weeks to discuss further treatments.

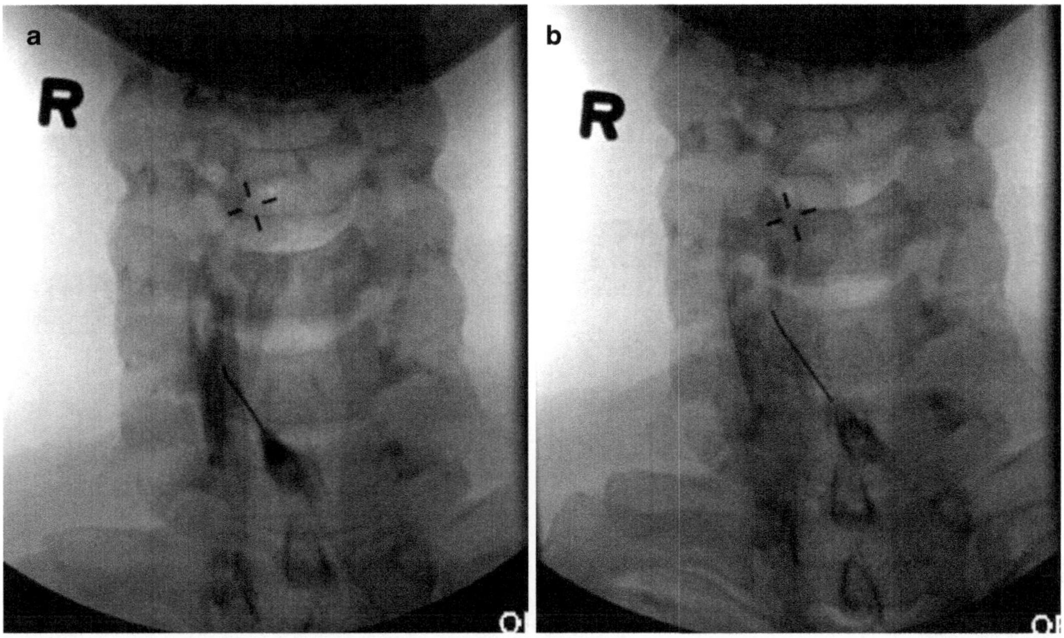

Fig. 15.1 Fluoroscopy-guided right stellate ganglion block at C6 following contrast injection (**a**) and medication injection (**b**)

In the clinic, the patient reported that he received about 70% pain relief for 1 week from his third block. He also stated Duloxetine at 60 mg QHS helped with his pain and mood. He continued physical therapy with some improvement in his right hand range of motion, but the muscle twitches and tightness remained. He weaned himself off of oxycodone/Acetaminophen due to the fear of addiction. He did not think Gabapentin provided any benefits. After discussion with the patient, the plan was to continue his home exercise program, Duloxetine, and add Baclofen (Table 15.2) for muscle twitches. Next he was instructed to wean off of Gabapentin by decreasing by 300 mg/day every 3 days. After being off of Gabapentin for a few days, he was to start Topiramate and increase to 100 mg twice a day (BID) (Table 15.2). He was also referred to pain psychology. At the same time, ketamine infusion and spinal cord stimulation (SCS) were discussed. Patient was hesitant about these two therapies.

At the patient's follow-up appointments, Topiramate was weaned off because of intolerable tingling in the hands and feet (Table 15.3). Baclofen was continued as it provided good relief of the muscle twitches and tightness without side effects. His pain remained and was rated as 8 on the VAS. At this point, the patient decided to proceed with a ketamine infusion.

After psychological evaluation, the patient was admitted to a regular ward for continuous intravenous low-dose ketamine infusion (Table 15.2) for 6 days. His pain and other symptoms resolved 3 days into the infusion therapy. He was able to use his hand to eat, comb hair, get dressed, etc. Sometimes his hand was still a little sensitive to touch. He had near complete relief for about 3 months, then the pain and other symptoms returned, and was back to baseline 4 months after the treatment. He subsequently received a repeat ketamine infusion therapy with similar relief lasting for only 1 month.

At the follow-up appointments, SCS was revisited, and patient became interested. After passing a psychological evaluation, the patient underwent permanent SCS trial (Fig. 15.2). During the 7-day trial, he had 80–90% pain relief and significant functional improvement. Subsequently, the patient received a spinal cord

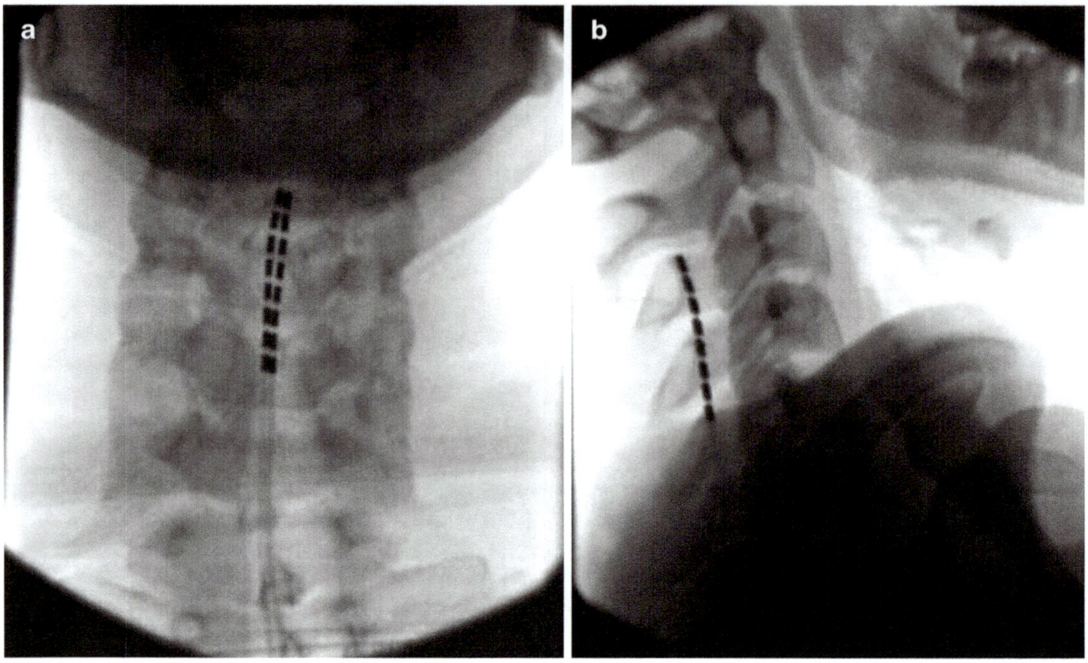

Fig. 15.2 Fluoroscopy-guided spinal cord stimulator leads placement. Two 8-contact leads entered at T3-4 interlaminar space with tips placed at C2 anterior-posterior view (**a**) and lateral view (**b**)

stimulator implant with substantial pain relief. At his next two follow-up appointments, the SCS programs were further optimized. He had nearly complete relief of pain and other symptoms. He was continued on Duloxetine, Baclofen, and home exercise. Instructions were provided for him to slowly wean down/off of the medications as tolerated. Four months later, his pain remained to be nearly completely relieved, his function was back to baseline, and he weaned off of both medications. He was very satisfied.

What Is the Prognosis of This Condition?

The outcome of CRPS is highly variable. Sandroni et al. reported that 74% of patients with CRPS underwent resolution, often spontaneously [28]. However, in another study by De Mos et al. [29], at an average of 6 years (range from 2.1 to 10.8 years) since onset, only 30% of CRPS patients considered themselves recovered, 54% were stable, and 16% still reported severe progressive disease. The disease also highly impacted patients' ability to work, with 31% incapable of work permanently and 28% requiring working adjustments. CRPS outcome was worse in patients with the involvement of the upper extremity, a precipitating injury other than fracture, and cold CRPS. If not well controlled, CRPS can spread to affect a wider area over time. The largest systematic study on spreading of CRPS showed 48% of 185 CRPS patients displayed spreading of CRPS to second limb or more, 49% contralateral spread, 30% ipsilateral spread, 14% diagonal spread, and spread triggered by additional trauma in 37–91% of the patients [30]. A recent review of studies on the outcome of CRPS type I concluded that many CRPS patients recovered within 6–13 months, but a significant number of patients experienced some lasting symptoms, and some experienced chronic pain and disability [31].

Discussion

Prevalence

There have been several studies on the epidemiological occurrence of CRPS in recent years, with varying results. The first study by Sandroni et al. showed the overall incidence of CRPS I to be 5.46 per 100,000 person years (0.55%) [28]. A subsequent study by de Mos et al. reported the overall incidence of CRPS to be 26.2 per 100,000 person years (2.62%) in the Netherlands [32]. More recently, Elsharydah et al. conducted a nationwide retrospective analysis of inpatient databases from 2007 to 2011, which showed an overall incidence of CRPS I to be 0.07% [33]. All these studies demonstrated that CRPS more commonly affected women than men and the upper extremity more than the lower extremity [28, 32, 33]. A variety of studies indicated that extremity fracture and surgery were common inciting events of CRPS I. Seven percent of patients who suffered a single fracture of the wrist or ankle developed CRPS I [34]. Following closed reduction of a distal radius fracture and casting, 32.2% of patients developed CRPS [35], 4.36% of patients developed CRPS I following elective foot and ankle surgery [36], and 8.3% following carpal tunnel release surgery [37]. All these studies were done in 2011 or prior on patients who were diagnosed with CRPS according to the IASP Criteria instead of the stricter Budapest Criteria. This indicates that the results from these studies may be falsely high.

Differential Diagnosis

The differential diagnoses include arthritis, Lyme disease, generalized muscle diseases, deep vein thrombosis, Raynaud's disease/phenomenon, nerve injury, infection, or neuropathy.

Predictive Value of CRPS Diagnostic Criteria

The diagnosis of CRPS relies on clinical manifestations, and can be challenging. The original International Association for the Study of Pain (IASP) Criteria proved to be able to identify most cases of CRPS with a sensitivity of 0.99, but had poor specificity and led to over-diagnosis [38]. The improved Budapest Criteria retains a sensitivity of 0.99, but has a specificity of 0.79, in contrast to the original IASP criteria's specificity of 0.41 [1]. Unfortunately, there is no confirmatory testing or imaging for diagnosing CRPS.

Strength of Evidence for Different Treatment Modalities

Although CRPS symptoms may spontaneously improve, aggressive treatment should not be delayed because progressive worsening of symptoms is associated with poor outcome. CRPS is a poorly understood and phenotypically variable disease. Treatment of CRPS is often very challenging and needs a multimodal approach including physical therapy, psychological therapy, medical management, and interventional procedures (Tables 15.4 and 15.5). Because research into medical therapies specifically in CRPS has been scarce, medical treatment for CRPS has

Table 15.4 Risks and complications of interventions

Intervention	Risks and complications
Stellate ganglion block	Infection, hematoma, trauma to carotid, vertebral artery, and internal jugular vein, injury to vagus nerve and brachial plexus roots, pneumothorax, hemothorax, chylothorax, esophageal perforation, intravascular injection, epidural and intrathecal injection, block of the brachial plexus, recurrent laryngeal nerve and phrenic nerve
Spinal cord stimulation	Infection, bleeding, dural puncture, nerve injury, spinal cord injury, defective lead, lead migration, lead fracture, battery failure, battery site discomfort
DRG stimulation	Infection, bleeding, dural puncture, nerve injury, temporary motor stimulation, defective lead, lead migration, lead fracture, device failure, battery site discomfort
Intrathecal drug therapy	Infection, bleeding, nerve injury, spinal cord injury, fractured catheter, pump failure, cerebrospinal fluid leak, hygroma, granuloma (from intrathecal opioid)

Table 15.5 Strength of evidence for different therapies

Therapy	Evidence-based conclusions
Physical therapy	Low-quality evidence suggests benefit of physical therapy in treating CRPS with a multimodal approach [42]
Anticonvulsants	There is moderate evidence for the effectiveness of gabapentin in treating pain in CRPS patients [43]
Antidepressants	TCA and SNRI have been used for the treatment of neuropathic pain, but no clinical trial aimed to treat CRPS has been performed [44, 45]
Anti-inflammatories	There is weak evidence for the effectiveness of steroid in the treatment of CRPS [43]
Alpha-2 adrenergic agonists	Weak evidence suggests the beneficial effect of alpha-2 agonists in treating CRPS [46]
Opioids	There is insufficient evidence to support that opioids are effective in treating neuropathic pain [43]
Vitamin C	Vitamin C provides no benefit in preventing CRPS after distal radius fractures [47]
Sympathetic block	Limited data suggests sympathetic blocks provide short-lasting relief in CRPS pain [48]
Immunoglobulin	High-quality evidence showed low-dose immunoglobulin treatment was not effective in relieving pain in patients with CRPS [49]
Ketamine	Moderate-quality evidence suggests subanesthetic dose of ketamine may be efficacious and safe in CRPS treatment [43, 50]
Spinal cord stimulation	High-quality evidence supports the role of SCS in improving pain relief and quality of life [51]

been largely based on therapeutic strategies adapted from neuropathic pain states.

Future Directions

The following treatment modalities can potentially be used for upper extremity CRPS in the future. Low-quality evidence supports the efficacy of bisphosphates in treating CRPS pain [39]. Recently there was a multicenter clinical trial on bisphosphate infusion in treating CRPS. The results are not known yet. There is high-quality evidence that DRG stimulation provides superior pain relief to SCS for CRPS in the lower limb, offering more posturally stable stimulation and precise paresthesia coverage [40]. DRG stimulation has not been used to treat upper extremity CRPS yet. Intrathecal drug therapy has been used to treat severe refractory CRPS, mostly in lower extremities, but very rarely in upper extremities. Evidence on intrathecal drug therapy is limited to lower extremity CRPS. Moderate-quality evidence supports that intrathecal baclofen decreases pain, improves dystonia, and improves quality of life [3]. There is low-quality evidence suggesting that intrathecal ziconotide relieves pain and symptoms of CRPS [41].

Summary

CRPS is a very complicated disabling disease that is far from being fully understood. Although, in recent years, discovery of its pathological mechanisms has resulted in much better understanding of the disease, the management of this disease remains challenging. A broad modalities of treatment have been used in treating CRPS clinically; however, most of the evidence for most treatments is of low or very low quality. This has led clinicians to adopt a trial and error approach toward managing this syndrome. More studies are needed to further advance our understanding of the pathophysiology. And well designed and meticulously conducted RCTs are needed to investigate the existing therapies, and therapies on the horizon. Society guidelines would be very helpful.

References

1. Harden RN, Bruehl S, Perez RS, Birklein F, Marinus J, Maihofner C, et al. Validation of proposed diagnostic criteria (the "Budapest criteria") for complex regional pain syndrome. Pain. 2010;150(2):268–74.
2. Birklein F, Schlereth T. Complex regional pain syndrome-significant progress in understanding. Pain. 2015;156(Suppl 1):S94–103.
3. Urits I, Shen AH, Jones MR, Viswanath O, Kaye AD. Complex regional pain syndrome, current concepts and treatment options. Curr Pain Headache

Rep. 2018;22(2):10. https://doi.org/10.1007/s11916-018-0667-7.
4. Bruehl S, Maihofner C, Stanton-Hicks M, Perez RS, Vatine JJ, Brunner F, et al. Complex regional pain syndrome: evidence for warm and cold subtypes in a large prospective clinical sample. Pain. 2016;157(8):1674–81.
5. Marinus J, Moseley GL, Birklein F, Baron R, Maihofner C, Kingery WS, et al. Clinical features and pathophysiology of complex regional pain syndrome. Lancet Neurol. 2011;10(7):637–48.
6. Shi X, Wang L, Li X, Sahbaie P, Kingery WS, Clark JD. Neuropeptides contribute to peripheral nociceptive sensitization by regulating interleukin-1beta production in keratinocytes. Anesth Analg. 2011;113(1):175–83.
7. Parkitny L, McAuley JH, Di Pietro F, Stanton TR, O'Connell NE, Marinus J, et al. Inflammation in complex regional pain syndrome: a systematic review and meta-analysis. Neurology. 2013;80(1):106–17.
8. Meacham K, Shepherd A, Mohapatra DP, Haroutounian S. Neuropathic pain: central vs. peripheral mechanisms. Curr Pain Headache Rep. 2017;21(6):28. https://doi.org/10.1007/s11916-017-0629-5.
9. Eisenberg E, Chistyakov AV, Yudashkin M, Kaplan B, Hafner H, Feinsod M. Evidence for cortical hyperexcitability of the affected limb representation area in CRPS: a psychophysical and transcranial magnetic stimulation study. Pain. 2005;113(1–2):99–105.
10. Kohr D, Tschernatsch M, Schmitz K, Singh P, Kaps M, Schafer KH, et al. Autoantibodies in complex regional pain syndrome bind to a differentiation-dependent neuronal surface autoantigen. Pain. 2009;143(3):246–51.
11. Goebel A, Blaes F. Complex regional pain syndrome, prototype of a novel kind of autoimmune disease. Autoimmun Rev. 2013;12(6):682–6.
12. Albrecht PJ, Hines S, Eisenberg E, Pud D, Finlay DR, Connolly MK, et al. Pathologic alterations of cutaneous innervation and vasculature in affected limbs from patients with complex regional pain syndrome. Pain. 2006;120(3):244–66.
13. Oaklander AL, Rissmiller JG, Gelman LB, Zheng L, Chang Y, Gott R. Evidence of focal small-fiber axonal degeneration in complex regional pain syndrome-I (reflex sympathetic dystrophy). Pain. 2006;120(3):235–43.
14. Bruehl S. An update on the pathophysiology of complex regional pain syndrome. Anesthesiology. 2010;113(3):713–25.
15. Harden RN, Duc TA, Williams TR, Coley D, Cate JC, Gracely RH. Norepinephrine and epinephrine levels in affected versus unaffected limbs in sympathetically maintained pain. Clin J Pain. 1994;10(4):324–30.
16. Kurvers H, Daemen M, Slaaf D, Stassen F, van den Wildenberg F, Kitslaar P, et al. Partial peripheral neuropathy and denervation induced adrenoceptor supersensitivity. Functional studies in an experimental model. Acta Orthop Belg. 1998;64(1):64–70.
17. Schattschneider J, Hartung K, Stengel M, Ludwig J, Binder A, Wasner G, et al. Endothelial dysfunction in cold type complex regional pain syndrome. Neurology. 2006;67(4):673–5.
18. Dayan L, Salman S, Norman D, Vatine JJ, Calif E, Jacob G. Exaggerated vasoconstriction in complex regional pain syndrome-1 is associated with impaired resistance artery endothelial function and local vascular reflexes. J Rheumatol. 2008;35(7):1339–45.
19. Koban M, Leis S, Schultze-Mosgau S, Birklein F. Tissue hypoxia in complex regional pain syndrome. Pain. 2003;104(1–2):149–57.
20. Baron R, Schattschneider J, Binder A, Siebrecht D, Wasner G. Relation between sympathetic vasoconstrictor activity and pain and hyperalgesia in complex regional pain syndromes: a case-control study. Lancet. 2002;359(9318):1655–60.
21. Reinersmann A, Maier C, Schwenkreis P, Lenz M. Complex regional pain syndrome: more than a peripheral disease. Pain Manag. 2013;3(6):495–502.
22. Moseley GL. Distorted body image in complex regional pain syndrome. Neurology. 2005;65(5):773.
23. Lewis JS, Kersten P, McCabe CS, McPherson KM, Blake DR. Body perception disturbance: a contribution to pain in complex regional pain syndrome (CRPS). Pain. 2007;133(1–3):111–9.
24. Azqueta-Gavaldon M, Schulte-Gocking H, Storz C, Azad S, Reiners A, Borsook D, et al. Basal ganglia dysfunction in complex regional pain syndrome - a valid hypothesis? Eur J Pain. 2017;21(3):415–24.
25. Cappello ZJ, Kasdan ML, Louis DS. Meta-analysis of imaging techniques for the diagnosis of complex regional pain syndrome type I. J Hand Surg Am. 2012;37(2):288–96.
26. Maihofner C, Handwerker HO, Neundorfer B, Birklein F. Patterns of cortical reorganization in complex regional pain syndrome. Neurology. 2003;61(12):1707–15.
27. Pleger B, Tegenthoff M, Ragert P, Forster AF, Dinse HR, Schwenkreis P, et al. Sensorimotor retuning [corrected] in complex regional pain syndrome parallels pain reduction. Ann Neurol. 2005;57(3):425–9.
28. Sandroni P, Benrud-Larson LM, McClelland RL, Low PA. Complex regional pain syndrome type I: incidence and prevalence in Olmsted county, a population-based study. Pain. 2003;103(1–2):199–207.
29. de Mos M, Huygen FJ, van der Hoeven-Borgman M, Dieleman JP, Ch Stricker BH, Sturkenboom MC. Outcome of the complex regional pain syndrome. Clin J Pain. 2009;25(7):590–7.
30. van Rijn MA, Marinus J, Putter H, Bosselaar SR, Moseley GL, van Hilten JJ. Spreading of complex regional pain syndrome: not a random process. J Neural Transm (Vienna). 2011;118(9):1301–9.
31. Bean DJ, Johnson MH, Kydd RR. The outcome of complex regional pain syndrome type 1: a systematic review. J Pain. 2014;15(7):677–90.
32. de Mos M, de Bruijn AG, Huygen FJ, Dieleman JP, Stricker BH, Sturkenboom MC. The incidence of

complex regional pain syndrome: a population-based study. Pain. 2007;129(1–2):12–20.
33. Elsharydah A, Loo NH, Minhajuddin A, Kandil ES. Complex regional pain syndrome type 1 predictors - epidemiological perspective from a national database analysis. J Clin Anesth. 2017;39:34–7.
34. Beerthuizen A, Stronks DL, Van't Spijker A, Yaksh A, Hanraets BM, Klein J, et al. Demographic and medical parameters in the development of complex regional pain syndrome type 1 (CRPS1): prospective study on 596 patients with a fracture. Pain. 2012;153(6):1187–92.
35. Jellad A, Salah S, Ben Salah Frih Z. Complex regional pain syndrome type I: incidence and risk factors in patients with fracture of the distal radius. Arch Phys Med Rehabil. 2014;95(3):487–92.
36. Rewhorn MJ, Leung AH, Gillespie A, Moir JS, Miller R. Incidence of complex regional pain syndrome after foot and ankle surgery. J Foot Ankle Surg. 2014;53(3):256–8.
37. da Costa VV, de Oliveira SB, Fernandes Mdo C, Saraiva RA. Incidence of regional pain syndrome after carpal tunnel release. Is there a correlation with the anesthetic technique? Rev Bras Anestesiol. 2011;61(4):425–33.
38. Bruehl S, Harden RN, Galer BS, Saltz S, Bertram M, Backonja M, et al. External validation of IASP diagnostic criteria for complex regional pain syndrome and proposed research diagnostic criteria. International Association for the Study of Pain. Pain. 1999;81(1–2):147–54.
39. Chevreau M, Romand X, Gaudin P, Juvin R, Baillet A. Bisphosphonates for treatment of complex regional pain syndrome type 1: a systematic literature review and meta-analysis of randomized controlled trials versus placebo. Joint Bone Spine. 2017;84(4):393–9.
40. Harrison C, Epton S, Bojanic S, Green AL, FitzGerald JJ. The efficacy and safety of dorsal root ganglion stimulation as a treatment for neuropathic pain: a literature review. Neuromodulation. 2018;21(3):225–33.
41. Kapural L, Lokey K, Leong MS, Fiekowsky S, Stanton-Hicks M, Sapienza-Crawford AJ, et al. Intrathecal ziconotide for complex regional pain syndrome: seven case reports. Pain Pract. 2009;9(4):296–303.
42. Smart KM, Wand BM, O'Connell NE. Physiotherapy for pain and disability in adults with complex regional pain syndrome (CRPS) types I and II. Cochrane Database Syst Rev. 2016;2:CD010853.
43. Zyluk A, Puchalski P. Effectiveness of complex regional pain syndrome treatment: a systematic review. Neurol Neurochir Pol. 2018;52:326.
44. Duong S, Bravo D, Todd KJ, Finlayson RJ, Tran Q. Treatment of complex regional pain syndrome: an updated systematic review and narrative synthesis. Can J Anaesth. 2018;65:658.
45. Harden RN, Oaklander AL, Burton AW, Perez RS, Richardson K, Swan M, et al. Complex regional pain syndrome: practical diagnostic and treatment guidelines, 4th edition. Pain Med. 2013;14(2):180–229.
46. Goh EL, Chidambaram S, Ma D. Complex regional pain syndrome: a recent update. Burns Trauma. 2017;5:2. https://doi.org/10.1186/s41038-016-0066-4. eCollection 2017.
47. Evaniew N, McCarthy C, Kleinlugtenbelt YV, Ghert M, Bhandari M. Vitamin C to prevent complex regional pain syndrome in patients with distal radius fractures: a meta-analysis of randomized controlled trials. J Orthop Trauma. 2015;29(8):e235–41.
48. Straube S, Derry S, Moore RA, Cole P. Cervico-thoracic or lumbar sympathectomy for neuropathic pain and complex regional pain syndrome. Cochrane Database Syst Rev. 2013;(9):CD002918.
49. Goebel A, Bisla J, Carganillo R, Frank B, Gupta R, Kelly J, et al. Low-dose intravenous immunoglobulin treatment for long-standing complex regional pain syndrome: a randomized trial. Ann Intern Med. 2017;167(7):476–83.
50. Connolly SB, Prager JP, Harden RN. A systematic review of ketamine for complex regional pain syndrome. Pain Med. 2015;16(5):943–69.
51. Visnjevac O, Costandi S, Patel BA, Azer G, Agarwal P, Bolash R, et al. A comprehensive outcome-specific review of the use of spinal cord stimulation for complex regional pain syndrome. Pain Pract. 2017;17(4):533–45.

A 75-Year-Old Woman with Hand Grip Weakness

16

Evan Goodman and Tariq Malik

Case Description

This is a 75-year-old woman with past medical history of hypertension, hyperlipidemia, and osteoarthitis who presents with complaint of numbness/tingling, grip weakness, and pain in her right hand roughly 6 months in duration. She is unsure what brought her symptoms on. At times she has noticed numbness in her thumb, index, and middle finger. She describes that during these episodes she often "shakes" her hand. The symptoms are most noticeable at late at night or early in the morning, but recently reported dropping objects with her right hand and at times difficulty with writing. She denies any tobacco products, and states one glass of red wine in the evening. On further questioning, she does admit to similar symptoms a few years ago while working as an administrative assistant prior to retiring. Physical examinations reveal symmetrical strength and reflexes in the upper limb, with possible weakness in the right hand.

E. Goodman (✉)
Department of Anesthesiology and Critical Care, University of Chicago, Chicago, IL, USA
e-mail: egoodman@dacc.uchicago.edu

T. Malik
Department of Anesthesia and Critical Care, University of Chicago, Chicago, IL, USA
e-mail: tmalik@dacc.uchicago.edu

What Is Your Preliminary Diagnosis?

The symptoms are suggestive of compression neuropathy. The distribution area of paresthesia in the lateral three digits suggests median nerve neuropathy or cervical radiculopathy affecting C6 or C7. But the absence of other accompanying features of radiculopathy, i.e., pain shooting from the shoulder down the arm or weakness in the muscles and intact reflexes, makes it an unlikely diagnosis. Median nerve can be entrapped at or around elbow either by two heads of pronator or an anomalous fibrous band. Wrist arthritis or that of carpometacarpal joint of the thumb can also present as wrist pain and weakness. Tendonitis or tenosynovitis of various tendons can behave similarly.

In the absence of any obvious swelling or focal tenderness, with symptoms confined to distal to the wrist, median nerve entrapment (also called carpal tunnel syndrome) at the wrist is the most likely diagnosis.

How Is Diagnosis Confirmed?

Diagnosis is confirmed by ruling out other conditions that can account for the patient's symptom as well as demonstrating positive findings on physical examination and testing if needed.

Carpal tunnel can be a seemingly straightforward presentation and is still largely considered

T. Malik (ed.), *Practical Chronic Pain Management*, https://doi.org/10.1007/978-3-030-46675-6_16

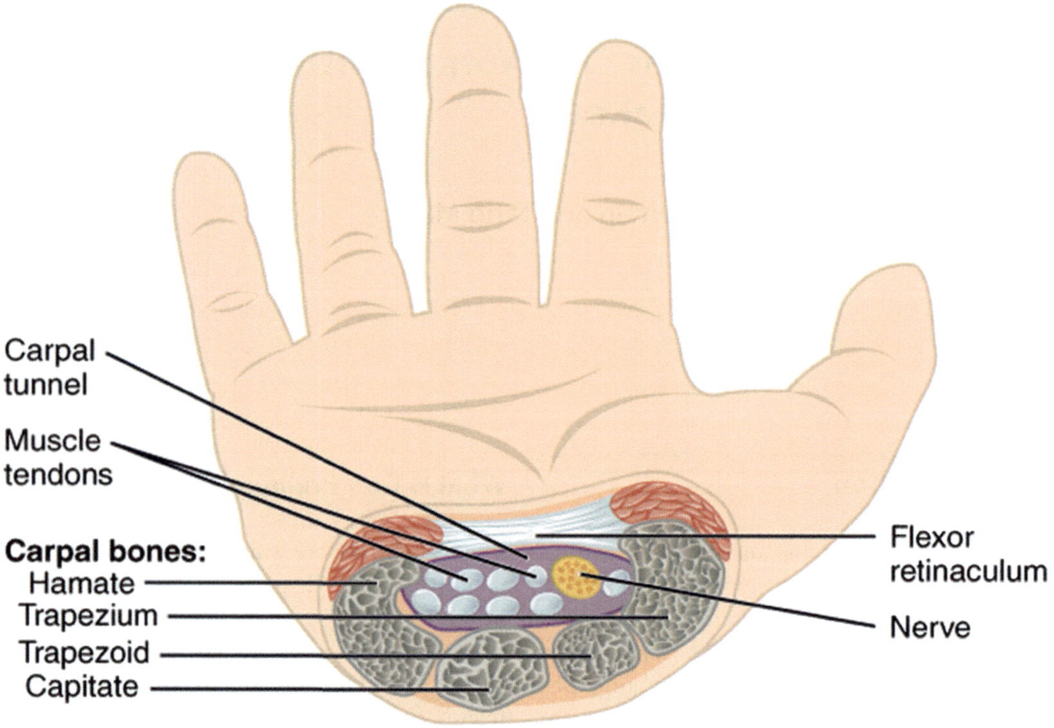

Fig. 16.1 Cross-section across the wrist. (From Gray [67])

a clinical diagnosis. However, according to the American Academy of Orthopedic Surgeons clinical guidelines and recommendations, history and physical exam bears only grade C evidence [1]. Even so, the clinical interview is still vital for gathering appropriate patient information, medical history, functional history, and occupational information. In the course of early CTS, sensory complaints are common within the distribution of the median nerve (Figs. 16.1 and 16.2). Patients may describe burning, numbness, or tingling classically in the thumb, index, middle, and radial ring finger [2–5]. Symptoms of paresthesia may be worse in the evening hours, though sensitivity (51–96%) and specificity (27–68%) of these features, when compared against conduction studies, are poor and range widely [2–5].

Patients may also complain of dropping items [6]. And though patients may state discomfort of the entire hand, the fifth digit is rarely involved [7].

Careful cervical spine examination is done to evaluate for the presence of radiculopathy or thoracic outlet problem. Elbow area is examined for any entrapment neuropathy of median (by the pronator teres or ligament of Struthers) or radial nerve at or around elbow joint.

Compression of median nerve will spare all forearm muscles as well as sensation over the thenar eminence. However, abductor pollicis brevis and opponens pollicis are affected. Thenar eminence atrophy is a strong evidence for ruling in carpal tunnel syndrome [1, 7]. This finding is very late in the course of chronic carpal tunnel syndrome. At this point, it is further advisable to check the abductor pollicis strength as it is commonly affected [7]. This is best performed with the patient's affected hand in the supine position. Ask the patient to bring their first digit straight upward toward the ceiling. The examiner then performs the test with resistance at the base of the first digit.

Regarding the use of special tests, the examiner should keep in mind that there are a plethora of special tests that have been documented. This chapter is not exhaustive regarding special tests, and below are some of the more common tests

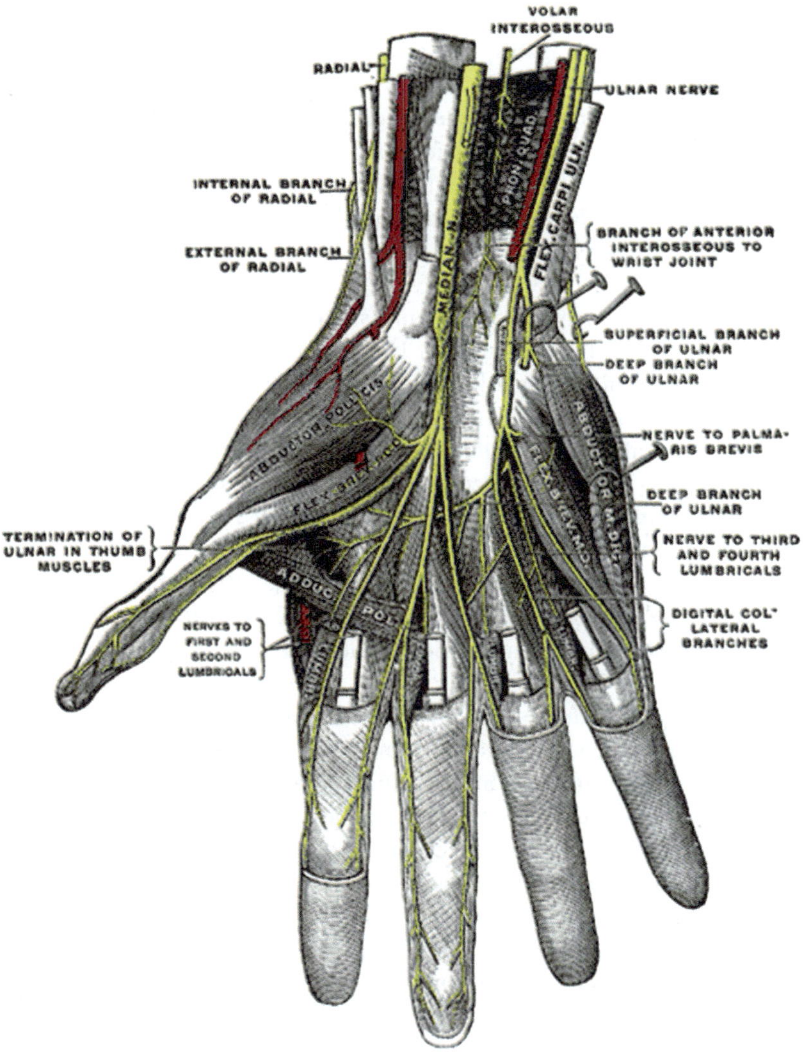

Fig. 16.2 Nerves of the hand. (From Sobotta [68])

highlighted. For increased accuracy they should be combined [7].

Tinel's test, originally described by Dr. J. Tinel to detect neuromas in 1915, involves tapping over the course of median nerve for about 2–3 cm starting the distal wrist crease in an attempt to elicit symptoms along the distribution of the median nerve. This test's precision is lacking, as the findings differ depending on the examiner and pressure applied. The range of sensitivities and specificities again varies (23–76% and 55–100%, respectively) [3, 4, 8–13].

With flexion at the wrist crease by bringing the hands together with palms facing, the patient is performing Phalen's test. This action causes supposed compression of the median nerve underneath the transverse carpal ligament. A positive test is elicited when symptoms present themselves in less than 1 minute along the median nerve distribution. The sensitivity is around 70% and specificity ranges from 20% to 80%. As above, not a strong independent testing measure [3, 4, 10, 11, 14–16].

Reverse Phalen's test is opposite of Phalen's test, where compression is achieved by complete dorsiflexion of the wrist for 1 minute with a lower sensitivity of around 43% and specificity of around 74%. Carpal compression test involves direct compression of the median nerve at the wrists using sustained pressure for up to a minute. The sensitivity and specificity of this test are both around 90%.

Kuhlman looked at six common physical findings comparing them against electromyography/nerve conduction velocity (EMG/NCV; Phalen's test, Tinel's test, numbness of index finger, weakness of abductor brevis, compression test, square-shaped wrist) and found each sign not sensitive but fairly specific. He found square-shaped wrist sign as the most sensitive feature.

Given the clinical suspicion for CTS, one may refer for complementary investigation including NCS/EMG examination. This chapter is not comprehensive regarding the diagnostic criteria for CTS. However, NCS/EMG studies are very helpful for determining the severity of carpal tunnel syndrome and confirming the site of nerve compression. One may see the sensory nerve affected prior to the motor nerve, and a decrease in conduction velocity [7]. It has been reported that sensory latencies measured by stimulating the palm and measuring at the wrist is a sensitive test [17].

According to a study from *Muscle & Nerve* 2010, the "CSI" (combined sensory index) may have the highest sensitivity and specificity [18]. The CSI is a summation of three comparison studies analyzing differences in sensory latencies of the median, ulnar, and radial nerves from three locales. Recordings are taken from the ring finger (median and ulnar), thumb (median and radial), and transplanar studies (median and ulnar). Even with considerable investigation to diagnose CTS, however, in mild cases there has been a reported 15% false negative [19].

US examination may be beneficial for evaluation depending on the skill of the examiner and is gaining popularity in its use. A meta-analysis examining 28 trials and just shy of 4000 wrists determined that a cross sectional area of the median nerve at the carpal tunnel inlet greater than 9 mm^2 is a significant diagnostic tool with odds ratio 40.4, sensitivity 87.3%, and specificity 83.3% [20].

Other sonographic studies have attempted to quantify mild, moderate, and severe carpal tunnel syndrome. One such study evaluated 164 patients measuring the inlet and outlet of the carpal tunnel using ultrasound. Their findings were in close agreement with using a cutoff value of 8.5 mm^2 at the inlet and outlet for carpal tunnel syndrome [21]. It is worth noting in this study the patients were diagnosed prior with NCS/EMG testing [21]. Nevertheless, they were unable to use sonographic assessment in the proper grading of mild, moderate, or severe CTS [21]. Another study by Klauser, Halpern, and De Zord et al. states a 99% sensitivity and 100% specificity for CTS if a 2 mm^2 cross-sectional difference exists at the median nerve between the carpal tunnel and pronator quadratus [22].

MRI of the wrist can show swelling/compression of the nerve. Rarely vascular studies of the area may reveal or confirm a vascular pathology causing compression neuropathy.

What Is the Pathophysiology of This Condition?

Carpal tunnel syndrome encompasses a constellation of symptoms secondary to compression of the median nerve affecting digits 1–3 and sometimes the radial half of digit 4. The pathophysiology is complex and continues to be investigated. The carpal tunnel is superiorly bordered by the flexor retinaculum, and inferiorly by the carpal bones. The four flexor superficialis tendons, four flexor profundus tendons, flexor pollicis longus tendon, and median nerve traverse this area. Symptoms arise as a result of compression and traction of the median nerve at the carpal tunnel, leading to a median mononeuropathy at the wrist [23]. The compression of the median nerve is thought to be secondary to fibrous hypertrophy of the flexor synovium due to repetitive wrist movements [23]. Interestingly, from a 1980s small study analyzing carpal pressures, they found increased pressure in neutral, flexion, and extension in symptomatic patients compared to control [24]. They also determined that, in symptomatic patients, pressure was elevated the most with wrist extension [24]. As an aside, acute and chronic trauma both to the lunate causing dislocation or subluxation have resulted in compression of the median nerve [25]. The two areas where median nerve commonly gets compressed are one under the proximal flexor retinaculum that is exacerbated by wrist flexion and the other distally at hook of the hamate [23].

With compression and traction of the median nerve, it is believed that intraneural microcirculation is altered [23]. Also, myelin and axonal injuries may result causing dysfunction of the nerve and supporting tissues [23].

How Is This Problem Managed?

The management depends upon the severity of the clinical feature. There are a variety of treatments available for CTS, ranging from bracing, alternative therapies, oral medications, and injections to surgical intervention. Non-surgical interventions are often offered to patients diagnosed with mild to moderate symptoms [26]. Whereas surgical intervention may be offered to patients who have failed conservative treatment or who have severe CTS with signs of acute denervation [27].

In a stepwise fashion, bracing and/or splinting is common, as patients suffering from carpal tunnel are recommended to immobilize the affected side with orthosis. There is strong evidence that outcomes are improved [6]. In one study of auto assembly workers, a 6 week trial of nocturnal splinting compared to ergonomic control cohort experienced significantly reduced discomfort, which was maintained a year out [28]. Interestingly, improvement occurred in the splinted group regardless of baseline impairment [28]. In another study, a Cochrane review of 21 trials and 884 included subjects found relief using a brace after only 4 weeks [26]. In terms of splinting positioning, there is not a conclusive recommendation for neutral vs. slight extension [29]. Wearing a brace full-time does not seem to benefit the patient more than at night [26, 29].

Besides bracing as an initial intervention, oral over-the-counter pain medication are commonly used – up to 50.8% NSAIDs seen in CTS treatment [30]. But Cochrane review did not find NSAIDs to be of benefit [26]. Regarding other PO medications, there has been moderate evidence of the short-term effectiveness of oral steroids with prednisolone 20 mg/d for 2 weeks and then 10 mg/d for 2 weeks compared to splinting alone regarding short-term function [31]. But when prednisolone as prescribed above was compared to prednisolone 20 mg daily for 2 weeks and then placebo for 2 weeks, there was no difference long term, up to 12 months [32]. And it was seen that the 2 weeks of oral steroid was as effective as the 4 week prescription in the short term [32]. The side effects of PO steroids must be heavily considered.

Regarding manual interventions, there has been small sampled evidence that carpal bone mobilization significantly improved symptoms after 3 weeks [26]. There is also limited evidence to the effectiveness of tendon and nerve gliding exercises [29].

Patients seem to benefit from injection for symptom relief. Per Cochrane, local corticosteroid injection provided greater relief than placebo injection at 1 month [33]. It was further seen that local injections provided greater benefit up to 3 months than oral steroids [33]. But, an injection does not have a significant improvement when compared to anti-inflammatory and splinting at 2 months [33]. No seen increased benefit from two injections [33]. It is important to remember that, with local steroid use, there is a risk of atrophy and injury to the median nerve and systemic absorption, preceding the potential for Cushing syndrome with steroid use [34].

Recently, the regenerative movement is gaining popularity. There are studies that have shown therapeutic benefit from platelet-rich plasma in neuropathies both in the laboratory and clinical setting [35–39].

Within the last few years, one such study of 14 participants investigated a single injection of PRP 1–2 ml under US guidance for mild CTS [40]. At 1 month follow-up, 8 patients had either "full" or "almost full" recovery on VAS and 3 with "great" improvement [40]. Then at 3 month follow-up, pain was not greatly improved in 3 patients [40].

For severe CTS, there is strong evidence for surgical intervention with evidence of median nerve denervation [27]. There may even be a place for surgery for moderate CTS [7]. However, it remains unclear whether surgical intervention should be offered earlier in the course [41]. But when it comes to choosing approach, there may not be a significant difference in the long term between open vs. endoscopic [7]. It has been stated in a systematic review by Huissted et al. 2010 that surgical intervention may be more effective than "prolonged" conservative interventions over time [41]. Some studies have shown better result from surgery over steroids and splinting for symptom relief and outcome [42, 43]. Prior to surgery, those patients who responded to steroid injection favorably seem to have a better response to surgery [44]. Like many surgical interventions, there is the risk for bleeding and infection. Regarding approach and risks from surgical intervention, endoscopic release was seen with possibly more neuropathic complaints, i.e., neuropraxia and sensory complaints [45]. Whereas with an open approach, there is potential for negative wound healing [45].

What Is the Prognosis of This Condition?

Given that CTS syndrome is a very common neuropathy, up to 90% of all neuropathies that present to a variety of clinic settings, prognostication of the condition is vital [7]. Burton et al. attempted to investigate prognostic factors in CTS patients who were treated conservatively vs. no treatment analyzing up to 16 cohort studies [46].

Of 9 conservatively treated patient studies, they found a wide range (23–89%) of studies with negative outcomes at 3 years [46–55]. Various studies defined negative outcomes differently with worsening symptoms, needing surgery, or missing work [46–55]. About 4 studies showed that surgical intervention was needed 57–66% of the time after conservative treatment between a 6 month and 3 year follow-up period [50, 56–58]. They did have consensus in 3 or more cohorts that symptom duration, positive Phalen, and thenar wasting was associated with decreased benefit of conservative treatment, but many studies were affected by various forms of bias, and this needs to be further studied [46]. They however were unable to substantiate NCS/EMG severity as a negative predictor for failed conservative treatment [46, 49, 54, 55, 57, 59].

With regard to no intervention, two studies of untreated CTS patients found negative outcomes between 32% and 58% at 1 year [48, 49]. Interestingly, the four studies of untreated patients displayed a percentage of 28–62% that stabilized or improved with no treatment [59–62]. Their analysis displays the course and prognosis of CTS to be highly variable [46].

Discussion

CTS is likely the most common nerve entrapment and neuropathy of the upper limb [63]. Depending on one's definition, CTS may be seen in 5.3% of women and 2.1% of men, or CTS affects women 3 times more than men [64, 65]. There is an estimated incidence of 1–3 cases per 100 subjects per year [63]. CTS has been linked to a variety of other medical conditions, including DM, thyroid disease, and pregnancy. Even if the clinical picture seems clear, one must be aware of other diagnosis that may have similar symptomatology; these include pronator teres syndrome, thoracic outlet syndrome, and anterior interosseous compression. The examiner should keep in mind the possibility of the double crush phenomenon including CTS at the wrist but perhaps including other pathology affecting the patient proximally (Table 16.1).

CTS presents initially with sensory manifestations early in the course, often most discomforting at night [2]. In more advanced cases the

Table 16.1 Differential diagnosis of CTS

Tendonitis	Pain and swelling along the tendons
Wrist arthritis	Tender along the joint, abnormal X-ray
Thumb CMC arthritis	Tender at joint, crepitus, X-ray findings
De Quervain's tenosynovitis	Tenderness and swelling along the radial aspect of the wrist joint
Ganglion cyst	Palpable mass, MRI
Wartenberg's syndrome	Superficial radial nerve entrapment at mid forearm causing pain at the wrist, ulnar deviation of the hand

Table 16.2 Diagnostic tests

Physical findings	Tinel's sign, Compression test, Phalen's test, reverse Phalen test, weakness in Abductor pollicis brevis
Diagnostic blocks	Injection at the compression site
MRI	Swelling of the nerve
Ultrasound	Swelling, compression, also helps in diagnostic block
EMG/NCV	Slow conduction, loss of axons
X-ray	Wrist arthritis, thumb CMC arthritis
Arteriography	Vascular malformation, aneurysm

patient may complain of weakness, and possibly even thenar atrophy [1, 7]. For improved sensitivity and specificity, the examiner should combine multiple special tests with the physical exam [7]. EMG/NCS is a good supplemental diagnostic tool, specifically to grade severity of CTS (Table 16.2). Keep in mind that one may need to perform the "CSI" if clinically concerned for CTS. Even still, false negatives up to 15% have been reported [19]. But using NCS/EMG as a prognostic factor for outcomes from conservative management remains inconclusive [46].

With symptomatic CTS, there is a wide range of patients that have stabilized or improved in a small group of studies without treatment [18–21]. Determining which patients will improve without intervention remains difficult[46]. Regardless, patients may benefit from bracing for a period of 4–6 weeks [26–28]. For a short period of symptom control, corticosteroid injection has shown symptom improvement [33]. If the patient has a favorable response and the patient goes on to have surgical intervention, they may have a better outcome [44]. Unfortunately prior studies have shown that even with conservative management, patients may eventually have surgery, 57–66% by 3 years [50, 56–58]. Surgery is recommended for severe CTS and for patients without benefit from prolonged conservative interventions [27]. Compared to conservative measures with splinting, one high-quality randomized control trial showed statistically significant benefit from surgery at 3 and 6 months up to a year [41, 66].

Even if the perception of carpal tunnel syndrome may seem simplistic, the challenge remains in its properly selected treatment. It still remains to be seen why certain individuals may improve with no intervention or with conservative measures. Still causing physician and patient frustration is why a significant percentage of people may need surgical intervention even after conservative measures. Various surgical interventions and approaches continue to be investigated as new technologies and techniques are created. Perhaps one eventually displays superiority. One particular aspect being explored, the timing of surgery, may have significant importance on management, particularly for those with moderate severity. Significant interest regarding the regenerative medicine movement using PRP/stem cell will most likely continue, and research into its efficacy and safety is needed as it may have a role in the treatment of CTS one day.

Conclusion/Summary

CTS is a common condition that can be easily misdiagnosed. Each case should be properly evaluated. Mild cases can be managed conservatively. Steroid injection provides only short-term relief. Surgery is the only definite treatment that should be considered if motor symptoms are present, pain is intense, or NCV/EMG show evidence of axonal loss.

References

1. American Academy of Orthopaedic Surgeons (AAOS). Clinical practice guideline on the treatment of carpal tunnel syndrome. Rosemont: American Academy of Orthopaedic Surgeons (AAOS); 2008. p. 76.
2. Szabo RM, Slater RR Jr, Farver TB, Stanton DB, Sharman WK. The value of diagnostic testing in carpal tunnel syndrome. J Hand Surg [Am]. 1999;24(4):704–14.
3. Buch-Jaeger N, Foucher G. Correlation of clinical signs with nerve conduction tests in the diagnosis of carpal tunnel syndrome. J Hand Surg (Br). 1994;19(6):720–4.
4. Katz JN, Larson MG, Sabra A, Krarup C, Stirrat CR, Sethi R, et al. The carpal tunnel syndrome: diagnostic utility of the history and physical examination findings. Ann Intern Med. 1990;112(5):321–7.

5. Gupta SK, Benstead TJ. Symptoms experienced by patients with carpal tunnel syndrome. Can J Neurol Sci. 1997;24(4):338–42.
6. American Academy of Orthopaedic Surgeons (AAOS). American Academy of Orthopaedic Surgeons clinical practice guideline on management of carpal tunnel syndrome. Rosemont: American Academy of Orthopaedic Surgeons (AAOS); 2016. p. 983.
7. Aroori S, Spence RAJ. Carpal tunnel syndrome. Ulster Med J. 2008;77(1):6–17.
8. Kuhlman KA, Hennessey WJ. Sensitivity and specificity of carpal tunnel syndrome signs. Am J Phys Med Rehabil. 1997;76(6):451–7.
9. Kuschner SH, Ebramzadeh E, Johnson D, Brien WW, Sherman R. Tinel's sign and Phalen's test in carpal tunnel syndrome. Orthopedics. 1992;15(11):1297–302.
10. Gerr F, Letz R, Harris-Abbott D, Hopkins LC. Sensitivity and specificity of vibrometry for detection of carpal tunnel syndrome. J Occup Environ Med. 1995;37(9):1108–15.
11. Golding DN, Rose DM, Selvarajah K. Clinical tests for carpal tunnel syndrome: an evaluation. Br J Rheumatol. 1986;25(4):388–90.
12. Heller L, Ring H, Costeff H, Solzi P. Evaluation of Tinel's and Phalen's signs in diagnosis of the carpal tunnel syndrome. Eur Neurol. 1986;25(1):40–2.
13. Mondelli M, Passero S, Giannini F. Provocative tests in different stages of carpal tunnel syndrome. Clin Neurol Neurosurg. 2001;103(3):178–83.
14. De Smet L, Steenwerckx A, Van den Bogaert G, Cnudde P, Fabry G. Value of clinical provocative tests in carpal tunnel syndrome. Acta Orthop Belg. 1995;61(3):177–82.
15. Kaufman MA. Differential diagnosis and pitfalls in electrodiagnostic studies and special tests for diagnosing compressive neuropathies. Orthop Clin North Am. 1996;27(2):245–52.
16. Bruske J, Bednarski M, Grzelec H, Zyluk A. The usefulness of the Phalen test and the Hoffmann-Tinel sign in the diagnosis of carpal tunnel syndrome. Acta Orthop Belg. 2002;68(2):141–5.
17. Huang JH, Zager EL. Mini-open carpal tunnel decompression. Neurosurgery. 2004;54:397–9.
18. Malladi N, Micklesen PJ, Hou J, Robinson LR. Correlation between the combined sensory index and clinical outcome after carpal tunnel decompression: a retrospective review. Muscle Nerve. 2010;41(4):453–7.
19. American Association of Electrodiagnostic Medicine, American Academy of Neurology, American Academy of Physical Medicine and Rehabilitation. Practice parameter for electrodiagnostic studies in carpal tunnel syndrome: summary statement. Muscle Nerve. 2009;25:918–22.
20. Tai T-W, Wu C-Y, Su F-C, Chern T-C, Jou I-M. Ultrasonography for diagnosing carpal tunnel syndrome: a meta-analysis of diagnostic test accuracy. Ultrasound Med Biol. 2012;38(7):1121–8.
21. Mohammadi A, Afshar A, Etemadi A, Masoudi S, Baghizadeh A. Diagnostic value of cross-sectional area of median nerve in grading severity of carpal tunnel syndrome. Arch Iran Med. 2010;13(6):516–21.
22. Klauser AS, Halpern EJ, De Zordo T, et al. Carpal tunnel syndrome assessment with US: value of additional cross-sectional area measurements of the median nerve in patients versus healthy volunteers. Radiology. 2009;250(1):171–7.
23. Aboonq MS. Pathophysiology of carpal tunnel syndrome. Neurosciences (Riyadh). 2015;20(1):4–9.
24. Gelberman RH, Hergenroeder PT, Hargens AR, Lundborg GN, Akeson WH. The carpal tunnel syndrome: a study of carpal canal pressures. J Bone Joint Surg. 1981;63(2):380–3.
25. Moore KL, Dalley AF, Agur AMR. Clinically oriented anatomy. Baltimore: Lippincott Williams & Wilkins; 2010.
26. O'Connor D, Marshall S, Massy-Westropp N. Non-surgical treatment (other than steroid injection) for carpal tunnel syndrome. Cochrane Database Syst Rev. 2003;(1):CD003219.
27. Page MJ, Massy-Westropp N, O'Connor D, Pitt V. Splinting for carpal tunnel syndrome. Cochrane Database Syst Rev. 2012;7:CD010003.
28. Werner R, et al. Randomized controlled trial of nocturnal splinting for active workers with symptoms of carpal tunnel syndrome. Arch Phys Med Rehabil. 2005;86(1):1–7.
29. Huisstede BM, Hoogvliet P, Randsdorp MS, Glerum S, Middelkoop MV, Koes BW. Carpal tunnel syndrome. Part I: effectiveness of nonsurgical treatments–a systematic review. Arch Phys Med Rehabil. 2010;91(7):981–1004.
30. Miller RS, Iverson DC, Fried RA, Green LA, Nutting PA. Carpal tunnel syndrome in primary care: a report from ASPN. Ambulatory Sentinel Practice Network. J Fam Pract. 1994;38:337–44.
31. Mishra S, Prabhakar S, Lal V, Modi M, Das CP, Khurana D. Efficacy of splinting and oral steroids in the treatment of carpal tunnel syndrome: a prospective randomized clinical and electrophysiological study. Neurol India. 2006;54:286–90.
32. Chang MH, Ger LP, Hsieh PF, Huang SY. A randomised clinical trial of oral steroids in the treatment of carpal tunnel syndrome: a long term follow up. J Neurol Neurosurg Psychiatry. 2002;73:710–4.
33. Marshall SC, Tardif G, Ashworth NL. Local corticosteroid injection for carpal tunnel syndrome. Cochrane Database Syst Rev. 2007;(2):CD001554.
34. Lambru G, Lagrata S, Matharu MS. Cutaneous atrophy and alopecia after greater occipital nerve injection using triamcinolone. Headache. 2012;52:1596–9.
35. Allampallam K, Chakraborty J, Robinson J. Effect of ascorbic acid and growth factors on collagen metabolism of flexor retinaculum cells from individuals with and without carpal tunnel syndrome. J Occup Environ Med. 2000;42:251–9.
36. Farrag TY, Lehar M, Verhaegen P, Carson KA, Byrne PJ. Effect of platelet rich plasma and fibrin sealant on facial nerve regeneration in a rat model. Laryngoscope. 2007;117:157–65.

37. Cho HH, Jang S, Lee SC, Jeong HS, Park JS, Han JY, Lee KH, Cho YB. Effect of neural-induced mesenchymal stem cells and platelet-rich plasma on facial nerve regeneration in an acute nerve injury model. Laryngoscope. 2010;120:907–13.
38. Anjayani S, Wirohadidjojo YW, Adam AM, Suwandi D, Seweng A, Amiruddin MD. Sensory improvement of leprosy peripheral neuropathy in patients treated with perineural injection of platelet-rich plasma. Int J Dermatol. 2014;53:109–13.
39. Park GY, Kwon DR. Platelet-rich plasma limits the nerve injury caused by 10% dextrose in the rabbit median nerve. Muscle Nerve. 2014;49:56–60.
40. Nikolaou V, Malahias M, Johnson E, Babis G. Single injection of platelet-rich plasma as a novel treatment of carpal tunnel syndrome. Neural Regen Res. 2015;10(11):1856–9.
41. Huisstede BM, et al. Carpal tunnel syndrome. Part II: effectiveness of surgical treatments—a systematic review. Arch Phys Med Rehabil. 2010;91(7):1005–24. https://doi.org/10.1016/j.apmr.2010.03.023.
42. Gerritsen AA, de Vet HC, Scholten RJ, et al. Splinting vs surgery in the treatment of carpal tunnel syndrome: a randomized controlled trial. JAMA. 2002;288:1245–51.
43. Hui AC, Wong S, Leung CH, et al. A randomized controlled trial of surgery vs steroid injection for carpal tunnel syndrome. Neurology. 2005;64:2074–8.
44. Edgell SE, McCabe SJ, Breidenbach WC. Predicting the outcome of carpal tunnel release. J Hand Surg Am. 2003;28:255–61.
45. Toussaint CP, Ali ZS, Zager EL. Distal entrapment syndromes: carpal tunnel, cubital tunnel, peroneal, and tarsal tunnel. In: Youmans and Winn neurological surgery. 7th ed. Philadelphia: Elsevier; 2017. p. 2019–2031e.4.
46. Burton CL, Chesterton LS, Chen Y, Windt DAVD. Clinical course and prognostic factors in conservatively managed carpal tunnel syndrome: a systematic review. Arch Phys Med Rehabil. 2016;97(5):836–852e.1.
47. DeStefano F, Nordstrom DL, Vierkant RA. Long-term symptom outcomes of carpal tunnel syndrome and its treatment. J Hand Surg [Am]. 1997;22:200–10.
48. Lian BT, Urkude R, Verma KK. Clinical profile, electrodiagnosis and outcome in patients with carpal tunnel syndrome: a Singapore perspective. Singap Med J. 2006;47:1049–52.
49. Kiylioglu N, Bicerol B, Ozkul A, Akyol A. Natural course and treatment efficacy: one-year observation in diabetic and idiopathic carpal tunnel syndrome. J Clin Neurophysiol. 2009;26:446–54.
50. Kaplan SJ, Glickel SZ, Eaton RG. Predictive factors in the non-surgical treatment of carpal tunnel syndrome. J Hand Surg (Br). 1990;15:106–8.
51. Muhlau G, Both R, Kunath H. Carpal tunnel syndrome—course and prognosis. J Neurol. 1984;231:83–6.
52. Katz JN, Lew RA, Bessette L, et al. Prevalence and predictors of long-term work disability due to carpal tunnel syndrome. Am J Ind Med. 1998;33:543–50.
53. Katz JN, Keller RB, Simmons BP, et al. Maine carpal tunnel study: outcomes of operative and nonoperative therapy for carpal tunnel syndrome in a community-based cohort. J Hand Surg [Am]. 1998;23:697–710.
54. Goodwill CJ. The carpal tunnel syndrome. Long-term follow-up showing relation of latency measurements to response to treatment. Ann Phys Med. 1965;8:12–21.
55. Kouyoumdjian JA, Morita MP, Molina AF, et al. Long-term outcomes of symptomatic electrodiagnosed carpal tunnel syndrome. Arq Neuropsiquiatr. 2003;61:194–8.
56. Boyd KU, Gan BS, Ross DC, Richards RS, Roth JH, MacDermid JC. Outcomes in carpal tunnel syndrome: symptom severity, conservative management and progression to surgery. Clin Invest Med. 2005;28:254–61.
57. Duckworth AD, Jenkins PJ, Roddam P, Watts AC, Ring D, McEachan JE. Pain and carpal tunnel syndrome. J Hand Surg [Am]. 2013;38:1540–6.
58. Miranda BH, Asaad K, Cerovac S. Carpal tunnel syndrome study: local corticosteroids, conversion to surgery and NHS implications. J Plast Reconstr Aesthet Surg. 2013;66:1432–3.
59. Padua L, Padua R, Aprile I, Pasqualetti P, Tonali P. Multiperspective follow-up of untreated carpal tunnel syndrome: a multicenter study. Neurology. 2001;56:1459–67.
60. Padua L, Padua R, Lo Monaco M, et al. Natural history of carpal tunnel syndrome according to the neurophysiological classification. Ital J Neurol Sci. 1998;19:357–61.
61. Ortiz-Corredor F, Enriquez F, Diaz RJ, Calambas N. Natural evolution of carpal tunnel syndrome in untreated patients. Clin Neurophysiol. 2008;119:1373–8.
62. Resende LA, Tahara A, Fonseca RG, Sardenberg T. The natural history of carpal tunnel syndrome: a study of 20 hands evaluated 4 to 9 years after initial diagnosis. Electromyogr Clin Neurophysiol. 2003;43:301–4.
63. Bickel KD. Carpal tunnel syndrome. J Hand Surg Am. 2010;35:147–52.
64. Shiri R, Miranda H, Heliovaara M, Viikari-Juntura E. Physical work load factors and carpal tunnel syndrome: a population-based study. Occup Environ Med. 2009;66:368–73.
65. Stevens J, Sun S, Beard C. Carpal tunnel syndrome in Rochester, Minnesota, 1961 to 1980. Neurology. 1988;38:134–8.
66. Gerritsen AA, de Vet HC, Scholten RJ, Bertelsmann FW, de Krom MC, Bouter LM. Splinting vs surgery in the treatment of carpal tunnel syndrome: a randomized controlled trial. JAMA. 2002;288:1245–51.
67. Gray H. Anatomy of the human body (See "book" section below). Bartleby.com: Gray's Anatomy, Plate 422; 1918.
68. Sobotta J. Atlas and text-book of human anatomy, volume III, vascular system, lymphatic system, nervous system and sense organs. Philadelphia: W. B. Saunders; 1908.

17 A 55-Year-Old Woman with Little Finger Numbness and Pain for 6 Months

Tariq Malik

Case Report

A 55-year-old woman is referred to the pain clinic for pain in her left hand. The pain started 6 months ago with no inciting event. She has a desk job and works on a computer all day. Her symptoms are the worst early in the morning and toward the end of the day. She has a history of diabetes and hypertension, but both are well controlled. She has tried a wrist-splint followed by an elbow-splint as suggested by her primary care physician, but despite trying it for a month, she has noticed no relief. She has been referred to the pain clinic for further evaluation and management of her symptoms.

On close questioning, she describes most of her symptoms confined to ring and little finger, but at times all over the hand. She denies any weakness but acknowledges easy fatigability when typing or writing. She also noticed weird feeling in her hand when she is driving for a long time. She has tried over-the-counter medication but with no relief. She is sleeping OK but wakes up infrequently with a sensation that her fingers are numb or dead.

T. Malik (✉)
Department of Anesthesia and Critical Care, University of Chicago, Chicago, IL, USA
e-mail: tmalik@dacc.uchicago.edu; TMuslim@dacc.uchicago.edu

What Is Your Diagnosis?

The patient has symptoms very suggestive of entrapment neuropathy. The common sites of nerve entrapment are at or around elbow and at the wrist. The median, ulnar, and radial nerves or their branches quite often get entrapped. The diagnosis of nerve entrapment requires localization of the nerve involved, site of entrapment, extent of nerve dysfunction, and the pathophysiology of nerve entrapment.

History and physical examination are quite important in localizing the site, nerve involved, and the extent of nerve dysfunction. The detailed knowledge of anatomy of the nerve course and its innervation is very helpful to make a clinical diagnosis. The median nerve has no motor or sensory branches in the arm, but it innervates the flexor and pronator muscles in the anterior compartment of the forearm (except the flexor carpi ulnaris and part of the flexor digitorum profundus, innervated by the ulnar nerve). It also supplies innervation to the thenar muscles and lateral two lumbricals in the hand. Its palmar cutaneous branch innervates the lateral aspect of the palm, and the digital cutaneous branch innervates the lateral three and a half fingers on the anterior (palmar) surface of the hand. The radial nerve innervates most of the skin of the posterior side of forearm, the dorsal surface of the lateral side of the palm, and dorsal surface of the lateral three and a half digits. It also provides the motor

T. Malik (ed.), *Practical Chronic Pain Management*, https://doi.org/10.1007/978-3-030-46675-6_17

innervation to the triceps brachii and the extensor muscles in the forearm. Ulnar nerve has no sensory or motor branches in the arm, but as it enters the forearm behind the medial epicondyle, it passes the two heads of the flexor carpi ulnaris, innervating it. Ulnar nerve supplies the medial half of flexor digitorum profundus and majority of the small muscles of the hand, and is the sensory nerve for the medial side of the hand.

The patient symptoms are confined to the ring and little finger. She denies any weakness in wrist flexor muscle group. She has noticed fatigability when she types or drives for long distance. This makes it more likely that ulnar nerve is dysfunctional most likely at or below the elbow after the branches to the forearm muscles have left the main nerve.

How Would You Prove Your Diagnosis?

The history is very suggestive of ulnar nerve dysfunction. A careful physical examination should focus on sensory and motor exam of each major nerve supplying the forearm and the hand. In case of ulnar nerve, the focus should be on testing flexor carpi ulnaris, hypothenar muscles, adduction/abduction of the fingers, and the sensory testing of hypothenar eminence and of the medial most two digits. The physical findings may or may not be positive depending upon the extent of nerve dysfunction. Special tests to evaluate nerve compression include Tinel's sign and Froment's sign. Froment's sign is a test of adductor pollicis function; to compensate for loss of this muscle function results in flexion of interphalangeal joint of the thumb, a positive Froment's sign. This is elicited when patient is asked to pinch a piece of paper between the thumb and index finger. Percussion of ulnar nerve at the site of compression can elicit paresthesia or tingling sensation along the nerve.

It is important to rule out other potential causes. Review of system is important to look for any rheumatological disorders, orthopedic joint–related issues, neurological problems, thoracic outlet syndrome, and cervical spine foraminal issues causing radicular pain, and any other disease like tumor irritating the brachial plexus and mimicking ulnar nerve neuropathy. It is extremely important to ensure that the patient does not have another coexisting nerve entrapment problem or masquerading as ulnar nerve pain.

Do You Need Any Testing?

Ulnar nerve entrapment is a clinical diagnosis. Part of the evaluation is to look for any contributing factors, confirm the exact site of entrapment, document the extent of nerve dysfunction for prognosis and recovery, and any underlying disease process causing or contributing to the problem, i.e., physical injury, infection, tumor, bone deformity, or any immune-mediated process.

Physical examination should include complete upper extremity examination including neck range of motion, shoulder and elbow joint examination, as well as hand examination. Physical examination is good at excluding other issues but still may not be able to rule out certain disease processes. X-ray of the elbow joint may exclude any bony problem. Blood work is not needed unless systemic disorder is suspected, in which case its better ordered and managed by the rheumatologist or the primary care physician.

EMG/NCV study is useful in localizing the site of nerve entrapment as well as type of lesion (demyelination vs. axonal loss). If the symptoms are mild (predominantly sensory and little to no motor dysfunction/weakness) electromyography study does not need to be done. In case of severe symptoms and when planning for surgery, it is very helpful to have the study done to localize the site of ulnar nerve entrapment as it would help to plan for the site and extent of nerve decompression. It is imperative to the study if the diagnosis is less than clear to rule out brachial plexopathy or any other neurological problem not only to avoid a futile surgery but also for proper management of the patient. The study is also helpful in tracking the recovery after surgery. Therefore, preoperative study is quite helpful for later comparison. Severe abnormalities in preoperative study are a marker of poor recovery.

Ultrasound of the nerve has also been found to be helpful. It is operator dependent, and data is still limited. The nerve is scanned along the length for any swelling or echogenic deformity. The sensitivity has been found to be better than EMG/NCV.

MRI is done to evaluate the nerve and any other pathology. T2 sequence is used to look for any swelling or deformity. It has reportedly extremely high sensitivity. It can also help in evaluating any other pathology around the nerve that could be causing the problem.

What Is the Pathophysiology of This Condition?

The nerve is damaged by either compression, traction, or stretching. Stretching seems to be the most common mechanism. The nerve has long tortuous course especially in and around elbow. When the elbow is moved from full extension to full flexion, the nerve needs to stretch around 30% from its baseline at rest. This traction can be worse if there is accompanying elbow joint pathology after fracture, dislocation, arthritis, or from valgus deformity. The stretch may compromise blood flow to the nerve causing demyelination and or axonal loss. The range of movement from extension to flexion can cause the nerve to dislocate in and of the ulnar groove causing mechanical irritation and damage. The movement also causes narrowing of the space between the medial epicondyle and olecranon process; the space is bridged by the origin of flexor carpi ulnaris muscle with the ulnar nerve underneath the muscle. The pressure around the nerve under the muscle has been measured at 200 mmHg either at full flexion or during isometric forearm muscle contraction.

The nerve is also exposed in the retro-epicondylar area and is open to direct trauma or to repetitive micro-trauma during a regular day's work.

How Do You Manage This Condition?

The management depends upon the underlying reason. Quite often, there is no secondary issue. The most common reason for ulnar nerve dysfunction is profession related (work or athletic). It is important to evaluate biomechanics of the work place environment. Avoiding extreme flexion of the elbow is helpful. In general, acetaminophen and NSADIs are attempted but there is no evidence they are helpful in case of chronic nerve entrapment. Role of membrane stabilizing drugs has also not been tested in any study. Splints are helpful in special situations. Unintentional prolonged elbow flexion like when asleep or at work can be avoided if an elbow splint is worn to remind and to prevent extreme flexion.

Any Role for Injection Therapy?

The role of injection therapy is not clear. In general, in the few studies that evaluated it, it was not very effective. Injection does have a diagnostic value in localizing the site of compression. Quite often, steroid is injected to treat any inflammatory component that could be making the nerve compression worse. If it helps, it is worth repeating it as long the relief is significant and for a long time without any worsening symptoms. Normally the relief is short lived and there is always a danger of making the matter worse by injuring the nerve with needle or intraneural injection. Ultrasound guidance is quite helpful though does not guarantee that it will not happen.

When Should the Patient Be Referred for Surgery?

A patient should be referred for surgery when the patient has failed 3–6 months of conservative therapy depending upon severity of the symptoms. When motor weakness is present, surgery should be done earlier than later. If the sign of axonal loss is present on initial evaluation, the patient should be referred for surgical evaluation right away. The surgical outcome is much better when done early. The most important step before surgical intervention is proper diagnosis as decompression at the wrong site will not help, and extensive decompression can jeopardize the health of the nerve by damaging its blood supply. Also, in the absence of nerve entrapment pathology, the surgery will not work. The surgical interventions vary from minimal decompression to anterior transposition.

Discussion

Ulnar neuropathy is the second most frequent entrapment neuropathy in adults [1]. In a study in the general population in Italy, incidence was 20.9%, with males affected more than females [2]. The nerve has long and tortuous course and can be compressed at many points from elbow to the wrist. The ulnar nerve comes from the lower trunk of the brachial plexus and its fibers come from C8 to T1 nerve roots. The nerve runs medial to the brachial artery in the upper arm, in close proximity to the median nerve. The nerve innervates no structure in the arm. The nerve runs between the medial head of the triceps and medial intermuscular septum on its way to the medial epicondyle. Close to the elbow, it runs through the retro-epicondylar groove between the medial epicondyle and olecranon process. It then passes under the humero-ulnar aponeurotic arcade (HUA), also called the Osborne ligament, which is a dense aponeurosis between the tendon attachments of the flexor carpi ulnaris (FCU). The area beneath the Osborn ligament is also called the cubital tunnel. The nerve then passes through the belly of the FCU muscle and out through the deep flexor-pronator aponeurosis. The nerve innervates the FCU and the flexor digitorum profundus (FDP) in the forearm. In the distal forearm, the palmar ulnar cutaneous branch (PUC) and the dorsal ulnar cutaneous (DUC) branch come off the ulnar nerve before it enters the hand ventral to the Guyon canal. The ulnar nerve then enters through the Guyon canal at the level of the distal wrist crease. The flexor retinaculum and hypothenar muscles define the floor, while the roof consists of the volar carpal ligament. The lateral (radial) border is defined by the hook of the hamate, while the pisiform, pisohamate ligament, and abductor digiti minimi muscle belly compose the medial (ulnar) border. The ulnar nerve passes through the Guyon canal with the ulnar artery.

In the canal, the nerve separates into the superficial sensory branch and the deep palmar motor branch. The superficial sensory branch provides sensory innervation to the palmar aspects of the medial half of the fourth digit and the fifth digit. Before the nerve exits through the pisohamate hiatus, the motor fibers branch off from the deep palmar motor branch to innervate the hypothenar muscles (abductor digiti minimi, flexor digiti minimi, opponens digiti minimi, and palmaris brevis). The deep palmar branch gives motor innervation to the adductor pollicis, the deep head of the flexor pollicis brevis, the third and fourth lumbricals, and the three palmar and four dorsal interossei muscles [3].

The anatomic factors put the nerve at risk of damage along its long course. Its exposed at the cubital tunnel and subject to trauma. The nerve is subject to compression at medial intermuscular septum, ulnar groove, cubital tunnel, and the flexor-pronator aponeurosis. Among all these compression points, cubital tunnel is the most common site of ulnar entrapment [4].

The pressure within the cubital tunnel increases [5], and the nerve needs to lengthen to accommodate for increase in the distance as the elbow goes from extension to flexion. Several anatomic variations of the HUA can contribute to ulnar nerve compression. The HUA retinaculum connecting medial epicondyle and olecranon may be either hypertrophied, compressing the nerve, or absent, allowing sub-luxation of the nerve from the groove during elbow flexion [6]. Displacement or dislocation of the ulnar nerve occurs in 5–30% of normal individuals and can be associated with nerve injury [7]. Dislocation usually occurs bilaterally and thus has no localizing significance. A unilaterally dislocated ulnar nerve can be an important clinical sign. The HUA retinaculum may be replaced by an accessory muscle, the anconeus epitrochlearis (5–30% in cadaver studies), which is proposed to cause ulnar neuropathy in some cases [8].

The ulnar nerve entrapment presents as intermittent numbness and tingling in the ulnar nerve distribution unless precipitating factor is a trauma. It is usually associated with elbow flexion, particularly at night. Pain is not a dominant feature, but patients may complain of pain due to overuse of the forearm flexors. The symptoms become continuous if the entrapment progressively gets severe. The natural history of entrapment is unknown. In general, patients with only sensory symptoms do not progress and did not require surgery at 100 months of follow-up [9]. Motor symptoms are a late presentation. The motor weakness affects pinching movement of the thumb, dexterity of fingers, and strength of grasp movement. The wrist flexion is not affected significantly due to preservation of flexi carpi radialis muscle. On physical examination, sensory deficit can be demonstrated in the ulnar nerve distribution. Motor sign of weakness is seen in the form of positive Froment's sign (due to weak adductor pollicis), clawing of hand due to unopposed extension at metacarpophalangeal joint, and unopposed flexion at the interphalangeal joints. Palmaris brevis wrinkle sign is positive, which is wrinkling of the skin over the hypothenar eminence when patient abducts the little finger. Forced flexion of the elbow and sustained pressure over the various points of ulnar nerve are equivalent to median nerve compression test and Phalen test. These two tests together have very high sensitivity (91%) in diagnosing ulnar nerve entrapment [10]. Weakness of the third palmer interosseous results in abduction posture of little finger, which is an early sign and called Wartenberg's sign. Compression at the wrist results in a variety of findings from pure sensory findings to mixture of motor and sensory signs to pure motor signs. The most common type of ulnar neuropathies at the wrist is compression of the deep palmar branch. Ulnar neuropathies of the wrist and hand are divided into three types. Type I lesion involves deep and the superficial branches of the ulnar nerve just proximal to or within the Guyon canal; this causes mixed motor and sensory deficits and weakness of hand muscles. Type II is from a lesion involving the deep branch which causes a pure motor deficit. Type III lesion is confined to the superficial branch, causing sensory deficits to the palmar aspect of the medial half of the fourth digit and the fifth digit. The sensory loss in type I and type III lesions spares the dorsal aspect of the hand and fingers and the hypothenar eminence [11].

Ulnar nerve entrapment is a clinical diagnosis, but the clinical features are not reliable and anatomical variations make any symptom or sign to be fool proof. The physical signs have low diagnostic accuracy [12]. This makes electrophysiological studies invariably needed. The study serves many purposes. It can document presence of mono-neuropathy, localize the site of entrapment, rule out other diseases like motor neuron disease, and type of damage (demyelination vs. axonal loss). The study has variable sensitivity from 37% to 90% with specificity at around 95% [13]. The sensitivity is low in mild cases and high in severe cases. The American Association of Neuromuscular and Electrodiagnostic Medicine (AANEM) Guidelines are frequently cited in most studies of ulnar neuropathy at the elbow. The AANEM guidelines [14] for the diagnosis of ulnar neuropathy at the elbow recommend performing ulnar sensory nerve conduction studies and motor nerve conduction studies to the abductor digiti minimi. Elbow position during testing (with flexion between 70° and 90° recommended) should be recorded and adequate warming maintained. A minimum of 10 cm should be present between the above-elbow and below-elbow sites of stimulation. The diagnosis of ulnar neuropathy at the elbow can be made when the conduction velocity across the elbow is greater than or equal to 10 m/s slower than the wrist to below-elbow segment. Other supportive findings include a drop in CMAP amplitude of greater than 20% across the elbow. The sensitivity can be improved if the 10 cm above and below the elbow distance is explored at 2 cm intervals. Needle electromyography is not as sensitive as velocity conduction studies but helps to confirm ulnar neuropathy by demonstrating normal activity in non-ulnar innervated muscles. Lately, the role of ultrasound is being evaluated in the diagnosis of ulnar entrapment. The focal enlargement is used to diagnose nerve pathology. The main issue is finding cut-off limits for the diagnostic purposes as the extent of normal size variation is not known. Beekman et al. proposed cross-sectional area of 10 mm^2 and diameter of 2.4 mm as upper limits of normal. Using these criteria, the ultrasound was found to have sensitivity similar to that to EMG/NCV (80%). Volpes et al. found CSA of 14.6 $mm^2 \pm 5$ mm in diseased nerve vs. 7.1 $mm^2 \pm 2$ mm in normal subjects. They also found that there was a correlation between the nerve surface area and severity of the nerve dysfunction as seen on electrophysiological study – larger the nerve size, more the severity of entrapment. The ultrasound imaging is also useful in excluding false negative NCV study. Mapping the nerve before the study can diagnose a dislocated ulnar nerve. This helps measure the exact length of the nerve when performing NCV study, which otherwise would have been spuriously fast due to nerve subluxation [15]. MRI is also a useful imaging modality [16]. The T2 sequence is used to look for any sign of hyperintensity at the site of nerve dysfunction. The size of the nerve can be measured more reliably than ultrasound, which is an operator-dependent technique. The MRI sensitivity has been found to be around 83–85%. MRI can help localize the lesion when EMG cannot localize its exact site. MRI can also help evaluate mild lesions when EMG study is negative as well as pick up false positive EMG study. There is a current trend to replace EMG/NCV study with either ultrasound or MRI but even though the studies are promising there is not enough information available for these imaging modalities to replace EMG/NCV test yet.

Various systems have been proposed to categorize ulnar nerve entrapment severity. McGowan proposed his grading system in 1950, which is still widely used (Table 17.1). Dellon proposed his 10-point system to categorize disease intensity using objective findings on physical examination. These grading systems are used to evaluate response of patients to therapy.

Management of the nerve entrapment is based on two basic principles: lower the pressure or decompress the nerve. The conservative approach is used in the absence of severe symptoms. This consists of patient education on biomechanics that increase pressure on the nerve at the elbow level. This includes educating the patient to avoid posture that requires extreme or prolonged elbow flexion like during reading or telephoning, helping him modify the work environment by optimizing the height of the work surface and to pad surfaces on which the elbow and the forearm rest, as well as, splinting the elbow during sleep to discourage prolonged flexion. Steroid injections have not been found to be helpful [17–19]. Surgery is the definite solution if done at the proper site of compression. Various surgical techniques are used from in situ release, to medial epicondylectomy, to anterior transposition. Despite an extensive body of literature, the preferred approach to decompress the ulnar nerve at the elbow is still unknown. The results of each technique are comparable. However, decompression with the nerve transposition is associated with more wound infections than simple decompression [20]. Simple decompression is associated with smaller incision, shorter operative time, less intraoperative manipulation of the nerve, and a lower risk of nerve devascularization. Campbell et al. have stressed the importance of the proper surgical approach by ensuring to localize the exact site of nerve entrapment [21].

Most reports in the surgical literature are optimistic with satisfactory improvement or complete recovery achieved in 80–90% of patients undergoing decompression by a variety of means. The duration of symptoms before surgery is an important predictor of surgical success. A history of trauma to the elbow, the presence of muscle atrophy, and epineural fibrosis found intra-operative correlate with poor outcome [22].

Table 17.1 McGowan classification of ulnar neuropathy at the elbow

GARDE	Sensory symptoms	Motor examination
1	Mild paresthesia or sensory loss	No weakness
2A	Moderate sensory loss	No intrinsic atrophy, mild weakness
2B	Moderate sensory loss	3/5 Intrinsic strength, moderate weakness
3	Severe sensory loss or paresthesia	Severe intrinsic atrophy and weakness

Data from Goldberg et al. [23]

Conclusion

Ulnar nerve is a very common mono-neuropathy due to its unique anatomical location, which exposes itself to nerve damage. Diagnosis is usually straightforward if proper physical examination is performed. However, due to anatomical variation, it could be challenging. Majority of cases resolve with conservative measures. If symptoms are severe or surgical intervention is planned, EMG/NCV should be done to find the exact site of compression. MRI and/or ultrasound can be useful in narrowing down the site of entrapment. Steroid injection is not helpful. Proper surgical technique depends upon identifying the exact site of compression before the surgery, otherwise it will fail. All surgical techniques are equally good options. Surgical outcome depends upon the duration of symptoms and severity of the symptoms before the surgery.

References

1. Miller RG. Ulnar nerve lesions. In: Brown WF, Bolton CF, editors. Clinical electromyography. Stoneham: Butterworths; 1987. p. 99–116.
2. Chang KV, Wu WT, Han DS, Özçakar L. Ulnar nerve cross-sectional area for the diagnosis of cubital tunnel syndrome: a meta-analysis of ultrasonographic measurements. Arch Phys Med Rehabil. 2018;99(4):743–57.
3. Depukat P, Mizia E, Klosinski M, et al. Anatomy of Guyon's canal - a systematic review. Folia Med Cracov. 2014;54(2):81–6.
4. Palmer BA, Hughes TB. Cubital tunnel syndrome. J Hand Surg Am. 2010;35(1):153–6.
5. Werner CO, Ohlin P, Elmqvist D. Pressure recorded in neuropathy. Acta Orthop Scan. 1985;56:404–6.
6. ODriscoll SW, Horii E, Carmichael SW, et al. The cubital tunnel and ulnar neuropathy. J Bone Joint Surg. 1991;73B:613–7.
7. Childress HM. Recurrent ulnar nerve dislocation at the elbow. Clin Orthop. 1975;108:168–73.
8. Masear VR, Hill JJ, Cohen SM. Ulnar compression neuropathy secondary to the anconeus epitrochlearis muscle. J Hand Surg Am. 1988;13A:720–4.
9. Dellon AL, Hament W, Gittelshon A. Non-operative management of cubital tunnel syndrome: an eight year prospective study. Neurology. 1993;43:1673–7.
10. Novak CB, Lee GW, MacKinnon SE, et al. Provocative testing for cubital tunnel syndrome. J Hand Surg Am. 1994;19A:817–20.
11. Robertson C, Saratsiotis J. A review of compressive ulnar neuropathy at the elbow. J Manip Physiol Ther. 2005;28(5):345.
12. Beekman R, Schreuder AH, Rozeman CA, Koehler PJ, Uitdehaag BM. The diagnostic value of provocative clinical tests in ulnar neuropathy at the elbow is marginal. J Neurol Neurosurg Psychiatry. 2009;80:1369–74.
13. Werner RA. Electrodiagnostic evaluation of carpal tunnel syndrome and ulnar neuropathies. PMR. 2013;5(5 Suppl):S14–21.
14. Thibault MW, Robinson LR, Franklin G, Fulton-Kehoe D. Use of the AAEM guidelines in electrodiagnosis of ulnar neuropathy at the elbow. Am J Phys Med Rehabil. 2005;84(4):267Y273.
15. Campbell WW, Carroll DJ, Greenberg MK, et al. Literature review of the usefulness of nerve conduction studies and electromyography in the evaluation of the patients with ulnar neuropathy at the elbow. Muscle Nerve. 1999;22(Suppl 8):S175–205.
16. Vucic S, Cordato DJ, Yiannikas C, et al. Utility of magnetic resonance imaging in diagnosing ulnar neuropathy at the elbow. Clin Neurophysiol. 2006;117:590–5.
17. Hong C, Long H, Kanakamedala V, et al. Splinting and local steroid injection for the treatment of ulnar neuropathy at the elbow: clinical and electrophysiological evaluation. Arch Phys Med Rehabil. 1996;77:573–7.
18. vanVeen KE, Alblas KC, Alons IM, Kerklaan JP, Siegersma MC, Wesstein M, Visser LH, Vankasteel V, Jellema K. Corticosteroid injection in patients with ulnar neuropathy at the elbow: a randomized, double-blind, placebo-controlled trial. Muscle Nerve. 2015;52(3):380–5.
19. Podnar S, Omejec G. Why do local corticosteroid injections work in carpal tunnel syndrome, but not in ulnar neuropathy at the elbow? Muscle Nerve. 2016;53(4):662–3.
20. Khedr EM, Fawi G, Allah Abbas MA, El-Fetoh NA, Zaki AF, Gamea A. Prevalence of common types of compression neuropathies in Qena Governorate/Egypt: a population-based survey. Neuroepidemiology. 2016;46(4):253–60.
21. Campbell WW, Pridgeon RM, Sahni KS. Short segment incremental studies in the evaluation of ulnar neuropathy at the elbow. Muscle Nerve. 1992;15:1050–4.
22. Chan RC, Paine KWE, Varughese G. Ulnar neuropathy at the elbow: comparison of simple decompression and anterior transposition. Neurosurgery. 1980;7:7545–50.
23. Goldberg BJ, Light TR, Blair SJ. Ulnar neuropathy at the elbow: results of medial epicondylectomy. J Hand Surg Am. 1989;14(2 Pt 1):182–8.

A 68-Year-Old Man with Chronic Wrist Pain

18

Evan Goodman and Tariq Malik

Case Description

A 68-year-old, right-hand-dominant man presents to the pain clinic with the chief complaint of right wrist pain with significant range of motion limitation. His pain has slowly progressed over the past 5 years, which has ultimately led to him retiring from his job in the auto industry, where he worked on an assembly line. His pain has previously been managed with NSAIDs. He describes the pain as being a constant 6/10 ache in his wrist which is worsened by activity. He denies any previous trauma but endorses that the nature of his work required him to partake in repetitive motions of his hands. On exam, he displays significant tenderness to palpation of the dorsal aspect of the hand with mild swelling and limitation of flexion, extension, and rotation due to pain.

What Is Your Preliminary Diagnosis?

In the absence of any red flag in the history, i.e., weight loss, fever, swelling, discoloration of the skin, or major trauma, chronic joint pain is most likely from wear and tear of the joint. The preliminary diagnosis in this patient would include either idiopathic or post-traumatic osteoarthritis of the wrist or thumb. Idiopathic causes include avascular necrosis of the carpal bones, congenital deformities of the wrist causing abnormal loading patterns of the carpal bones, and localized scaphotrapezium-trapezoid arthritis. Post-traumatic osteoarthritis is the result of damage to the ligaments and bones of the wrist, which ultimately leads to distorted loading patterns of the carpal bones causing progressive arthrosis of the joints, which can be described in a staging format [1–3].

How Is Diagnosis Confirmed?

The confirmation of diagnosis first begins with a thorough history focusing on the age of the patient, hand dominance, time course of symptoms, hobbies and occupation, as well as activities or specific motions which exacerbate symptoms. This is then followed by a physical exam focusing on limitations in range of motion, loss of strength, exercises which reproduce symptoms and palpation for areas of tenderness,

E. Goodman
Department of Anesthesiology and Critical Care, University of Chicago, Chicago, IL, USA
e-mail: egoodman@dacc.uchicago.edu

T. Malik (✉)
Department of Anesthesia and Critical Care, University of Chicago, Chicago, IL, USA
e-mail: TMuslim@dacc.uchicago.edu; tmalik@dacc.uchicago.edu

T. Malik (ed.), *Practical Chronic Pain Management*, https://doi.org/10.1007/978-3-030-46675-6_18

crepitus, erythema, and/or swelling. The focus of the physical exam should be to pinpoint the specific joints involved in producing the patient's symptoms and to rule out any other diagnosis. Specific exams include Watson's test which assesses scaphoid lunate instability in patients with SLAC wrist (scapholunate advanced collapse), tenderness over the anatomical snuff box, and pain with pronation and supination, which are associated with SNAC wrist (scaphoid nonunion advanced collapse). Following a detailed history and physical exam, radiographic X-ray imaging plays the role in identifying the cause of wrist osteoarthritis as well as establishing joint involvement and extent of pathology [4]. More extensive exams with CT or MRI are rarely performed; however a CT arthrogram has utility prior to limited wrist fusions to evalaute the joint spaces of the joint at the writs as well as quality of the bones that would be fused. MRI is only indicated in patients with Keinbock's disease (carpal avascular necrosis) when evaluating for the utility of a proximal row carpectomy [4]. Additionally, local anesthetic/steroid joint injections play a role in diagnosis as they may assist in pinpointing the specific joints involved.

What Is the Pathophysiology of This Condition?

The wrist is a complex joint made up of 7 carpal bones and more than 30 ligaments arranged into proximal and distal rows with connections with the distal radius and ulna or metacarpal bones, respectively. Although the osteoarthritic processes that affecting these joint spaces share the same pathophysiology, the ultimate etiology that begins the process is what differs. Osteoarthritis of the wrist can be categorized as occurring either as the result of an idiopathic or traumatic process. Idiopathic conditions include Keinbock's disease resulting in avascular necrosis of the lunate and congenital malformations of the carpal bones causing altered joint kinematics. Any trauma to the carpal bones or their associated ligaments may result in altered kinematics and loading conditions of the carpal bones facilitating an osteoarthritic process. Watson and Ballet described a progressive osteoarthritic process as a result of chronic scapholunate tears known as scaphoid lunate advanced collapse of the wrist (SLAC), which starts at the radial styloid-scaphoid junction and then progresses to involve each carpal joint [1]. Additionally, fracture and nonunion of the scaphoid bone has also been described to result in a similar progression of osteoarthritis of the wrist, and this has been termed scaphoid nonunion advanced collapse (SNAC). Regardless of the inciting event, the pathophysiology behind the osteoarthritic process is the same.

The pathophysiology of osteoarthritis begins in the cartilage surrounding the joint space. With mechanical stress and injury, chondrocytes undergo altered gene expression producing increased amounts of inflammatory cytokines including IL-1B and TNF alpha and matrix degrading enzymes such as collagenase and ADAMTS-5, which break down the cartilage surface. As collagen fragments are released, more cytokines and chemokines become present as an inflammatory process occurs, thus continuing to promote an environment of cartilage catabolism. Early stages of osteoarthritis are characterized by abnormalities in the cartilage surface. With progression of disease, this then results in erosion, which can progress all the way to the subchondral bone, which becomes activated and thickens. Osteophytes also develop at the margins of the joint spaces, which can be seen on X-ray images. These are areas of new cartilage formation, which ultimately ossifies due to neurovascular invasion from bone [5].

How Is This Problem Managed?

The management of osteoarthritis of the wrist is focused on relief of pain and improving function. Most patients are disturbed by pain and less by loss of functionality from losing range of motion. Key aspect of the management is to assess the effect of wrist pain on patient's life. Various interventions are available, but none reverses the underlying pathology. Most interventions are treating the symptoms only. A stepwise approach to the management of osteoarthritis of the wrist begins with non-surgical interventions such as activity modification, physical and occupational therapy, and splinting. Analgesics such as topical and oral non-steroidal anti-inflammatory agents are the first line agents for pain relief as recommended by both the American College of Rheumatology and the National Institute for Health and Care Excellence. These medications include Diclofenac, Indomethacin, Ibuprofen, and Naproxen. Although a meta-analysis supports the efficacy of oral NSAIDs with a moderate effect size of 0.29 (95% CI 0.22–0.35) [6], chronic use is associated with gastrointestinal, cardiovascular, and renal toxicity. Special consideration needs to be taken when prescribing these agents to patients as those with a history of peptic ulcer disease may benefit from a selective COX-2 inhibitor while an individual with a history of cardiovascular disease may benefit from a non-selective COX inhibitor, as selective COX-2 inhibitors are associated with increased risk of myocardial infarction, stroke, and mortality. The European Society for Clinical and Economic Aspects of Osteoporosis and Osteoarthritis (ESCEO) developed a treatment algorithm (Fig. 18.1) for assisting in the prescribing of appropriate NSAID agents to patients with osteoarthritis and can be an invaluable tool when prescribing NSAID agents to patients with risk factors [7]. Given the risks associated with oral NSAID therapy, topical preparations of NSAIDs are now playing a larger role in the treatment of osteoarthritis as their risk profile is less significant than their oral counterparts, and their pooled effect size from a meta-analysis published by Zhang et al. was greater at 0.44 (95% CI 0.27, 0.62).

The next step to consider in the management of osteoarthritis is the utility of intra-articular injections of a mixture of a local anesthetic and steroid. These injections play a role in being diagnostic and therapeutic in part that, if the correct joint is injected, the patient will experience immediate relief from the local anesthetic and lasting relief from the long acting steroid. Most evidence in support of the efficacy of joint injections for the treatment of osteoarthritis of the wrist is anecdotal; however, an RCT by Meenagh et al. showed no clinical benefit gained from intra-articular steroid injections to the first CMCJ patients with moderate to severe osteoarthritis in comparison to a placebo injection [8]. Interestingly, although VAS scores were not reduced in either group, beneficial effects on the patient's general well-being were observed in both groups. Although this study focused on injection of the first CMJ joint, other joints which can be injected under ultrasound guidance include the radiocarpal joint, distal radioulnar joint, and carpal joints. The magnitude of relief as well as the time course is variable between patients. The goal of the injection is to provide a period of relief to both increase the mobility of the infected joint and allow the patient to continue to participate in physical therapy and occupational therapy to strengthen the supporting muscles and ligaments around the affected joint. Repeat injections can occur every 3 months; however, if the injections and medical management provide minimal relief, the patient may require surgical intervention. Complications associated with intra-articular and periarticular injections include bleeding, infection, pain, trophic changes in the skin, and failure to provide relief.

Should medical management and injections fail to provide the patient with relief of symptoms, the next step is surgical intervention. The goal of surgery is to preserve as much mobility of the joint as possible while providing pain relief. The surgical techniques involved are selected based upon the progression of the disease, age of the patient, current joint mobility, and functional demands of the patient. The mobility-preserving surgical techniques include total wrist arthroplasty, proximal row carpectomy, partial fusion, and wrist denervation. The non-mobility preserving technique is a total wrist fusion, which is undertaken in patients with severe disease [9]. Although preservation of wrist mobility is important, a study by Laulan et al. revealed that 59% of patients are willing to sacrifice mobility for pain relief and that after surgery persistent pain is the main source of dissatisfaction with the procedure [10].

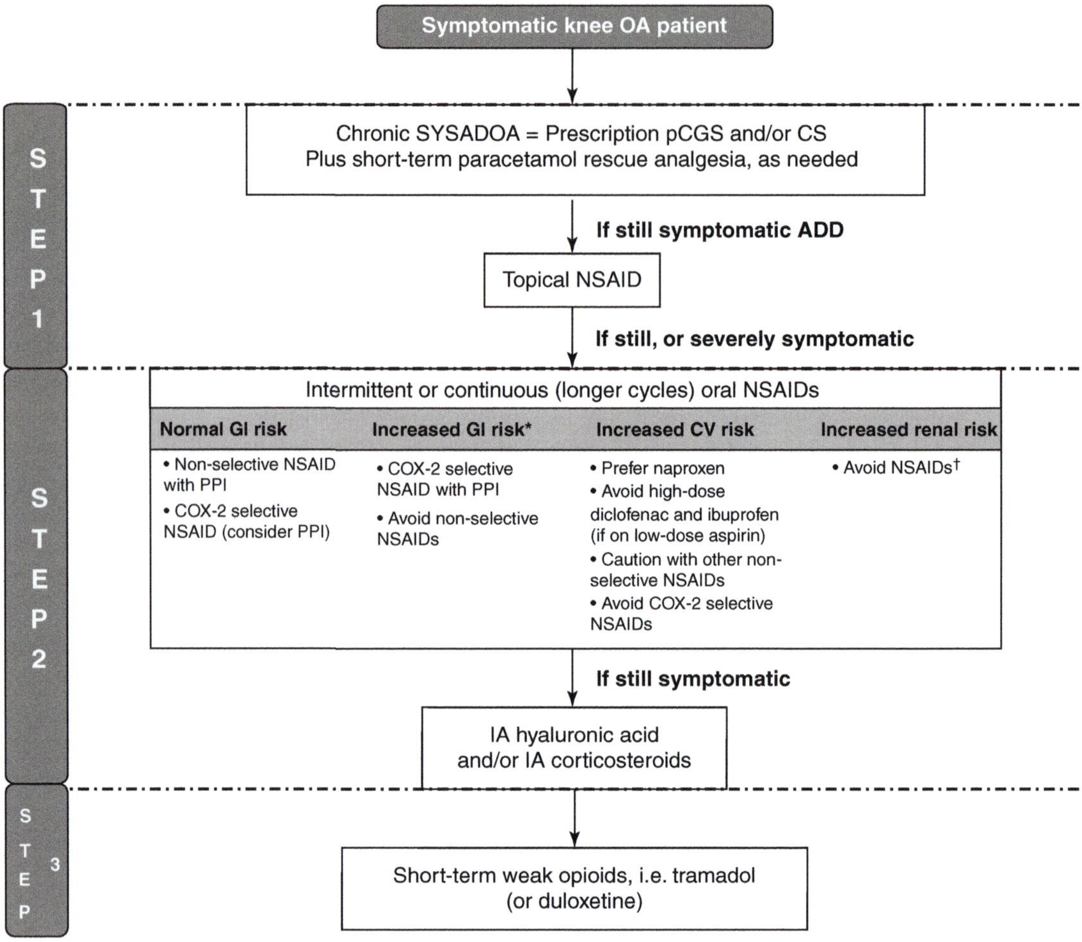

Fig. 18.1 European Society for Clinical and Economic Aspects of Osteoporosis and Osteoarthritis (ESCEO) developed a treatment algorithm. (From Bruyère et al. [7], with permission)

What Is the Long-Term Outcome – Complete Cure or Recurrent/Chronic Persistent Problem?

Osteoarthritis of the wrist is progressive disease process, which may be asymptomatic in its early stages with pain not presenting until later stages when significant joint damage has occurred or multiple joints have become involved. Early conservative management is often only temporary as wear and tear continues to be imparted on affected joints and oral and topical analgesics and local anesthetic/steroid injections become less effective. Surgical interventions become the next method of treatment; however, these too are only palliative. Mobility-preserving procedures using implantable hardware eventually begin to break down ultimately necessitating the patient to a total wrist fusion or wrist denervation as definitive therapy.

Discussion

Prevalence

Due to the progressive nature of the disease process where early stages may be asymptomatic or tolerable, the prevalence is difficult to determine. It also varies with age and with occupation. Among manual workers, it is the most common complaint along with back pain. A systematic review of 4000 radiographs found a prevalence of 5% [1], and a randomized cross-sectional national prevalence survey found a lifetime prevalence of 3.58% in employed individuals [2].

Differential Diagnosis

The wrist is a complex joint formed by the distal radius, distal ulna, seven carpal bones with multiple ligamentous attachments, and the base of the five metacarpal bones. It also forms the carpal tunnel containing the median nerve. The common generators of pain include the multiple articular surfaces of the carpal and metacarpal bones and their associated ligaments, the median nerve, and the tendon and muscular attachments of the first digit. Given the complexity of the joint and its diverse structural contents, there may be interrelating etiologies of a patient's wrist pain. In addition to osteoarthritis, the multiple articular surfaces contained within the wrist are also susceptible to rheumatoid arthritis and rarely gout and pseudogout. RA is an inflammatory process usually involving both wrist joints and may also result in deformity of the joint. Although rare, gouty arthritis and pseudo gout can affect the joints of the wrist [11]. It is the result of the deposition of uric acid and calcium pyrophosphate dihydrate crystals, respectively, in the joint space. Symptoms include an acute mono-arthritis with significant joint pain, erythema, and swelling.

The carpal bones themselves and their associated ligaments are also susceptible to injury secondary to trauma or metabolic processes such as Keinbock's disease, which results in avascular necrosis of the lunate. Another common generator of pain in the wrist includes an overuse injury of the first carpal metacarpal joint, which can result in both an osteoarthritis and/or de Quervain's tenosynovitis affecting the abductor pollicis longus and extensor pollicis brevis tendons. Entrapment of the median nerve in the carpal tunnel is another generator of wrist pain and weakness of thumb abduction. Lastly, the presence of ganglion cysts, which are fluid-filled collections of modified synovial or mesenchymal cells that occur at the synovial-capsular interfaces of the joints of the wrist, which occur in response to repetitive minor injury should also be in the diffrential of causes resulting in wrist pain [12].

Predictive Value of Different Clinical Features (Both on History and Physical Exam), and Lab Testing/Imaging

Predictive factors for diagnosing osteoarthritis of the wrist include age, gender (M vs. F), previous injury, right vs. left handedness, occupation or hobbies requiring repetitive motion, and the time course of symptoms. Physical exam findings such as pain with motion or palpation over specific joint spaces, limitation in range of motion, or erythema and/or swelling over joints are also predictive. Imaging findings of joint changes, including reduced joint space and the presence of osteophytes, are also predictive factors of a diagnosis of osteoarthritis.

Strength of Evidence for Different Treatment Modalities

Currently, the management of osteoarthritis begins with conservative therapy, which includes medication management with oral and topical regimens of NSAIDs, occupational and physical therapy, and splinting. With persistence in pain and limitation in joint range of motion, the next step to therapy involves intra-articular joint injections. Given the progressive nature of osteoarthritis of the wrist, these treatment modalities often become less effective over time, thus necessitating surgical interventions, which include total wrist arthroplasty, proximal row carpectomy, partial fusion, and wrist denervation. Currently, there is no literature comparing the effectiveness of conservative medical management vs. joint injections and surgical interventions of the management of osteoarthritis for the wrist. Most of the evidence is anecdotal and extrapolated from studies involving osteoarthritis of major joints such as the knee and shoulder.

Future Directions or Clinical Trials in Progress

As stated previously, evidence for intra-articular steroid injections is anecdotal. The first RCT published by Meenagh et al. investigating the effect of intra-articular steroid injection of the first CMCJ, which was underpowered and ended early due to recruitment issues, did not find any benefit of steroid injection over placebo [9]. Future clinical trials are necessary to evaluate the efficacy of intra-articular steroid injections as well as other injectable regenerative interventions such as prolotherapy and platelet-rich plasma, which are currently gaining interest for the treatment of osteoarthritis. Prolotherapy was described by George Hackett in the 1940s and consists of injecting dextrose into the ligaments and tendons around an affected joint to stimulate the development of fibrous tissue and bone cells, thus strengthening the joint [13]. A retrospective uncontrolled observational study by Hauser et al. evaluating 31 patients who underwent phototherapy for chronic wrist pain found that 90% achieved greater than 50% relief and 88% felt improvement in stiffness levels at an average of 22 months following their last treatment, which necessitates the need for future randomized clinical trials [12]. PRP therapy is the process of injecting a solution of concentrated autologous platelets into joint spaces with the goal of reducing the inflammatory process and modifying the balance of anabolism and catabolism in the affected joint space [14]. A non-controlled pilot study by Loibl et al. found that in 10 patients who underwent PRP therapy for osteoarthritis of the trapeziometacarpal joint, there was a statistically significant decrease in VAS scores from 6.2 ± 1.6 to 5.4 =/− 2.2 at 6 month follow-up ($P < 0.05$) and that Mayo Wrist scores also improved from 46.5 ± 18.6 to 67.5 ± 19.0 at 6 month follow-up [9]. This again points to a necessity for future clinical trials of another injectable therapy, which may provide analgesia while maintaining or improving mobility.

Conclusion/Summary

Osteoarthritis of the wrist is a non-inflammatory process, which results in the destruction of cartilage of the affected joint, eventually resulting in mechanical pain, reduced strength, and range of motion. The etiology of osteoarthritis of the wrist can be separated into traumatic and idiopathic causes. A stepwise approach to diagnosis includes starting with a thorough history paying special attention to hand dominance, occupational risk factors, functional requirements and the progression of pain, and any limitations in range of motion. The next step includes a physical exam pinpointing the pain-generating joints. Radiographic imaging is then used to detect the location and pattern of degenerative changes and therefore guiding management. The first steps in management begin with conservative management such as physical and occupational therapy, splinting, and oral analgesics. Although most of the evidence for intra-articular steroid/local anesthetic injections are anecdotal, they have provided patients with symptomatic relief while preserving function temporarily. As the disease process advances, definitive surgical interventions are often required, which are selected based upon the joints involved, the age of the patient, and functional requirements. Investigation into the efficacy of joint injections and the use of alternative injectable agents such as prolotherapy and hyaluronic acid are what represents the future of the management of wrist osteoarthritis with the goal of reducing pain while preserving function.

References

1. Watson HK, Ballet FL. The SLAC wrist: scapholunate advanced collapse pattern of degenerative arthritis. J Hand Surg Am. 1984;9A:358–65.
2. Dillon C, et al. Self-reported hand and wrist arthritis and occupation: data from the U.S. National Health Interview Survey-Occupational Health Supplement. Am J Ind Med. 2002;42(4):318–27. https://doi.org/10.1002/ajim.10117.

3. Weiss KE, Rodner CM. Osteoarthritis of the wrist. J Hand Surg Am. 2007;32(5):725–46. https://doi.org/10.1016/j.jhsa.2007.02.003.
4. Laulan J, et al. Wrist osteoarthritis. Orthop Traumatol Surg Res. 2015;101(1):S1–10. https://doi.org/10.1016/j.otsr.2014.06.025.
5. Felson DT. Osteoarthritis. In: Harrison's principles of internal medicine, vol. 2. 19th ed. New York, NY: McGraw-Hill; 2015. p. 2226–33.
6. Zhang W, et al. OARSI recommendations for the management of hip and knee osteoarthritis part III: changes in evidence following systematic cumulative update of research published through January 2009. Osteoarthr Cartil. 2010;18:476–99. https://doi.org/10.1016/j.joca.2010.01.013.
7. Bruyère O, et al. A consensus statement on the European Society for Clinical and Economic Aspects of Osteoporosis and Osteoarthritis (ESCEO) algorithm for the management of knee osteoarthritis—from evidence-based medicine to the real-life setting. Semin Arthritis Rheum. 2016;45(4):S3. https://doi.org/10.1016/j.semarthrit.2015.11.010.
8. Meenagh GK. A randomised controlled trial of intra-articular corticosteroid injection of the carpometacarpal joint of the thumb in osteoarthritis. Ann Rheum Dis. 2004;63(10):1260–3. https://doi.org/10.1136/ard.2003.015438.
9. Talwalkar SC, et al. Wrist osteoarthritis. Scand J Surg. 2008;97(4):305–9. https://doi.org/10.1177/145749690809700406.
10. Laulan J, Bacle G, de Bodman C, et al. The arthritic wrist. II – the degenerative wrist: indications for different surgical treatments. Orthop Traumatol Surg Res. 2011;97:S37–41.
11. Jacobs CL, Stern PJ. An unusual case of gout in the wrist: the importance of monitoring medication dosage and interaction. A case report. Chiropr Osteopat. 2007;15(1):16. https://doi.org/10.1186/1756-1340-15-16.
12. Minotti P, Taras JS. Ganglion cysts of the wrist. J Am Soc Surg Hand. 2002;2(2):102–7. https://doi.org/10.1053/jssh.2002.33318.
13. Hauser R, et al. Dextrose prolotherapy for unresolved wrist pain. Pract Pain Manag. 2009;9(9):72–89.
14. Loibl M, Lang S, Dendel LM, et al. Leukocyte-reduced platelet-rich plasma treatment of basal thumb arthritis: a pilot study. Biomed Res Int. 2016;2016:9262909.

A 45-Year-Old Patient with Chronic Chest Wall Pain

19

Daneel M. Patoli and Tariq Malik

Case Description

A 45-yr-old man is referred to the pain clinic for intractable chest wall pain, which is unresponsive to conventional therapy. He has no medical issues, never had any surgery or trauma to his chest wall area. He denies any history of illness, sickness, or any other issues in the past. He describes the pain as a vague, dull sensation, extending from the right side of his middle back, and extending along to the side of the chest wall. There is no skin discoloration, and his previous work up by his primary care physician is negative for any cardiac, pulmonary, or gastrointestinal disorder. The pain is aggravated by any type of physical activity, and he states there are no alleviating factors. Sleeping has not been an issue in general, but lately the pain has been keeping him up at night. He likes to exercise but has been cutting back on it as it is uncomfortable to exercise with the pain.

D. M. Patoli
Department of Anesthesiology and Critical Care, University of Chicago, Chicago, IL, USA
e-mail: Daneel.Patoli@dacc.uchicago.edu

T. Malik (✉)
Department of Anesthesia and Critical Care, University of Chicago, Chicago, IL, USA
e-mail: tmalik@dacc.uchicago.edu; TMuslim@dacc.uchicago.edu

What Is Your Preliminary Diagnosis?

A detailed history and physical exam is the cornerstone of managing any chronic pain disorder. It is important to rule out serious conditions that may require emergent medical or surgical treatment. This is especially true in a patient with chronic chest pain. With a broad differential diagnosis ranging from myocardial infarction to costochondritis, the history should focus on ruling out emergent pathology by asking key questions including presence of dyspnea on exertion, fevers, night sweats, unexpected weight loss, and past cardiac/pulmonary history. It is important to ask and look for other joints' involvement to account for any rheumatological disorder. Next, the goal should be to try to elicit any inciting event that may have led to the start of this pain, namely any trauma including minor falls, fights, and history of fever or flu-like symptoms. Furthermore, the patient's activity routine including exercise and the job function should be ascertained in detail. The idea is to determine any aggravating or relieving factors that can point toward the source of pain generator. In general, if pain is mechanical in nature, i.e., gets worse with activity, it tends to come from the musculoskeletal system. Pain that is dermatomal in distribution tends to point to nerve root irritation from various pathologies. There is always a possibility that he has post-herpetic neuralgia even in the absence of a rash and young age.

T. Malik (ed.), *Practical Chronic Pain Management*, https://doi.org/10.1007/978-3-030-46675-6_19

Physical exam should reveal any element of nerve dysfunction like sensory loss or excitability like allodynia or hyperalgesia favoring neuropathic pain as a cause of pain. Presence of tenderness in the intercostal area, at the costochondral junction, along the ribs or paraspinal area favors musculoskeletal etiology as the source of pain. The absence of any radicular or musculoskeletal symptoms, with the predominance of vague back and chest wall pain, would lead to the preliminary diagnosis of thoracic discogenic pain syndrome without nerve impingement.

How Is Diagnosis Confirmed?

Cardiac, pulmonary, and gastrointestinal issues should be ruled out with the help of a medical specialist. In their absence, a chest X-ray or CT of the chest should be done to rule out rib fracture, or an intra-thoracic malignancy. Patients with prior history of rheumatologic disorders should consult with their rheumatologist to rule out a rheumatologic cause for their pain. Studies may include plasma levels of ESR and CRP along with checking for multiple immunologic markers such as anti-neutrophil antibodies (ANA). Once cardiac, pulmonary, infectious, malignant, and immunological disorders have been actively ruled out, the most likely etiology would be degenerative disorder of the discs or other parts of the musculoskeletal system. An MRI of the thoracic spine would be required to confirm the diagnosis, showing mild to moderate herniation of one or multiple intervertebral discs impinging on the nerve roots leading to the intercostal nerves (Fig. 19.1).

What Is the Pathophysiology of This Condition?

While more rare than both lumbar and cervical disc herniations, a thoracic disc herniation is possible and is the root cause of thoracic disc pain syndrome leading to chronic chest wall pain. It is believed that when the thoracic vertebrae are stressed, with either repeated physical activity or any type of trauma, the outer ring of the disc, called the annulus fibrosis, herniates posteriorly into the spinal canal. While this herniation may lead to impingement of the intercostal nerve roots, this is not always the case. Because of the sensory innervation of the annulus fibrosis from nociceptive fibers, lack of nerve impingement can still cause pain secondary to the disc herniation itself. This is seen as a more vague, dull pain sensation in the middle of the back, and may cause some radiation to the chest wall, such as seen with our patient. If herniation persists lead-

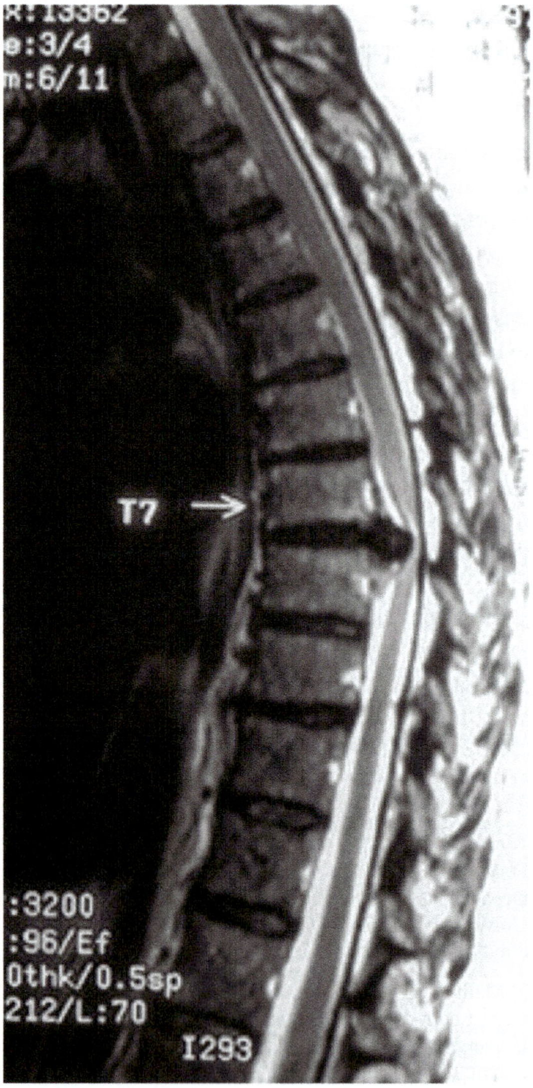

Fig. 19.1 Herniation of the T7-8 intervertebral disc seen on a sagittal section of a thoracic MRI

ing to further swelling, impingement of the intercostal nerve roots can occur, leading to the classic radicular pain.

How Is the Problem Managed?

There are generally two approaches to management of chronic pain, and they include the conservative and invasive approaches. This is also true for patients with non-radicular thoracic discogenic pain syndrome.

Conservative Management

1. *Identification and elimination of aggravating factors:* With thoracic discogenic pain, oftentimes there will be identifiable aggravating factors. These include but are not limited to poor posture, poor form when performing exercise routines, and supra physical work expectations. Identification of these factors and then taking steps to avoid the cause is the first step in preventing further propagation of the pain and disease process.
2. *Physical therapy:* Disc herniations, with and without nerve impingement, can resolve on their own time. However, pain is often a limiting factor and usually leads to restrictions to activities of daily living. Physical therapy should be used in these patients to alter their current regimen, and overcome their pain. Therapy regimens include incorporating back stretches and core muscle training to improve and stabilize the back. Electrical stimulation should be used only initially as it can disrupt the proper restoration of back function if used for prolonged periods of time.
3. *Anti-inflammatory medication:* Patients with disc herniation can often have debilitating pain leading to avoidance of daily activities including physical therapy. Therefore, it is recommended to use low to medium dose anti-inflammatory medications such as Ibuprofen to overcome the pain and continue to remain active. However, it is important to note that if the pain does not resolve after more than 6 weeks, anti-inflammatory medication should be discontinued and a different treatment option should be considered, given the increasing risks associated with long-term use of such medications, including GI bleeds.
4. *Heat/Ice Packs:* Can help relax paraspinal muscles that will spasm as a reflex protective mechanism in the setting of disc herniations.
5. *Opioids, muscle relaxants:* Medications such as Oxycodone, Hydrocodone, Tramadol, and Cyclobenzaprine should only be used sparingly and for uncontrollable pain. High risk for addiction is seen with these medications.

Invasive Interventions

If conservative management fails to provide adequate pain relief, a stepwise approach should be taken when considering invasive interventions. Prior to initiating invasive interventions, a detailed conversation with the patient should take place discussing the risks/benefits of all the procedures, and thorough understanding of the outcomes of these interventions. The patients should be made aware that most procedures come with their own downfalls, and that if the pain is tolerable, conservative management should continue instead of pushing forward with invasive interventions. If invasive interventions are chosen, the following are the considerations, though all of them have weak evidence to support their cause:

1. *Thoracic epidural steroid injection* – Typically done under fluoroscopic guidance in an accredited pain clinic, thoracic epidurals are quick procedures in which a needle is guided into the epidural space, and a solution containing a long-acting steroid and short-acting local anesthetic is used to both diagnose and confirm the pathology. Immediate relief points to a positive diagnosis.
2. *Intercostal nerve blocks* – Performed at the level of the offending rib. It is done both for diagnostic and for therapeutic reasons. A significant pain releif after the injection help. Procedure performed by finding inferior border of the offending rib and injection of local anesthetic solution along the inferior border to saturate the intercostal nerve. The procedure can also be performed by isolating the inter-

costal nerve root at its origin near the spinal cord and performing the block there.

3. *Microdiscectomy* – Performed in the operating room, a microdiscectomy is a minimally invasive procedure under fluoroscopic guidance in which portions of the offending thoracic disc are removed to relieve impingement, leading to resolution of symptoms.
4. *Spinal cord stimulation* – Operates by sending a constant stimulation signal to the spinal cord to impede the afferent pain pathways that are causing the patient to feel chest pain. Initially a stimulator trial is placed in the OR under moderate sedation and trialed for approximately 1–4 weeks. If good resolution of symptoms is seen, and the patient is able to resume normal activities of daily living, a permanent stimulator can then be placed under fluoroscopic guidance.
5. *Radiofrequency/Cryoablation* – Performed either in the operating room or in a pain clinic, the procedure consists of using high-frequency radio waves to ablate the offending nerve roots. Similarly, cryoablation utilizes the concept of extreme cold (−60 °F) to destroy the offending nerve root at the level of its origin.
6. *Laminectomy* – Invasive surgical procedure used in severe refractory cases of thoracic discogenic pain syndrome in which the thoracic lamina are removed to decompress the spinal canal and relieve impingement. Due to the anatomy of the thoracic vertebrae including narrow spinal canal, small epidural space, and thick spinal cord traversing through, there is a high risk for spinal cord injury with this operation. Typical approaches to the procedure include the anterior trans-sternal or transthoracic approach, the lateral costrotransversectomy approach, and the posterolateral transpedicular or trans facet with pedicular sparing approach [1].

Long-Term Outcome

Due to the rare incidence of thoracic disc herniations when compared to cervical and lumbar disc herniations, there is limited data on the long-term prognosis of the condition. Most data seems to suggest that prognosis for patients with this condition vary tremendously. Younger patients with a traumatic cause of thoracic disc herniation may later progress to having myelopathy; although, they are also the more favorable group in terms of full recovery. Middle-age to older patients who tend to get this disease secondary to disc degeneration have a more protracted, progressively worsening course. Oftentimes, these patients require surgical intervention to relieve the symptoms, though relief is not guaranteed. Overall, most patients without myelopathic symptoms should receive just conservative treatment including physical therapy, and NSAIDs, with around 80% recovering to previous activity levels.

Discussion

Prevalence

Thoracic disc herniations are significantly rarer than their counterparts, cervical and lumbar disc herniations. Interestingly, most thoracic disc herniations are found incidentally on MRI scans intended for other purposes. According to Malanga et al., autopsy studies have found asymptomatic disc herniations in 7–15% of patients that were examined, while Wood et al. found asymptomatic disc herniations on MRI scans in up to 37% of patients [2, 3]. Symptomatic disc herniation is much less common, and according to Fogwe et al., make up approximately 0.25–0.75% of all disc ruptures [4]. Of these patients, 80% of patients usually present in the third or fourth decades of their life [5]. In addition to being rarer than cervical and lumbar discectomies, the intervention upon these herniations is less common as well. Approximately 0.2–0.4% of all discectomies performed in the United States are upon thoracic intervertebral discs [3].

Differential Diagnosis

The differential diagnosis for patients with chest wall pain syndrome must include both diseases involving the chest wall and associated neurovascular bundles along with non-chest wall pathologies that can lead to chest pain. A comprehensive list of differential diagnoses should include but not be limited to the following [6]:

- *Cardiac* – Acute myocardial infarction, angina pectoris, aortic regurgitation, mitral valve prolapse, HOCM, pericarditis, sickle cell crisis, thoracic aortic dissection/aneurysm
- *Pulmonary* – Tracheal bronchitis, bronchiectasis, pulmonary embolism, pneumonia, pneumothorax, pleurisy, lung abscess, atelectasis, and carcinoma
- *GI* – Esophagitis, GERD, sphincter of Oddi dysfunction (referred chest pain), esophageal laceration, carcinoma, hiatal hernia, esophageal dysmotility disorder, peptic ulcer disease, perforated ulcer, biliary colic, cholecystitis, pancreatitis
- *Neurologic* – Intramedullary/extramedullary lesion, epidural spinal cord compression, herpes zoster infection/post herpetic neuralgia, nerve compression/radiculopathy, neurogenic tumors, CRPS, intercostal neuralgia
- *Bone* – Rib/sternal fracture, neoplasm, arthritis, ankylosing spondylitis, costochondritis, Tietze syndrome, unidentified inflammatory diseases, slipped rib syndrome
- *Muscle* – Myofascial pain syndrome, muscle spasms, contractures, dermatomyositis, polymyositis
- *Skin* – Burns, postoperative pain, mastodynia, post mastectomy syndrome, post thoracotomy syndrome, scleroderma, psoriatic arthritis
- *Psychiatric* – Conversion disorder, anxiety, depression, hypochondriasis
- *Extrathoracic disorders* – Posterolateral/anterolateral/posterior thoracic disc protrusion, osteoarthritis, thoracic outlet syndrome, Pancoast tumor and syndrome, gas entrapment syndrome, post radiotherapy chest pain, subphrenic abscess

Predictive Value of Different Clinical Features

Due to the nature of the disease process, with incidence of symptomatic pathology being very rare, and the association of symptoms to a wide variety of potential diagnoses, the sensitivity and specificity of each exam is not entirely known or beneficial. Rather, the diagnoses should be made after a comprehensive workup including history and physical exam, pertinent lab workup, and imaging studies are performed and reviewed. Some key signs/symptoms to be aware of include the following.

History and Physical Exam

Pain is a common symptom patients with thoracic discogenic pain syndrome complain of, and is seen in approximately 60% of patients. Radicular pain symptoms in a thoracic dermatomal distribution point highly to a disc herniation with radiculopathy. Patients with myelopathy including hyperreflexia, muscle weakness, and absence of pain sensation in the lower extremities with clear demarcation at the thoracic dermatomal regions should be highly suspicious for myelopathy secondary to cord compression. Furthermore, patients with annular tears may have referred pain despite compression of nerve roots based on the location of the tear. According to Schellhas et al., anterior annular tears may refer pain to the ribs, chest wall, sternum, or visceral structures, while lateral tears can produce radicular pain to visceral structures, and posterior tears can produce back pain in a localized or diffuse pattern [7, 8]. Provocative maneuvers such as the Spurling maneuver (cervical compression, extension, and ipsilateral rotation) to rule out cervical radiculopathy and the straight leg raise test to rule out lumbosacral radiculopathy may aid in ruling out other etiologies of chest wall pain, and point more toward a thoracic discogenic pain syndrome [7].

Lab Tests

There are no specific lab tests to rule in or out thoracic discogenic pain syndrome, although other lab tests should be ordered to rule out other causes of chest pain. These include but are not limited to complete blood count, comprehensive metabolic panel including LFTs, troponin assay, lipase, amylase, ESR, and CRP. Cultures from blood, urine, and sputum can be obtained to rule out an infectious process as well.

Imaging

The gold standard for diagnosing thoracic disc herniations is an MRI of the thoracic spine. It is an extremely sensitive test when searching for disc abnormalities, and a negative MRI essentially rules out thoracic disc herniation. However, a common downfall seen with MRI imaging is over reading the extent of thoracic disc herniation. A study by Brown et al. evaluating 55 patients with MRIs of the thoracic spine showing disc herniation went on to show that 40 of those patients did well with simple conservative management, while 15 patients required surgery [9]. Other imaging tests include chest X-ray looking for particular disc space narrowing and osteophyte formation in the thoracic vertebra, CT myelograms to look for cord compression, and thoracic discograms.

Strength of Evidence for Treatment Modalities

In short, because of the rarity of symptomatic thoracic disc herniations, it is difficult to measure the strength of different treatment modalities due to the lack of power for these respective studies. For example, only one study has looked at the efficacy of thoracic epidural steroid injections in the treatment of thoracic discogenic pain syndrome. The study by Manchikanti et al. looked more at the efficacy of epidural local anesthetic injection alone vs. steroid plus local anesthetic [10]. While the study showed both groups to have pain relief greater than 50%, the study was not designed to characterize the strength of the treatment in and of itself. More invasive treatment options such as laminectomy and discectomy have shown more promise but are counteracted by dangers of the procedure, such as risk for cord injury and damage to cardiovascular and pulmonary structures in the thorax. Haufe et al. looked at percutaneous laser disc decompression in their study as a minimally invasive approach to discectomy for thoracic disc herniations, hoping to avoid major surgical complications [2]. Conclusions of the study included no adverse events such as pneumothorax, discitis, and nerve injury, while 6 out of 10 patients reported a significantly lower pain level at 18–31 months. Spinal cord stimulation has been brought up as an intervention to limit pain from thoracic radiculopathy as it has been shown to do in cervical and lumbar pain, but studies are still being conducted at this time.

Future Directions

The goal of the future would be to find an appropriate, minimally invasive, low-risk procedure to eliminate thoracic discogenic pain. Up and coming procedures such as spinal cord stimulation and percutaneous laser disc decompressions offer a promising treatment option, but further studies must be done to truly quantify the efficacy of these procedures. This is of course limited by the lack of large numbers of patients with symptomatic thoracic disc herniations. Eventually, enough small studies performed can be reviewed in a meta-analysis to attain strong-enough data to bring these treatment options to the forefront.

Conclusion

To wrap up, thoracic discogenic pain syndrome secondary to disc herniations is a condition significantly more rare than lumbar and cervical disc herniations. Therefore, studies explaining the disease process and measuring the efficacy of certain treatment options are in their infancy. A standard approach to chest wall pain secondary to thoracic discogenic pain syndrome should take place in a stepwise manner. More serious cardiac, pulmonary, and GI disorders should be ruled first. Imaging studies such as CXR, CT, and MRI scans can be attained to aid in the diagnosis of thoracic disc herniation. Initial treatment options should focus on non-invasive measures such as physical therapy, anti-inflammatory medications, hot/cold compresses, and sparing use of muscle relaxants and opioids. If pain continues to persist, more invasive interventions can then be discussed. While data regarding the efficacy of interventions such as thoracic epidural steroid injections, spinal cord stimulation, and surgical discectomy/laminectomy is still being derived, there are small studies to support the use of these interventions, and can be considered on a case by case basis.

References

1. Quint U, Bordon G, Preissl I, Sanner C, Rosenthal D. Thoracoscopic treatment for single level symptomatic thoracic disc herniation: a prospective followed cohort study in a group of 167 consecutive cases. Eur Spine J. 2011;21(4):637–45.
2. Haufe SM, Mork AR, Pyne M, Baker RA. Percutaneous laser disc decompression for thoracic disc disease: report of 10 cases. Int J Med Sci. 2010;7:155–9.
3. Wood KB, Schellhas KP, Garvey TA, Aeppli D. Thoracic discography in healthy individuals. Spine. 1999;24(15):1548.
4. Sari H, Misirlioglu TO, Palamar D. Regression of a symptomatic thoracic disc herniation with a calcified intervertebral disc component. Acta Orthop Traumatol Turc. 2016;50(6):698–701.
5. Göçmen S, Çolak A, Mutlu B, Asan A. Is back pain a diagnostic problem in clinical practices? A rare case report. Agri. 2015;27(3):163–5.
6. Oken JE, Hanyu-Deutmeyer A. Chest wall pain syndrome [Internet]. PMR KnowledgeNow. [cited 15 Apr 2019]. Available from: https://now.aapmr.org/chest-wall-pain-syndrome/.
7. Malanga GA, Alladin I, Tai Q, Talavera F, White RD. Thoracic discogenic pain syndrome [Internet]. In: Ho S, editor. Background, epidemiology, functional anatomy; 2018. [cited 15 Apr 2019]. Available from: https://emedicine.medscape.com/article/96284-overview.
8. Schellhas KP, Pollei SR, Dorwart RH. Thoracic discography. Spine. 1994;19(18):2103–8.
9. Brown CW, Deffer PA, Akmakjian J, Donaldson DH, Brugman JL. The natural history of thoracic disc herniation. Spine. 1992;17(Suppl):S97.
10. Manchikanti L, Cash KA, McManus CD, Pampati V, Benyamin RM. Thoracic interlaminar epidural injections in managing chronic thoracic pain: a randomized, double-blind, controlled trial with a 2-year follow-up. Pain Physician. 2014;17:E327–38.

A 45-Year-Old Woman with Persistent Pain After Mastectomy

20

Arjun Ramesh, Jonathan Church, Adam C. Young, and Tariq Malik

Case Presentation

A 38-year-old woman is diagnosed with breast cancer and after oncologic workup undergoes mastectomy with primary reconstruction along with lymph node removal. She has history of general anxiety disorder and a 20 pack year history of smoking. Her post-operative period is complicated by pain issues but does well overall. She follows up with her oncologist and surgeon who eventually refers her to pain clinic as pain at the surgical site is not abating. In the pain clinic, she describes the pain as a persistent, dull, burning sensation at the surgical site and in the axilla. She notes that her left arm has been difficult to move and activities such as combing her hair is challenging. On physical examination, the surgical scar has healed well, but she has areas of allodynia and hyperalgesia in and around the surgical area along with numbness in the axilla. There is no area of discoloration. Shoulder movement is limited by pain but arm strength and sensations are intact. The pain can be extreme at its worst, rated at 10/10, and is exacerbated by movements of the left arm. Current alleviating factors include avoiding use of her left arm, ice, and amitriptyline. She presents to your pain clinic for further workup.

A. Ramesh
Department of Anesthesiology, Rush University, Chicago, IL, USA

J. Church
Department of Anesthesiology, Chicago, IL, USA

A. C. Young (✉)
Pain Management Divison, Illinois Bone and Joint Institute, Morton Grove, IL, USA
e-mail: ayoung@ibji.com; Adam_Young@Rush.Edu

T. Malik
Department of Anesthesia and Critical Care, University of Chicago, Chicago, IL, USA
e-mail: tmalik@dacc.uchicago.edu; TMuslim@dacc.uchicago.edu

What Is the Most Likely Diagnosis?

The patient is a young female who had surgery with poor pain control postoperatively, without any regional anesthesia, and has anxiety disorder. Her recovery is uneventful but tissues have healed well. On physical examination she shows elements of somatosensory nerve dysfunction. In the absence of any nociceptive tissue damage (recurrence of tumor, infection, rib damage, etc.), she has developed chronic postsurgical pain syndrome, which is a type of neuropathic pain.

How Can the Diagnosis Be Confirmed?

Most chronic pain conditions are diagnosed clinically. There is no lab test or imaging that can clinch the diagnosis. In case of cancer patients, it

T. Malik (ed.), *Practical Chronic Pain Management*, https://doi.org/10.1007/978-3-030-46675-6_20

is imperative that recurrence of tumor is ruled out conclusively. This should be done with the help of the oncologist. In the presence of negative tumor recurrence or infection workup, the diagnosis of chronic past mastectomy pain is confirmed. Clinical symptoms and signs associated with neuropathic pain have been studied over the decades. Common symptoms reported by the patients are pain (burning, sharp, shooting), dysesthesia (pins, needles, numbness, tingling), and sensitivity to touch. In one study of about 500 patients, the most common symptoms were burning pain (65%), paroxysmal sharp pain (57%), and pain to touch (55%).

Is There Any Role for Testing?

All neuropathic pain conditions are diagnosed clinically. A good history and physical examination is key to establishing diagnosis. According to Neuropathic Pain Special Interest Group, pain is neuropathic if history and physical examination correlate and corroborate with a nerve lesion. Symptoms-based questionnaires are used to screen for and diagnose neuropathic pain (Leeds Assessment of Neuropathic Symptoms and Signs, the Neuropathic Pain Questionnaire, Pain DETECT). Imaging, neurophysiologic testing, punch biopsy, and quantitative sensory testing (QST) are important research tools that may help in confirming pathology but cannot explain cause of pain or help decide a treatment plan or help with prognosis of the condition. Imaging can rule out cause (rib fracture, recurrence of tumor, infection), electrophysiological testing can evaluate weakness by testing large fibers, QST can objectively evaluate small fibers by testing touch and pain threshold, and punch biopsy can identify small fiber loss.

What Is the Pathophysiology of the Condition?

The exact etiology of PMPS is unknown. It is a neuropathic pain disorder. Poorly controlled pain in the immediate post-operative period can lead to sensitization of the peripheral nerves due to neuroplasticity resulting in chronic pain. Damage to the nerves during surgical dissection, like intercostobrachial nerve, can lead to the loss of peripheral nerve fibers resulting in a de-afferentation pathophysiology with sprouting of new connections with the spinal cord producing hyperalgesia and allodynia along with numbness. Damage to the nerves can lead to neuroma development causing persistent pain. Phantom breast pain is purely a central pain phenomenon. In general, pathophysiology varies among patients and may change over the course of time.

How Is the Condition Managed?

The condition is best managed using a multidisciplinary approach. The most important intervention is patient education and developing a trusting relationship with the patient. Focus is on rehabilitating functional status. By the time the patient comes to the pain clinic, they have tried NSAIDs, Tylenol, and various other remedies. It is important to compile a list of interventions that have been tried and failed. It is also crucial to find out why a therapy has failed (i.e., due to side effect or improper dose was tried).

Multidisciplinary approach includes occupational therapy to improve shoulder function and use of physical modalities like massage, TENS unit, tissue ultrasound, acupuncture to help regain upper extremity function. There are no RCT to back them up. Patients with pain catastrophizing symptoms should be referred to pain psychologist for cognitive behavior therapy.

Neuro-SIG of the IAPS, Canadian Pain Society, and the European Federation of Neurological Societies (EFNS) all have published evidence-based guidelines for the pharmacological management of neuropathic pain, which are quite similar in general (Tables 20.1, 20.2, and 20.3).

The role of injection therapies in managing neuropathic pains is not well defined. The interventions (nerve block, epidural steroid injections,

Table 20.1 Neuro-SIG (IASP) guidelines for the pharmacological management of neuropathic pain

First line	TCA (amitriptyline) SNRI (Venlafaxine, Duloxetine) Anticonvulsant (gabapentin, pregabalin) Topical lidocaine 5%
Second line	Tramadol Opioid (low dose)
Third line	Bupropion, Paroxetine, Citalopram Carbamazepine, Lamotrigine, Oxcarbazepine, Topiramate, Valproic acid) Topical low-concentration capsaicin, dextromethorphan, memantine, Mexiletine

Table 20.2 Canadian Pain Society guidelines for the pharmacological management of neuropathic pain

First line	Anti-depressants (TCA) Anticonvulsant (gabapentin, pregabalin)
Second line	SNRI (Venlafaxine, Duloxetine) Topical lidocaine 5%
Third line	Tramadol Long-acting opioid
Fourth line	Cannabinoids Methadone Lamotrigine, Oxcarbazepine, Topiramate, Valproic acid)

neuromodulation therapy, intrathecal therapy) commonly employed by pain physicians were reviewed by IAPS and found that they were backed by poor-quality evidence and none got strong recommendation from the IAPS. There is renewed interest in managing PMPS with neuromodulation therapy but the evidence for the effectiveness of spinal cord stimulation is lacking and there is just one case report for the successful treatment of PMPS using dorsal root ganglion technique.

Discussion

Breast cancer is the most common malignancy in women worldwide, and treatment often requires surgery [1, 2]. Breast cancer can be treated with radical mastectomy, modified radical mastectomy, or lumpectomy with possible axillary dissection or sentinel node biopsy [2, 3]. Although treatment has improved survival rates, postoperative complications such as post mastectomy pain syndrome (PMPS) can greatly diminish patients' quality of life. PMPS results in chronic

Table 20.3 Stepwise approach to treating patients with neuropathic pain

Step 1
- (a) Establish diagnosis
- (b) Identify external and internal stresses
- (c) Identify co-morbidities
- (d) Patient education

Step 2
- (a) Treat underlying disease contributing or causing neuropathic pain
- (b) Initiate treatment with first line drugs (TCA, SSNI, gabapentin, pregabalin)
- (c) Lidocaine if pain localized to one spot
- (d) Initiate nonpharmacological interventions (OT, CBT, etc.)

Step 3
- (a) Reassess pain and functional improvement frequently
- (b) If significant pain relief (e.g., average pain reduced to ≤3/10) and tolerable adverse effects, continue treatment; if partial pain relief (e.g., average pain remains ≥5/10) titrate doses of the first line drugs.
- (c) If no or inadequate pain relief (e.g., <30% reduction) at target dosage after an adequate trial, switch to an alternative first-line medication.
- (d) If first-line drugs fail, switch to first-line drugs in combination.

Step 4
- (a) If first-line drugs fail alone or in combination, try second- and then third-line drugs.
- (b) Referral to interventional pain clinic for injection therapy.

post-operative neuropathic pain and has a reported incidence ranging from 25% to 60% [4]. As with other neuropathic pain syndromes, pain from PMPS will present as burning, tingling, shooting, stinging, or stabbing [2]. Pain is localized to the chest wall, axilla, and upper extremity ipsilateral to the breast surgery. It is often related to injury of the intercostobrachial nerve (ICBN), but also the medial pectoral, lateral pectoral, thoracodorsal, long thoracic nerves [5]. The most common location for pain is the medial arm with an incidence of 70%, followed by the shoulder and anterior surface of the chest, with incidences of 55% and 52%, respectively [6]. Pain can be moderate to severe with a negative impact on activity and quality of life [7]. To make the diagnosis, pain must be present for 3 months or more. If inadequately treated, patients can develop lymphedema or adhesive capsulitis of the ipsilateral shoulder as a result of immobility.

Risk factors for PMPS are numerous and multifactorial. Risk factors have been identified in the preoperative, intraoperative, and postoperative periods. In the *preoperative* period, risk factors include young age (<50 years old) [8], presence of preoperative breast pain or other chronic pain syndromes, and obesity. The most significant *intraoperative* risk factor has been identified as performance of axillary lymph node dissection [9]. These procedures commonly include stretch, ligation, or division of the ICBN, which has been theorized to lead to the ultimate development of PMPS in vulnerable patients [10]. In the *postoperative* period, uncontrolled acute postoperative pain, cancer recurrence, local metastasis, lymphedema, implant-related pain, and muscle spasm have been indicated as risk factors. Adjuvant therapy with radiation can lead to plexopathy, neuritis, or local necrosis/myositis. Adjuvant chemotherapy can lead to the development of neuropathy. Surgical complications play a role as infection or hematoma can lead to inflammation or irritation of both muscle and fascial planes leading to somatic symptoms. Psychological factors, including anxiety, depression, and catastrophizing have been described as increasing the development of PMPS [2, 8].

Differential Diagnosis

The differential diagnosis for PMPS is numerous and includes any other injury that can cause shoulder or chest wall pain. As PMPS is a diagnosis of exclusion, it is essential to rule out other pathologies prior to making the diagnosis. Other etiologies of pain which can mimic that of PMPS include the following:

- Shoulder musculoskeletal disorders such as bursitis, adhesive capsulitis, tendonitis, or rotator cuff injury
- Cervical radiculopathy
- Chemical neuropathy
- Herpes zoster
- Local infection
- Breast cancer bone metastasis lymphedema
- Rib necrosis
- Complex regional pain syndrome of the upper extremity
- Axillary hematoma
- Breast cancer recurrence (although it should be noted pain is not a common presenting symptom)

Confirming the Diagnosis

PMPS should be entertained when a patient complains of neuropathic symptoms, sharp or lancinating pain, burning pain, or hypersensitivity across the surgical incision or surgical site. It has been suggested that the pain must be at least 4 on a 10 point pain scale and be present for at least 3 months. Pain symptoms can affect any or all of the ipsilateral chest wall, arm, axilla, and are present at least 50% of the time [10]. Patients endorse poor sleep and difficulty performing activities of daily living. A thorough physical exam should be undertaken to rule out alternate causes of pain in the region. An examination of the surgical site can inspect for signs of local infection or tumor recurrence. The scar should be investigated for possible neuroma. Attention should be paid to the shoulder, as sub-acromial bursitis, adhesive capsulitis, and rotator cuff injury can mimic the pain of PMPS. Physical examination is quite useful in ruling out shoulder pathologies. Physical exam should also be used to evaluate for specific nerve injuries to the previously mentioned nerves. Although pain from PMPS often presents with symptoms in the distribution of the ICBN (axilla and medial aspect of proximal upper extremity), other nerve injuries must be ruled out as well. The long thoracic nerve (C5, C6, C7) innervates the serratus anterior, and injury can be identified by a winged scapula. A winged scapula can be identified by applying an inline force against a forward outstretched arm. Lateral (C5, C6, C7) and medial (C8, T1) pectoral nerves innervate the pectoralis major and minor. Injuries to the pectoral nerves may present with pectoralis muscle atrophy and weakness. The thoracodorsal nerve (C6, C7, C8) supplies the latissimus dorsi, and injury may present with atrophy and weakness of the muscle. If rotator cuff injury or cervical radiculopathy is suspected, further testing with magnetic resonance imaging (MRI) or electromyography (EMG) will more accurately characterize and localize the site of injury [11]. Plain radiographs of the chest and/or shoulder can demonstrate rib or shoulder invasion or fracture, positron emission tomographic scans can show recurrence or metastasis, MRI neurography can reveal injuries to the brachial plexus, and ultrasound can show fluid collections such as abscess or hematoma in the axilla. In the absence of alternate explanation for the pain, a diagnosis of PMPS can be made.

Treatment

Physical therapy (PT) is an important aspect of treating PMPS. PT should be targeted at preserving range of motion of the ipsilateral shoulder, increasing strength, and minimizing limitations. It is useful when started immediately after surgery in order to prevent the development of PMPS. However, the exact timing of initiation of therapy is a topic of debate. Early physical therapy has been associated with increased wound drainage and seroma formation, which could potentially trigger pain via compression of the ICBN. However, in the group of patients with pain secondary to lymphedema, early physical therapy has been shown to improve outcomes. An appropriate treatment plan could include passive range of motion exercises until drains are removed, at which time active stretching and strengthening can be initiated. Initiation of physical therapy in the postoperative period is also useful to prevent bursitis and adhesive capsulitis, which may complicate diagnosis of PMPS in patients with persistent pain after breast surgery [2].

Treating PMPS also includes a multimodal medical regimen, with attention to neuropathic pain medications. Anticonvulsants, such as gabapentin or pregabalin, should be instituted at low dose, and escalated gradually until symptoms are better controlled, or side effects preclude increasing the dosage. A suggested starting dose is 300 mg per day for gabapentin [12] and 75 mg per day for pregabalin. Treatment with tricyclic antidepressants, as well as serotonin-norepinephrine reuptake inhibitors, has been shown to reduce pain scores in this patient population, and should be started at low doses and increased as tolerated. Studies have shown improvement in PMPS pain with amitriptyline at 25 mg per day, increasing to 100 mg per day over 4 weeks and with venlafaxine 18.75 mg per day [4]. Non-steroidal anti-inflammatory medications as well as acetaminophen may be added to the therapy as they may help with some of the inflammatory pain that accompanies PMPS in local muscles and ipsilateral shoulder. Topical lidocaine or capsaicin can be considered as these both treat superficial symptoms such as allodynia or hyperesthesia, but will likely have little or no effect on deeper or more complex symptoms.

PMPS is a disease of the nervous system, so it should come as no surprise that these patients will often respond to blockade of multiple targets. Although large, formal, well-designed trials are lacking to support any one specific intervention, there are several reports of peripheral nerve blocks that help these patients. Blocks targeting the ICBN are attractive as injury to the ICBN is felt to be the inciting event for the development of PMPS. ICBN blocks have been described by locating the intercostal nerve as it exits the thorax via the second intercostal space with ultrasound. In a series of six patients, half experienced greater than 50% reduction in pain. Although expected to have short-term effects, three patients in this study reported that their pain was improved from baseline even 1 week after injection [13]. If a patient does respond to ICBN block, radiofrequency ablation or cryoneurolysis of the nerve may provide sustained relief. At present, there is a lack of evidence to support this practice aside from anecdotal reports. Serratus plane blocks (SPB) have recently gained some traction as a treatment for PMPS. SPB targets cutaneous branches of intercostal nerves 2–6 as they pass through the serratus anterior muscle, which covers the T2 branches that contribute to the intercostobrachial nerve [14]. Zocca et al. found that PMPS treated with serratus plane blocks showed 25% to complete relief in all eight patients included for a duration ranging from 2 days to 12 weeks. Although blockade of the serratus plane is anticipated to be of short duration, many of these patients claimed their pain improved from baseline or were using less breakthrough medication. The study also found serratus plane blocks particularly useful for patients suffering chronic pain as a result of a reconstructive implant. They attributed inconsistency of the magnitude of effect in their study to scarring in the planes of the targeted nerves from radiation [15]. It has been suggested that neurolysis within the serratus plane may be useful in end of life situations but is limited in other situations due to possible inclusion of the long thoracic nerve, resulting in scapular winging [14, 15]. Intercostal nerve blocks have limited evidence to support their use [16]. Intercostal blocks targeting the regions of the patient's pain symptoms appears to be a reasonable strategy, as opposed to targeting the first and second intercostal nerves (the contributions to the ICBN). Of the four case series reporting on intercostal nerve blocks to treat PMPS, half of patients achieved complete pain relief from local anesthetic alone [16]. Should the pain return, it would be reasonable to consider cryoneurolysis or radiofrequency denervation of the intercostal nerves. Should a patient have bilateral PMPS, it is strongly suggested that a thoracic epidural injection with a larger volume (e.g., 8 mL) be attempted, as opposed to bilateral intercostal nerve blocks, to achieve a multi-level bilateral intercostal block. The latter of which could predispose a serious situation should the patient suffer pneumothoraces. The lone study investigating paravertebral blocks (PVB) was underpowered but still demonstrated complete relief of PMPS pain symptoms in two of the ten patients included. Scar neuroma injections can be easily performed in the office as well and have the potential to improve pain that is localized to the incisional scar only.

As the pain from PMPS is at least partially mediated by the sympathetic nervous system, diagnostic and therapeutic stellate ganglion blocks (SGB) have been considered [16, 17]. However, at this time there is not enough compelling evidence to recommend the routine use of these blocks in the management of these patients. If a patient does receive relief from a diagnostic stellate ganglion block, repeat blocks can be considered to prolong relief. It should be noted that in one of the two published studies on SGB for treatment of PMPS, gabapentin provided better relief than SGB.

Other treatment modalities that have shown promise include acupuncture and pulsed laser therapy [3]. The same goes for local infiltration of the pectoralis muscle with botulinum toxin, which has been described in one case report to have decreased pain and increased ROM of the arm at the shoulder, but no large trials have been conducted to further support this practice [18]. Operative fat grafting has been a topic of research in the treatment of PMPS. It has been shown to improve scar softness and improve pain control in other neuropathically mediated pain states. In the setting of PMPS, it has been shown to provide a significant reduction in pain scores, but the mechanism is poorly understood. It is thought that infusion of mesenchymal stems cells can aid in pain control by improving loose connective tissue regeneration, with subsequent release of nerve entrapment, and by reducing radiation-induced inflammation with concomitant reduction in pain [2]. In theory, the application of neuromodulation, in the form of spinal cord stimulation (SCS), could provide patients with PMPS a chance at durable relief. SCS is approved to treat chronic, neuropathic pain states that have failed to respond to more conservative treatment, which on its surface would appear to include PMPS.

The use of opioid medications to treat PMPS is a topic of debate. While opioids have shown utility in controlling acute postoperative pain following breast surgery, routine and long-term use of these medications has not been shown to provide significant benefit [2, 7, 19]. Additionally, with the current concerns over opioid misuse and abuse, caution should be used when instituting long-term opioid therapy. The benefits of opioids for the treatment of chronic, non-cancer pain should be weighed carefully against the risks of long-term use, addiction, and misuse.

All chronic pain states include a psychological component; a formal mental health evaluation can be useful in the management of PMPS. Cognitive behavioral therapy, with an emphasis on self-management training, has been shown to be beneficial in this patient population. Self-management training focuses on helping the patient develop problem-solving and symptom management skills, while also building self-confidence. The ultimate goal is to allow the patient to manage and handle their pain in a way that is beneficial, without the need for provider input. These sessions can be carried out one on one or in a group therapy setting at the discretion of the mental health professional [2].

References

1. Fam BN, El-Sayed GGE, Reyad RM, Mansour I. Efficacy and safety of pulsed radiofrequency and steroid injection for intercostobrachial neuralgia in postmastectomy pain syndrome - a clinical trial. Saudi J Anaesth. 2018;12(2):227–34.
2. Tait RC, Zoberi K, Ferguson M, Levenhagen K, Luebbert RA, Rowland K, et al. Persistent post-mastectomy pain: current status and future directions. J Pain. 2018;19:1367.
3. Ebid AA, El-Sodany AM. Long-term effect of pulsed high-intensity laser therapy in the treatment of post-mastectomy pain syndrome: a double blind, placebo-control, randomized study. Lasers Med Sci. 2015;30(6):1747–55.
4. Larsson IM, Ahm Sorensen J, Bille C. The post-mastectomy pain syndrome-a systematic review of the treatment modalities. Breast J. 2017;23(3):338–43.
5. Brackstone M. A review of the literature and discussion: establishing a consensus for the definition of post-mastectomy pain syndrome to provide a standardized clinical and research approach. Can J Surg. 2016;59(5):294–5.
6. Couceiro TC, Valenca MM, Raposo MC, Orange FA, Amorim MM. Prevalence of post-mastectomy pain syndrome and associated risk factors: a cross-sectional cohort study. Pain Manag Nurs. 2014;15(4):731–7.
7. Steyaert A, Forget P, Dubois V, Lavand'homme P, De Kock M. Does the perioperative analgesic/anesthetic regimen influence the prevalence of long-term chronic pain after mastectomy? J Clin Anesth. 2016;33:20–5.
8. Alves Nogueira Fabro E, Bergmann A, do Amaral ESB, Padula Ribeiro AC, de Souza Abrahao K, da Costa Leite Ferreira MG, et al. Post-mastectomy pain syndrome: incidence and risks. Breast. 2012;21(3):321–5.
9. Couceiro TC, Menezes TC, Valenca MM. Post-mastectomy pain syndrome: the magnitude of the problem. Rev Bras Anestesiol. 2009;59(3):358–65.
10. Waltho D, Rockwell G. Post-breast surgery pain syndrome: establishing a consensus for the definition of post-mastectomy pain syndrome to provide a standardized clinical and research approach - a review of the literature and discussion. Can J Surg. 2016;59(5):342–50.
11. Woodward TW, Best TM. The painful shoulder: part I. Clinical evaluation. Am Fam Physician. 2000;61(10):3079–88.
12. Amr YM, Yousef AA. Evaluation of efficacy of the perioperative administration of Venlafaxine or gabapentin on acute and chronic postmastectomy pain. Clin J Pain. 2010;26(5):381–5.
13. Wijayasinghe N, Duriaud HM, Kehlet H, Andersen KG. Ultrasound guided intercostobrachial nerve blockade in patients with persistent pain after breast cancer surgery: a pilot study. Pain Physician. 2016;19(2):E309–18.
14. Takimoto K, Nishijima K, Ono M. Serratus plane block for persistent pain after partial mastectomy and axillary node dissection. Pain Physician. 2016;19(3):E481–6.
15. Zocca JA, Chen GH, Puttanniah VG, Hung JC, Gulati A. Ultrasound-guided serratus plane block for treatment of postmastectomy pain syndromes in breast cancer patients: a case series. Pain Pract. 2017;17(1):141–6.
16. Wijayasinghe N, Andersen K, Kehlet H. Neural blockade for persistent pain after breast cancer surgery. Reg Anesth Pain Med. 2014;39:272–8.
17. Nabil Abbas D, Abd El Ghafar EM, Ibrahim WA, Omran AF. Fluoroscopic stellate ganglion block for postmastectomy pain: a comparison of the classic

anterior approach and the oblique approach. Clin J Pain. 2011;27(3):207–13.
18. Dessy LA, Maruccia M, Mazzocchi M, Scuderi N. Treatment of post mastectomy pain syndrome after mastopexy with botulinum toxin. J Plast Reconstr Aesthet Surg. 2014;67(6):873–4.
19. Hojan K, Wojtysiak M, Huber J, Molinska-Glura M, Wiertel-Krawczuk A, Milecki P. Clinical and neurophysiological evaluation of persistent sensory disturbances in breast cancer women after mastectomy with or without radiotherapy. Eur J Oncol Nurs. 2016;23:8–14.

Chronic Pain and Postherpetic Neuralgia

21

Beth VanderWielen and Alaa Abd-Elsayed

Case Description

A 75-year-old woman presents with persistent chest pain of 8 months duration. It started after she developed a rash which lasted few weeks. She was diagnosed with shingles by her primary care physician and was treated with antiviral medicines. The rash healed but pain never way. Pain is severe, persistent and keeps her up at night. There are no other symptoms. The skin in the painful part is sensitive to touch and she is having hard time wearing clothes. She is referred to the pain clinic for pain management.

What Is Your Preliminary Diagnosis?

She has most likely chronic pain from postherpetic neuralgia, which is especially common especially after age 50. History of shingles followed by pain usually clinches the diagnosis. It is always important to rule out other causes. Pain can be from a fractured rib, an underlying chest wall tumor, or radicular pain from nerve root irritation from any other pathology. It is important to rule out other pathologies using history and physical examination including imaging if needed.

How Is Diagnosis Confirmed?

Diagnosis of postherpetic neuralgia is made based on clinical presentation.

Since this disease is actually a resurgence of the varicella zoster virus (VZV) which clinically presents as chicken pox, it is important to first discuss the original clinical diagnosis of infection as history can often be helpful to inform a diagnosis of subsequent sequela.

Chicken pox is diagnosed based on clinical symptoms which presents as a diffuse, pruritic, fluid-filled, vesicular rash which typically lasts 5–7 days after which the lesions crust over and become scabs [1]. Transmission occurs with direct contact of the fluid from the vesicles which contains VZV or through droplets from nasopharyngeal secretions from infected individuals [1]. Patients are considered contagious from 48 hours prior to onset of rash and until the lesions have fully crusted over. Bacterial super-infection of lesions, encephalitis, or Reye's syndrome are known complications of infection [1].

B. VanderWielen
Department of Anesthesiology, University of Wisconsin-Madison Hospitals and Clinics, Madison, WI, USA

A. Abd-Elsayed (✉)
Department of Anesthesiology, University of Wisconsin School of Medicine and Public Health, Madison, WI, USA

T. Malik (ed.), *Practical Chronic Pain Management*, https://doi.org/10.1007/978-3-030-46675-6_21

After this systemic illness resolves, later resurgence of symptoms often years after the initial infection includes pain, fever, and/or malaise, followed by painful or pruritic skin lesions. The skin lesions, commonly referred to as shingles, generally start as erythematous papules or macules which progress from vesicles to pustules, followed by crusted lesions which occur 14–21 days post infection [2]. Shingles is due to the reactivation of the VZV virus. Unlike the original chickenpox infection which is spread diffusely across the body, shingles presents in one or two dermatomes and does not cross midline [3].

Postherpetic neuralgia is the most common sequela of VZV infection, affecting approximately 20 percent of individuals who present with shingles with pain existing beyond 1–3 months after the resolution of the skin lesions [2–4]. The presentation of postherpetic neuralgia varies based on the particular nerves affected (Table 21.1) [2, 5]. Factors which contribute to the intensity of postherpetic neuralgia include rash severity, age, immunosuppression, and co-existing inflammation [2].

Pain from postherpetic neuralgia can be described as severe and can dramatically affect a person's ability to perform activities of daily living, impair sleep, and potentially trigger depression [2]. Concurrent bacterial infection by common organisms including staphyloccous aureus or streptococcus pyogenes can also exacerbate the pain [2].

Table 21.1 Characteristic physical exam findings

Cranial nerve involved	Syndrome	Symptoms
Ophthalmic division of the trigeminal nerve (V1 branch)	Herpes zoster ophthalmicus	Visual loss; can be preceded by vesicles on the tip or lateral side of the nose called Hutchinson's sign
Facial nerve[a]	Ramsay Hunt syndrome	Facial nerve palsy, otalgia, vesicular eruptions in the auricle
Auditory nerve[a]		Vertigo, sensorineural hearing loss, tinnitus

[a]Often occur concurrently due to close proximity

What Is the Pathophysiology of This Condition?

Though not entirely understood, the reactivation of VZV is the cause of shingles ,while the initial infection with VZV causes chickenpox [3]. Once the initial chickenpox lesions resolve, VZV can hide within the sensory dorsal root ganglion stealthily avoiding immune attack. In healthy, immunocompetent individuals, T-cell lymphocytes are activated and form "memory" during the initial infection to subsequently provide protection against resurgence of the virus [2]. However, this "memory" or activation, proliferation, and protection of the T lymphocytes can wane over time leading to an unfortunate resurgence of symptoms in approximately 30% of affected individuals [6]. Additionally, as other conditions or circumstances are acquired which hinder the immune system such as human immunodeficiency virus (HIV), concomitant immunosuppressive disease, cancer, inflammatory bowel disease, or use of immunosuppressive drugs, the dormant herpes zoster virus is allowed to escape the watchful T lymphocytes. The virus then tracks along the nerve root reaching the epidermis and causes the skin vesicles to form. These skin vesicles contain viral particles and can be transmitted to others when exposure occurs [2].

For unclear reasons, the thoracic level is most commonly affected followed by the lumbar, cervical, and sacral dermatomes [2]. In severe disease, systemic dissemination can be fatal occur and involve any organ system including the nervous, cardiovascular, gastrointestinal, and/or pulmonary systems [2].

How Is This Problem Managed?

While it has been shown that antivirals help to heal vesicular herpetic lesions and decrease symptomatology, efficacy in the prevention of postherpetic neuralgia remains unclear. Prompt treatment with antiviral medications within 72-hours of initial infection is recommended to shorten the duration of rash and therefore the infective phase of the disease [2] (Table 21.2)

[7–10]. If acyclovir resistance develops, second-line antivirals may be used including foscarnet and cidofovir [2].

Systemic corticosteroids in combination with an antiviral agent have been shown to be effective in reducing the duration of dermatomal pain, recovery of hearing impairment, and improvement of facial nerve function in the case of Ramsay Hunt syndrome [2]. Unfortunately, systemic corticosteroids not been shown to be effective in preventing postherpetic neuralgia [11].

Other multimodal agents to help manage the pain from postherpetic neuralgia are frequently utilized for symptomatic pain control (Table 21.3) [12–24].

Invasive interventional treatments remain experimental but have been trialed with limited success for postherpetic neuralgia pain

Table 21.2 Antiviral medications for herpes zoster. All medications and formulations require renal adjustment for decreased glomerular filtration rate

Antiviral medication	Dosage	Common side effects ≥ 5% prevalence
Acyclovir	PO: 800 mg 5 times/day × 7–10 days IV: 10 mg/kg q8h × 8 days	PO: malaise, nausea IV: nausea/vomiting, phlebitis, increase of BUN/Cr
Famciclovir	500 mg q8h × 7 days	Headache, nausea/vomiting, fatigue, diarrhea, dysmenorrhea
Valacyclovir	1000 mg q8h × 7 days	Headache, nausea/vomiting, abdominal pain, increased ALT/AST, nasopharyngitis, fatigue, depression, skin rash, dysmenorrhea, arthralgia

Data from references [6–10]

PO per os, *IV* intravenous, *q8h* every 8 hours, *BUN* blood urea nitrogen, *Cr* creatinine, *ALT* alanine transaminase, *AST* aspartate aminotransferse

Table 21.3 Pharmacologic treatments of postherpetic neuralgia

Treatment modality	Recommended dose	Common side effects	Evidence
Gabapentin	Immediate release: 300–1800 mg qday Titrated to effect, BID or TID Extended release: 300–1800 qday Titrated to effect	>10% frequency: dizziness, drowsiness, ataxia, fatigue	Lexicomp® Online [12]; Rauck et al. [13], Fan et al. [14]
Pregabalin	Immediate release: 150–600 mg qday Titrated to effect, BID or TID dosing Extended release: 165–660 mg qday Titrated to effect	>10% frequency: peripheral edema, dizziness, drowsiness, headache, fatigue, weight gain, xerostomia, visual field loss, blurred vision	Lexicomp® Online [15]
Amitriptyline[a]	10–25 mg qhs or BID; increase dose 10–25 mg every 2–7 days; max dose 200 mg/day	Frequency not defined: arrhythmias, CNS dysfunction, rash, diabetes, SIADH, hepatitis, weakness, tremor, NMS, serotonin syndrome	Lexicomp® Online [16]
Nortriptyline[a]	10–20 mg qhs, may increase every 3–5 days in 10 mg qday increments; max 160 mg/day	Frequency not defined: arrhythmias agitation, anxiety, dizziness, drowsiness, SIADH, weight changes, ileus, thrombocytopenia, agranulocytosis, increased LFTs, tremor, visual changes	Lexicomp® Online [17]

(continued)

Table 21.3 (continued)

Treatment modality	Recommended dose	Common side effects	Evidence
Desipramine[a]	12.5–25 mg qday or BID, increase dose every 2–7 days up to max 150 mg/day	Frequency not defined: arrhythmias, stroke, ataxia, confusion, fatigue, diaphoresis, skin rash, SIADH, weight changes, urinary retention, constipation or diarrhea, thrombocytopenia, agranulocytosis, increased LFTs, tremor, visual changes	Lexicomp® Online [18]
Capsaicin 8% patch (Qutenza®)	Apply patch to painful area for 60 mins (up to 4 patches for coverage); repeat ≥3 months for symptom control	>10% frequency: localized erythema, local pain	Lexicomp® Online [19]
Lidocaine 5% patch	Apply to most painful area, can stay on up to 12 hrs over a 24-hr interval; up to 3 patches at once may be applied	>10% frequency: erythema, petechia	Lexicomp® Online [20]
Cobalamin[b]	1.00 mg/2 ml local subcutaneous injection × 28 days	Bleeding/bruising at injection site	Xu et al. [21]
Ascorbic Acid[b] (Pascorbin®)	IV: 7.5 g/50 ml; 2–4 treatments/week × 2 weeks	Itching/burning at injection site, paresthesia, urticaria	Schencking et al. [22]
Zinc sulfate[b]	IV 10–20 mg IV qday or 35 mg 3x/week × 3 weeks followed by oral elemental zinc 10–20 mg/day × 2 months	No noted side effects in case reports; frequency not defined, though dizziness, headache, nausea, vomiting have all been reported	Lexicomp® Online [23], Lin et al. [24]

qday daily, *BID* twice daily dosing, *TID* three times daily dosing, *CNS* central nervous system, *SIADH* syndrome of inappropriate antidiuretic hormone secretion, *NMS* neuroleptic malignant syndrome, *LFTs* liver function tests
[a]Off label or experimental use
[b]Adjuvant therapy to neuromodulators and antivirals + off label use

(Table 21.4) [25–30]. Generally invasive methods are considered a treatment of last resort due to the limited evidence and higher risk of complications.

Vaccination

The luxury of vaccination against herpes zoster has afforded an opportunity to discuss prevention of postherpetic neuralgia rather than treatment. The CDC recommends the VZV vaccine for all children 12 months of age or older who lack immunity to VZV [3]. It is important to recognize that children who have received the VZV vaccine remain at risk to develop subsequent herpes zoster, though their risk is significantly lower than those children who endured infection [3]. Per the Center for Disease Control and Prevention, 99.5% of individuals born in 1978 or earlier have been infected with wild-type (or non-vaccine acquired) VZV [3]. It is estimated that 33% of the US population will develop herpes zoster over the course of their lifetime with approximately one million new cases annually [6]. Per the CDC, herpes zoster rates are increasing in the USA for unclear reasons [3].

To proactively prevent herpes zoster infection, adults aged 50 years and older should receive two doses 2–6 months apart of shingles vaccine (Shingrix®). Shingrix® is new 2017 FDA-approved vaccine formulation and is recom-

Table 21.4 Interventional treatments of postherpetic neuralgia

Intervention	Inclusion group	Outcomes	Common risks	Evidence
Intrathecal and epidural injections				
2 mg of midazolam (IT[a]) + 60 mg of methylprednisolone (EP) single shot	Patients w/ persistent allodynia for 3–6 months	Analgesia ≤1 month	Sedation, PDPH	Dureja et al. [25]
80 mg methylprednisolone acetate +10 mg bupivacaine (EP) single shot	Acute herpes zoster (rash <7 days)	Analgesia ≤1 month; ineffective for prevention of PHN	Dizziness, flushing, headache, backache	Van Wijck et al. [4]
IV acyclovir 10 mg/kg TID × 9 days + prednisolone 60 mg q/day w/ taper for 21 days vs. 6–12 cc 0.25% bupivacaine q6-8h or 12 h + methylprednisolone 40 mg q3–4 days via EP catheter for 7–21 days	Acute herpes zoster (rash <7 days)	22.2% incidence of pain after 1 year in acyclovir +steroids vs. 1.6% after epidural +steroids	Acyclovir + steroids: nausea, vomiting, diarrhea, dyspepsia Steroids+ epidural: sweating, fainting, neck pain, paresis, oliguria	Pasqualucci et al. [26]
Nerve blocks and epidural injections				
PVB vs. stellate ganglion block vs. single epidural steroid injection vs. continuous epidural	Heterogeneous mix; meta-analysis	PVB and continuous or repeated epidurals decreased duration of pain and incidence of PHN at 3, 6, and 12 months; no improvement of pain w/stellate ganglion or single epidural injection	Dizziness, headache, backache, PDPH	Kim et al. [27]
Cryotherapy 30 second liquid nitrogen spray in affected dermatome weekly ranging from 1–20 treatments	Heterogeneous mix; PHN 1 week to >1 month of symptoms	Reduction in pain by ≥70% achieved in 75% of patients, unclear duration of sustained pain relief	None cited	Calandria [28]
Spinal cord stimulation	PHN >2 years	82% achieved long-term pain relief (median 29; range 9–38.5 months)	None cited; though lead failure, migration, infection, pain, wound breakdown all cited with stimulators [29]	Harke et al. [30]

IT intrathecal, *EP* epidural, *PDPH* post-dural puncture headache, *PVB* paravertebral block, *PHN* postherpetic neuralgia, *qday* dosed once daily, *BID* twice daily dosing, *TID* three times daily dosing

[a]Off label use, preservative free hydrochloride solution

mended even if patients received the previous live attenuated Zostavax® vaccine [3]. Shingrix® is 90% effective compared to 51% effective for Zostavax [3, 29]. Furthermore, Shingrix has sustaining efficacy over time, while Zostavax wanes to 18% effective in persons greater than 80 years old [3, 31]. In addition, Shingrix® contains an adjuvant component called AS01B, which helps to boost the immune system to increase duration of effectiveness [32].

What Is the Prognosis of This Condition?

Debilitating pain from postherpetic neuralgia is well documented and of variable duration [2, 3, 5]. Permanent complications from herpes zoster infection vary and are associated with the location of the affected dermatome and type of medical care received at symptom onset. It is estimated that 6% of cases that affect the eye result in permanent visual loss [33]. Other common complications of eye involvement include conjunctivitis, keratitis, scleritis, uveitis/iridocyclitis, and anterior uveitis [34]. Herpes zoster affecting the facial nerve may leave permanent palsies in 50% of patients. Secondary infection affects up to 30% of individuals [34]. Several other known complications of herpes zoster includes, but not limited to, myositis, Guillian-Barré syndrome, limb paresis, foot drop, voiding dysfunction, stroke, and jaw osteonecrosis [34]. Mortality from herpes zoster is estimated to be 0.017–0.465/100,000 person-years [33].

Discussion

Prevalence

Herpes zoster is extremely common with one third of all people developing infection during their lifetime; 20% of these affected individuals will develop postherpetic neuralgia [2, 3].

Differential Diagnosis

The differential diagnosis of herpes zoster includes impetigo, contact dermatitis, folliculitis, scabies, insect bites, papular urticaria, candida infection, dermatitis herpetiformis, drug eruptions, or vesicular exanthemas caused by coxsackie or echo virus. Zoster is also often confused with the rash of herpes simplex virus (HSV), including eczema herpeticum [6, 35].

Predictive Value of Different Clinical Features (History and Physical Exam) and Lab Testing/Imagining

Herpes zoster is considered to be a clinical diagnosis based on symptoms and presence of a vesicular rash in a dermatomal distribution. While techniques including electron microscopy and the Tzanck smear can confirm the diagnosis of herpes viral infection, these techniques are rarely used clinically due to cost and accessibility. A Tzanck smear has a sensitivity of ≥80% and specificity of ≥90% with a positive predictive value of ≥0.88 and negative predictive value of ≥0.82. However, these methods cannot distinguish the difference between herpes simplex virus and varicella zoster virus [2, 35].

Other confirmatory techniques which are more commonly used clinically for disseminated disease include polymerase chain reaction (PCR), direct immunofluorescense assay, skin biopsy, or viral culture [2]. PCR has a high sensitivity (95%) and specificity (100%) due to the detection of viral DNA and is often readily available if the clinical diagnosis is in question [6].

Strength of Evidence for Different Treatment Modalities

Evidence for capsaicin 8% patches, gabapentin, pregabalin, amitriptyline, nortriptyline, and desipramine have consistent, good-quality patient-oriented evidence for clinical use, also known as a grade A rating as determined by the American Academy of Family Physicians (AAFP). Antivirals including acyclovir, valacyclovir, and famciclovir have inconsistent or limited-quality patient-oriented evidence in decreasing the duration of symptoms and severity of pain related to postherpetic neuralgia, consistent with a grade B rating [6].

Role of Sympathetic Block

Often commonly practiced and suggested, sympathetic blocks have no proven role in preventing or treating postherpetic neuralgia. There is no randomized study, few outcome studies, or retrospective reports published. Level of evidence is reported at level 2C.

Role of Neuromodulation

Kurklinksy et al. [36] published a review of literature on this topic. In his article, he found 20 original reports that described 309 patients with

PHN who were treated with SCS. Sixteen reports had a permanent implantation of SCS, with a total of 255 patients, out of which 120 had long-term pain relief. There were six reports of subcutaneous PNS for PHN (in a thoracic area). Four reports provided data on success rates where all five patients received complete pain relief. Pulsed radiofrequency has also been reported in case reports as an effective intervention by applying the modality at DRG level. Overall, the strength of evidence for neuromodulatory therapy is 2C.

Future Directions or Clinical Trials in Progress

Future topics for investigation include delineating sustained duration of vaccination effectiveness, especially in light of the newly released Shingrix vaccine. In addition, the factors related to triggers of zoster infection remain largely unknown. While we know that age has a clear link to emergence of the herpes zoster virus, it remains unclear if recommendations for earlier vaccination should occur in specific groups of younger individuals. Immunocompromised individuals have been identified to be at high risk of zoster infection, yet it remains unclear what triggers the disease in healthy individuals.

Despite a significant number of medications available to treat postherpetic neuralgia, many of these medications have significant side effects which preclude their use in certain individuals. As of May 2018, 146 trials investigating new treatments for postherpetic neuralgia are registered with ClinicalTrials.gov[36]. Six of these clinical trials are actively enrolling patients; three are investigating drug treatments and three are investigating invasive treatment modalities. The drug treatment groups include EMA401, a competitive antagonist of the angiotensin II receptor, 3VM1001 Cream, which includes a low concentration of copper, as well as ABX-1431 affecting neuromodulation. Invasive techniques undergoing evaluation include transcranial magnetic simulation for facial pain related to HSV affecting the trigeminal nerve, performance of a lumbar sympathetic block under fluoroscopy, and effectiveness of electroacupuncture for intractable neuropathic pain [37].

Conclusion/Summary

Herpes zoster is a pervasive, debilitating disease which disproportionally affects older individuals and those suffering from immunosuppression. It can affect eyesight and neurological function, and cause such severe pain that quality of life can suffer immensely. While new technology and vaccination availability is continually improving, many people around the globe do not have access to these medical therapies or they remain cost prohibitive. Even among infected individuals with access to treatment, medication side effects can limit their use. Further investigation into more favorable and easily tolerated treatment methods is ongoing and details regarding the long-term efficacy of the new herpes zoster vaccination remains unclear.

References

1. Albrecht M. Clinical features of varicella-zoster virus infection: chickenpox. In: UpToDate, Post TW (editors). UpToDate. Waltham. Accessed on 09 May 2018.
2. Koshy E, Mengting L, Kumar H, Jianbo W. Epidemiology, treatment and prevention of herpes zoster: a comprehensive review. Indian J Dermatol Venereol Leprol. 2018;84:251–62.
3. CDC.gov. Shingles (Herpes Zoster): for health care professionals. CDC. [Internet] 2018. [Accessed 25 May 2018.] Available from: https://www.cdc.gov/shingles/hcp/clinical-overview.html.
4. Van Wijck A, Opstelten W, Moons K, Van Essen G, Stolker R, Kalkman C, Verheij T. The PINE study of epidural steroids and local anaesthetics to prevent postherpetic neuralgia: a randomized controlled trial. Lancet. 2006;367(9506):219–24.
5. Shailesh G, Parikh V, Parikh R. Herpes zoster oticus: a rare clinical entity. Contemp Clin Dent. 2010;12(2):127–9.
6. Saguil A, Kane S, Mercado M. Herpes zoster and postherpetic neuralgia: prevention and management. Am Fam Physician. 2017;96(10):656–63.
7. Harpaz R, Ortega-Sanchez I, Seward J. CDC: prevention of herpes zoster: recommendations of the advisory committee on immunization practices (ACIP). MMWR Recomm Rep. 2008;57(05):1–30.

8. Lexicomp® Online. Acyclovir (systemic): drug information. Hudson: Lexi-Comp, Inc; 2018.
9. Lexicomp® Online. Famciclovir: drug information. Hudson: Lexi-Comp, Inc; 2018.
10. Lexicomp® Online. Valacyclovir (systemic): drug information. Hudson: Lexi-Comp, Inc; 2018.
11. Han Y, Zhang J, Chen N, He L, Zhou M, Zhu C. Corticosteroids for prevention postherpetic neuralgia. Cochrane Database Syst Rev. 2013;3:1–31.
12. Lexicomp® Online. Gabapentin: drug information. Hudson: Lexi-Comp, Inc; 2018.
13. Rauck R, Irving G, Wallace M, Vanhove G, Sweeney M. Once-daily gastroretentive gabapentin for postherpetic neuralgia: integrated efficacy, time to onset of pain relief and safety analyses of data from two phase 3, multicenter, randomized, double-blind placebo-controlled studies. J Pain Symptom Manag. 2013;46(2):219–28.
14. Fan H, Yu W, Zhang Q, Cao H, Li J, Wang J, Shao Y, Hu X. Efficacy and safety of gabapentin 1800mg treatment for post-herpetic neuralgia: a meta-analysis of randomized controlled trials. J Clin Pharm Ther. 2014;39(4):334–42.
15. Lexicomp® Online. Pregabalin: drug information. Hudson: Lexi-Comp, Inc; 2018.
16. Lexicomp® Online. Amitriptyline: drug information. Hudson: Lexi-Comp, Inc; 2018.
17. Lexicomp® Online. Nortriptyline: drug information. Hudson: Lexi-Comp, Inc; 2018.
18. Lexicomp® Online. Desipramine: drug information. Hudson: Lexi-Comp, Inc; 2018.
19. Lexicomp® Online. Capsiacin: drug information. Hudson: Lexi-Comp, Inc; 2018.
20. Lexicomp® Online. Lidocaine (topical): drug information. Hudson: Lexi-Comp, Inc; 2018.
21. Xu G, Zhong-Wei L, Feng Y, Tang W, Xu G. A single-center randomized controlled trial of local methylcobalamin injection for subacute herpetic neuralgia. Pain Med. 2013;14:884–94.
22. Schencking M, Vollbracht C, Weiss G, Lebert J, Biller A, Goyvaerts B, Kraft K. Intravenous vitamin C in the treatment of shingles: results of a multicenter prospective cohort study. Med Sci Monit. 2012;18(4):215–24.
23. Lexicomp® Online. Zinc sulfate: drug information. Hudson: Lexi-Comp, Inc; 2018.
24. Lin Y, Lan K, Want L, Chen J. Treatment of postherpetic neuralgia with intravenous administration of zinc sulfate: a case report. A A Pract. 2018;11(1):8–10.
25. Dureja G, Usmani H, Khan M, Tahseen M, Jamal A. Efficacy of intrathecal midazolam with or without epidural methylprednisolone for management of post-herpetic neuralgia involving lumbosacral dermatomes. Pain Physician. 2010;13(3):213–21.
26. Pasqualucci A, Pasqualucci V, Galla F, De Angelis V, Marzocchi V, Coulssi R, et al. Prevention of post-herpetic neuralgia: acyclovir and prednisolone versus epidural local anesthetic and methylprednisolone. Acta Anaesthesiol Scand. 2000;44:910–8.
27. Kim H, Ahn H, Lee J, Choi S, Cheong Y, Kwon K, Yoon S, Leem J. Effects of applying nerve blocks to prevent postherpetic neuralgia in patients with acute herpes zoster: a systemic review and meta-analysis. Korean J Pain. 2017;30(1):3–17.
28. Calandria L. Cryoanalgesia for post-herpetic neuralgia: a new treatment. Int J Dermatol. 2011;50(6):746–50.
29. Eldabe S, Buschser E, Duarte R. Complications of spinal cord stimulation and peripheral nerve stimulation techniques: a review of the literature. Pain Med. 2016;17(2):325–36.
30. Harke H, Gretenkort P, Ladleif H, Koester P, Rahman S. Spinal cord stimulation in postherpetic neuralgia and in acute herpes zoster pain. Anesth Analg. 2002;94(3):694–700.
31. Merck. [Internet]. Merck.com. 2018 [cited 11 May 2018]. Available from: https://www.merck.com/product/usa/pi_circulars/z/zostavax/zostavax_pi2.pdf.
32. Drug and device news. P T. 2017;42(12):726–63.
33. Kawai K, Gebremeskel B, Acosta C. Systematic reviews of incidence and complications of herpes zoster: towards a global perspective. BMH Open. 2014;4(6):E 004833.
34. Chen L, Arai H, Chen L, Chou M, Djauzi S, Dong B, et al. Looking back to move forward: a twenty-year audit of herpes zoster in Asia- Pacific. BMC Infect Dis. 2017;17(213):2–39.
35. Oranje A, Folkers E. The Tzanck Smear: old, but still of inestimable value. Pediatr Dermatol. 1988;5(2):127–9.
36. Kurklinsky S, Palmer SC, Arroliga MJ, Ghazi SM. Neuromodulation in postherpetic neuralgia: case reports and review of the literature. Pain Med. 2018;19(6):1237–44.
37. National Institute of health: US. National Library of Medicine. [Internet] 2018. ClinicalTrials.gov. [Accessed 01 May 2018]. Available from: https://www.clinicaltrials.gov/ct2/results?cond=Postherpetic+Neuralgia&term=&cntry=&state=&city=&dist=.

22 Functional Abdominal Pain (Chronic Abdominal Pain)

Tariq Malik

Case Description

An 18-year-old woman presents to the pain management clinic with complaints of recurrent abdominal pain for the past 1 year. She describes her pain as central abdominal pain, non-radiating, crampy in nature, accompanied by nausea but no vomiting. Pain is worsened by eating and last from few minutes to few hours, nothing helps when its severe and she often end up going to the ER where intravenous analgesic helps. She has been going to the ER more often lately and has also missed many school days. She does not remember if there was a triggering event such as infection, surgery, or trauma. It came on insidiously and has not left since it started. The pain is not associated with certain foods or with a change in bowel habits. She was previously evaluated by her pediatrician who reported that an abdominal ultrasound and CBC were unrevealing for an obvious cause. She was referred to a gastroenterologist who did upper gastrointestinal scope and did not find any pathology. She was found to have no food allergy and rest of her labs done over the years by various consultants has been consistently negative. She does not take any medications and is otherwise healthy. She is a senior in high school and has been very worried about college acceptance and picking a career path. She is concerned about how this abdominal pain will affect her quality of life at school.

T. Malik (✉)
Department of Anesthesia and Critical Care, University of Chicago, Chicago, IL, USA
e-mail: TMuslim@dacc.uchicago.edu

What Is Your Preliminary Diagnosis?

The patient has been extensively evaluated by various consultants and all her laboratory tests and imaging have been negative. She is not losing weight and has no constitutional symptoms such as fever, blood in stools, or night sweats. Her symptoms are consistent with gut dysmotility and functional bowel disorder. The preliminary diagnosis is most consistent with functional abdominal pain (FAP), also known as centrally mediated abdominal pain syndrome. Abdominal pain can vary widely in etiology and presentation; however, recurrent pain without obvious cause and associated with stress is likely functional abdominal pain. FAP is pain that persists for at least 6 months, without evidence of structural or metabolic disease, has no relationship to events (digestion, menstruation, bowel movements), and interferes with daily functioning [1]. The pain is constant or frequently recurring. It has a higher comorbidity with psychiatric disorders; and would even satisfy a pain criterion toward that diagnosis of a somatization disorder [2].

T. Malik (ed.), *Practical Chronic Pain Management*, https://doi.org/10.1007/978-3-030-46675-6_22

How Is Diagnosis Confirmed?

A detailed HPI should be obtained on presentation, including pain location, quality, frequency, duration, and any exacerbating/alleviating factors. The physical exam should review vital signs (noting tachycardia, presence of fever), and obtain a thorough abdominal exam (presence of peritoneal findings). FAP is not usually associated with physical exam findings consistent with organic causes of abdominal pain such as fever, jaundice, abdominal masses, blood in stool, etc.

Description of Pain

FAP patients often describe their pain in emotional terms [2], as constant, not relating to any physiological process (eating, defecation), and in a large area of the abdomen vs a precise location. It is constant or very frequent, pain is often severe and compromises daily functioning. There may also be descriptions of other extraintestinal pain.

Symptom Behavior

These behaviors are typical of FAP patients but are neither sensitive nor specific and have limited diagnostic values. They include urgent reporting of intense symptoms, minimizing potential role for psychosocial contributors, seeking healthcare frequently, requesting narcotics, wanting complete symptom relief, requesting diagnostic studies, and taking limited personal responsibility for self-management [2].

Psychosocial Features and Assessment

It is helpful to evaluate psychosocial history and identify any stressors (death, divorce, or trauma/abuse). Patients may exhibit anxiety, depression, or somatization. However, unlike patients with these primary diagnoses, patients with FAP do not often want to accept that these could contribute to their prevention [2].

In addition, the ROME IV criteria can be used to diagnose FAP (Table 22.1). It should be noted that the most recent edition of the ROME criteria published in 2016, refers to FAP as "Centrally mediated abdominal pain syndrome" to highlight its strong central component and lack of evidence for abdominal structural/mechanical/metabolic disease process [3]. The ROME IV criteria allow for a clinical diagnosis of FAP and related functional conditions (irritable bowel syndrome, functional dyspepsia, abdominal migraine). As a change from the prior Rome III criteria, FAP can be diagnosed based on symptoms "after appropriate medical evaluation the symptoms cannot be attributed to another medical condition" rather than the previous criteria's requirement that there "is no evidence for organic disease" [4].

Table 22.1 Diagnostic criteria for FAP, based on ROME IV

ROME IV criteria
Continuous or nearly continuous abdominal pain
No or only occasional relationship of pain with physiological events (eating, defection, menses)
Pain limits some aspects of daily functioning
Pain is not feigned
Pain is not explained by another structural or functional GI disorder or other medical condition

Must include ALL of the above; criteria fulfilled for the last 3 months with symptom onset at least 6 months before diagnosis

Diagnostic studies may also be done to exclude organic and physiological causes, but may not always be necessary in the absence of alarming symptoms. Imaging studies such as ultrasound, CT, or endoscopic studies or laboratory studies (CBC, liver panel, lipase, urinalysis) can determine if there is a potential abdominal process at work (Table 22.2).

What Is the Pathophysiology of This Condition?

Like many chronic pain conditions, the etiology and pathophysiology of FAP is not well understood [2], but is thought to be due to impaired nociception involving a central process resulting in visceral hyperalgesia. The condition is best explained using biopsychosocial model. The condition may be precipitated by some event that initiates a hypersensitivity which is then sustained. The sensitivity could come from low grade inflammation affecting nerve endings, or

Table 22.2 Chronic abdominal pain algorithm

1. Does pain improves with defecation? Does patient has altered stool consistency or frequency	
a. If yes, then	Irritable bowel syndrome
b. If no	Move to next question
2. Is pain upper abdominal along with sensation of satiety or fullness or feeling of heart burn with eating	
a. Yes	Functional dyspepsia
b. No	Next question
3. Constant or frequent vague or crampy abdominal pain with no evidence of malingering	
a. Yes	Functional abdominal pain
b. No	Look for
4. Increased pain with contraction or palpation of the abdominal wall muscles (Carnett's sign)	
a. Yes	Muscle wall pathology/ somatic pain
b. No	See if
5. Increased pain with opioid use	
a. Yes	Narcotic bowel

repeated chemical irritation from the breakdown products of food/bile acids, or repeated bowel distention. The increased sensitivity leads to persistent sensory neuronal input in the dorsal horn of the spinal cord which may become abnormally excitable and hyperalgesic due to several factors including persistent activation of NMDA receptor [1]. There may be alterations in endogenous pain modulation systems, including dysfunction of descending pain modulation and cortical pain modulation circuits [2]. Whatever the mechanism, the presence of this sensitization leads to complaints of pain along with symptoms of bloating or indigestion and/or altered bowel frequency [4]. Role of enteric plexus cannot be discounted. In normal gut, serotonin is released from enetrochromaffin cell and activates peristaltic reflex. Vagal and spinal afferent are also involved in modulating bowel peristalsis. The eneteric reflex involves release of excitatory (acetylcholine, tachykinins) or inhibitory neurotransmitters (vasoactive intestinal peptides, nitric oxide). Imbalance in these neurotransmitters either from serotonergic dysfunction or food mediated release of these chemicals in maladaptive neuronal circuitry can account for many symptoms of functional abdominal pain. Belief systems and coping mechanisms typically seen in FAPS patients are consistent with the possibility of altered influences of cortical networks (including prefrontal and parietal cortical regions) on limbic and pain modulation circuits. Early life stresses (parental loss, physical or verbal abuse) or adult life psychological stresses (divorce, bereavement) can affect brain-gut axis, creating hypersensitive gut by facilitating afferent transmission by lowering activity in the descending inhibitory pathways [2]. There is no proof that these psychological traits have any causal relation. At the very least, they contribute to behavior which involve preoccupation with symptoms, catastrophization, and frequent use of healthcare resources.

Repeated injury can cause abdominal nerve receptors to become overly sensitized. Patients who have had multiple abdominal surgeries, procedures, or insults (e.g., infection), can perceive a later painful experience as more painful/out of proportion to what is expected.

Psychological factors are thought to play a role in amplifying pain signals and causing perception of pain with low-level inputs and persistence of pain after the inputs have ended. Stressors such as death, divorce, or abuse can precipitate episodes, and times of added stress can make symptoms worse. Furthermore, the pain itself may act as a stressor, participating in a positive feedback loop.

Diagnostic testing should be limited. In the absence of alarming symptoms, the risk of missing an organic cause is less than 5%. Celiac disease can be ruled out using blood test (tissue tranglutaminase antibodies) or duodenal mucosal biopsy. Somehow celiac disease is more uncommon in patients with functional gut disorder than in the general population. Inflammatory bowel disease is highly unlikely(less than 1% chance) if C-reactive protein level or fecal calprotectin levels are low along with clinical features of functional symptoms. Colorectal cancer is also very unlikely if there are no accompanying alarming symptoms (weight loss, blood in the stool).

Table 22.3 Medications for treating functional abdominal psain

Medication	Serotonin effects (5-HT)	Histamine effects (H-1)	Acetylcholine effects	Initial dose (mg)	Dose range (mg)
Amitriptyline	++	++	++++	10	25–150
Imipramine	++	++	++++	10	25–150
Desipramine	++++	++	+	10	25–150

How Is This Problem Managed?

Treatment is often very difficult and frustrating. Most patients seek care from multiple physicians and seek validations of their sickness as all tests tend to come back within normal range. There is no treatment modality to cure FAP. However, there are helpful ways that clinicians can provide relief. Management is based on a therapeutic, trusting physician-patient relationship and can also include medications that act centrally [2] (Table 22.3). Treatment is best when multi-faceted and can include both psychological and pharmacological approaches. The best intervention is extensive education of the patients on the pathophysiology and nature of functional abdominal pain. It is important to stress the benign nature of the disease. Many physicians start by encouraging patients to keep a diary to identify possible triggers (emotional or situational) that precipitate worsening of symptoms.

Psychological treatment options include cognitive behavioral therapy or psychotherapy, relaxation techniques, or hypnosis. Furthermore, reassurance and education on dietary modifications, stress reduction, and coping mechanisms also help.

Pharmacologically, antidepressants, particularly, low-dose daily tricyclic antidepressants (TCAs) or SSRI/SNRIs, can help provide symptomatic relief for chronic abdominal pain [2]. The mechanism by which these medications to relieve FAP is not understood [4]. One proposed mechanism is serotonin-mediated effects on the GI tract, such as increased motility, another, for TCAs, is a norepinephrine-mediated decrease in pain sensitivity as is hypothesized for their use in other pain disorders, and a third potential mechanism is through their anticholinergic effects on the GI system [4]. In a Cochrane meta-analysis, 59% of the patients improved on TCA vs 39% in the control group. Amitriptyline was found to be most helpful in dose range 25–150 mg daily. The beneficial effects may take 4–6 weeks to show up. In cases where a psychiatric disorder is also present, antidepressants can alleviate depression or anxiety contributing to symptoms, providing additional benefit. SSRIs have not shown to make a difference in abdominal pain but do help by improving sense of well-being and have better side-effect profile compared to TCA. SRNIs (venlafaxine/duloxetine) have shown to improve pressure tolerance of colonic balloon distention but no effect on abdominal pain. They are used in refractory abdominal cases. Opioids do not have a role in managing FAP, and can lead to addiction, dependence, or narcotic bowel syndrome.

What Is the Prognosis of This Condition?

As stated above, FAP is not curable, but treatments are aimed at improving symptoms and overall quality of life. FAP does have a chronic course. FAP can negatively affect general health, personal relationships, psychological well-being, with patients often developing or having co-existing psychiatric disorders. Distress and disability overall is a concern in these patients.

Discussion

Prevalence

The epidemiology of FAP is difficult to determine. It is generally considered less common than other functional gastrointestinal disorders such as irritable bowel syndrome or functional dyspepsia. Reported prevalence figures in North America range from 0.5% to 2% [6]. FAP is quite common in children, with an estimated worldwide prevalence of 13.5% in the pediatric population [4]. The disorder is more common in females (Female:male = 3:2), with prevalence peaking in the fourth decade of life [2]. Clinical evidence suggests that there is a strong association of negative early life events and certain psychosocial stressors with increased pain reports among patients with functional gastrointestinal disorders [2].

Furthermore, FAP has a large economic healthcare burden. FAP patients in the United States missed work a mean of 11.8 days in a year, 3 times more than subjects without abdominal symptoms, and "felt too sick to go to work" at the moment of the survey in 11.2% of cases, about 3 times more frequently than respondents without functional gastrointestinal disorders [4].

Differential Diagnosis

FAP is a diagnosis of exclusion. The differential diagnosis includes irritable bowel syndrome (pain with abnormal bowel movements), functional dyspepsia (pain in upper abdomen, associated with symptoms of indigestion), and abdominal migraine (sudden onset of severe pain associated with other migraine-like symptoms such as sweating, dizziness, light sensitivity). FAP differs from IBS in that pain is the central complaint, rather than abnormal bowel movements. Pain associated with CAPS may be colicky in nature, as in IBS, although it tends to be more prolonged and widespread [5]. Patients with abdominal migraines describe their pain as cyclical, rather than constant or near-constant in FAP.

Predictive Value of Different Clinical Features (Both on History and Physical Exam) and Lab Testing/Imaging

Since FAP is a diagnosis of exclusion, a detailed clinical evaluation is the most helpful in making a diagnosis. This is best achieved with the use of the ROME criteria. Evaluation of symptom behavior and psychosocial features can be helpful, but are neither sensitive nor specific for diagnosing FAP. In the absence of alarming signs or symptoms, laboratory testing or imaging studies may not be necessary.

Strength of Evidence for Different Treatment Modalities

There are no randomized control trials to evaluate the effectiveness of various pharmacological drugs. Most studies were single center, with small sample size, and with heterogeneous methodology, and still most interventions were shown to be better than placebo. Based on a systemic review and a meta-analysis, the NNT for TCA to show improvement in abdominal pain is 5, and for overall improvement, NNT is 4.

Nonpharmacological interventions have not been studied specially in chronic abdominal pain but have been studied in patients with other functional gut disorders. Cognitive behavior disorder, hypnotherapy, and stress management have all found to be useful in those conditions. These interventions may not affect the intensity of pain but the overall global score improves.

Future Directions

More research is needed to better characterize patients with FAP, implement diagnostic criteria with improved specificity, and further understand the central pathophysiological process involved.

Conclusion/Summary

In conclusion, FAP, is a centrally mediated pain process that can have a huge impact of patients' quality of life. It is a clinical diagnosis and one of exclusion, using a detailed clinical evaluation with the help of the ROME IV criteria. FAP can be distinguished from other functional, non-centrally mediated, GI disorders such as IBS, functional dyspepsia, and abdominal migraines. The mainstay of treatment involved both pharmacological and psychological approaches to improve symptom management and overall quality of life.

References

1. Greenberger NJ. Chronic abdominal pain and recurrent abdominal pain - gastrointestinal disorders [Internet]. Merck Manuals Professional Edition. Merck Manuals; 2018.
2. Clouse RE, Mayer EA, Aziz Q, Drossman DA, Dumitrascu DL, Mönnikes H, et al. Functional abdominal pain syndrome. Gastroenterology. 2006;130(5):1492–7.
3. Schmulson MJ, Drossman DA. What is new in Rome IV. J Neurogastroenterol Motil. 2017;23(2):151–63.
4. Drossman DA, Hasler WL. Rome IV—functional GI disorders: disorders of gut-brain interaction. Gastroenterology. 2016;150(6):1257–61.
5. Keefer L, Drossman DA, Guthrie E, Simrén M, Tillisch K, Olden K, et al. Centrally mediated disorders of gastrointestinal pain. Gastroenterology. 2016;150(6):1408–19.

A 35-Year-Old Man with Chronic Abdominal Pain (Chronic Pancreatitis)

23

Sumit Jain and Dalia H. Elmofty

Case Description

A 35-year-old man with a history of alcohol abuse presents to his primary care physician for chronic abdominal pain. The pain began approximately 1 year prior and has been relatively unchanged in quality since its onset. During this time, he has had approximately 35 pounds of unintentional weight loss. The pain is mid-epigastric and he describes it as a nagging, constant, and dull in nature that worsens approximately 30 minutes after meals. The pain radiates to his back and associated with nausea following meals. He has tried antacids (e.g., tums, omeprazole, ranitidine) and pain medications (e.g., tylenol, ibuprofen, naproxen) with some relief of symptoms. He reports that leaning forward or sitting straight sometimes relieves his discomfort. He denies any associated fevers, chills, changes in his bowel habits, diarrhea, constipation, melena, hematochezia, dysuria, or polyuria.

S. Jain
Department of Anesthesiology, Northshore University, Evanston, IL, USA

D. H. Elmofty (✉)
Department of Anesthesia, University of Chicago, Chicago, IL, USA
e-mail: delmofty@dacc.uchicago.edu

What Is Your Preliminary Diagnosis?

The differential diagnosis of mid-epigastric pain is quite broad, and therefore it is essential to gather a thorough history to narrow the diagnosis. There are several elements in this case presentation that points toward a potential diagnosis of CP. The main complaint in patients with CP is abdominal pain, with incidence of approximately 81.7% [1]. Patients with alcoholic CP have two distinguished patterns of abdominal pain. The first pattern that is described is of intermittent pain episodes that typically last <10 days followed by periods without pain, which can last greater than 1 year [2]. The second pattern is characterized by chronic pain complaints with intermittent exacerbations. As the disease progresses the pain can change from pattern one to two, and in some patients the pain can eventually stop as the disease burns out and glands are destroyed [3]. The pain is epigastric, radiates to the back, and occurs 15–30 minutes following meals. Although abdominal pain is the most common complaint, it may not be present in up to 20% of patients [1, 4]. These patients may present with exocrine dysfunction without abdominal pain. Other common complaints include loss of weight, dyspepsia, nausea, anemia, and new onset diabetes [1].

As seen in the case above, one of the most common etiologies of CP that can be identified on history is alcohol use. In males, alcohol use

T. Malik (ed.), *Practical Chronic Pain Management*, https://doi.org/10.1007/978-3-030-46675-6_23

represents the most common etiology for CP [1]. For females, biliary disease is the most common etiology [1]. When all patients are considered, biliary disease is the most common cause (38.5%) for CP [1].

What Is the Pathophysiology of This Condition?

The major hallmarks seen in CP is a combination of glandular atrophy, ductal changes, fibrosis, and inflammation [5]. Several theories have been postulated to provide a unifying synthesis of the pathophysiology of CP with the four major traditional theories being the oxidative stress, toxic metabolic, stone and duct obstruction, and necrosis-fibrosis models [5]. The oxidative stress model postulated by Braganza states that the root cause of CP is due to the by-product of hepatic oxidases, which in excess result in oxidative stress to the pancreas [6]. This leads to inflammation and tissue damage [6]. The major limitation of this theory is that there is no evidence that the oxidative stress initiates the disease process [5]. The toxic-metabolic theory proposed by Bordalo et al. states that alcohol directly damages the acinar cell leading to alterations in cellular metabolism [7]. However, there is limited literature to support that steatopancreatitis seen in alcoholics is a precursor of fibrosis [5, 8]. The stone and ductal theory emphasized by Sarles et al. states that CP is a separate entity from acute pancreatitis [8]. The CP pathogenesis is initiated by increased pancreatic exocrine function modulated by alcohol [9]. This in turn leads to increased pancreatic fluid lithogenicity resulting in stone and protein plug formation [5, 9]. This can cause stasis and obstruction resulting in atrophy and fibrosis [5, 9]. One of the major flaws within this study is that in early stages of pancreatitis, mild fibrosis protein plugs were found in less than half of the patients [10]. Additionally, causality between protein plugs and pancreatic fibrosis has not been well established in the literature. The necrosis-fibrosis theory states that recurrent episodes of acute pancreatitis result in inflammation and necrosis leading to scarring, obstruction, and stone formation within the tubules [5].

Newer concepts include the primary duct hypothesis proposed by Cavallini. Within this theory, the major etiology of ductal destruction is an immunologic attack causing fibrosis and scarring [11]. Alcohol may play a role in modulating target antigens resulting in this autoimmune attack [5, 11]. The sentinel acute pancreatitis event (SAPE) hypothesis by Whitcomb et al. incorporates several prior theories (necrosis-fibrosis, toxic-metabolic, oxidative stress) in order to provide a unifying mechanism for the development of CP [5, 12, 13]. Within this theory, the sentinel event is an episode of acute pancreatitis that sensitizes the pancreas. If the inciting factors are removed, the pancreas can heal. However, if there are repeated bouts of pancreatitis, the acinar cells continue to secrete cytokines resulting in inflammation and deposition of collagen leading to fibrosis [12, 13].

Currently, the pathogenesis of CP appears to be multifactorial. It is likely that different etiologies result in CP through various mechanisms [5]. For example, the pathogenesis of CP secondary to obstruction may be different than that due to alcohol.

How Is the Diagnosis Made?

History

Early diagnosis of CP is essential as advanced CP has a poor prognosis with a mortality rate twofold higher than the general population. Obtaining key information from a patient's history can direct a physician toward the diagnosis of CP [14]. Approximately 60–80% of cases are related to alcohol consumption, usually between 80–120 g/day [14–16]. Epidemiological studies have shown that there is also a dose response relationship between the amount of daily alcohol use and risk for developing CP [16]. Smoking was also found to have a higher prevalence in patients with CP, with a multicenter study reporting that nearly half of patients with CP were current smokers [17]. Other risk factors include chronic renal failure, hypercalcemia, hyperlipidemia, autosomal disease (i.e., CFTR and SPINK mutations), recurrent acute pancreatitis, and sphincter of oddi disorders.

Laboratory Tests

No single laboratory test is diagnostic for early pancreatitis. In acute pancreatitis, measurement of pancreatic enzymes is useful. There can be elevations in lipase and amylase that are greater than three times the upper limit of normal [18, 19]. However, in CP there is typically loss of exocrine function secondary to fibrosis. Therefore, the serum concentrations of these enzymes may be normal to mildly elevated [19]. Other laboratory tests that can assist in the diagnosis of CP include elevated total bilirubin, alkaline phosphatase, hepatic transaminase, fasting serum glucose, low fecal elastase, and low trypsinogen [20]. These tests have low utility as they are neither strongly sensitive nor specific. The secretin stimulation test is the most sensitive available option but currently is not commonly available [20]. There are no biomarkers that have been well established to aid in diagnosis of CP.

Imaging

Endoscopic retrograde cholangiopancreatography remains the gold standard in detecting early changes [21]. However, this procedure requires a specialized gastroenterology physician who can evaluate for ductal changes and is invasive. Therefore, it is typically reserved for patients with inconclusive testing [21]. The initial imaging modality that can assist in diagnosis of CP is a contrast-enhanced computerized tomography (CT) scan. Findings of the CT scan include dilation of the main pancreatic duct, pancreatic atrophy, pseudocysts, and intraductal calcifications. Studies show that the degree of calcifications is directly proportional to disease duration [22, 23]. CT imaging has a specificity 80–90% and sensitivity between 74 and 100% for detecting advanced disease [24].

Other imaging modalities that have a role in diagnosing CP include magnetic resonance cholangiopancreatography (MRCP) and endoscopic ultrasound (EUS). The benefit of MRCP is that there is no radiation exposure and has the ability to detect parenchymal and ductal changes [25]. In combination with the secretin secretion test, MRCP has a useful role in diagnosing early CP (sensitivity of 77% and specificity of 83%) [26]. EUS has an emerging role in the diagnosis of early pancreatitis with a sensitivity of 97% and a specificity of 60% [20]. Furthermore, the complication rates with EUS are low in comparison to ERCP [20]. The role of EUS has been limited by the low interobserver agreement [27].

How Is This Problem Managed?

Management options for CP can be separated into lifestyle, medical, endoscopic, interventional pain, and surgical treatment options. The major initial emphasis in management of CP focuses on having the patient implement lifestyle changes. These include alcohol cessation, tobacco cessation, and low-fat diets with vitamin supplementation and antioxidants [28]. Support groups are essential as patients with CP can oftentimes become socially isolated as a result of their disease [29].

Medical Management

Medical management of CP focuses on the chronic disabling pain which plagues patients. One analysis showed that over 85% of patients reported pain during their disease course [29]. Increasing evidence shows that the pain in CP is secondary to peripheral and central sensitization. This evolves over time in the setting of chronic inflammation and fibrosis triggering nociceptive afferent receptors [30]. Pancreatic enzyme supplementation has been postulated for the treatment of pain related to its negative feedback on the pancreas resulting in lower pancreatic stimulation and CCK levels [30]. High CCK levels have previously been found in patients with pain secondary to CP [30]. However, the use of pancreatic enzyme supplementation was questioned in a recent systemic review. This meta-analysis of five trials found that pancreatic enzyme supplementation did not relieve abdominal pain compared to placebo [31]. The Cochrane review also found no benefit in quality of life, pain, or steatorrhea in patients receiving pancreatic enzyme supplementation [32]. The most common side effect of these medications is related to development of gastrointestinal (GI) symptoms including diarrhea, flatulence, nausea, and constipation.

Antioxidants have also been evaluated in the treatment of CP, as there are often deficiencies in several micronutrients including selenium, vitamin A, vitamin E, beta-carotene, and xanthine [33]. Deficiencies in these antioxidants can result in increased oxidative stress, which may worsen symptoms. Several systemic reviews have been performed on this subject with mixed findings on effectiveness. Zhou et al. performed a meta-analysis of 573 patients and found that antioxidants were associated with significant pain relief and decreased need for analgesics [34]. A Cochrane review on this subject also found slight improvement in pain control in individuals receiving antioxidants [35]. Other meta-analyses have found no significant improvement in pain compared to placebo [36, 37]. The major drawback associated with antioxidant use was the side-effect profile with approximately one out of six patients reporting mild adverse effects (e.g., headache, GI symptoms) [35]. These side effects were sufficient for patients to stop being compliant with use [35]. Currently, there is not sufficient literature to draw a conclusion regarding the use of antioxidants.

The next line of therapy that has been advocated in use of CP is non-opioid analgesics. This aligns with the World Health Organization analgesic ladder established in 1986 for cancer pain, which has relevance in providing a framework of how to approach a CP patient [38]. The first step in the ladder advocates use of medications including paracetamol, acetaminophen, and nonsteroidal anti-inflammatory drugs (NSAIDs). NSAIDs are better equipped at managing musculoskeletal pain than the visceral pain typically seen in CP. Additionally, the side-effect profile in long-term use of NSAIDs is well established with GI complications [39]. This mainly results from the inhibition of the COX-1 inhibitor that is found throughout the GI tract [39]. Additionally, outside of aspirin, NSAIDs also have shown to increase the risk of cardiovascular events [39]. The major problem with first-ladder medications is that they are typically not strong enough to manage the pain of patients with CP.

Physicians often employ the use opioid analgesics to manage pain complaints in patients with CP. The first choice for treatment of pain in CP is typically tramadol at a dose of 25–50 mg given its safety profile and weak μ-OR agonist activity [30]. Additionally, tramadol has shown to have SNRI properties that result in decreased pain transmission at the level of the spinal cord [30]. Physicians should proceed with caution prior to proceeding to stronger opioids. There has been no study which has identified that patients on chronic opioids have better pain control in CP. If opioids are prescribed, they should be the lowest dose possible and for the shortest interval.

The focus on treatment of CP has shifted to centrally acting drugs. Medications including nortriptyline and gabapentin have shown efficacy in treating neuropathic pain, and therefore, may have a role in patients with CP. Olesen et al. performed a randomized, controlled trial of 64 patients with escalating doses of pregablin and found statistically significant improvement in pain control at 3 weeks in the treatment group compared to control [40]. Tricyclic antidepressants (TCAs) have an extensive side-effect profile including anticholinergic (altered mental status, dry mouth, mydriasis), CNS (myoclonus, syncope), cardiac (tachycardia, orthostatic hypotension), and gastrointestinal (deceased bowel motility) effects which both clinicians and patients should be aware of before prescribing. Other medications which have shown efficiency for treating neuropathic pain, but not specifically chronic pancreatitis, include serotonin and norepinephrine reuptake inhibitors (SNRIs) (i.e., venlafaxine, milnacipran, duloxetine) and norepinephrine and dopamine reuptake inhibitor (NDRIs) (i.e., bupropion) [41]. Medications such as selective serotonin reuptake inhibitors (SSRIs) (i.e., fluoxetine, paroxetine, citalopram, escitalopram, sertraline, fluvoxamine) have not shown to be as efficacious as TCAs in treatment of neuropathic pain [41].

Endoscopic

When medical management fails, it may be necessary to proceed with more invasive measures to achieve adequate pain control. Therapeutic indications to proceed with ERCP include treatment of ductal strictures, obstructive stones, and pseudocysts. However, there is no established guidelines of when to proceed with ERCP, and currently it is partially based on subjective judgment taking into account prior treatment attempts and individual patient factors [42]. ERCP ductal decompression with sphincterotomy or placement of stents has shown to provide sustained pain relief that can last up to 12 years in some patients [43]. For pseudocysts, endoscopic drainage has shown to be equivalent to surgical intervention [44]. Extracorporeal shock wave lithotripsy (ESWL) with or without ERCP has also shown to be effective in patients with significant number of obstructive stones [44].

Interventional Pain

Several interventional pain procedures exist that can assist in controlling pain for patients with CP. For patients with chronic abdominal wall pain (CAWP) secondary to CP, interventional pain strategies include transverse abdominis plane (TAP) block and trigger point injections (TPIs). TPIs contain local anesthetics such as bupivacaine or ropivacaine in combination of steroids. The combination of these medications results in decreasing localized inflammatory response and eliminating abdominal muscle spasms [45]. TPIs are performed in a sterile protocol typically under ultrasound guidance with a 25–27 g needle to minimize the risk of penetrating too deep with the needle into the peritoneal cavity. TPI is usually safe, especially with use of ultrasound, but complications do include intravascular injection leading to local anesthetic toxicity, subcutaneous/intramuscular hematoma, infection, and lipodystrophy [46]. The local anesthetic is injected between the internal oblique and transversus abdominis muscles, above the iliac crest and below the costal margin at the level of the anterior axillary line. This in turn provides pain relief to the anterolateral abdominal wall extending down from the costal margin to the inguinal ligament [46, 47].

The celiac plexus block (Fig. 23.1) involves placement of the needle in the anterior and lateral aspect of the L1 vertebral body, and it is the preferred interventional pain procedure for controlling pain from CP [45, 48, 49]. In a study by Leung et al. approximately half of patients had complete analgesia following the block with a mean period of relief lasting approximately 2 months [49]. This injection consists of local anesthetic and steroids and is typically performed under fluoroscopy with advancement of a 22 g 6–7 inch needle using oblique, anterior-

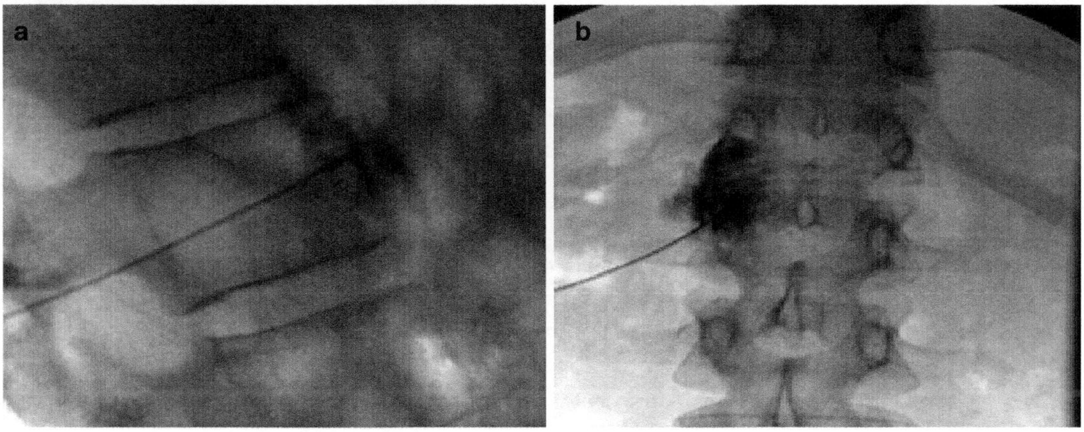

Fig. 23.1 (**a**, **b**) Celiac plexus block with lateral/AP fluoroscopic view showing spread of contrast on lateral side of L1 vertebrae

posterior, and lateral views [45]. Approaches can also be taken via EUS with similar improvement of pain control in comparison to fluoroscopy [50]. Rare serious side effects seen in celiac plexus blocks include pneumothorax and diarrhea [45]. Neurolytic blocks with alcohol or phenol can be administered for prolonged duration of relief.

Bilateral T11 splanchnic block has been shown to provide longer lasting pain relief compared to the celiac plexus block (Fig. 23.2) [51]. If patients have relief with the block, the decision can be made to proceed with radiofrequency ablation. Splanchnic radiofrequency ablation provided prolonged relief of symptoms in 11 out of 18 patients in one study with the median relief lasting greater than three and a half years [52]. The major concern with T11 splanchnic nerve block is risk of pneumothorax [52].

Several clinical trials are in progress to determine more effective treatment regimens for CP. Currently, a study in the Netherlands looking at patients with large duct CP is evaluating early surgical intervention versus a combination of endoscopic and medication management [53]. Medication management includes the use of central acting medications including gabapentin and pregabalin [53]. Studies are also looking at the usefulness of S-ketamine which also is a central acting medication that acts on the *N*-methyl-D-aspartate (NMDA) receptor. A small blinded crossover trial of nine patients showed significant modulation of hyperalgesia in patients who received S-ketamine, and therefore a larger study is in progress [54]. In interventional pain, future studies are looking at the role of spinal cord stimulation (SCS) which has been utilized for treating several pain syndromes in the past [45]. Several case reports at this time have shown the utility of SCS in treatment of chronic visceral abdominal pain [55, 56]. There are no randomized trials on the use of SCS for CP at this time and further studies are needed. From a surgical standpoint, the use of islet auto-transplant is still in its infancy and has potential to be a revolutionary therapeutic option in the future.

Surgical Intervention

Nearly half of the patients with CP will have surgery during their disease course [53]. Surgery is often performed to alleviate the abdominal pain that plagues patients. It is also used to prevent or cure further pancreatic or other organ damage typically via biliary, duodenal, or vascular decompression [54]. The major surgeries that are performed are pancreatic duct drainage and surgical resection of inflamed pancreatic tissue [54]. For pancreatic duct disease, the most

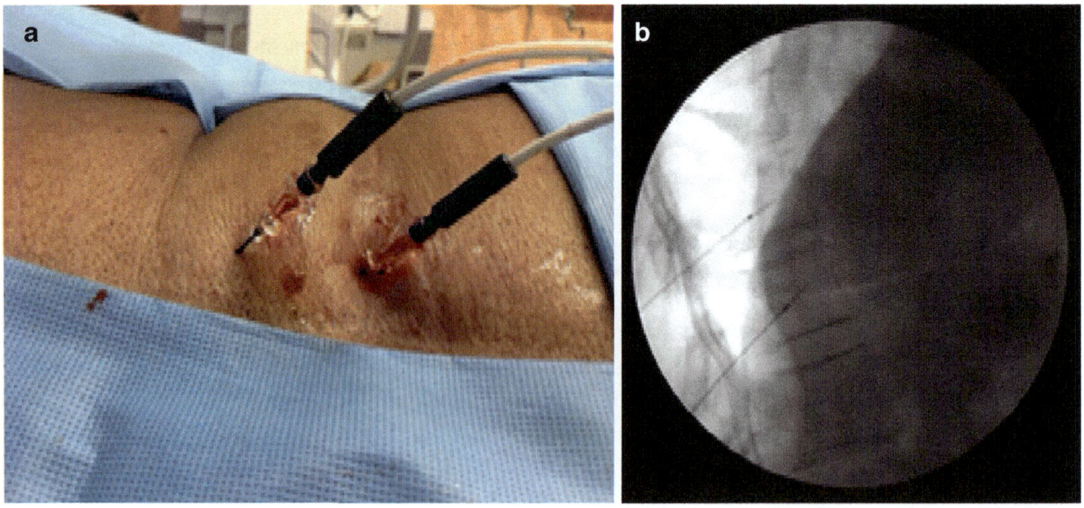

Fig. 23.2 (**a**) The lateral fluoroscopic view shows the placement of the two needles placed at T11 and T12 (**b**) with corresponding X-ray. (From Kapural and Jolly [45], with permission)

common surgery performed is a lateral pancreaticojejunostomy, which has been shown to provide relief in excess of 60% of patients [55]. Few studies have compared surgical versus endoscopic intervention, but two small randomized controlled trials found that surgery had superior long-term outcomes in regard to pain control than endoscopy [56, 57]. Resection procedures commonly focus on the pancreatic head, which is often the site of obstructive complications (Fig. 23.3) [54]. The Whipple procedure, which involves resection of the duodenum and pancreas, was previously widely performed, but has fallen out of favor for duodenum-preserving pancreatic head resections [54]. For patients with end-stage CP, duodenum- and spleen-preserving total pancreatectomy may be indicated [54]. For patients with persistent severe pain, a new surgical modality recently developed is coupling total pancreatectomy and islet auto-transplant [58]. Following a total pancreatectomy, islets are isolated from the resected pancreas and placed into the patient's liver. This allows for monitoring of ambient blood glucose monitoring and appropriate secretion of insulin [58]. Initial results have shown improved quality of life in most patients with improved patient survival compared to total pancreatectomy alone [58].

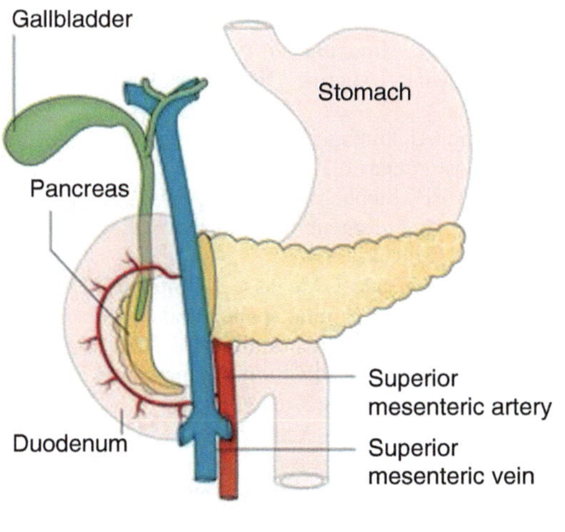

Fig. 23.3 The image above represents the Beger procedure in which the pancreatic head is resected, and the duodenum is preserved. (From Kleeff et al. [59], with permission)

Discussion

The incidence of CP is estimated to be 50–75 cases per 100,000 patients per year [59]. Diagnosing early CP can be difficult but can result in improved mortality. The differential diagnosis for CP is broad because patients often present with upper abdominal pain. The differential diagnosis to consider for CP includes chronic gastritis, peptic ulcer disease, cholelithiasis/cholecystitis, inflammatory bowel disease, myocardial infarction, or mesenteric artery ischemia.

It is therefore essential for physicians to gather a thorough history focusing on risks factors that increase a patient's chances of having CP. This can be done by keeping in mind the TIGAR-O mnemonic. The physical examination does not have much of a role as it lacks sensitivity or specificity in identifying CP. The lab test with the highest sensitivity is the secretin stimulation test, but it is difficult to obtain [20]. Imaging can significantly aid physicians in diagnosing CP with CT, MRI, and EUS all having high sensitivity. ERCP has a positive predictive value of 77% and can be used in circumstances where imaging and pancreatic enzyme testing is inconclusive [60].

Once the diagnosis of CP has been made, the initial focus should be lifestyle changes. Patients should be aggressively counseled on minimizing controllable risk factors with emphasis on halting alcohol and tobacco use. Even with halting of these risk factors, some patients will continue to have persistent pain. Medical management focuses on using central acting medications such as pregabalin with avoidance of opioids when possible. Interventional pain and endoscopic procedures may need to be considered in conjunction with medical management to adequately handle pain symptoms. Endoscopic procedures including ductal stent placement with or without ESWL can provide extended relief in several patients. Interventional pain procedures with proven efficacy in managing pain include celiac plexus and splanchnic blocks. Even with aggressive management, approximately 50% of patients will require surgery at some point in their disease process [53]. Newer techniques such as the Beger procedure (Fig. 23.3) are being used with increasing frequency.

Conclusion

CP is a debilitating disease that can dramatically impact a patient's morbidity and mortality. Obtaining a thorough history focusing on the chronicity of medical complaints, location of pain, and trigger risk factors can narrow down the differential diagnosis, enabling the early diagnosis of CP. Early imaging studies such as an abdominal CT with contrast can aid in diagnosis and allow for early intervention. A multimodal approach consisting of aggressive lifestyle modifications and non-opioid medications should be utilized. If these interventions prove to be unsuccessful, endoscopic and/or interventional pain procedures can be considered given their proven efficacy. Even with these measures, patients may continue to have symptoms and surgical intervention should be considered after.

References

1. Chen WX, Zhang WF, Li B, et al. Clinical manifestations of patients with chronic pancreatitis. Hepatobiliary Pancreat Dis Int. 2006;5(1):133–7.
2. Ammann RW, Muellhaupt B. The natural history of pain in alcoholic chronic pancreatitis. Gastroenterology. 1999;116(5):1132–40.
3. Enweluzo C, Tlhabano L. Pain management in chronic pancreatitis: taming the beast. Clin Exp Gastroenterol. 2013;6:167–71.
4. Layer P, Yamamoto H, Kalthoff L, Clain JE, Bakken LJ, Dimagno EP. The different courses of early- and late-onset idiopathic and alcoholic chronic pancreatitis. Gastroenterology. 1994;107(5):1481–7.
5. Stevens T, Conwell DL, Zuccaro G. Pathogenesis of chronic pancreatitis: an evidence-based review of past theories and recent developments. Am J Gastroenterol. 2004;99(11):2256–70.
6. Braganza JM. Pancreatic disease: a casualty of hepatic "detoxification"? Lancet. 1983;2:1000–2.
7. Bordalo O, Goncalves D, Noronha M, et al. Newer concept for the pathogenesis of chronic alcoholic pancreatitis. Am J Gastroenterol. 1977;68:278–85.
8. Sarles H, Bernard JP, Johnson C. Pathogenesis and epidemiology of chronic pancreatitis. Ann Rev Med. 1989;40:453–68.
9. Sarles H. Pathogenesis of chronic pancreatitis. Gut. 1990;31:629–32.
10. Ammann RW, Heitz PU, Kloppe G. Course of alcoholic chronic pancreatitis: a prospective clinicomorphological long-term study. Gastroenterology. 1996;111:224–31.
11. Cavallini G. Is chronic pancreatitis a primary disease of the pancreatic ducts? A new pathogenetic hypothesis. Ital J Gastroenterol. 1993;25:400–7.
12. Whitcomb DC, Gorry MC, Preston RA, et al. Hereditary pancreatitis is caused by a mutation in the cationic trypsinogen gene. Nat Genet. 1996;14:141–5.
13. Whitcomb DC, Schneider A. Hereditary pancreatitis: a model for inflammatory disease of the pancreas. Best Pract Res Clin Gastroenterol. 2002;16:347–63.
14. Yamabe A, Irisawa A, Shibukawa G, et al. Early diagnosis of chronic pancreatitis: understanding the factors associated with the development of chronic pancreatitis. Fukushima J Med Sci. 2017;63(1):1–7.
15. Talamini G, Bassi C, Falconi M, et al. Alcohol and smoking as risk factors in chronic pancreatitis and pancreatic cancer. Dig Dis Sci. 1999;44:1303–11.
16. Lin Y, Tamakoshi A, Hayakawa T, et al. Associations of alcohol drinking and nutrient intake with chronic pancreatitis:findings from a case-control study in Japan. Am J Gastroenterol. 2001;96:2622–7.
17. Yadav D, Hawes RH, Brand RE, et al. Alcohol consumption, cigarette smoking, and the risk of recurrent acute and chronic pancreatitis. Arch Intern Med. 2009;169(11):1035–45.
18. Etemad B, Whitcomb DC. Chronic pancreatitis: diagnosis, classification, and new genetic developments. Gastroenterology. 2001;120:682–707.
19. Chase CW, Barker DE, Russell WL, Burns RP. Serum amylase and lipase in the evaluation of acute abdominal pain. Am Surg. 1996;62:1028–33.
20. Nair RJ, Lawler L, Miller MR. Chronic pancreatitis. Am Fam Physician. 2007;76(11):1679–88.
21. Lew D, Afghani E, Pandol S. Chronic pancreatitis: current status and challenges for prevention and treatment. Dig Dis Sci. 62(7):1702–12.
22. Sharma R Imaging in chronic pancreatitis. Pancreapedia; Exocrine Pancreas Knowledge Base. 2015.
23. Dimagno MJ, Dimagno EP. Chronic pancreatitis. Curr Opin Gastroenterol. 2005;21(5):544–54.
24. Luetmer PH, Stephens DH, Ward EM. Chronic pancreatitis: reassessment with current CT. Radiology. 1989;171(2):353–7.
25. Balci NC, Alkaade S, Magas L, Momtahen AJ, Burton FR. Suspected chronic pancreatitis with normal MRChronic pancreatitis: findings on MRI in correlation with secretin MRChronic pancreatitis. J Magn Reson Imaging. 2008;27(1):125–31.
26. Conwell DL, Lee LS, Yadav D, et al. American pancreatic association practice guidelines in chronic pancreatitis: evidence-based report on diagnostic guidelines. Pancreas. 2014;43(8):1143–62.
27. Wallace MB, Hawes RH, Durkalski V, et al. The reliability of EUS for the diagnosis of chronic pancreatitis: interobserver agreement among expe-

rienced endosonographers. Gastrointest Endosc. 2001;53(3):294–9.
28. Goulden MR. The pain of chronic pancreatitis: a persistent clinical challenge. Br J Pain. 2013;7(1):8–22.
29. Ammann RW, Buehler H, Muench R, Freiburghaus AW, Siegenthaler W. Differences in the natural history of idiopathic (nonalcoholic) and alcoholic chronic pancreatitis. A comparative long-term study of 287 patients. Pancreas. 1987;2(4):368–77.
30. Singh VK, Drewes AM. Medical management of pain in chronic pancreatitis. Dig Dis Sci. 2017;62(7):1721–8.
31. Yaghoobi M, Mcnabb-baltar J, Bijarchi R, Cotton PB. Pancreatic enzyme supplements are not effective for relieving abdominal pain in patients with chronic pancreatitis: meta-analysis and systematic review of randomized controlled trials. Can J Gastroenterol Hepatol. 2016;2016:8541839.
32. Shafiq N, Rana S, Bhasin D, et al. Pancreatic enzymes for chronic pancreatitis. Cochrane Database Syst Rev. 2009;(4):CD006302.
33. Morris-stiff GJ, Bowrey DJ, Oleesky D, Davies M, Clark GW, Puntis MC. The antioxidant profiles of patients with recurrent acute and chronic pancreatitis. Am J Gastroenterol. 1999;94(8):2135–40.
34. Zhou D, Wang W, Cheng X, Wei J, Zheng S. Antioxidant therapy for patients with chronic pancreatitis: a systematic review and meta-analysis. Clin Nutr. 2015;34(4):627–34.
35. Ahmed Ali U, Jens S, Busch OR, et al. Antioxidants for pain in chronic pancreatitis. Cochrane Database Syst Rev. 2014;(8):CD008945.
36. Talukdar R, Murthy HV, Reddy DN. Role of methionine containing antioxidant combination in the management of pain in chronic pancreatitis: a systematic review and meta-analysis. Pancreatology. 2015;15(2):136–44.
37. Cai GH, Huang J, Zhao Y, et al. Antioxidant therapy for pain relief in patients with chronic pancreatitis: systematic review and meta-analysis. Pain Physician. 2013;16(6):521–32.
38. World Health Organization. Analgesic ladder. Geneva: World Health Organization; 1986.
39. Brune K, Patrignani P. New insights into the use of currently available non-steroidal anti-inflammatory drugs. J Pain Res. 2015;8:105–18.
40. Olesen SS, Bouwense SA, Wilder-smith OH, Van Goor H, Drewes AM. Pregabalin reduces pain in patients with chronic pancreatitis in a randomized, controlled trial. Gastroenterology. 2011;141(2):536–43.
41. Dworkin RH, O'Connor AB, Backonja M, et al. Pharmacologic management of neuropathic pain: evidence-based recommendations. Pain. 2007;132:237–51.
42. Gachago C, Draganov PV. Pain management in chronic pancreatitis. World J Gastroenterol. 2008;14(20):3137–48.
43. Rösch T, Daniel S, Scholz M, et al. Endoscopic treatment of chronic pancreatitis: a multicenter study of 1000 patients with long-term follow-up. Endoscopy. 2002;34(10):765–71.
44. Adler DG, Baron TH, Davila RE, Egan J, Hirota WK, Leighton JA, et al. for the Standards of Practice Committee of American Society for Gastrointestinal Endoscopy. ASGE guideline: the role of ERChronic pancreatitis in diseases of the biliary tract and the pancreas. Gastrointest Endosc. 2005;62:1–8.
45. Kapural L, Jolly S. Interventional pain management approaches for control of chronic pancreatic pain. Curr Treat Options Gastroenterol. 2016;14(3):360–70.
46. Narouze S. Chronic abdominal wall pain: diagnosis and interventional treatment. In: Kapural L, editor. Chronic abdominal pain: an evidence-based, comprehensive guide to clinical management. New York: Springer; 2015. p. 189–95.
47. Soilman LM, Narouze S. Ultrasound-guided transversus abdominus plan block for the management of abdominal pain: an alternative to differential epidural block. Tech Reg Anesth Pain Manag. 2009;13:117–20.
48. Kapural L, Puyalert M, Walsh M, Sweiss G. Interdisciplinary treatment of the pain from chronic pancreatitis. In: Hayek S, Shah BJ, Desai MJ, Chelimsky TC, editors. Pain medicine, an interdisciplinary case-based approach. New York: Oxford University Press; 2015. p. 289–97.
49. Leung JW, Bowen-wright M, Aveling W, Shorvon PJ, Cotton PB. Coeliac plexus block for pain in pancreatic cancer and chronic pancreatitis. Br J Surg. 1983;70(12):730–2.
50. Gress F, Schmitt C, Sherman S, Ciaccia D, Ikenberry S, Lehman G. Endoscopic ultrasound-guided celiac plexus block for managing abdominal pain associated with chronic pancreatitis: a prospective single center experience. Am J Gastroenterol. 2001;96(2):409–16.
51. Badhey HS, Jolly S, Kapural L. Bilateral splanchnic block T11 provides longer pain relief than celiac plexus block from non-malignant abdominal pain. Miami: Abstracts from the American Society of Regional Anesthesia and Pain Medicine 14 annual pain medicine meeting; 2015. 11/21/2015; Abs 140.
52. Verhaegh BP, van Kleef M, Geurts JW, et al. Percutaneous radiofrequency ablation of the splanchnic nerves in patients with chronic pancreatitis: results of single and repeated procedures in 11 patients. Pain Pract. 2013;13:621–6.
53. Ahmed Ali U, Issa Y, Bruno MJ, et al. Early surgery versus optimal current step-up practice for chronic pancreatitis (ESCAPE): design and rationale of a randomized trial. BMC Gastroenterol. 2013;13:49.
54. Bouwense SA, Buscher HC, van Goor H, et al. *S*-ketamine modulates hyperalgesia in patients with chronic pancreatitis pain. Reg Anesth Pain Med. 2011;36:303–7.
55. Khan I, Raza S, Khan E. Application of spinal cord stimulation for the treatment of abdominal visceral pain syndromes: case reports. Neuromodulation. 2005;8:14–27.

56. Kapural L, Nagem H, Tlucek H, Sessler DI. Spinal cord stimulation for chronic visceral abdominal pain. Pain Med. 2010;11:347–55.
57. Steer ML, Waxman I, Freedman S. Chronic pancreatitis. N Engl J Med. 1995;332:1482–90.
58. Bellin MD, Freeman ML, Gelrud A, et al. Total pancreatectomy and islet autotransplantation in chronic pancreatitis: recommendations from PancreasFest. Pancreatology. 2014;14(1):27–35.
59. Kleeff J, Whitcomb DC, Shimosegawa T, et al. Chronic pancreatitis. Nat Rev Dis Primers. 2017;3:17060.
60. Ahmad SA, Wray C, Rilo HL, Choe KA, Gelrud A, Howington JA, et al. Chronic pancreatitis: recent advances and ongoing challenges. Curr Probl Surg. 2006;43:127–238.

Pain in the Pelvis

24

Naveed Mameghani and Tariq Malik

Case Description

A 35-year-old woman is referred to the pain clinic for pelvic pain of 1 year duration. She has history of intermittent pelvic pain for many years, but the pain has become more intense and constant for the last 1 year. She denies any history or trauma, infection, surgery, or any other psychosocial stresses in her life. She has been worked by her primary care physician and by a gynecologist. All the diagnostic workup has been negative so far. She has tried nonsteroid anti-inflammatory medicines, acetaminophen, and even marijuana but has found no relief. Pain is intense enough that she cannot concentrate on her work and has called in sick quite a few times. She is sleeping poorly and is feeling down quite a lot. She has developed low back pain for the last few months which is localized, nonradiating, and unaccompanied by any other symptom. There are no relieving or worsening factors. She does notice increase in pain when she is walking or sitting for a long time, but no relation to bladder or bowel movement. She has been suggested a diagnostic laparoscopic surgery, but she is not sure if to go ahead with that plan as she has been told it may not help and there is a chance pain may get worse.

N. Mameghani · T. Malik (✉)
Department of Anesthesia and Critical Care, University of Chicago, Chicago, IL, USA
e-mail: TMuslim@dacc.uchicago.edu; tmalik@dacc.uchicago.edu

What Is Your Preliminary Diagnosis?

The patient is suffering from a chronic pain in her lower abdomen and pelvic area. Despite going on for a long time, there are no other symptoms suggestive of any malignancy, inflammation, or any organ dysfunction. Her symptoms are suggestive of pelvic in origin with no obvious pathology. Negative workup by her primary care and by her gynecologist led credence to the idea that she is suffering from chronic pelvic pain syndrome.

How Is the Diagnosis Confirmed?

Chronic pelvic pain has been historically difficult to diagnose as there are several potential causes, and they frequently have symptoms that overlap [1]. It is defined as pain in the lower abdomen or pelvis that has occurred for at least 6 months and does not exclusively occur around the menstrual cycle or sexual intercourse. The diagnosis requires detailed history and physical examination especially pelvic exam by an expert physician who specializes in treating chronic pelvic pain conditions. The chronic pelvic pain syndrome is differentiated from chronic pelvic pain which is diagnosed if patient has some underlying pathology that might be contributing to the pelvic pain. The most common causes are irritable bowel syndrome, interstitial cystitis, endometriosis, adhesions, and pelvic inflammatory

T. Malik (ed.), *Practical Chronic Pain Management*, https://doi.org/10.1007/978-3-030-46675-6_24

disease [1]. Dysmenorrhea and dyspareunia have higher prevalence in women with chronic pelvic pain then those without [1].

Stress, anxiety, sleep disorders, and depression are also common in these patients and patients with other chronic pain states [1, 2]. It is thought that an integrative multidisciplinary approach to diagnosis is superior to an approach where organic causes of the pain are totally excluded before other causes such as psychological, environmental, and dietary causes are considered [3]. Practitioners that should be involved in an integrative approach include gynecologists, pain specialists, physical therapists, psychologists, and nutritionists. Being fixated on a somatic diagnosis is more likely with a nonintegrative approach [3]. After a period of 1 year, it was shown that patients with the integrative approach had significantly greater pain relief than the standard treatment group. History and physical exam are very important to the diagnosis of this condition. Special attention should be given to location, quality, intensity, and presence of radiation of pain as well as history of prior pregnancies, sexually transmitted diseases, sexual abuse, or surgeries. Any pain with sexual intercourse or menses should be noted as should signs of depression, anxiety, or decreased quality of life. Depression is a predictor of pain severity in this patient population and can be an indicator of response to treatment [4]. Red flag findings of postcoital bleeding, postmenopausal bleeding, hematuria, pelvic mass, or unintended weight loss should prompt evaluation for systemic disease and malignancy [5]. A pain diary kept for several menstrual cycles can be useful to discover provoking and alleviating factors as well as temporal relationships [6]. Time should be spent documenting the patients' baseline functional status and pain levels so improvement can be monitored over time. Physical exam should attempt to recreate the pain by palpation or positioning and should evaluate the gastrointestinal, musculoskeletal, reproductive, urinary, and neurological systems [4]. Exam should include a complete abdominal and pelvic exam as well an attempt to localize trigger points, sacroiliac joint or symphysis pubis tenderness. If findings are constant with a specific disorder, then that specific disorder should be evaluated and treated. There is no one set of diagnostic tests or labs that should be run on every patient with chronic pelvic pain as this has not been shown to be effective [4]. Tests should only be performed as indicated by history and physical exam, and they will change the diagnosis or management of the condition [4]. Common tests that are ordered include complete blood count with differential, erythrocyte sedimentation rate, urinalysis, Chlamydia and gonorrhea testing, and pregnancy testing [5]. Transvaginal ultrasound can be used to detect pelvic masses that cannot be palpated on exam, adenomyosis, and hydrosalpinx which is an indicator of pelvic inflammatory disease [5]. MRI can be used to further characterize abnormalities found on ultrasound such as adenomyosis but is costly and is not always effective in finding endometriosis. Laparoscopy is very common in the workup of patients with severe pain and unclear diagnosis. In the past, it was considered the "gold standard" for workup but now has become second line and is reserved for when other interventions fail [6]. The most common diagnoses that result from it include endometriosis and adhesions [5]. If endometriosis is suspected as the cause of pain, then confirmation with laparoscopy is not needed and a trial of medical therapy is indicated as discussed later in this chapter [7]. It is important to remember that a negative laparoscopy does not automatically mean that the patient does not have an active disease process or basis for their pain [4]. Pain mapping is a technique where laparoscopy is done under local anesthesia and tissues are pulled and probed with surgical instruments while the patient is asked if pain is reproduced [5]. This is done in an effort to localize the source of pain to a particular organ or tissue and has been shown to be successful with certain cases [8]. Consultations where the patients' ideas and concerns are elicited have been shown to result in a better doctor-patient relationship and improved concordance with evaluation and treatment [6].

What Is the Pathophysiology of This Condition?

Exact pathophysiology is unknown. It is considered a functional pain syndrome where because of neuroplasticity the peripheral afferent signaling along with central signal processing has been altered. Patients with functional disorders have been found to have lower threshold to visceral stimuli, increased sensitivity during normal organ function, and tenderness in the expanded areas of somatic referral. These phenomena are explained by sensitization of non-nociceptive mechanoreceptors, awakening of silent nociceptors in combination with sensitization of central processing at the spinal cord, mid-brain, and limbic system level. These phenomena have been seen in the experimental setting but hard to find proof of their presence in clinical setting. What trigger such phenomenon is unknown, but it could be triggered by minor nociceptive events.

Nociceptive, neuropathic, and inflammatory pain all have roles in chronic pelvic pain [9]. Studies have shown increased nerve fibers including sensory and sympathetic fibers in women with endometriosis which highlights the role of nociception [9]. Inflammatory pain is associated with cross-sensitization where repeated pain signaling from one organ can lead to false pain sensation from another organ that is supplied by the same dorsal root ganglion [9]. This phenomenon could potentially explain the link between chronic pelvic pain with irritable bowel and painful bladder syndromes. Tumor necrosis factor (TNF), an inflammatory mediator involved with chronic pelvic pain, has been shown to have higher levels in the peritoneal fluid of women with endometriosis, and trials using infliximab (monoclonal antibody against TNF with side effects of infections and reactivation of tuberculosis) in patients with endometriosis showed improvement in their pain [9]. Prostaglandins E2 and F2 also play a role by mediating inflammation directly and by causing increased levels of other mediators such as histamine, serotonin, and nerve growth factors. Studies have shown higher COX2 levels, an enzyme involved in synthesis of prostaglandins, in women with endometriosis [9]. Estrogen also increases COX2 activity so it is thought that estrogen antagonists can lower prostaglandin levels. Nerve growth factor (NGF) plays a role by increasing pain receptors, sympathetic ganglia, small nerve fibers, and release of substance P [9]. High NGF levels were also seen in patients with endometriosis [9]. Mast cells store inflammatory mediators and release these factors that go on to cause pain and they increase in tissues with endometriosis [9]. Some studies have shown high levels of mast cells in patients with irritable bowel syndrome and interstitial cystitis, and this may be another link between these diseases and mast cell-mediated chronic pelvic pain and can be a potential target for developing new drugs to treat chronic pelvic pain [9]. Neuropathic pain can be related to injury to either central or peripheral nervous systems. Central sensitization is a phenomenon where the central nervous system continues to receive pain signals even once the source of the pain is removed and can manifest in hyperalgesia and allodynia which are very common in patients with chronic pelvic pain [9].

How Is This Problem Managed?

Chronic pelvic pain is hard to manage. A multidisciplinary approach is employed at the outset. Like any other chronic medical condition, each patient should be an active participant in the management of her pain condition.

[6]. Goals should include improving quality of life and allowing the patient to take an active role in their care. Evidence-based practice in treating chronic pelvic pain is often lacking, and many times the focus is on improvement of symptoms. Even if there is a disease process that can be treated, this may not always resolve the pain the patient is experiencing [5]. Nevertheless, if a possible contributing disease process is found it should be treated. For instance, if a patient is thought to have irritable bowel syndrome with gas, bloating, and abdominal pain, then a trial of anti-spasmodics would be indicated. If the cause of pain remains unknown, then a trial of acetaminophen (CNS COX activity inhibition with side effects of liver toxicity at high doses) or nonsteroidal anti-inflam-

matory drugs (COX inhibitors with side effects of gastrointestinal bleeding and renal dysfunction) is indicated. If this does not help the patient and the pain has a cyclical component, then hormone therapy with oral contraceptives, depot medroxyprogesterone, or gonadotropin-releasing hormone agonists should be tried [5]. These are especially useful in patients with endometriosis.

If there is a neuropathic component suspected and the patient does not have an underlying mood disorder, then medications such as the gabapentinoids (such as gabapentin or pregabalin, which reduce calcium currents and have a side effect of sedation), tricyclic antidepressants (blocks serotonin and norepinephrine transporters thereby increasing the levels of these neurotransmitters with side effects of weight loss, sexual dysfunction, dry mouth, drowsiness, tachycardia, and arrhythmias), or serotonin-norepinephrine reuptake inhibitors (blocks reuptake of serotonin and norepinephrine thereby increasing their levels with side effects of weight loss, sexual dysfunction, and drowsiness) can be used. There is no strong evidence for effectiveness of any pharmacotherapy in managing chronic pelvic pain. Membrane stabilizers and antidepressants are used as they have been found to be effective in other chronic pain conditions with neuropathic components.

In a small randomized pilot study, gabapentin decreased pain and improved mood compared to placebo and it was sustained at 6 months of follow-up. In another study comparing amitriptyline to gabapentin, patients taking gabapentin (alone or combined with amitriptyline) had superior pain reduction with lower VAS scores. Side effects were lowest in the gabapentin-only group. Selective serotonin reuptake inhibitors should be reserved for patients with underlying mood disorders as they are more effective for this indication rather than neuropathic pain [5]. Opioids are not ideal for chronic pelvic pain and best avoided, and should only be used for patients as a bridge to surgery or for postoperative pain. Surgery is generally a last resort as it is thought to have limited benefit, and many patients will have persistent pain even after the procedure [5, 10]. Injection of local anesthetic and steroid mixtures can be diagnostic and therapeutic for issues with peripheral nerves. Various injection techniques are reported in the literature based on case reports or observational studies but none are based on evidence. Superior hypogastric plexus and ganglion impair blocks can also be effective in a select few and in carefully selected patients. Neuromodulation can be used if there is sacral nerve involvement; however, studies are still ongoing to determine its role in treating chronic pelvic pain [5]. Common non-pharmacologic interventions for chronic pelvic pain include pelvic floor physical therapy, dietary changes, TENS, acupuncture, cognitive behavioral therapy (CBT), and mindfulness training. There is lack of data on appropriate selection of treatment options and patient counseling.

Patients who underwent weekly physical therapy and visits with psychologists over a 10-week period experienced significant and long-term improvement in pain and ability to work [7]. Somatosensory stimulation using acupuncture along with psychotherapy has been shown to reduce pain in women with endometriosis [11].

What Is the Prognosis of This Condition?

The prognosis of chronic pelvic pain can vary greatly. If there is a specific disease process that is thought to be causing the patients pain and it is appropriately treated, this can sometimes resolve the pain. In other instances, the pain is related to several different diagnoses and has several different contributing factors which all need evaluation, and in these cases treatment is often not curative [4]. It is still unknown why some of these disorders lead to a chronic pain state in some patients while in other patients they are cured with initial treatment. Central sensitization and psychosocial factors do seem to play a major role in patient outcome.

Discussion

Prevalence

Chronic pelvic pain is actually more common than most would think with up to one in six women experiencing this disorder [6]. Population-based survey in the USA reveals prevalence of 12% and life time incidence of 33%. Worldwide prevalence has been reported at 2–24%. It accounts for 10% of referrals to gynecology clinics, 33% of laparoscopies, and 12–16% of hysterectomies. Its prevalence is at par with migraine and back pain. In over half of the reported cases, there is more than one etiology of the chronic pelvic pain for that particular patient. There is also a large psychosocial component to this disorder with about half of the patients experiencing it also reporting prior sexual, physical, or emotional trauma and about one-third showing signs of posttraumatic stress disorder [5, 12]. Patients with posttraumatic stress disorder are more likely to report their pain as severe compared to patients without this disorder even when there is no medical basis for the difference in perceived pain levels [13]. It is estimated that every year in the USA chronic pelvic pain has medical costs of 2.8 billion dollars and a total loss of productivity of 15 billion dollars [14].

Differential Diagnosis

The differential diagnosis for chronic pelvic pain consists of a large number of diverse diagnoses. For most patients, the root cause of the pain is due to several different sources and not a single disease process. This is why it can be difficult to diagnose and treat. Nevertheless, some of the most common etiologies will be reviewed in this section. Irritable bowel syndrome (IBS) is one of the most common causes of chronic pelvic pain. Up to 30% of chronic pelvic pain patients have IBS, and 40% of this subgroup goes undiagnosed [15]. It is associated with abdominal pain and changes in the patient's normal bowel movements and can be diagnosed with the Rome criteria. Patients can experience constipation, diarrhea, both together or neither condition. The cause is not clear but the diagnosis should only be made in the absence of red flag symptoms such as weight loss, blood in the stool, personal or family history of inflammatory bowel disease, or onset of symptoms past the age of 50. While there is no cure, this disease is typically treated with dietary modifications to increase fiber intake, medications such as laxatives for constipation and loperamide (opioid receptor agonist at the level of the myenteric plexus of the large intestine with side effects of cramping, nausea, and dizziness) for diarrhea, probiotics, and psychotherapy. Endometriosis, the presence of endometrial tissue outside of the endometrial cavity is another frequent cause of chronic pelvic pain. It is most accurately diagnosed with histopathology, and there is up to a 33% prevalence of endometriosis in patients with chronic pelvic pain. On the other hand, many patients who are found to incidentally have endometriosis do not have pelvic pain. A type of endometriosis known as deep infiltrating endometriosis where there is a penetration of the peritoneum of more than a 5 millimeter depth is most associated with pelvic pain [9]. The pain related to this is typically from dyspareunia, dysuria, dysmenorrhea, or dyschezia. Transvaginal ultrasound is the best tool for diagnosis and is much more cost-effective than MRI. Adenomyosis is the presence of endometrial glands in the myometrium. This is a similar but separate entity from endometriosis. It can be either localized or spread diffusely throughout the entire uterus. When diffusely spread, it can cause the uterus to become bulky and heavy. It can also be diagnosed with transvaginal ultrasound, MRI, or histopathology. Intraperitoneal adhesions are another common cause of chronic pelvic pain and are frequently diagnosed with laparoscopy. Previous abdominal or pelvic surgeries, pelvic inflammatory disease, or endometriosis can predispose patients to form adhesions. Surgical trauma disrupts mast cells which release histamine and kinins that in turn increase vascular permeability [16]. Fibrin deposits then form and if they are not removed by absorption or fibrinolysis, then fibroblasts and blood vessels will form [16]. Usually, the fibrin exudates are broken down; however, the surgical trauma causes a reduction in peritoneal fibrinolysis which will lead to formation of adhesions [16]. It is thought that adhesions cause visceral pain through reduction in organ mobility [17]. In many cases, surgical lysis of adhesions has not been shown to have a significant reduction in pain compared to conservative management [9]. Laparoscopy alone was also shown to be superior to lysis of adhesions in reducing pain due to a placebo effect and reduced risk of operative complications [18]. Pelvic inflammatory disease is an infection involving the uterus, ovaries, and fallopian tubes and is another cause of chronic pelvic pain. Bacteria spread from the vagina and cervix and most commonly involve Chlamydia or gonorrhea. Patients may present with fever, uterine or adnexal tenderness, and vaginal discharge. It may be diagnosed with ultrasound, MRI, laboratory tests such as nucleic acid amplification tests or enzyme-linked immunosorbent assays to detect the pathogens involved, histopathology, or laparoscopy. It can lead to chronic pelvic pain potentially through the formation of adhesions. Interstitial cystitis is a disorder where the patient experiences pain in the bladder without any organic causes. This disease is poorly understood and the cause of it remains elusive. Patients often have symptoms of urinary frequency, urgency, and dyspareunia along with bladder pain. It is a diagnosis of exclusion and there is no cure. Symptoms are typically treated with lifestyle changes such as stress reduction and diet modification along with medications such as NSAIDs and neuropathic medications such as amitriptyline. These patients often have coexisting psychosocial issues and tend to believe they have lower social support than control patients, possibly showing a role for counseling and close support these patients [19]. Myofascial physical therapy, which includes internal and external muscle and connective tissue manipulation of the abdomen, hip girdle, and pelvic floor, has also been shown to be useful in this group of patients [20]. Lastly, there can be musculoskeletal causes to chronic pelvic pain such as trigger points, pelvic muscle spasms, nerve entrapment, or lumbar degenerative disk disease [21, 22].

Predictive Value of Different Clinical Features (History and Physical Exam) and Lab Tests/Imaging

Given the wide range of contributing factors to chronic pelvic pain, there can be a variety of signs from the history and physical exam that can be of predictive value. While the following is certainly not an exhaustive list, we will review common history and physical exam findings. On history, crampy abdominal pain can be related to irritable bowel syndrome (IBS) or inflammatory bowel disease. Pain that fluctuates with the menstrual cycle can be due to endometriosis or adenomyosis, while pain unrelated to the menstrual cycle could be from adhesions, interstitial cystitis, IBS, or a musculoskeletal issue. Pain with urinary urgency can point to interstitial cystitis. Postcoital or postmenopausal bleeding and unexpected weight loss can potentially be findings of malignancy. Prior abdominal or pelvic surgery or infections make adhesions more likely. Moving on to the physical exam, the finding of an enlarged tender uterus could be due to adenomyosis. Lack of uterine mobility on bimanual examination could be from adhesions or endometriosis. Pelvic floor muscle tenderness is a sign of interstitial cystitis. Adnexal or uterine masses could represent malignancy. Basic laboratory testing such as complete blood count with differential, erythrocyte sedimentation rate and urinalysis are nonspecific but can hint at an underlying abnormality. A positive chlamydia or gonorrhea test is seen in pelvic inflammatory disease. Ultrasound can be used to detect masses and adenomyosis with good predictive value. Laparoscopy, while reserved for cases of severe and refractory pain, is also very predictive when adhesions or endometriosis are seen.

Strength of Evidence for Different Treatment Modalities

While there are many different treatments for chronic pelvic pain, there are varying degrees of evidence for their use. Use of acetaminophen for somatic pain has grade A and level 1A evidence [23]. Evidence shows support for gabapentin and pregabalin in treating neuropathic pain (level 1A, grade A evidence); however, studies on their use for chronic pelvic pain are limited [23]. It has been shown that gabapentin along with amitriptyline in combination is more effective than amitriptyline alone [24]. Use of tricyclic antidepressants and SNRIs in chronic pelvic pain is mostly evidence based on neuropathic pain, and studies are limited on their use for chronic pelvic pain; however, their use for neuropathic pain has level 1A and grade A evidence [23]. SSRIs have been shown to be beneficial for depression but not for pain and thus should not be used first line for pain [5]. Oral contraceptives, progestogens, and gonadotropin-releasing hormone agonists have been shown to be beneficial for endometriosis and cyclic pelvic pain [25]. Women taking goserelin (GnRH agonist) had better pain scores after once year than those taking progestrogen [25]. A Cochrane review shows evidence for use of NSAIDs for inflammatory processes (level 1A, grade A evidence) such as dysmenorrhea but states that they lack effectiveness for endometriosis [23, 26]. Women who underwent reassurance ultrasound scans and had counseling were more likely to report improved pain compared to a "wait and see" policy [25]. Opioid usage in chronic nonmalignant pain remains controversial and should not be used in most patients [27]. Use of transcutaneous electrical nerve stimulation has a level 1B and grade B of evidence and there is no good evidence for or against its use [23]. Neuromodulation for pelvic pain currently has a level 3 and grade C evidence with its role currently developing with further research needed [23]. Nerve blocks also have a level 3 and grade C evidence, and they do have a role as part of a broad management plan [23]. Surgery should be reserved for women with severe and refractory pain after trying conservative and medical management. Local excision of endometriosis has had good short-term outcomes but in the long term has had a high reoperation rate (level 2 evidence) [28].

Future Directions and Clinical Trials

Chronic pelvic pain is a problem that affects a large number of patients and has potentially debilitating consequences. It can severely impact a person's quality of life and self-worth and has a prominent psychosocial component. It is frequently multifactorial in regard to etiology and remains difficult to diagnose and treat because of this. While there are many available therapies which have strong levels of evidence, most of these therapies have not yet been extensively studied specifically for patients with chronic pelvic pain. This is needed so practitioners can select the most effective and appropriate therapies for their patients. Further work in the area of neuromodulation for treatment of chronic pelvic pain also needs to be done as this has the possibility of helping these patients. This is a disorder which needs a multidisciplinary approach, and practitioners need to be educated about this fact so they can make the appropriate specialist referrals in order to best serve the patient. While significant work remains to be done, with further education, research, and awareness we have the potential to improve the lives of many.

Conclusion/Summary

Chronic pelvic pain remains an entity that is difficult to diagnose and affects more people than most would think. This is both due to a lack of education and awareness among providers and the fact that the differential diagnosis is wide and spans several different organ systems. Many patients with this disease suffer greatly from pain, worsened quality of life, and potentially depression stemming from these problems. Many patients go undiagnosed. Due to the nature of this disease, a multidisciplinary approach is key. Counseling and psychosocial support can empower these patients and help improve their symptoms. Keeping the patient informed and involved in their treatment process also improves outcomes and patient satisfaction. There are several medical and interventional therapies available to patients; however, most of these therapies have not been extensively studied in this patient population specifically. Likely a combination of medical and interventional therapies along with counseling, physical therapy, and psychiatric care will be of most benefit to patients compared to any one of these single entities alone. Further research and improvement in available therapies will aid in improving the diagnosis, treatment, and patient outcomes related to this disease.

References

1. Zondervan KT, Yudkin PL, Vessey MP, Jenkinson CP, Dawes MG, Barlow DH, Kennedy SH. Chronic pelvic pain in the community—symptoms, investigations, and diagnoses. Am J Obstet Gynecol. 2001;184(6):1149–55.
2. Meissner K, Schweizer-Arau A, Limmer A, Preibisch C, Popovici RM, Lange I, de Oriol B, Beissner F. Psychotherapy with somatosensory stimulation for endometriosis-associated pain. Obstet Gynecol. 2016;128(5):1134–42.
3. Peters AA, Jellis B, Hermans J, Trimbos JB. A randomized clinical trial to compare two different approaches in women with chronic pelvic pain. Obstet Gynecol. 1991;77(5):740–4.
4. Howard FM. Chronic pelvic pain. Obstet Gynecol. 2003;101(3):594–611.
5. Zondervan KT, Yudkin PL, Vessey MP, Jenkinson CP, Dawes MG, Barlow DH, Kennedy SH. Chronic pelvic pain in the community – symptoms, investigations, and diagnoses. Am J Obstet Gynecol. 2001;184:1149–55.
6. Speer LM, Mushkbar S, Erbele T. Chronic pelvic pain in women. Am Fam Physician. 2016;93(5):380–7.
7. Williams RE, Hartmann KE, Sandler RS, Miller WC, Savitz LA, Steege JF. Recognition and treatment of irritable bowel syndrome among women with chronic pelvic pain. Am J Obstet Gynecol. 2005;192(3):761–7.
8. Rapkin AJ, Kames LD, Darke LL, Stampler FM, Naliboff BD. History of physical and sexual abuse in women with chronic pelvic pain. Obstet Gynecol. 1990;76(1):92–6.
9. Yosef A, Ahmed AG, Al-Hussaini T, Abdellah MS, Cua G, Bedaiwy MA. Chronic pelvic pain: pathogenesis and validated assessment. Middle East Fertil Soc J. 2016;21(4):205–21.
10. Molegraaf MJ, Torensma B, Lange CP, Lange JF, Jeekel J, Swank DJ. Twelve-year outcomes of laparoscopic adhesiolysis in patients with chronic abdominal pain: a randomized clinical trial. Surgery. 2017;161(2):415–21.
11. Gyang A, Hartman M, Lamvu G. Musculoskeletal causes of chronic pelvic pain: what a gynecologist should know. Obstet Gynecol. 2013;121(3):645–50.
12. Stovall TG, Ling FW, Crawford DA. Hysterectomy for chronic pelvic pain of presumed uterine etiology. Obstet Gynecol. 1990;75(4):676–9.
13. Howard FM, El-Minawi AM, Sanchez RA. Conscious pain mapping by laparoscopy in women with chronic pelvic pain. Obstet Gynecol. 2000;96(6):934–9.
14. Shakiba K, Bena JF, McGill KM, Minger J, Falcone T. Surgical treatment of endometriosis: a 7-year follow-up on the requirement for further surgery. Obstet Gynecol. 2008;111(6):1285–92.
15. Brown J, Crawford TJ, Allen C, Hopewell S, Prentice A. Nonsteroidal anti-inflammatory drugs for pain in women with endometriosis. Cochrane Database Syst Rev. 2017;(1):CD004753.
16. Gambone JC, Mittman BS, Munro MG, Scialli AR, Winkel CA, Chronic Pelvic Pain/Endometriosis Working Group. Consensus statement for the management of chronic pelvic pain and endometriosis: proceedings of an expert-panel consensus process. Fertil Steril. 2002;78(5):961–72.
17. Practice Committee of the American Society for Reproductive Medicine in Collaboration with the Society of Reproductive Surgeons. Pathogenesis, consequences, and control of peritoneal adhesions in gynecologic surgery. Fertil Steril. 2007;88(1):21–6.
18. Fitzgerald MP, Payne CK, Lukacz ES, Yang CC, Peters KM, Chai TC, Nickel JC, Hanno PM, Kreder KJ, Burks DA, Mayer R. Randomized multicenter clinical trial of myofascial physical therapy in women with interstitial cystitis/painful bladder syndrome and pelvic floor tenderness. J Urol. 2012;187(6):2113–8.
19. Duffy DM. Adhesion controversies: pelvic pain as a cause of adhesions, crystalloids in preventing them. J Reprod Med. 1996;41(1):19–26.
20. Nickel JC, Tripp DA, Pontari M, Moldwin R, Mayer R, Carr LK, Doggweiler R, Yang CC, Mishra N, Nordling J. Psychosocial phenotyping in women with interstitial cystitis/painful bladder syndrome: a case control study. J Urol. 2010;183(1):167–72.
21. Royal College of Obstetricians and Gynacologists. The initial management of chronic pelvic pain. Green top guideline 41. 2012. p. 1–18.
22. Nolan TE, Metheny WP, Smith RP. Unrecognized association of sleep disorders and depression with chronic pelvic pain. South Med J. 1992;85(12):1181–3.
23. Oikawa Y, Ohtori S, Koshi T, Takaso M, Inoue G, Orita S, Eguchi Y, Ochiai N, Kishida S, Kuniyoshi K, Nakamura J. Lumbar disc degeneration induces persistent groin pain. Spine. 2012;37(2):114–8.
24. Cheong YC, Smotra G, Williams ACDC. Non-surgical interventions for themanagement of chronic pelvic pain. Cochrane Database Syst Rev. 2014;3:CD008797.
25. Engeler D, Baranowski AP, Borovicka J, Cottrell A, Dinis-Oliveira P, Elneil S, Hughes J, Messelink EJ, Van Ophoven A, Reisman Y, de C Williams AC. EAU guidelines on chronic pelvic pain. EAU guidelines, edition presented at the 27th EAU Annual Congress, Paris; 2012.
26. Sator-Katzenschlager SM, Scharbert G, Kress HG, Frickey N, Ellend A, Gleiss A, Kozek-Langenecker SA. Chronic pelvic pain treated with gabapentin and amitriptyline: a randomized controlled pilot study. Wien Klin Wochenschr. 2005;117(21–22):761–8.
27. Fall M, Baranowski AP, Elneil S, Engeler D, Hughes J, Messelink EJ, Oberpenning F, Williams AC. EAU guidelines on chronic pelvic pain. Eur Urol. 2010;57(1):35–48.
28. Meltzer-Brody S, Leserman J, Zolnoun D, Steege J, Green E, Teich A. Trauma and posttraumatic stress disorder in women with chronic pelvic pain. Obstet Gynecol. 2007;109(4):902–8.

25 Interstitial Cystitis/Bladder Pain Syndrome

Paul K. Cheng and Tariq Malik

Case Description

A 65-year-old man presents to your pain management clinic with 6 months of pelvic pain worsened when his bladder feels full and is relieved after he urinates. He reports increased frequency of urination without change in the appearance or consistency of his urine. He was previously evaluated by his primary care doctor who informed him that his urinalysis did not show any abnormalities and his prostate was normal. He does not take any medications that would affect his urination and his only other medical problems are hypertension, hyperlipidemia, and depression.

What Is Your Preliminary Diagnosis?

The preliminary diagnosis is interstitial cystitis (IC), also known as bladder pain syndrome (BPS). Comprising one part of the spectrum of chronic pelvic pain, IC/BPS has been historically hard to define as various professional society guidelines, including those from the American Urologic Association, National Institute of Diabetes and Digestive and Kidney Diseases, and European Association of Urology, describe different diagnostic criteria [1–5]. However IC/BPS generally consists of an unpleasant sensation or chronic pressure, discomfort, or suprapubic pain associated with filling of the bladder that is accompanied by urinary symptoms such as urge to void, frequency, or nocturia [1]. BPS is a chronic condition, though the specific minimum time frame for diagnosis varies from 6 weeks to 6 months based on different guidelines [2, 3]. Additionally, it is a diagnosis of exclusion and care must be taken to rule out the many diseases which may present in a similar fashion [1–4].

How Is Diagnosis Confirmed?

Diagnostic Criteria

The diagnostic criteria for IC/BPS differ based on the professional society and are summarized as follows:

A. American Urologic Association (AUA) – an unpleasant sensation of pain or pressure perceived to be related to the urinary bladder. It is associated with lower urinary tract symptoms of more than 6 weeks. Patient should have no urinary tract infection or other identifiable causes of symptoms [4, 5]. Cystoscopy is not required for diagnosis but should be considered [4].

P. K. Cheng (✉)
Department of Anesthesiology and Pain Medicine, UC Davis Medical Center, Sacramento, CA, USA
e-mail: pcheng2@dacc.uchicago.edu

T. Malik
Department of Anesthesia and Critical Care, University of Chicago, Chicago, IL, USA

T. Malik (ed.), *Practical Chronic Pain Management*, https://doi.org/10.1007/978-3-030-46675-6_25

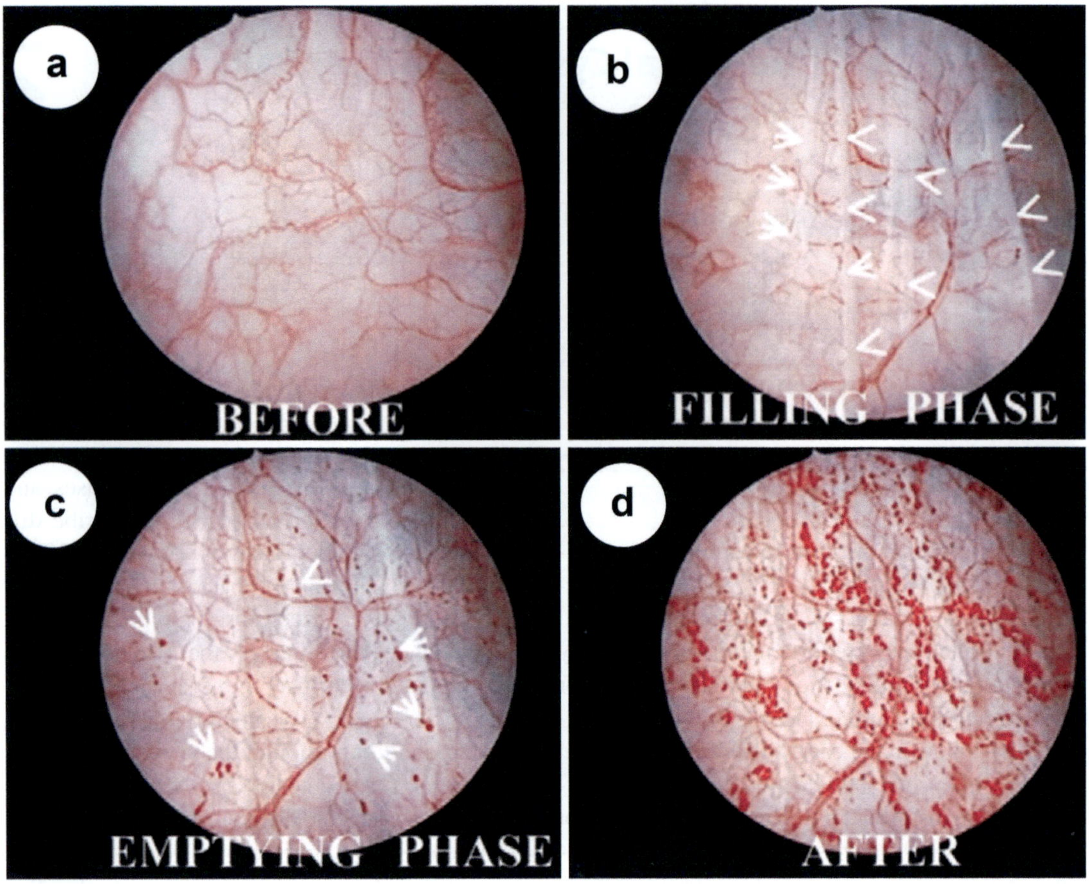

Fig. 25.1 Cystoscopic image of glomerulations in the bladder urothelium. This figure demonstrates the appearance of the bladder wall/urothelium, before (**a**), during (**b** and **c**), and after (**d**) hydrodistension. Glomerulations are petechia which develop from distal capillaries and are best seen in image **d**. (From Tamaki et al. [6], with permission)

B. National Institute of Diabetes and Digestive and Kidney Diseases (NIDDK) – in addition to the clinical symptoms of suprapubic pain or discomfort associated with either bladder filling or urinary urgency, the patient must have glomerulations (punctate petechial bladder wall hemorrhages) or classic Hunner's ulcers on cystoscopy (Figs. 25.1 and 25.2) [6, 7]. Specifically, the patient must have 10 glomerulations per quadrant of the bladder wall in at least 3 quadrants after distention of bladder to 80–100 cm of water pressure for 1–2 minutes [3, 5].
C. International Society for the Study of Bladder Pain syndrome – IC/BPS is defined as chronic pelvic pain, pressure, or discomfort perceived to be related to the urinary bladder. It is accompanied by at least one other urinary symptom (persistent urge to void or urinary frequency). Other diseases which may cause similar symptoms must be excluded by history and physical, urinalysis, urine culture, uroflowmetry, post-void residual, cystoscopy, and biopsy [5].
D. European Association of Urology (EAU) – The EAU separates IC and BPS into two distinct entities. BPS refers to the syndrome of suprapubic pain related to bladder filling which is persistent or recurrent over a 6-month period, worsened with increased bladder volume, and relieved by voiding. This suprapubic pain sometimes radiates to

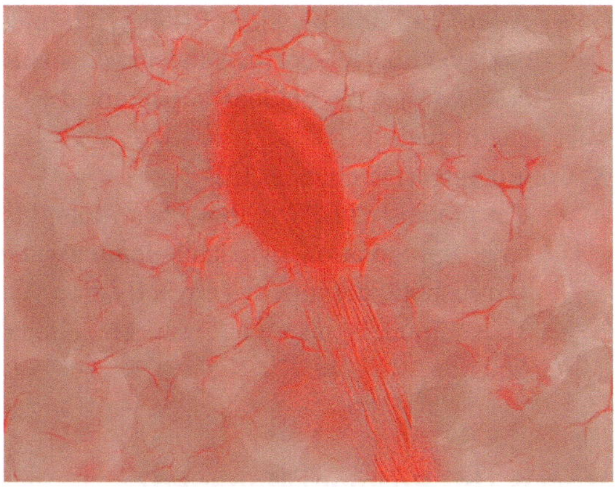

Fig. 25.2 Illustration of Hunner's lesions within the bladder urothelium. Hunner's lesions are superficial ulcerations in the bladder mucosa with small vessels radiating toward the discrete central scar. Water-fall like bleeding is described around the ulcer [1, 2, 7, 8]. (Original illustration by chapter author)

the groin, vagina, rectum, or sacrum. Patients typically have urinary frequency and always have nocturia. The term "interstitial cystitis" should be reserved only for the subset of BPS patient with signs of chronic inflammation extending submucosally on cystoscopy with hydrodistention and bladder biopsy [5].

All ages are affected by BPS though middle-aged women are the most affected group, particularly those from a lower socioeconomic status [3–5]. There is a strong female predominance with female to male ratios ranging from 5:1 to 10:1 [4]. BPS generally presents during the 40th decade or after, though a significant number of patients younger than 30 are affected and interestingly, symptoms tend to vary by age [3, 4]. Patients younger than 30 more commonly experience daytime frequency compared to dysuria and urinary urgency. Additionally, those younger than 30 are more likely to complain of dyspareunia and vulvar pain. For patients 30–50-years old, nocturia is much more common than daytime frequency and dysuria [4, 5, 8]. Symptoms are aggravated by certain foods including citrus, tomatoes, vitamin C, artificial sweeteners, coffee, tea, carbonated alcoholic beverages, and spicy food [5]. Generally foods high in acidic content, potassium, and caffeine exacerbate BPS. Sodium bicarbonate and calcium glycerophosphate can improve symptoms [3, 8].

What Is the Pathophysiology of This Condition?

Like many chronic pain conditions, BPS has an etiology which is poorly understood [2, 3]. BPS first appeared in medical literature more than 200 years ago and the term "interstitial cystitis" was first used in 1876 by Samuel Gross, an academic surgeon in Philadelphia who wrote about diseases of the bladder, and again in 1914 by gynecologist Guy Hunner in 1914 when he first described bladder epithelial damage and ulceration, now known as Hunner's lesions [1, 8].

There are multiple components thought to be related to the pathophysiology:

1. Urothelial and epithelial dysfunction [1, 3, 5, 9]
   - The bladder urothelium has protective layer of dense glycosaminoglycans (GAG) which is reduced in IC/PBS patients.
   - GAGs are a family of polysaccharide molecules forming the framework of extracellular matrix along with other components such as collagen, elastin, fibronectin, and laminin.
   - The GAG layer acts as a hydrated gel cushion in the bladder wall and helps for selective exchange of certain electrolytes and non-electrolytes in urine.
   - Impairment of the GAG layer leads to imbalance in urine storage which is thought to cause frequent urination, reduced urine capacity, bladder pain, and increased urothelial permeability.
   - The most common GAG molecules in the bladder include hyaluronate, keratin sulfate, dermatan sulfate, chondroitin sulfate, heparin, and heparin sulfate.
   - This theory is supported by the finding of glomerulations and/or Hunner's ulcers on cystoscopy which are signs of epithelial dysfunction and damage.

2. Tamm-Horsfall glycoprotein [5]
   - The Tamm-Horsfall glycoprotein (THP) is an anionic protein found abundantly in urine that binds and neutralizes urinary toxins.
   - Abnormal or low THP is thought to contribute to the pathophysiology of BPS.
3. Mast cell activation [3, 5, 9]
   - Inflammatory mediators in mast cells such as histamine, leukotrienes, serotonins, and cytokines are thought to play a role of frequency, pain, and fibrosis.
   - Bladder wall biopsies show an increased number of mast cells in BPS patients and activation of these cells.
4. Infection [3, 5]
   - Many patients with BPS note that their pain started with an acute urinary tract infection, but their symptoms never resolved with antibiotics.
   - It is possible that the urinary bladder gets sensitized from the inflammation of a UTI or the infection itself causes modifications in GAGs.
5. Anti-proliferative factor [5]
   - Anti-proliferative factor is a glycopeptide found to be elevated in urine of BPS patients.
   - APF inhibits proliferation of normal bladder epithelial cells and causes epithelial thinning.
   - APF also decreases heparin-binding epidermal growth factor, a factor which facilitates cell migration for epithelial repair.
6. Genetics [3, 5]
   - Twin studies show higher concordance of IC among monozygotic twins compared to dizygotic twins; therefore, a genetic component of the disease is likely.
   - Additionally, adult first-degree relatives of patients with BPS have a 17-time higher rate of developing IC.
7. Central sensitization of the spinal cord or sensory processing abnormality [5]
   - Like most chronic pain conditions, BPS is thought to have some contribution from central sensitization of the spinal cord or abnormality of sensory processing.
   - This would also explain the increased incidence of different concurrent chronic pelvic pain syndromes in BPS patients.
   - Additional non-bladder-related syndromes can potentially sensitize the lower spinal cord so that the bladder is perceived as a site of pain.
8. Neuroendocrine changes [3]
   - Cat models of BPS/IC have been found to have upregulation of catecholamines and sympathetic nervous system activation.
   - These models also had reduced adrenal function.

How Is This Problem Managed?

Treatment for IC/BPS can be divided into four general categories – non-medication management, oral medications, intravesicular therapy, and interventions/surgeries.

Non-medication Management

Patients with IC/BPS should be educated about the condition, instructed on dietary changes such as avoiding food triggers, and taught stress management. Care should be taken to get baseline voiding symptoms and pain levels in order to measure the effectiveness of subsequent treatments. Physical therapy, development of coping strategies, and cognitive behavior therapy are also crucial to management [2, 4, 8]. Any psychologic comorbidities should be appropriately treated [2]. There are two common misconceptions in non-medication management of IC. First, some patients drink cranberry juice thinking it would help their pain such as in bacterial cystitis; however, the acidification of the urine caused by cranberry worsens BPS symptoms [1]. Second, some patients do Kegel exercises to strengthen the pelvic floor thinking that it can relieve symptoms; however, increased pelvic tone can worsen the pain of BPS. The reverse strategy of relaxing pelvic wall muscles, called Thiele's exercises, are more helpful [1].

Oral Medications

Multiple oral medications exist for the treatment if IC/BPS including the classically described "triple therapy" of amitriptyline (tricyclic antidepressant), hydroxyzine (antihistamine), cimetidine (histamine H2 receptor antagonist) [2, 8]. Pentosan polysulfate, a heparin-like carbohydrate derivative used frequently as an oral therapy, is thought to adhere to the bladder wall mucosal membrane and act as a buffer to control cell permeability to prevent irritating solutes in the urine from reaching the cells of the bladder wall [1, 2]. Cyclosporine, a potent immunosuppressant which interferes with T-cell function, is used after failing other oral therapies [1, 4]. Opioid medications are generally not recommended for treatment of IC and gabapentinoids, though useful for neuropathic pain, are not effective for IC/BPS [2, 8].

Intravesicular Therapy

One key treatment modality for IC/BPS is intravesicular instillation of medication during cystoscopy. Commonly used medications include heparin, lidocaine, hyaluronic acid, chondroitin sulfate, hyaluronic acid and chondroitin in combination, and dimethyl sulfate [2, 9]. By applying medication directly to the bladder mucosal, you can achieve high local drug concentration, reduced systemic side effects, and reduced drug-drug interaction. Additionally, some injectates are thought to directly repair urothelial defects. Some downsides of intravesicular therapy include the relative impermeability of urothelial cells for medication uptake, short duration of action, need for frequent administration, and risk of infection [9, 10]. Of note hydrodistention, or filling the bladder with water in the absence of any medication, constitutes a treatment modality as well [1].

Common intravesicular pharmacologic therapies include the following:

- *Heparin* – mimics the GAG lining itself and has anti-inflammatory properties as it can inhibit fibroblast proliferation, angiogenesis, and smooth muscle cell proliferation [9, 10].
- *Lidocaine* – a local anesthetic provides symptomatic relief as it is applied directly to the bladder mucosa [9].
- *Hyaluronic acid* – also a component of GAG layer thought to help rebuild the connective tissue of the bladder wall. Hyaluronic acid can also inhibit chemotactic and phagocytic functions of leukocytes [8–10].
- *Chondroitin sulfate* – another component of GAG layer [8–10].
- *Pentosan polysulfate* – a heparin analog that reinforces GAGs and reduces urothelial injury [9]. Also both pentosan polysulfate and heparin are thought to also neutralize toxic factors in the urine which may cause urothelial damage [5].
- *Dimethyl sulfoxide (DMSO)* – an anti-inflammatory molecule which also serves as a scavenger of intracellular hydroxyl radicals, blocks nerve transmission, and causes both smooth muscle relaxation and collagen inhibition. It is also thought to cause nitric oxide release with desensitization of nociceptive pathways [9, 10].
- *Triamcinolone* – synthetic glucocorticoid with anti-inflammatory properties [1].
- *Botulinum toxin A* – potent neurotoxin produced from clostridium botulinum and prevents neurotransmission at the presynaptic membrane of the neuromuscular junction causing flaccid paralysis of the detrusor muscle and providing symptomatic relief of bladder pain [8–11].

Interventions/Surgery

If more-conservative therapies fail to control the symptoms of IC/BPS, advanced procedures and surgeries can be performed. Cystoscopies with fulguration/destruction of Hunner's lesions can be effective for patients with one study reporting 76% improvement in symptoms with destruction of Hunner's lesions [1, 2]. Neuromodulation, including sacral or pudendal nerve stimulation, has been shown to cause a significant reduction in pelvic pain as well as improve symptoms of daytime frequency and nocturia though the literature is somewhat scant at the moment [8, 12, 13]. Finally if all other therapies fail, cystectomy can be considered [2].

Guidelines

The various professional society guidelines differ on the treatment of IC/BPS. The AUA, RCOG/BSUG, and EAU guidelines are summarized as follows:

American Urological Association (AUA) 2014 Guidelines [1, 4]

These guidelines define six levels of treatment:

1. Patient education/self-care/behavior modifications/stress management
2. Physical therapy and pain management. Oral pharmaceutical treatment – amitriptyline, cimetidine, pentosan polysulfate, hydroxyzine. Vesicular pharmaceutical treatment – dimethyl sulfoxide, heparin, lidocaine
3. Endoscopic interventions – bladder hydrodistention (short-duration/low pressure), fulguration of Hunner's lesions followed by triamcinolone injection
4. Intravesicular botulinum A toxin or trial of neurostimulation followed by permanent implantation
5. Oral cyclosporine
6. Major surgery – urinary diversion with or without cystectomy

AUA does not recommend the following – pelvic floor exercises, long-term antibiotics, Bacille Calmette-Guerin (BCG) intravesicular therapy, oral glucocorticoid, or high-pressure/long-duration hydrodistention. Overall no single treatment benefits all or even most patients with BPS except for fulguration of Hunner's lesions.

Royal College of Obstetricians and Gynaecologists (RCOG)/ British Society of Urogynaecology (BSUG) 2016 Guidelines [1]

- Conservative measures should be done first such as patient education/stress management and pain symptom management.
- Oral medications are the next step with emphasis on amitriptyline and cimetidine.
- The third step is intravesicular therapy should conservative measures and oral medications fail. The strongest evidence exists for lidocaine, heparin, and botulinum toxin.
- Pain clinic consultation and multidisciplinary team discussion is recommended prior to more advanced options including fulguration of Hunner's lesions, neuromodulation, cyclosporine A, cystoscopic hydrodistention, and major surgery.

European Association of Urology (EAU) 2017 Guidelines [1]

- Overall these guidelines emphasize a holistic patient-centered approach and are less didactic for a treatment algorithm instead providing general guiding principles.
- Patient education is prioritized at the onset followed by physical therapy including transvaginal manual therapy of pelvic floor muscles, myofascial therapy, then finally levator muscle trigger point injection.
- Female patients may benefit from early referral for sexual counseling.
- Limited evidence exists for following therapies which are not recommended – electromagnetic, microwave, extracorporeal shockwave therapies, transcutaneous electrical nerve stimulation (TENS), hyperbaric oxygen therapy.
- Most patients will not have control with monotherapy and should have multimodal therapy targeted toward symptoms.
- Amitriptyline is the primary recommend oral therapy with nortriptyline as the alternative choice should the patient develop side effects to amitriptyline.
- Oral pentosan polysulfate has shown subjective improvement, and its effect is enhanced with treatment duration and concomitant use of subcutaneous heparin.
- Azathioprine can reduce pain and LUTS while cyclosporine A and methotrexate can help pain but have no benefit for urgency or frequency.
- Oral corticosteroids are not recommended.
- Intravesicular treatments can be used for medications which are not active orally for to obtain high intravesicular concentration and minimize systemic side effects though one should always consider the risks of repeated catheterization including infection as well as high costs. Recommended intravesicular agents include local anesthetic, hyaluronic acid, chondroitin sulfate, and heparin.
- In particular, a combination of intravesicular lidocaine, sodium bicarbonate, and heparin has been show to be effective and cause sustained relief in a high proportion of patients.
- Evidence for injected hyaluronic acid or chondroitin sulfate is limited.

- Overall, there is limited evidence for the following oral and/or vesicular pharmacotherapies – cimetidine, prostaglandins, L-arginine, oxybutynin, duloxetine, clorpactin, DMSO, BCG.
- Hydrodistention is recommended as a diagnostic, not therapeutic, tool. When used therapeutically it has greater benefits when used in conjunction with botox.
- Transurethral resection, fulguration, or lasering of Hunner's lesions is effective overall.
- Major surgery should be the last resort. Surgeries include urinary diversion without cystectomy, supratrigonal cystectomy with bladder augmentation, subtrigonal cystectomy, and cystectomy with ileal conduit formation.

What Is the Prognosis of This Condition?

BPS/IC is not curable with treatments aimed at improving symptoms and quality of life [1]. Unfortunately, IC/BPS is known to negatively affect work life, psychological well-being, personal relationships, and general health [4]. Patients suffering from this disorder often develop depression, sleep dysfunction, catastrophizing, anxiety, stress, social functioning difficulties, and sexual dysfunction [4, 8].

Discussion

Prevalence

Overall, the disease prevalence for BPS/IC ranges significantly due to different clinical definitions. One study estimates that in the United States, BPS affects 45/100,000 women and 8/100,000 men, with joint prevalence being 10.6/100,000 [3]. Another studying using US census data from 2006, which included 131,691 adult females, shows a female-specific prevalence ranging from 2.7% to 6.5% based on self-reported symptoms, translating to 3.3–7.9 million US women 18 years or older with BPS. Interestingly, only 9.7% of these patients were actually given a formal diagnosis of BPS/IC [5, 9]. The disease prevalence is thought to be increasing over the past few decades with some population studies showing disease rates of 10/100000 (0.01%) in 1975, then 30/100000 (0.03%) in 1987, and 510/100000 (0.5%) in 1994 [5]

Very few population studies have been done outside the United States; however, one recent study by Lee et al. (2018) evaluated the prevalence in Taiwan of BPS to be 21.8–40.2/100000. Of note that mean age in this population was 48 with a 78.7% female predominance [14].

Differential Diagnosis

BPS is a diagnosis of exclusion which is obtained through careful history-taking and various tests including urine dipstick, renal tract ultrasound, and cystoscopy [1, 2, 4]. The differential diagnosis includes the following – malignancy, infection, overactive bladder, cystitis caused by radiation or drugs, bladder outlet obstruction, irritable bowel syndrome, diverticular disease, urinary tract stones, urethral diverticulum, pelvic organ prolapse, endometriosis, and pudendal nerve entrapment [2, 4, 8]. Interestingly UTI is a common concurrent disease and many patients actually develop BPS following a UTI, though careful attention should be paid toward differentiating BPS symptoms from infectious symptoms [2]. Another area of diagnostic confusion is differentiating BPS and overactive bladder syndrome (OAB), as both cause urinary frequency. However urinary frequency due to fear of incontinence is generally OAB, while frequency due to pain with filling of the bladder is BPS [1]. For patients it may be helpful to keep a bladder diary or a log of daily voiding frequency and urinary volume as well as pain, sexual activity, and analgesic use [1, 2, 8].

BPS/IC can often present concurrently with other pain syndromes such fibromyalgia 9–12%, chronic fatigue 9.5%, and irritable bowel syndrome 7–48%, as well as a variety of gynecologic pain disorders including vulvodynia, genital pain, and endometriosis [3, 5].

Predictive Value of Different Clinical Features and Lab Testing/Imaging

Overall 100% of BPS patients have pelvic pain and voiding frequency is almost universal, affecting 92% of patients. Urinary urgency is also quite common at 84% [4]. Cystoscopy, though frequently done for BPS patients especially to exclude other diagnoses, is not in itself diagnostic unless Hunner's lesions are found [1, 2, 8].

To aid in diagnosis, the National Institute of Diabetes and Digestive and Kidney Diseases (NIDDK) lists exclusion criteria for IC/BPS diagnosis, which are shown below. However due to the diversity of symptoms in IC/BSP, using this exclusion criteria too strictly can miss up to 60% of patients regarded by experienced clinicians as definitely or likely having IC [5].

1. Bladder capacity greater than 350 mL on awake cystometry using either a gas or liquid filling medium
2. Absence of an intense urge to void with the bladder filled to 100 mL gas or 150 mL water during cystometry, using a fill rate of 30–100 mL per minute
3. The demonstration of phasic involuntary bladder contractions on cystometry using the fill rate described previously
4. Duration of symptoms less than 9 months
5. Absence of nocturia
6. Symptoms relieved by antimicrobials, urinary antiseptics, anticholinergics, or antispasmodics
7. A frequency of urination, while awake, of less than 8 times a day
8. A diagnosis of bacterial cystitis or prostatitis within a 3-month period
9. Bladder or ureteral calculi
10. Active genital herpes
11. Uterine, cervical, vaginal, or urethral cancer
12. Urethral diverticulum
13. Cyclophosphamide or any type of chemical cystitis
14. Tuberculous cystitis
15. Radiation cystitis
16. Benign or malignant bladder tumors
17. Vaginitis
18. Age less than 18 years

Strength of Evidence for Different Treatment Modalities

Table 25.1 summarizes the strength of evidence for different treatment modalities based on evaluation from AUA, EUA, the Royal College of Obstetricians and Gynaecologists/British Society of Urogynaecology (RCOG/BSUG), and Canadian Urological Association (CUA) [1, 2, 4, 5, 15].

Future Directions or Clinical Trials in Progress

Future Oral Therapies

Pharmacologic agents currently being researched involve drugs that target specific components of the inflammatory cascade. Such agents include anti-nerve growth factor, anti-tumor necrosis factor, and antagonists of Toll-like receptors [16].

Future Intravesicular Therapies

A large proportion of current research focuses on novel intravesicular therapies. One agent of particular interest is the liposome – concentric phospholipid bilayers enclosing aqueous interior. Injection of the empty liposome into the bladder has been shown in recent studies to reduce bladder hyperactivity induced by protamine sulfate, potassium chloride, or acetic acid in an IC/BPS rat model. Liposomes are thought mechanistically to use surface ligands to attach to injured urothelium and assist in repair [9, 10, 16]. Liposomes can also be used to carry drugs more effectively to the urothelium. Recent research involves the use of liposome mediated-botulinum toxin, tacrolimus, lidocaine, and pentosan polysulfate as intravesicular therapies [9, 16].

Additional intravesicular therapies being studied revolve around immunomodulation or cellular regeneration. In one case study, autologous platelet-rich plasma injected into the bladder demonstrated significant improvement in pain with an increase in urinary IL-8 and vascular endothelial growth factor. PRP is thought to augment urothelial wound healing since it is a

Table 25.1 Efficacy of treatment based on medical Literature

IC/BPS treatment	EAU grade of recommendation	AUA grade of recommendation	RCOG/BSUG grade of recommendation
Opioids	NR	Should be initiated with multimodal therapy (no grade assigned)	NR
Amitriptyline	A	B	B
Cimetidine	NR	B	B
Hydroxyzine	A	C	B
Pentosan polysulfate	A	B	A
Antibiotics	NR	NR	NR
Gabapentinoids	NR	NR	NR
Cyclosporine A	A	C	D
Intravesicular heparin	NR	C	D
Intravesicular hyaluronic acid	B	NR	B
Intravesicular lidocaine	NR	B	B
Intravesicular DMSO	A	C	C
Intravesicular botulinum toxin	NR	C	B
Intravesicular chondroitin sulfate	B	NR	D
Intravesicular BCG	NR	NR	NR
Hydrodistension	C	C	D
Electrocautery	Recommended for Hunner's lesions (no grade assigned)	C	Recommended (no grade assigned)
Major surgery	NR	C	D

Data from [1, 2, 4, 5, 15]

This table lists the therapies used for IC/BPS and the grade of recommendation from various professional societies

A = Good scientific evidence suggest benefits substantially outweigh risk. B = At least fair scientific evidence suggest benefits outweigh risk. C = At least fair scientific evidence suggest that there are benefits but the balance between benefits and risks are too close to make general recommendations. D = At least fair scientific evidence suggests that the risks of the clinical service outweigh the potential benefits. NR = no recommendation

source of growth factors and promote angiogenesis, increased blood flow, and oxygenation in the wound. It recruits macrophages and neutrophils which induce neural hypersensitivity of the wound then switch to an anti-inflammatory phenotype to release anti-inflammatory factors overall causing repair of the urothelium and decreasing pain [11]. PRP is also thought to treat neuropathic pain by releasing platelet and stem cell-released factors initiating a complex cascade of wound healing events in which it initiates wound healing, tissue remodeling, and axon regeneration [11]. Mesenchymal stem cell intravesicular therapy has also shown promise with studies demonstrating that injection of cord-blood-derived MCSs into bladder of an IC rat model showed improvement of urothelium layer. MSCs differentiated into epithelial cells and stimulated the epithelial growth factor signaling cascade [3].

Future Interventions

From an intervention standpoint, the main treatment currently being evaluated is superior hypogastric plexus radiofrequency ablation. Pulsed RF treatment of superior hypogastric plexus provides nondestructive neuromodulation to the nerve plexus which transmits the majority of pain signals from pelvic viscera including the bladder [17]. The procedure is done by guiding a needle under fluoroscopy anterior to the L5 vertebral body bilaterally to the superior hypogastric

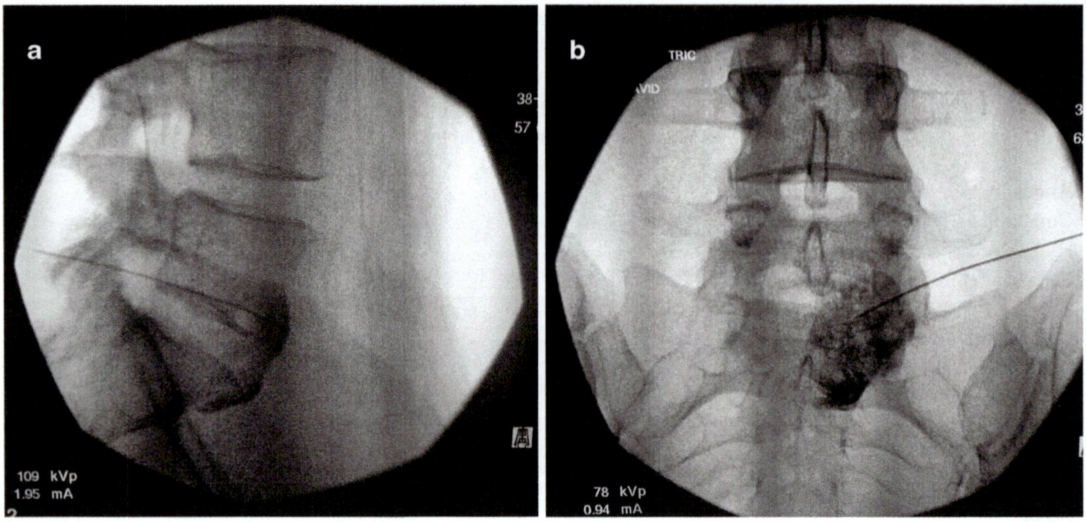

Fig. 25.3 (**a**, **b**) Radiofrequency ablation of superior hypogastric plexus. (Original images from chapter author). These fluoroscopic images of an RF ablation of the superior hypogastric plexus show needle placement and appropriate contrast dye spread anterior to the L5 vertebral body from a right-sided approach in the sagittal view (**a**) and the coronal view (**b**)

plexus then injecting local anesthetic for a diagnostic block followed by the RF ablation (see Fig. 25.3a, b). One case report from Korea demonstrated a 2.5-year improvement in a 35-year-old female with BPS unresponsive to regular intravesicular chondroitin and oral medications (gabapentin, pentosan polysulfate) following two pulsed radiofrequency treatments of the superior hypogastric plexus [17].

Biomarkers

Much of the recent research has focused on finding biomarkers for diagnosis of BPS/IC. None of the biomarkers have been completely validated to the point of being included in diagnostic guidelines; however, many hold promise. APF (antiproliferative factor) is the most widely studied and elevation of urinary APF has been found to be highly specific and sensitive for diagnosis of BPS/IC; however, there has been no evidence of APF expression during early phases of IC/PBS [3, 8]. Pro-inflammatory chemokines and interleukins are increased in IC/PBS, particularly interleukin-6. Research shows that increased urine levels of IL-6 has a sensitivity of 70%, specificity of 72.4%, positive predictive value of 77.8%, and negative predictive value of 63.6% [3]. Urinalysis of patients with IC/BPS also shows high levels of EGF, insulin-like growth factor-1, insulin-like growth factor-binding protein-3, and uroplakin III-delta4 while showing a significantly decreased levels of heparin-binding epidermal growth factor. Finally, some animal studies suggest that inflammatory markers including fibroblast growth factor 7 and chemokine ligand 21 are particularly altered in bladder wall biopsy samples from IC/PBS patients with mRNA levels correlating with disease severity; however, more studies need to be done to further evaluate these biomarkers [3].

Conclusion/Summary

Interstitial cystitis or bladder pain syndrome is a chronic pelvic pain condition exacerbated by bladder distention and accompanied by lower urinary tract symptoms. The diagnosis and treatment of IC is informed by guidelines from various professional societies including the AUA,

NIDDK, EAU, RCOG, and BSUG and can vary significantly. Overall, IC/BPS remains a clinical diagnosis with research currently being done to evaluate potential biomarkers to aid in diagnosis. Management involves both non-pharmacologic therapy (patient education, lifestyle changes, physical therapy) and oral/intravesicular medications with more advanced interventions including neuromodulation and bladder surgery reserved for the proportion of patients that do not respond to conservative measures. Further research is being done to develop additional pharmacotherapies and interventions to help treat IC/BPS.

References

1. Douglas-Moore JL, Goddard J. Current best practice in the management of cystitis and pelvic pain. Ther Adv Urol. 2018;10(1):17–22.
2. Goddard J. Cystitis and pelvic pain management: guidelines versus real-world practice. Urologia. 2017;84(Suppl 1):1–4.
3. Patnaik SS, Lagana AS, Vitale SG, Buttice S, Noventa M, Gizzo S, et al. Etiology, pathophysiology and biomarkers of interstitial cystitis/painful bladder syndrome. Arch Gynecol Obstet. 2017;295(6):1341–59.
4. Hanno PM, Burks DA, Clemens JQ, Dmochowski RR, Erickson D, Fitzgerald MP, et al. AUA guideline for the diagnosis and treatment of interstitial cystitis/bladder pain syndrome. J Urol. 2011;185(6):2162–70.
5. McLennan MT. Interstitial cystitis: epidemiology, pathophysiology, and clinical presentation. Obstet Gynecol Clin N Am. 2014;41(3):385–95.
6. Tamaki M, Saito R, Ogawa O, Yoshimura N, Ueda T. Possible mechanisms inducing glomerulations in interstitial cystitis: relationship between endoscopic findings and expression of angiogenic growth factors. J Urol. 2004;172(3):945–8.
7. Fall M, Logadottir Y, Peeker R. Interstitial cystitis is bladder pain syndrome with Hunner's lesion. Int J Urol. 2014;21 Suppl 1:79–82.
8. Chrysanthopoulou EL, Doumouchtsis SK. Challenges and current evidence on the management of bladder pain syndrome. Neurourol Urodyn. 2014;33(8):1193–201.
9. Meng E, Hsu YC, Chuang YC. Advances in intravesical therapy for bladder pain syndrome (BPS)/interstitial cystitis (IC). Low Urin Tract Symptoms. 2018;10(1):3–11.
10. Ha T, Xu JH. Interstitial cystitis intravesical therapy. Transl Androl Urol. 2017;6(Suppl 2):S171–S9.
11. Jhang JF, Wu SY, Lin TY, Kuo HC. Repeated intravesical injections of platelet-rich plasma are effective in the treatment of interstitial cystitis: a case control pilot study. Low Urin Tract Symptoms. 2019;11(2):O42–7.
12. Wang J, Chen Y, Chen J, Zhang G, Wu P. Sacral neuromodulation for refractory bladder pain syndrome/interstitial cystitis: a global systematic review and meta-analysis. Sci Rep. 2017;7(1):11031.
13. Tirlapur SA, Vlismas A, Ball E, Khan KS. Nerve stimulation for chronic pelvic pain and bladder pain syndrome: a systematic review. Acta Obstet Gynecol Scand. 2013;92(8):881–7.
14. Lee MH, Chang KM, Tsai WC. Morbidity rate and medical utilization in interstitial cystitis/painful bladder syndrome. Int Urogynecol J. 2018;29(7):1045–50.
15. Lusty A, Kavaler E, Zakariasen K, Tolls V, Nickel JC. Treatment effectiveness in interstitial cystitis/bladder pain syndrome: do patient perceptions align with efficacy-based guidelines? Can Urol Assoc J. 2018;12(1):E1–5.
16. Andersson KE, Birder L. Current pharmacologic approaches in painful bladder research: an update. Int Neurourol J. 2017;21(4):235–42.
17. Kim JH, Kim E, Kim BI. Pulsed radiofrequency treatment of the superior hypogastric plexus in an interstitial cystitis patient with chronic pain and symptoms refractory to oral and intravesical medications and bladder hydrodistention: a case report. Medicine (Baltimore). 2016;95(49):e5549.

Chronic Pain After Hernia Repair

26

Nicholas Kirch and Maunak V. Rana

Case Description

A 35-year-old male presents to the pain clinic for evaluation of groin pain 3 months after a successful indirect inguinal hernia procedure. His surgery, performed under general anesthesia, with mesh repair, was uncomplicated and he was noted to be doing well until 2 weeks after the surgery, at which time the patient developed burning pain in the scar region radiating down into the ipsilateral testicle [1–4]. Physical activity is painful resulting in a sharp pain, rated 8/10. He has tried rest and acetaminophen with hydrocodone without benefit.

Examination reveals a well-developed, well-nourished male in discomfort while seated. His gait is antalgic due to pain in the left inguinal region. Evaluation reveals a 2 cm diagonal scar in the inguinal region, which is tender to light touch. This region is not indurated, warm, or erythemic. The patient has been seen by his surgeon and has been told that he has healed well. There is no evidence of hernia or palpable mass. The patient has a noticeable area of discomfort over the scar, with radiating pain into the groin and into the testicle. There is no tenderness to palpation over the pubic tubercle and no tenderness at the anterior superior iliac spine. Genital exam reveals normal bilateral, descended testes.

What Is Your Preliminary Diagnosis?

Chronic post-surgical pain is very common after hernia repair. There are three nerves (ilioinguinal, iliohypogastric, and genitofemoral nerve) in the surgical field that makes this surgery as one of the most common surgery associated with chronic post-surgical pain. The patient meets the criteria for the diagnosis of chronic post-surgical pain as defined by the International Association for the Study of Pain, which defines chronic post-surgical pain as pain persisting more than 3 months after surgery. History and physical examination is very suggestive of neuropathic pain. There is no obvious pathology, the wound has healed well, and there are no other clinical findings explaining his condition. Neuropathic pain is often described by patients as sharp, shooting, stabbing, or burning in nature. There may be finding of allodynia, hyperalgesia, or hypoesthesia on physical examination. The pain distribution or sensory disturbances on exam may be in a particular nerve distribution, which may help to narrow down the pain to one nerve. It is important to exclude non-neuropathic elements

N. Kirch
Department of Anesthesiology and Critical Care, University of Chicago, Chicago, IL, USA

M. V. Rana (✉)
Department of Anesthesia and Critical Care, University of Chicago, Chicago, IL, USA
e-mail: mrana@dacc.uchicago.edu

T. Malik (ed.), *Practical Chronic Pain Management*, https://doi.org/10.1007/978-3-030-46675-6_26

of pain including recurrence of hernia, tumor, myofascial pain, or entrapped bowel.

In this patient, the most likely diagnosis is neuropathic pain, most likely involving ilioinguinal nerve.

How Is the Diagnosis Confirmed?

The diagnosis of chronic post herniorrhaphy pain is made based on the clinical history, location of pain, as well as ruling out alternative sources of pain. Ilioinguinal neuralgia often arises after abdominal surgery, pelvic surgery, or inguinal hernia surgery. The physical examination of the patient allows for the opportunity to differentiate between the potential sources of pain. The presence of allodynia leads to a neuropathic pain entity and steers the practitioner away from trigger point–related pain. As to the location of the discomfort, the patient has pain over the scar in the inguinal region. This could be due to neuroma or nerve entrapment either from scar tissue, mesh, or sutures. The lack of pain in the pubic tubercle region leads away from the diagnosis of genitofemoral neuralgia. The lack of discomfort over the anterior superior iliac spine would lead away from the diagnosis of meralgia paresthetica, as would the location of the pain.

As mentioned above, CPIP can result from other etiologies, which must be ruled out. Hernia recurrence, while rare, is a possibility. Excessive scar formation can result in pain at the site of incision that does not follow specific nerve pathways. Local factors related to mesh interactions with tissues, from tacking suture to the mesh itself, can lead to a meshoma or even adhesions to surrounding structures like intestines or spermatic cord as the source of pain.

Ultrasound is a useful noninvasive imaging modality that is very sensitive for the diagnosis of occult hernia (Fig. 26.1). It can help differentiate any swelling in the area as fluid collection due to seroma/infection or recurrence of hernia, but is often limited by pain during examination and operator's experience. The presence of anatomical defects, additional herniation, or development of a neuroma, which would appear on ultrasound with a characteristic feature around a cut/accessed nerve, can easily be assessed [5]. CT is more sensitive than US in exploring anatomy of the area and is fewer operators dependent. It can also differentiate seroma from infection. MRI is the most sensitive imaging option to evaluate anatomical pathology. It is much better at evaluating post-surgical scarring and can also evaluate the status of mesh and surgical repair.

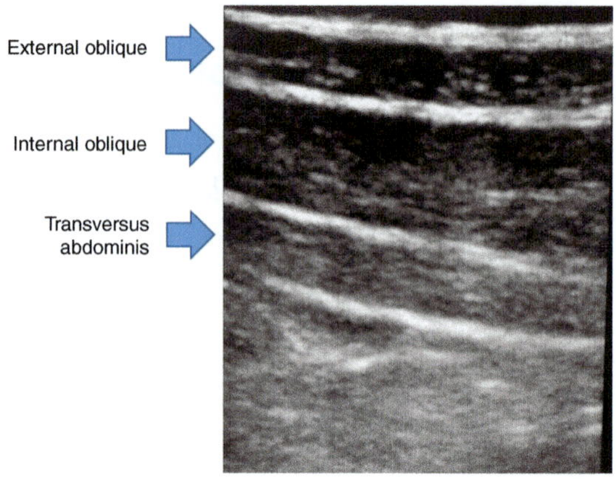

Fig. 26.1 Ultrasound of muscle layers of the abdominal wall, from top to bottom: external oblique, internal oblique, transversus abdominis

Quite often the imaging is done primarily to rule out pathologies like infection, breakdown of repair, excessive scarring, or recurrence of hernia and not to rule in neuropathic pain. At the end of the day, it is a clinical diagnosis and a diagnosis of exclusion.

If no other causes of pain can be identified, a diagnostic and potentially therapeutic block of the nerve can be done. But the injection is primarily done to identify which nerve is most likely involved as the source of neuropathic pain.

What Is the Pathophysiology of This Condition?

The development of pain after hernia surgery is multifactorial in origin. The underlying mechanism is the same as in other chronic post-surgical pains. Damage or prolonged activation of the nerve fibers lead to peripheral and/or central sensitization that often involves transcriptional changes in the cell bodies of the neuron leading to altered ion channel receptors expression and altered neurotransmitters release. Prolonged NMDA activation leads to apoptosis. The cell death leads to sprouting of non-noxious nerve fibers into the noxious pathways. This leads to the development of allodynia and hyperalgesia. The release of chemokines, ATP, NO, cytokines by the activated astrocytes, and microglia also contribute to the maintenance of hypersensitivity. Predisposition due to underlying medical conditions may occur due to pre-existing neuropathy and medical conditions including diabetes mellitus. The concept of hyperalgesic priming, related to the inflammatory response to surgery, demonstrates a possible cause for the development of chronic pain in subsets of patients. A multivariate analysis highlighted the role of preoperative pain, type of pain, type of anesthesia, among other factors including type of mesh utilized that may play a role in the development of pain after surgery [6]. Additional risk factors identified in studies include young age and female sex (Table 26.1) [7].

Additionally, iatrogenic causes after surgery include tissue injury due to aberrant anatomy, nerve injury, or entrapment. This neurotrauma may lead to chronic long-term pain, as has been suggested based on the literature review [8–11]. Based on the theoretical role of nerve injury, and in many cases the development of neuroma as a causative factor, it has been suggested that neuromodulation or even a purposeful resection of the ilioinguinal nerve may lead to a decrease in postoperative pain and is considered a treatment for recalcitrant, chronic pain [12].

Table 26.1 Risk factors for developing chronic pain post hernia repair

Risk Factors for developing chronic pain post hernia repair [6–8]:
Young age
Female sex
Preoperative chronic pain
Operation for recurrent hernia
Less experienced surgeon
Heavyweight mesh
Mesh fixation
Postoperative complications (infection, hematoma, neuroma)
Severe early postoperative pain

How Is This Problem Managed?

The problem requires multimodal and multidisciplinary approach. It is very important to assess psychological stresses that work on pain-coping skills at the outset. The most important intervention in the management of any chronic pain condition is education of the patient.

In the absence of quality randomized controlled trials, pharmacological and interventional pain management strategies are based on small studies, case series, and extrapolation of evidence from other neuropathic conditions. There are general guidelines by the various pain societies to treat neuropathic pain but no society has specifically provided guidelines for post-herniorrhaphy pain. These pain societies categorize calcium channel modulators (gabapentin/pregabalin), topical lidocaine, tricyclic antidepressants (amitriptyline, nortriptyline, desipramine), and SSRI (duloxetine, venlafaxine) as first line of therapy.

These medications are started after patient has failed to respond to over-the-counter analgesics (NSAIDS, acetaminophen). Each medication should be assessed based on patient-specific comorbidities/concerns as well as tolerance to medication side effects. Effective dose of gabapentin ranges from 600 to 1200 mg three times a day; pregabalin dose ranges from 50 to 200 mg three times a day. Renal adjustment is needed for both drugs. Lidocaine cream or patch is effective for managing allodynia. Amitriptyline effective dose ranges from 25 to 150 mg per day. Duloxetine is started at 30 mg a day and dose titrated up to 120 mg a day if needed. Tramadol is a weak mu opioid with SSRI and weak NMDA antagonist properties and has been effective in many neuropathic pain conditions. Patients who fail to respond to these drugs can be tried on other channel blockers (Lamotrigine, topiramate, carbamazepine, oxcarbazepine, and mexiletine) or antidepressants (bupropion, citalopram, and paroxetine). They have been found to be variably effective in various neuropathic conditions.

In the setting of pain refractory to conservative treatment, more invasive techniques including nerve blocks have been used. While traditionally performed in a field block format, the use of nerve stimulator and now the use of ultrasound to directly identify tissue planes and neurovascular structures have greatly improved fidelity and success of this technique. While preprocedure nerve blocks to decrease the development of pain after the procedure has also been evaluated, in a triple-blinded, placebo controlled trial of patients undergoing inguinal hernia repair, intraoperative infiltration of local anesthetic did not have an effect on postoperative pain [13]. Post-procedural nerve blocks serve as diagnostic and short-term therapeutic interventions [14].

If a nerve block has successfully been performed to isolate the causative nerve, neurolysis, or neuroablation using cryoablation, radiofrequency ablation or chemical neurolysis has been used to achieve longer pain control [15, 16].

As the indications for neuromodulation continue to expand, peripheral nerve field stimulation and spinal cord stimulation are increasingly utilized to treat refractory pain. While there are no large studies treating CPIP, there have been case reports and papers showing promise [17, 18]. With these techniques, patient selection is thought to play a role in their success, having highly motivated patients who have passed a psychiatric evaluation. An additional benefit to neuromodulation is that they are nonpermanent in nature, leading to minimal long-term morbidity.

In the surgical literature, neurectomy has been advocated with varying results with some patients receiving benefit for post-surgical pain and others persisting with pain or developing new, distinct pain [19]. Due to anatomical differences and the complex course of nerves in the groin, it is often difficult to isolate a single nerve to alleviate the pain, which has led to the technique of triple neurectomy, or removal of iliohypogastric, ilioinguinal, and genital branch of genitofemoral nerve, in addition to mesh extraction or tack removal [20]. Some surgeons advocate for doing a repeat open procedure to best have access to all of these structures in a single staged procedure (Fig. 26.2) [21].

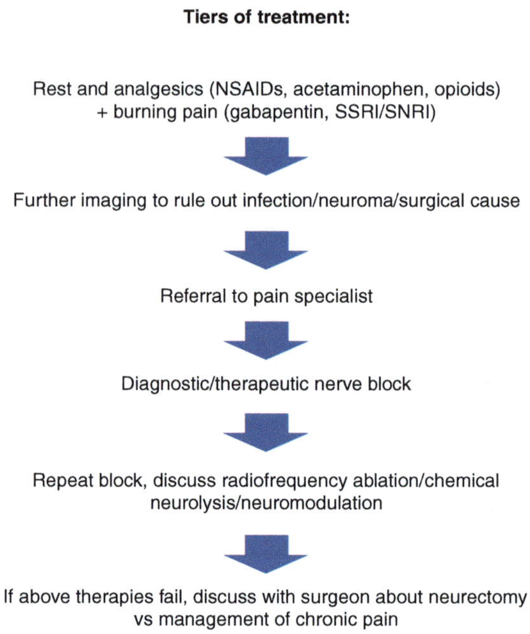

Fig. 26.2 Tiers of treatment

What Is the Prognosis of This Condition?

Pain before and immediately after surgery is seemingly important in the development and analysis of prognosis. Patients who have higher postoperative pain scores early in recovery are likely to continue with chronic pain in this surgical population [21, 22]; in addition, patients with preoperative pain were found to have increased risk for postoperative pain by a factor of 1.5 [23]. On evaluation, 26.9% without preoperative pain developed chronic pain vs. 76.7% of patients with preoperative pain developed chronic post-surgical pain [6]. In another study, 88% of patients with preoperative pain went on to develop chronic pain after surgery [24]. Therefore, it is important to make chronic pain patients aware of their increased risks prior to surgery, as well as to aggressively treat post-herniorrhaphy pain [25].

Ultimately, these cases significantly reduce quality of life, increase direct and indirect socioeconomic burdens, as well as increase likelihood of being diagnosed with associated affective disorders, such as anxiety and depression [21, 22, 25].

Discussion

Prevalence

With an annual 800,000 inguinal hernia repairs conducted alone in the United States with more than 20 million performed around the world, the treatment of post-herniorrhaphy inguinal pain has become ever more in focus. Studies differ in the prevalence of chronic post-surgical pain, ranging from 8% to 16%; even some studies are as low as 0.2% [1, 3, 6, 22]. These studies differ due to definitions of how long one must have pain postoperatively to have chronic pain (between 3 and 6 months) and what constitutes chronic pain (any pain vs. the degree it impacts the patient's life), as well as the methods of their studies. However, based on these numbers in the United States alone 64,000–128,000 patients and even based on the most conservative numbers 1600 patients annually are impacted in some capacity.

Differential Diagnosis

The differential diagnosis of post-herniorrhaphy pain includes scar tissue, neuroma, recurrent hernia, myalgia/trigger points, and neuralgias.

Predictive Value of Different Clinical Features and Lab Testing/Imaging

As previously mentioned, there is an increased likelihood of developing chronic pain after hernia surgery if chronic pain is present prior to surgery [23]. However there are no specific tests/imaging studies that can be done to help predict which non-chronic pain population is more prone to develop this condition. There exists variability in the literature regarding the age of the patient and the development of chronic pain after hernia surgery, with a few studies noting no influence of age and some evaluations noting a discernible effect of age on the presence of chronic pain after surgery [1, 6, 18]. Pre-emptive analgesia has not been clearly shown to affect the outcome of chronic pain [23]. Additionally, intraoperative injection of local anesthetic at the site of surgery did not lead to a decrease in pain during the subsequent days after surgery [24]. It is also unclear based on multiple studies whether the type of repair, open or endoscopic, correlates to the occurrence of postoperative pain. In the surgical community, many people have speculated whether the type of mesh and fixation used in the procedure can help mitigate the occurrence of chronic pain; however, none of these studies are definitive.

Strength of Evidence for Different Treatment Modalities

As mentioned above, data for pre-emptive infiltration of local anesthesia has not demonstrated consistent results for affecting the development/persistence of chronic pain. The use of nerve blocks after the development of chronic pain also has shown conflicting efficacy. There are few randomized, controlled trials available for evaluation of efficacy of nerve blocks.

Additionally, though advocated by surgeons, reoperation has not demonstrated significant efficacy. In one evaluation [21], 6 out of 40 patients studied still persisted with pain despite re-exploration of the surgical site.

The use of analgesics too is difficult to analyze as the type of pain described is variable. Whereas for neuropathic pain, a membrane stabilizer would be a first-line choice, as patients differ in presentation as highlighted previously. There are no current studies comparing the efficacy of different classes of analgesics for chronic post-inguinal surgery pain.

Future Directions or Clinical Trials in Progress

Current directions for preventing the development of CPIP focus mostly on improving surgical techniques; as surgeries continue to become less invasive, there is a theoretical benefit to less tissue damage. Additionally, there is ongoing research around the best type of mesh to avoid development of postoperative pain. Treatment of post hernia repair chronic pain continues to evolve as neuromodulatory techniques continue to improve, as well as neuroablative techniques. Additional trials will need to be undertaken to determine the optimal role of peripheral stimulation. In some European countries the treatment of CPIP is done in dedicated hernia centers, where experts in pain management utilize a uniform scaled intervention system from conservative management to neuroablative and ultimately surgical intervention. This both results in early standard of care treatment for these patients as well as it allows for data collection for further studies [4].

Conclusion/Summary

The management of chronic pain following inguinal hernia surgery should start with a thorough physical exam, which may include imaging, to rule out alternative causes of pain as well as possible recurrence of the hernia. However, once other causes have been excluded, the mainstay initial treatment of this condition includes rest and analgesics. If refractory to conservative management, more invasive techniques like nerve blocks, nerve ablation, peripheral nerve stimulation, and ultimately neurectomy may need to be provided. Patients who have chronic pain prior to hernia repair are more likely to develop postoperative chronic pain, as well as patients who develop severe postoperative pain early are more likely to continue to transition from acute to chronic pain. There are no tests that are currently available to determine who is susceptible to having chronic pain nor are there preprocedural treatments to decrease the likelihood of developing long-term pain. There is a need for studies performed by experts at dedicated hernia centers to determine future best practice guidelines regarding surgical techniques as well as to continue to develop novel treatment options for patients refractory to current therapies.

References

1. Donati M, Brancato G, Giglio A, Biondi A, Basile F, Donati A. Incidence of pain after inguinal hernia repair in the elderly. A retrospective historical cohort evaluation of 18-years' experience with a mesh & plug inguinal hernia repair method on about 3000 patients. BMC Surg. 2013;13(Suppl 2):S19.
2. Condon RE. Groin pain after hernia repair. Ann Surg. 2001;233(1):8.
3. Callesen T, Bech K, Kehlet H. Prospective study of chronic pain after groin hernia repair. Br J Surg. 1999;86(12):1528–31.
4. Andresen K, Rosenberg J. Management of chronic pain after hernia repair. J Pain Res. 2018;11:675–81.
5. Lawande AD, Warrier SS, Joshi MS. Role of ultrasound in evaluation of peripheral nerves. Indian J Radiol Imaging. 2014;24(3):254–8.
6. Manangi M, Shivshankar S, Vijayakumar A. Chronic pain after inguinal hernia repair. Int Sch Res Notices. 2014;2014:839681. https://doi.org/10.1155/2014/839681. eCollection 2014.
7. Bay-Nielsen M, Perkins FM, Kehlet H. Pain and functional impairment 1 year after inguinal herniorrhaphy: a nationwide questionnaire study. Ann Surg. 2001;233:1–7.
8. Bjurstrom MF, et al. Pain control following inguinal herniorrhaphy: current perspectives. J Pain Res. 2018;7(2014):277–90. *PMC*. Web.
9. Reinpold WM, Nehls J, Eggert A. Nerve management and chronic pain after open inguinal hernia repair: a prospective two phase study. Ann Surg. 2011;254(1):163–8.
10. Hakeem A, Shanmugam V. Inguinodynia following Lichtenstein tension-free hernia repair: a review. World J Gastroenterol. 2011;17(14):1791–6.
11. Emekisz S, Ozden H, Guven G. Effects of variable courses of inguinal nerves on pain in patients undergoing Lichtenstein repair for inguinal hernia: preliminary results. Acta Chir Belg. 2013;113(3):196–202.
12. Johner A, Fauldis J, Wiseman SM. Planned ilioinguinal nerve excision for prevention of chronic pain after inguinal hernia repair: a meta-analysis. Surgery. 2011 Sep;150(3):534–41.
13. Kurmann A, Fischer H, Dell-Kuster S, Rosenthal R, Audige L, Schupfer G, Metzger J, Honigmann P. Effect of intraoperative infiltration with local anesthesia on the development of chronic pain after inguinal hernia repair: a randomized, triple-blinded, placebo controlled trial. Surgery. 2015;157(1):144–54.
14. Willschke H, Marhofer P, Bosenberg A, Johnston S, Wanzel O, Cox SG, Sitzwohl C, Kapral S. Ultrasonography for ilioinguinal/iliohypogastric nerve blocks in children. Br J Anaesth. August 2005;95(2):226–30.

15. Rozen D, Ahn J. Pulsed radiofrequency for the treatment of ilioinguinal neuralgia after inguinal herniorrhaphy. Mt Sinai J Med. 2006;73:716–8.
16. Fine PG. Long-term consequences of chronic pain: mounting evidence for pain as a neurological disease and parallels with other chronic disease states. Pain Med. 2011;12:996–1004.
17. Parsons B, Schaefer C, Mann R, et al. Economic and humanistic burden of post-trauma and post-surgical neuropathic pain among adults in the United States. J Pain Res. 2013;6:459–69.
18. Aasvang EK, Gmaehle E, Hansen JB, et al. Predictive risk factors for persistent post herniotomy pain. Anesthesiology. 2010;112(4):957–69.
19. Andresen K, Burcharth J, Fonnes S, et al. Chronic pain after inguinal hernia repair with the ONSTEP versus the Lichtenstein technique, results of a double-blinded multicenter randomized clinical trial. Langenbeck's Arch Surg. 2017;402(2):213–8.
20. Poobalan AS, Bruce J, Smith WC, King PM, Krukowski ZH, Chambers WA. A review of chronic pain after inguinal herniorrhaphy. Clin J Pain. 2003;19:48–54.
21. Courtney CA, Duffy K, Serpell MG, O'Dwyer PJ. Outcome of patients with severe chronic pain following repair of groin hernia. Br J Surg. 2002;89(10):1310–4.
22. Bay-Nielsen M, Perkins FM, Kehlet H. Pain and functional impairment 1 year after inguinal herniorrhaphy: a nationwide questionnaire study. Ann Surg. 2001;233(1):1–7.
23. Dahl JB, Mathiesen O, Møiniche S. 'Protective premedication': an option with gabapentin and related drugs? A review of gabapentin and pregabalin in the treatment of postoperative pain. Acta Anaesthesiol Scand. 2001;48(9):1130–6.
24. Cybulka B. Inguinal pain syndrome. The influence of intraoperative local administration of 0.5% bupivacaine on postoperative pain control following Lichtenstein hernioplasty. A prospective case-control study. Pol Przegl Chir. 2017 Apr 30;89(2):11–25.
25. Kalliomaki ML, Sandblom G, Gunnarsson U, Gordh T. Peristent pain after groin hernia surgery: a qualitative analysis of pain and its consequences for quality of life. Acta Anaesthesiol Scand. 2009;53:236–46.

A 65-Year-Old Woman with Chronic Hip Pain

27

Khyrie Jones and Tariq Malik

Case Description

An elderly, obese, and sedentary female presents to a local clinic with chronic unilateral hip pain. The pain, onset years ago, has gradually worsened over time, and is described as a deep, dull, and aching soreness that occasionally radiates to the groin. Symptoms improve with rest and worsen throughout the day after physical activities with repetitive motions, prolonged standing, and walking long distances. Associations include brief morning stiffness in the hands (<30 min), swelling of the knees, and exacerbated pain when rising from a seated position. The patient denies recent falls and joint warmth or redness. Past medical and surgical histories are noncontributory, and family history is unremarkable. Physical exam is significant for enlarged bony deformities of the distal and proximal interphalangeal joints of the hands, crepitus of the knees, and limited range of motion of the ipsilateral hip with groin tenderness while flexed and externally rotated [8, 10].

K. Jones
Schwab Rehabilitation Hospital & Care Network/
University of Chicago, Chicago, IL, USA

T. Malik (✉)
Department of Anesthesia and Critical Care,
University of Chicago, Chicago, IL, USA
e-mail: TMuslim@dacc.uchicago.edu;
tmalik@dacc.uchicago.edu

What Is Your Preliminary Diagnosis?

The clinical and physical findings suggest osteoarthritis of the hip, especially considering the predisposing risk factors of the patient. Certain lifestyles (inactivity, heavy manual labor, etc.), prior joint injury or trauma, and family history of joint disease would have also supported osteoarthritis [3–5]. Additional symptoms may also include function-limiting hip pain (such as diminished walking distance) and mechanical instability (examples include a 'locking' or 'catching' sensation, shortening of the affected leg, or abnormal gait). The pain from osteoarthritis of the hip typically radiates to the groin; however, direct pressure over the groin does not increase pain. Concomitant findings may include neck pain associated with limited lateral rotation due to osteoarthritis of the cervical spine, lower back pain that radiates to the buttocks due to osteoarthritis of the lumbar spine, and localized knee pain due to osteoarthritis of the knee.

How Is Diagnosis Confirmed?

Osteoarthritis of the hip is typically diagnosed on the basis of clinical and radiographic evidence [2, 6, 7]. Although osteoarthritis is a clinical diagnosis, anteroposterior plain radiography (XR) of the hip/pelvis is recommended for confirmation and to determine disease progression and severity, and

T. Malik (ed.), *Practical Chronic Pain Management*, https://doi.org/10.1007/978-3-030-46675-6_27

characteristic findings include joint space narrowing, osteophytes (bony outgrowths due to bone remodeling), joint mice (sloughed articular cartilage and subchondral bone forming loose bodies), and subchondral sclerosis (bone eburnation) or cysts [3–5]. Magnetic resonance imaging (MRI) is not necessary in most patients with osteoarthritis unless additional pathology amenable to surgical repair is suspected [2]; however, MRI can identify osteoarthritis at the earlier stages of disease before radiographic changes (cartilage defects, bone marrow lesions) become apparent [8]. No specific laboratory abnormalities are associated with osteoarthritis; acute phase reactants such as serum erythrocyte sedimentation rate (ESR) and c-reactive protein (CRP) are within normal limits.

What Is the Pathophysiology of This Condition?

Osteoarthritis is a disease that affects all structures of the joint: the hyaline articular cartilage, subchondral bone, ligaments, capsule, synovium, and periarticular muscles (Fig. 27.1). The pathogenesis involves a combination of mechanical, inflammatory, and metabolic factors, resulting in structural destruction and painful joints. Osteoarthritis is characterized by chondrocyte-mediated excessive degradation and inadequate repair of articular cartilage at joint surfaces due to overactive proteolytic enzymes (e.g., matrix metalloproteases) in response to a compromised extracellular matrix (disorganized type II collagen, increased water content, decreased proteoglycans) and the accumulative presence of inflammatory cytokines (e.g., IL-1, IL-6, IL-17, TNF-α, TGF-β) in the synovium over time as the disease progresses [4, 5]. However, the pathophysiology of osteoarthritis is not fully understood, and the role of inflammation has been acknowledged and generally accepted only in recent years. Osteoarthritis is a heterogeneous disease with a wide range of underlying pathways, which lead to similar outcomes of joint destruction. A number of subtypes have been proposed on the basis of specific pathological processes, which include inflammatory type, mechanical overload, metabolic alterations, and premature cell death, but most likely it is a combination of all these present in varying degrees in different patients.

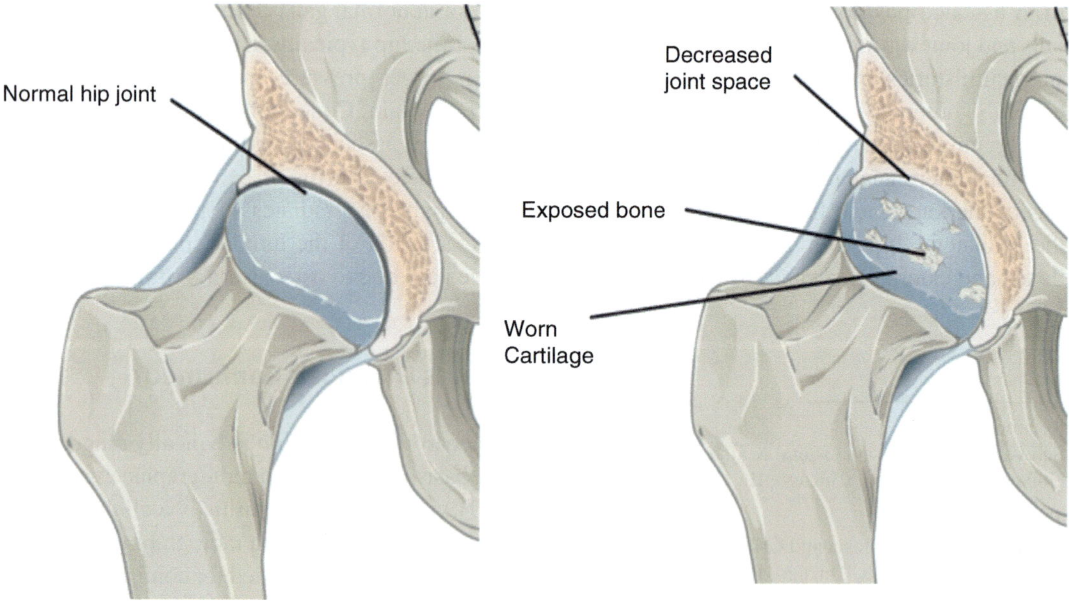

Fig. 27.1 (**a**, **b**) Osteoarthritis of a synovial joint results from aging or prolonged joint wear and tear. These cause erosion and loss of the articular cartilage covering the surfaces of the bones, resulting in inflammation that causes joint stiffness and pain. (From OpenStax College [9])

Mechanisms of pain in osteoarthritis include periosteal elevation, vascular congestion of subchondral bone leading to increased intraosseous pressure, synovitis, fatigue in muscles that cross the joint, overall joint contracture, joint effusion and stretching of the joint capsule, inflammation of periarticular bursae, and more [2]. Peripheral nociceptive mechanism does not explain pain in many patients with osteoarthritis as seen from discrepancy between the morphology of joints seen on X-ray images and intensity of pain experienced by patients. This is explained by the presence of neuropathic pain element, which involves neuroplastic changes affecting peripheral nerves or alerted pain processing affecting nerve pathways in the central nervous system. The presence of hypersensitization in patients with osteoarthritis, measured objectively by quantitative sensory testing (QST), has been been seen and they corelate with pain intensity and functional disability. The extent of sensitization seems to correlate with the extent of symptoms severity. Using self-reported questionnaire, the prevalence of neuropathic pain contribution is around 23% in patients with osteoarthritis. Pain sensitization seems to correlate with the presence of synovitis and effusion.

How Is This Problem Managed?

The initial management of osteoarthritis emphasizes conservative measures such as aerobic exercise (balance, land-based, aquatic), weight loss (for those with BMI >25), and activity modification with the goal to alleviate pain and improve functional status [2]. A cane or walker can be used for the contralateral hand in order to decrease the joint reaction force on the affected hip [5], and with assistance from physical and occupational therapy, the patient can benefit from joint-protection and energy-conservation techniques [2]. Long-term adherence to supervised physical activity regimens is needed to maintain the benefits of exercise, which are sustained for at least 3–6 months [11, 12].

Analgesics such as acetaminophen and nonsteroidal anti-inflammatory drugs (NSAIDs) are generally indicated as needed for persistent symptoms of mild-moderate pain in patients who do not adequately respond to conservative treatment [2] (Table 27.1). Although NSAIDs have been proven more effective than acetaminophen for pain relief [2, 13, 14], neither alter disease progression, and both must be considered due to the increased risk of gastrointestinal ulcers and bleeding from NSAIDs and liver injury from acetaminophen [2, 8]. Alternatives include celecoxib; a selective cyclooxygenase (COX)-2 inhibitor designed to alleviate the increased risk of gastrointestinal side effects; diclofenac, a topical NSAID for localized or limited symptoms [2]; and an adjuvant proton-pump inhibitor can be considered. Opioids, such as tramadol, are used judiciously and are generally not recommended due to substantial risk of adverse events (nausea, dizziness, drowsiness) and small clinical benefit as an efficacious alternative to acetaminophen and NSAIDs [15, 16]. Other commonly prescribed medications include topical capsaicin and naproxen for pain relief, and skeletal muscle relaxants (baclofen, tizanidine, cyclobenzaprine). The lowest effective dose is recommended for all pharmacologic therapy [2], and periodic clinical

Table 27.1 Pharmacologic recommendations for the initial management of hip osteoarthritis

We conditionally recommend that patients with hip osteoarthritis should use one of the following:
Acetaminophen
Oral NSAIDs
Tramadol
Intraarticular corticosteroid injections
We conditionally recommend that patients with hip osteoarthritis should not use the following:
Chondroitin sulfate
Glucosamine
We have no recommendation regarding the use of the following:
Topical NSAIDs
Intraarticular hyaluronate injections
Duloxetine
Opioid analgesics

From Hochberg et al. [21], with permission

[a]No strong recommendations were made for the initial pharmacologic management of hip osteoarthritis. For patients who have an inadequate response to initial pharmacologic management, please see the Results for alternative strategies.

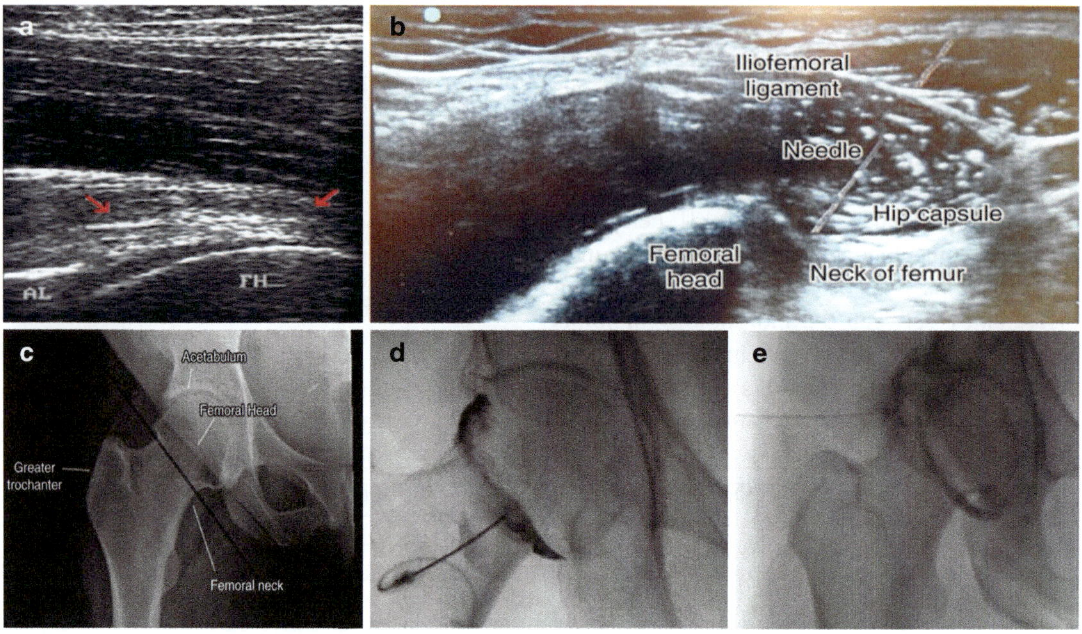

Fig. 27.2 Normal hip joint anatomy under ultrasound (**a**) and fluoroscopy (**c**); ultrasound-guided intraarticular hip injection (**b**); fluoroscopy-guided intraarticular hip injection, anterior approach (**d**) and lateral approach (**e**). (From Brown [23])

assessments should be performed regularly every 3 months to assess the effects of treatment on symptoms, functionality, and status [17].

Intra-articular corticosteroid injection under ultrasound or fluoroscopic guidance is a nonoperative therapeutic option that is indicated for short-term pain relief of moderate-severe symptomatic osteoarthritis of the hip (Fig. 27.2). Although this option is less utilized and studied for use at the hip than the knee, up to three injections to any individual osteoarthritic joint is generally recommended per year, and each injection variably effective between 4 weeks and 3 months [18–20]. Controversial evidence exists regarding frequent steroid injections and subsequent damage to cartilage (chondrodegeneration) [2]. Other nonoperative therapies include injections of intra-articular sodium hyaluronate (viscosupplementation) and platelet-rich plasma, which studies have shown beneficial in regard to pain relief; however, these are not currently recommended due to cost-effectiveness, limited evidence, and lack of clinical efficacy for osteoarthritis of the hip [2, 17, 18, 21–23]. Mesenchymal stem cells are an investigational treatment of knee osteoarthritis; however, they have not yet been cleared by the FDA for human clinical application to musculoskeletal diseases [2, 24].

Surgical intervention is indicated for patients with severe advanced symptomatic osteoarthritis who are unresponsive to conservative, pharmacologic, and nonoperative therapy and who have significant impairment in their quality of life due to osteoarthritis [2, 8]. Total hip arthroplasty (replacement) is the preferred treatment for older patients with advanced structural changes [2, 4, 5, 8]. Other noteworthy surgical options include hemiarthroplasty for the elderly with femoral neck fractures, total hip resurfacing for young and active male patients, and hip (periacetabular, femoral) osteotomy in select cases of hip developmental dysplasia or impingement [2, 4, 5, 8].

Chronic pain management is recommended for nonsurgical candidates. Duloxetine, thought to modulate endogenous pain inhibitory pathways by desensitizing central nociceptive processing, has been widely used for chronic musculoskeletal pain and osteoarthritis in multiple joints when other analgesics are inadequate or contraindicated [8, 26]. Radiofrequency ablation (rhizotomy) of articular branches of the femoral and obturator nerves is a minimally invasive neuromodulative procedure that several studies have also successfully shown to be effective for relief of chronic hip pain [27–29].

What Is the Prognosis of This Condition?

The prognosis in patients with osteoarthritis depends on the joints involved and on the severity of the condition, and although joint replacement is very favorable, a joint prosthesis may have to be revised 10–15 years after placement depending on the activity level of the patient [2]. Preoperative levels of pain, the presence of comorbidities and depression, and the presence of concomitant pain at other joints are associated with an increased risk of an unfavorable pain outcome after surgery [18, 25]. Complications of osteoarthritis generally include pain, bone deformity, and functional impairment [3, 4].

Discussion

The prevalence of hip osteoarthritis has been estimated to be between 1% and 10% [17, 30]. The incidence of symptomatic hip osteoarthritis, though variable, has been reported at 88 per 100,000 per year [5]. The CDC reports that arthritis affects 54.4 million adults in the United States, osteoarthritis being the most common form [1].

Osteoarthritis is diagnosed based on presentation and plain radiography. The differential diagnosis may include inflammatory arthritis (rheumatoid or septic), avascular necrosis (osteonecrosis), trochanteric bursitis, crystalline arthropathy (gout or pseudogout), or trauma (fracture, dislocation). All of the above are distinguished by their clinical picture and characteristics on imaging. The earliest affected movement of hip osteoarthritis is frequently internal rotation, while typical end-stage deformity affects external rotation [8]. The FABER (flexion, abduction, external rotation) test is a physical examination maneuver for hip pathology, and with osteoarthritis present, groin pain on external rotation has been elicited with a sensitivity of 57%, specificity of 71%, and positive likelihood ratio of 1.9 [32]. Studies have found that hip pain (groin and/or anterior thigh, with/without internal rotation) is discordant with radiographic evidence of hip osteoarthritis [31]. Radiographs of hip osteoarthritis from patients with frequent hip pain in the Framingham Osteoarthritis Study showed a sensitivity of 15.6%, specificity of 90.9%, and positive predictive value was 20.7% [31]; the Osteoarthritis Initiative showed a sensitivity of 9.1%, specificity of 94.3%, and positive predictive value of 23.8% [31]. The disease is best managed using biopsychosocial model of chronic diseases, i.e., in a multidisciplinary manner that encompasses non-pharmacological, pharmacological, and interventional therapies.

Non-pharmacological methods such as education and self-management, exercise, weight loss if overweight or obese, and walking aids as indicated are unanimously agreed by all guidelines as a first-line treatment.

Exercise therapy has been proven to be helpful by high-quality studies in decreasing pain and improving joint motion, with an effect sizes of 0.4–0.5 for hip osteoarthritis and knee osteoarthritis. Somehow weight loss is more effective for knee arthritis than for hip joint. Acetaminophen though used as first line of pharmacological intervention, in 2017 a meta-analysis concluded that given the very small effect sizes (less than 0.2) compared with placebo, it is of little use. Topical NSAIDs are effective for pain relief in osteoarthritis compared with placebo, with (corrected) mean effect sizes of 0.30 for pain relief and 0.35 for function. If acetaminophen is insufficient for pain relief, NSAIDs may be more efficacious. Diclofenac and etoricoxib (cox-2 inhibitor) are the most efficacious NSAIDs for pain relief in hip osteoarthritis, producing moderate to large effects. Topical rubefacients are not effective and glucosamine or chondroitin products are not recommended. Intraarticular steroid injection therapy is effective but benefit is short-term, for 4–6 weeks only. They are best used as adjuvant. It is most effective when signs of inflammation are present. Repeated injection may accelerate cartilage erosion or increase risk of infection if done before hip replacement surgery. There is little evidence for the clinical use of hyaluronic acid injections in the hip joints. Acupuncture has little or no effect in reducing pain compared with sham treatment. Duloxetine, a serotonin and norepinephrine reuptake inhibitor with antidepressant, central pain inhibitory, and anxiolytic activities, is recommended for neuropathic pain component. Opioids are not recommended as risks outweigh the benefit.

Radiofrequency ablation of the nerve innervating hip joint has been effective in many studies; review of the data by Bhatia et al. found available evidence mostly based on observational, non-randomized trials with inconsistent description of technique, anatomic landmarks for nerve block, and patient selection. They concluded that the therapy is safe and has a great potential to relieve pain in patients who are not a candidate for surgery because of coexisting medical conditions or does not want surgery.

Arthroscopy of hip joint provides temporary relief and is associated with a high conversion rate to THA (9.5–50%). Total hip replacement is done when all treatments fail. It is a proven effective and durable intervention with as many as 95% of prostheses remaining functional at 10 years. Early hip surgery is suggested when indicated as failure rate increases with delay. Hip resurfacing is suitable for a very specific subset of patients, usually young active men with large femoral heads, as an alternative to THA but overall it is not an alternative to hip replacement.

Conclusion/Summary

Osteoarthritis is a major source of bone deformity, chronic pain, and functional impairment. An individualized multidisciplinary approach, with both pharmacologic and non-pharmacologic intervention, best manages osteoarthritis in order to reduce morbidity and prevent complications. Unfortunately, no disease-modifying or structure-modifying intervention has been proved effective in osteoarthritis [2]. A significant limitation to treating osteoarthritis is the unknowingness of the exact etiology or underlying cause of osteoarthritis, as the literature has only recently identified the role of inflammation. Further research is needed to determine the effectivity of intra-articular injections (sodium hyaluronate, platelet-rich plasma), muscle relaxants (baclofen, tizanidine, cyclobenzaprine), and nutraceuticals (glucosamine, chondroitin sulfate). Analgesics, especially with opioids (tramadol), continue to be a sensitive and guarded issue, thus underappreciated. Future directions include the use of chondroprotective drugs (MMP inhibitors and growth factors) and mesenchymal stem cell therapy.

References

1. Arthritis [Internet]. Osteoarthritis (OA). Centers for Disease Control and Prevention; 2019. Available from: https://www.cdc.gov/arthritis/basics/osteoarthritis.htm.
2. Lozada C, Culpepper-Pace S. Osteoarthritis [Internet]. Overview. Medscape; 2019. Available from: https://emedicine.medscape.com/article/330487-overview.
3. Dominguez M. Osteoarthritis [Internet]. Osteoarthritis. Medbullets; 2019. Available from: https://step1.medbullets.com/msk/112032/osteoarthritis.
4. Dominguez M. Osteoarthritis [Internet]. Osteoarthritis. Medbullets; 2019. Available from: https://step2.medbullets.com/orthopedics/120529/osteoarthritis.
5. Watts E, Karadsheh M, Incavo S. Hip osteoarthritis [Internet]. Hip Osteoarthritis. Orthobullets; 2019. Available from: https://www.orthobullets.com/recon/5005/hip-osteoarthritis.
6. Jewell FM, Watt I, Doherty M. Plain radiographic features of osteoarthritis. In: Osteoarthritis. Oxford: Oxford University Press; 1998. p. 217–37.
7. Hunter DJ. Advanced imaging in osteoarthritis. Bull NYU Hosp Jt Dis. 2008 Jan;66(3):251.
8. Doherty M, Abhishek A. Clinical manifestations and diagnosis of osteoarthritis [Internet]. Clinical manifestations and diagnosis of osteoarthritis. UpToDate; 2017. Available from: https://www.uptodate.com/contents/clinical-manifestations-and-diagnosis-of-osteoarthritis?topicRef=106097&source=see_link#H3222307137.
9. OpenStax College. Anatomy & physiology - synovial joints [Internet]. Anatomy & physiology - synovial joints. OpenStax CNX; 2013. Available from: https://

cnx.org/contents/FPtK1zmh@7.30:bFtYymxt@4/Synovial-Joints.
10. Altman R, Alarcon G, Appelrouth D, Bloch D, Borenstein D, Brandt K, Brown C, Cooke TD, Daniel W, Feldman D, Greenwald R. The American College of Rheumatology criteria for the classification and reporting of osteoarthritis of the hip. Arthritis Rheum. 1991;34(5):505–14.
11. Fransen M, McConnell S, Hernandez-Molina G, Reichenbach S. Exercise for osteoarthritis of the hip. Cochrane Database Syst Rev. 2014;(4):CD007912.
12. Osteoarthritis [Internet]. Cochrane complementary medicine. Cochrane; [cited 2009 Jun 10]. Available from: https://cam.cochrane.org/osteoarthritis.
13. Chou R, McDonagh MS, Nakamoto E, Griffin J. Analgesics for osteoarthritis: an update of the 2006 comparative effectiveness review.
14. Towheed T, Maxwell L, Judd M, Catton M, Hochberg MC, Wells GA. Acetaminophen for osteoarthritis. Cochrane Database Syst Rev. 2006;(1):CD004257.
15. April KT, Bisaillon J, Welch V, Maxwell LJ, Jüni P, Rutjes AW, Husni ME, Vincent J, El Hindi T, Wells GA, Tugwell P. Tramadol for osteoarthritis. Cochrane Database Syst Rev. 2019;(5):CD005522.
16. da Costa BR, Nüesch E, Kasteler R, Husni E, Welch V, Rutjes AW, Jüni P. Oral or transdermal opioids for osteoarthritis of the knee or hip. Cochrane Database Syst Rev. 2014;(9):CD003115.
17. Alle-Deveza L, Eyles J. Management of hip osteoarthritis - UpToDate [Internet]. Management of hip osteoarthritis. UpToDate; 2019. Available from: https://www.uptodate.com/contents/management-of-hip-osteoarthritis.
18. Alle-Deveza L. Overview of the management of osteoarthritis - UpToDate [Internet]. Overview of the management of osteoarthritis. UpToDate; 2017. Available from: https://www.uptodate.com/contents/overview-of-the-management-of-osteoarthritis.
19. McCabe PS, Maricar N, Parkes MJ, Felson DT, O'Neill TW. The efficacy of intra-articular steroids in hip osteoarthritis: a systematic review. Osteoarthr Cartil. 2016;24(9):1509–17.
20. Lambert RG, Hutchings EJ, Grace MG, Jhangri GS, Conner-Spady B, Maksymowych WP. Steroid injection for osteoarthritis of the hip: a randomized, double-blind, placebo-controlled trial. Arthritis Rheum. 2007;56(7):2278–87.
21. Hochberg MC, Altman RD, April KT, Benkhalti M, Guyatt G, McGowan J, Towheed T, Welch V, Wells G, Tugwell P. American College of Rheumatology 2012 recommendations for the use of nonpharmacologic and pharmacologic therapies in osteoarthritis of the hand, hip, and knee. Arthritis Care Res. 2012;64(4):465–74.
22. Zhang W, Nuki G, Moskowitz RW, Abramson S, Altman RD, Arden NK, Bierma-Zeinstra S, Brandt KD, Croft P, Doherty M, Dougados M. OARSI recommendations for the management of hip and knee osteoarthritis: part III: changes in evidence following systematic cumulative update of research published through January 2009. Osteoarthr Cartil. 2010;18(4):476–99.
23. Brown MN. Intra-articular joint injections [Internet]. Intra-articular injections of hip joint. Anesthesia Key; 2017. Available from: https://aneskey.com/intra-articular-joint-injections/.
24. Chu CR, Rodeo S, Bhutani N, Goodrich LR, Huard J, Irrgang J, LaPrade RF, Lattermann C, Lu Y, Mandelbaum B, Mao J. Optimizing clinical use of biologics in orthopaedic surgery: consensus recommendations from the 2018 AAOS/NIH U-13 conference. J Am Acad Orthop Surg. 2019;27(2):e50.
25. Hawker GA, Badley EM, Borkhoff CM, Croxford R, Davis AM, Dunn S, Gignac MA, Jaglal SB, Kreder HJ, Sale JE. Which patients are most likely to benefit from total joint arthroplasty? Arthritis Rheum. 2013 May;65(5):1243–52.
26. duloxetine (Rx) [Internet]. Dosing & uses - dosage forms & strengths. Medscape; 2019. Available from: https://reference.medscape.com/drug/cymbalta-irenka-duloxetine-342960.
27. Vanaclocha-Vanaclocha V, Sáiz-Sapena N, Herrera JM. Percutaneous radiofrequency denervation in the treatment of hip pain secondary to osteoarthritis. EC Orthopaedics. 2016;4(6):657–80.
28. Chye CL, Liang CL, Lu K, Chen YW, Liliang PC. Pulsed radiofrequency treatment of articular branches of femoral and obturator nerves for chronic hip pain. Clin Interv Aging. 2015;10:569.
29. Bhatia A, Hoydonckx Y, Peng P, Cohen SP. Radiofrequency procedures to relieve chronic hip pain: an evidence-based narrative review. Reg Anesth Pain Med. 2018;43(1):72–83.
30. Murphy NJ, Eyles JP, Hunter DJ. Hip osteoarthritis: etiopathogenesis and implications for management. Adv Ther. 2016;33(11):1921–46.
31. Kim C, Nevitt MC, Niu J, Clancy MM, Lane NE, Link TM, Vlad S, Tolstykh I, Jungmann PM, Felson DT, Guermazi A. Association of hip pain with radiographic evidence of hip osteoarthritis: diagnostic test study. BMJ. 2015;351:h5983.
32. Reiman MP, Goode AP, Hegedus EJ, Cook CE, Wright AA. Diagnostic accuracy of clinical tests of the hip: a systematic review with meta-analysis. Br J Sports Med. 2013;47(14):893–902.

A 75-Year-Old Man with Chronic Knee Pain

28

Tariq Malik

Case Description

A 75-year-old male is referred to the pain clinic for chronic right knee pain. Pain is localized to the knee, worse in the morning, gets a little better with walking. He complains of intermittent swelling but no discoloration. No history of direct trauma or fall. He was quite athletic when in high school and college and remembers having few knee sprains but that never bothered him after college. He is an avid jogger but has been cutting down on his run quite a bit due to pain and stiffness. He has history of hypertension, which is well controlled. He is managing his pain with over-the-counter medications. He is referred to the pain clinic for an injection therapy as the medications are not helping enough.

What Is Your Diagnosis?

The patient is an elderly man with localized knee pain. Pain is mechanical in nature, which is very suggestive of pain related to knee joint structures. There is no history of infection, trauma, or tumor. In the absence of any constitutional symptoms and red flags in the history (fever, weight loss), the most likely disease process is one of degeneration [1]. All synovial joints have the tendency to develop arthritic changes. In this context, the patient most likely has osteoarthritis of the right knee joint [2]. It is important to be thorough when evaluating the patient to look for secondary causes of osteoarthritis. These include trauma, congenital or developmental disorders, calcium pyrophosphate dihydrate deposition disease, and other bone and joint disorders such as osteonecrosis, rheumatoid arthritis, gouty arthritis, septic arthritis, and Paget's disease of the bone [3]. In the absence of any contributing factor, the condition is called primary osteoarthritis. It is important to properly and thoroughly evaluate the joint: range of motion, joint line tenderness, joint swelling, neuromuscular intactness, and crepitus [4]. But no single clinical feature is absolutely sensitive or specific to clinch the diagnosis.

How Should the Diagnosis Be Confirmed?

Osteoarthritis can only be confirmed with an image study; however, the American College of Rheumatology suggests that a clinician can make a secure diagnosis of knee osteoarthritis (OA) without radiologic evidence. Clinical features may be very suggestive, but an image study is required to confirm it and to grade the extent of arthritis. Two view X-ray (AP and lateral view)

T. Malik (✉)
Department of Anesthesia and Critical Care, University of Chicago, Chicago, IL, USA
e-mail: TMuslim@dacc.uchicago.edu; tmalik@dacc.uchicago.edu

T. Malik (ed.), *Practical Chronic Pain Management*, https://doi.org/10.1007/978-3-030-46675-6_28

Table 28.1 The American College of Rheumatology clinical criteria for osteoarthritis

Clinical feature	Clinical plus imaging	Clinical plus laboratory
Knee pain for most days of the prior month, in addition to at least three of the following: 1. Crepitus 2. Morning stiffness less than 30 minutes duration 3. Age > 50 years 4. Bony prominence of the knee on examination 5. Tenderness of the knee joint line 6. No warmth on palpation	Knee pain for most days of the prior month, plus osteophytes on joint margins on X-ray, in addition to one of the following: 1. Crepitus 2. Morning stiffness less than 30 minutes duration 3. Age > 50 years	1. Crepitus 2. Morning stiffness less than 30 minutes duration 3. Age > 50 years 4. Tender to palpation 5. Enlarged joint 6. No warmth on palpation 7. ESR < 40 mmHg 8. Rheumatoid factor less than 1:40 9. Synovial fluid (cell count/ crystals – negative)

From Altman et al. [8], with permission

of the knee is obtained to evaluate and confirm the diagnosis. Sunrise view of the joint is obtained to evaluate patellofemoral arthritis. The presence of osteophytes is considered diagnostic; and joint space narrowing, an indirect measure of loss of joint cartilage, is used to quantify OA as mild, moderate, or severe [5]. Joint space is also affected by meniscal pathology and is therefore not a true representative of severity of joint arthritis. X-ray also helps rule out any other pathology that may be causing pain. Imaging should be obtained earlier if there is history of tumor in the past or there is a suspicion of tumor as bones are common sites for metastasis. If any irregularity or lesion is seen, it may need evaluation with CT or MRI. MRI is very sensitive and evaluates every part of the knee including bone marrow, ligaments, and other soft tissue structures. At times, bone scan is used to evaluate bone turnover changes seen with osteophyte formation, subchondral sclerosis, subchondral cyst formation, and bone marrow lesions as well as sites of synovitis [6].

Blood workup (CBC, ESR, C-reactive protein level, RF titer, and synovial fluid chemistry) is negative in primary osteoarthritis. The European League Against Rheumatism recommends the use of three symptoms (persistent pain, limited morning stiffness, and reduced function) and three signs (crepitus, restricted range of motion, and bony enlargement) for making the diagnosis of knee OA. As more factors are present, the likelihood of having a diagnosis of OA increases. When all six signs and symptoms are present, the probability of seeing OA on radiographs is 99% [7]. The American College of Rheumatology developed clinical criteria in 1998 to standardize the diagnosis of osteoarthritis using a combination of clinical features, lab test, and imaging (Table 28.1) [8].

What Is the Pathophysiology of the Disease?

The pathophysiology of this is disease is not completely understood. It used to be considered primarily a disease of hyaline cartilage with secondarily bone involvement, caused by overload or overuse, but the development of osteoarthritis has been found to be much more complicated. The role of synovitis and pro-inflammatory mediators in the pathogenesis of OA is increasingly being appreciated [9, 10]. The role of synovial inflammation is critical in producing the symptoms and structural progression of OA [11]. It also correlates with symptom severity, rate of cartilage degeneration, and osteophyte development [12, 13]. A number of pathways and immune mediators are involved in the degeneration of articular cartilage, synovial immunopathogenesis, and in subchondral bone degeneration. The interaction of these pro-inflammatory cytokines, reactive oxygen species (ROS), nitric oxide, matrix degrading enzymes, and biomechanical stress are ultimately responsible for the progression of OA in synovial joints. Improved understanding of the mechanisms promoting synovial inflammation in OA will eventually lead to novel therapeutic targets for controlling symptoms and slowing structural destruction of the joints. The measurement of inflammatory markers may also be useful in future as surrogate markers of disease activity or progression when evaluating effectiveness of an intervention [14].

How Is the Disease Managed?

It is a chronic joint disorder. The underlying pathology is elusive in most patients. There is no consistent correlation with the degree of pathology and extent of pain. The main aim is functional improvement [15]. Part of the clinical evaluation is to evaluate the extent of the disease burden. This can be done using WOMAC questionnaire. This questionnaire is also an important tool in gauging the extent of improvement after an intervention, and also to see progression of the disease over time.

The basic principles of management are the same as for any other chronic pain condition; it starts with conservative management, then medication, injection therapy, and surgery as a last resort.

The American Academy of Orthopedic Surgeons (AAOS), in 2013, published second edition of a comprehensive clinical practice guidelines for the treatment of knee osteoarthritis. The guidelines are quite comprehensive and each recommendation is backed by level of evidence.

The knee pain is best managed in a holistic fashion starting with lifestyle modification with focus on adjusting risk factors that can worsen osteoarthritis [16]. It is recommended that patient loses weight [17] if overweight (BMI > 25), and engage in low-impact exercise (biking, swimming) improving knee muscles strength [18]. There is plenty of evidence that many physicians underutilize nonpharmacological interventions when treating knee osteoarthritis [17]. There is no good evidence that TENS unit, massage therapy, knee braces, foot insole, or oral chondroitin or glucosamine is helpful. The analgesic effect of acetaminophen is poor, and NSAIDs (oral and topical) are much more effective [19]. Opioid use in controlling pain is not supported by evidence. There is strong evidence against the use of acupuncture in managing knee pain in OA [20, 21].

If these interventions are ineffective, especially physical therapy and NSAIDs, then injection therapies are offered. There is variable evidence that intraarticular steroid and hyaluronic acid injection are effective but the evidence for platelet-rich plasma injection is lacking. Total knee arthroplasty is needed when function activity does not improve despite conservative management and injection therapy [22].

Discussion

Knee osteoarthritis (OA) is a common and progressive joint disease affecting more than 250 million people worldwide. It affects 33% of the population aged 65 and above [1]. Women are affected more than men. African-Americans are more likely to develop painful knees. Obesity and strenuous physical activity involving kneeling, squatting, or prolonged standing are risk factors for developing osteoarthritis [16]. It has significant effects on function and considerable societal costs in terms of work loss, early retirement, and joint replacement. Osteoarthritis is a leading indication for the use of prescription drugs, which costs about $3000 per year per patient.

Pain intensity varies from mild to agonizing, intermittent or constant, dull, achy to sharp, with or without swelling. Physical examination may reveal decreased range of motion, crepitus, tender joint line, weakness, and difficult ambulation, especially when climbing steps up or down. Patients feel increased stiffness and pain at night or after prolonged rest that eases up within 30 minutes of activity. The diagnosis of osteoarthritis is based on clinical findings and imaging. The European League against Rheumatism and the American College of Rheumatology each describe list of criteria to diagnose osteoarthritis of the knee. The most frequent radiographic grading system is described by Kellgren and Lawrence. In this system, Grade 1 is characterized by doubtful joint space narrowing (JSN) and possible osteophytic lipping; Grade 2, by definite osteophytes and possible JSN on anteroposterior weight-bearing radiograph; Grade 3, by multiple osteophytes, definite JSN, sclerosis, and possible bony deformity; and Grade 4, by large osteophytes, marked JSN, severe sclerosis, and definite bony deformity.

The treatment guidelines recommend weight loss and exercise as first line of treatment followed by non-opioid analgesics orally, which include acetaminophen and NSAIDs. The benefit from acetaminophen is quite small and so is the analgesic effect of Celebrex. The NSAIDs are in general more effective than acetaminophen and Celebrex. Despite the extensive use of the intraarticular steroid, its benefits are transient, still debatable, and often patient dependent. Intraarticular hyaluronic acid injection is also effective but not recommended by AAOS. It is still recommended by others. It works best in mild to moderate OA, usually well tolerated, with minimal side effects. The intraarticular PRP injection has been shown effective when compared to steroid or HA, but studies were poorly done. Injection of PRP can lead to serious side effects though the incidence is low [23–25]. Use of botulism in knee has been tried but studies were of poor quality and not recommended by any society [26, 27]. In general, steroid injection can cause better relief than intraarticular hyaluronic acid injection in the short term, but at 3–6 months hyaluronic acid has better analgesic profile. The functional improvement is equivalent.

Patients who fail to respond to conservative therapy and are not a candidate for total knee replacement or do not wish to have surgery are offered thermal ablation of sensory articular nerves [28, 29]. The three nerves targeted are two on the medial side (superior and inferior genicular nerves) and one on the lateral side (lateral superior genicular nerve). The locations of the nerves have been described well and can be reliably located and destroyed using fluoroscopic guidance. They are purely afferent nerves and their destruction causes no motor weakness [30]. Patients are good candidate if they get more than 50% relief, preferably 70% relief, after a diagnostic block with a low-volume local anesthetic [31]. Open label trials have shown better analgesia at 3 months compared to control. Cooled radiofrequency (RF) by creating larger lesion increases the likelihood of complete destruction of these nerves and have shown in case series and a trial better clinical outcome compared to regular RF [32, 33].

Strength of Various Recommendations

The American College of Orthopedic Surgeons published a list of recommendations and graded the strength of recommendations as strong, moderate, limited, consensus opinion, and inconclusive based on the quality of evidence.

They gave strong recommendation to physical activity, and to the use of NSAIDs in symptomatic knee osteoarthritis. They also recommended strongly against the use of acupuncture, and the use of glucosamine and chondroitin due to proven lack of benefit. All patients with symptomatic osteoarthritis are recommended to lose weight; the strength of this recommendation is moderate.

The evidence for the use of knee brace, TENS units, or manual therapy to treat pain is inconclusive as the evidence comes from low-quality studies. There is no proven benefit from the use of acetaminophen to treat knee pain and is not suggested. The evidence for the use of intraarticular steroid injection is inconclusive, while the society recommended against the use of viscosupplementation injection into the joint .They could not recommend for or against the use of platelet-rich plasma or any other growth factor due to lack of good evidence. The document does not contain any evaluation of genicular nerve ablative treatment for chronic knee pain as the treatment arrived on the scene more recently. Multiple small trials have shown benefits of RF or cooled RF in relieving knee pain but trials are small, methodology and assessment inconsistent, and follow-up is usually for 3–6 months only.

Future Directions

Knee pain is a ubiquitous complaint in the elderly population. It is a cause of great disability. Available treatments are not very effective or do not last for long. Total knee replacement does not solve the problem in every patient; in fact, chronic post-surgical knee pain is a serious problem in about 20% of patients after surgery. There are no evidence-based guidelines to treat chronic post-surgical pain.

The common reason for ineffective treatment of chronic knee pain before or after surgery is poor understanding of the mechanism of pain generation. The problem is intertwined with every other chronic pain condition. It maybe that chronic knee pain is a syndrome and not a disease and therefore has various mechanisms of generation, explaining poor outcome in many patients despite every effort.

References

1. Lawrence RC, Felson DT, Helmick CG, et al.; National Arthritis Data Workgroup. Estimates of the prevalence of arthritis and other rheumatic conditions in the United States: part II. Arthritis Rheum. 2008;58(1):26–35. https://doi.org/10.1002/art.23176.
2. Stitik T, Kim JH, Stiskal D, et al. Osteoarthritis. In: Delisa J, Frontera W, editors. Delisa's physical medicine and rehabilitation: principles and practices. 5th ed. Philadelphia: Lippincott Williams & Wilkins; 2010. p. 781–810.
3. Kuyinu EL, Narayanan G, Nair LS, Laurencin CT. Animal models of osteoarthritis: classification, update, and measurement of outcomes. J Orthop Surg Res. 2016;11:19. https://doi.org/10.1186/s13018-016-0346-5.
4. Goldberg C. A practical guide to clinical medicine. San Diego: University of California San Diego School of Medicine; updated 2015 Oct [cited 2017 Jul 12]. Available from: https://meded.ucsd.edu/clinicalmed/joints.htm.
5. Sarwark MD. Arthritis of the knee. In: Sarwark JF, editor. Essentials of musculoskeletal care. 4th ed. Rosemont: American Academy of Orthopedic Surgeons; 2010. p. 650–6.
6. Bureau NJ, Kaplan PA, Dussault RG. MRI of the knee: a simplified approach. Curr Probl Diagn Radiol. 1995;24(1):1–49.
7. Zhang W, Doherty M, Peat G, et al. EULAR evidence-based recommendations for the diagnosis of knee osteoarthritis. Ann Rheum Dis. 2010;69(3):483–9. https://doi.org/10.1136/ard.2009.113100.
8. Altman R, Asch E, Bloch D, et al. Development of criteria for the classification and reporting of osteoarthritis. Classification of osteoarthritis of the knee. Diagnostic and Therapeutic Criteria Committee of the American Rheumatism Association. Arthritis Rheum. 1986;29(8):1039–49. https://doi.org/10.1002/art.1780290816.
9. Berenbaum F. Osteoarthritis as an inflammatory disease (osteoarthritis is not osteoarthrosis!). Osteoarthr Cartil. 2013;21(1):16–21.
10. Sellam J, Berenbaum F. The role of synovitis in pathophysiology and clinical symptoms of osteoarthritis. Nat Rev Rheumatol. 2010;6(11):625–35.
11. Ayral X, Pickering EH, Woodworth TG, Mackillop N, Dougados M. Synovitis: a potential predictive factor of structural progression of medial tibiofemoral knee osteoarthritis -- results of a 1 year longitudinal arthroscopic study in 422 patients. Osteoarthr Cartil. 2005;13:361–7.
12. Hill CL, Hunter DJ, Niu J, Clancy M, Guermazi A, Genant H, Gale D, Grainger A, Conaghan P, Felson DT. Synovitis detected on magnetic resonance imaging and its relation to pain and cartilage loss in knee osteoarthritis. Ann Rheum Dis. 2007;66:1599–603.
13. Torres L, Dunlop DD, Peterfy C, Guermazi A, Prasad P, Hayes KW, Song J, Cahue S, Chang A, Marshall M, Sharma L. The relationship between specific tissue lesions and pain severity in persons with knee osteoarthritis. Osteoarthr Cartil. 2006;14:1033–40.
14. Scanzello CR, Goldring SR. The role of synovitis in osteoarthritis pathogenesis. Bone. 2012;51(2):249–57.
15. AAOS: American Academy of Orthopaedic Surgeons. Treatment of osteoarthritis of the knee: evidence-based guideline. 2nd ed [Internet]. Rosemont: American Academy of Orthopaedic Surgeons; 2013. Available from: www.aaos.org/research/guidelines/treatmentofosteoarthritisofthekneeguideline.pdf.
16. Heidari B. Knee osteoarthritis prevalence, risk factors, pathogenesis and features: part I. Caspian J Intern Med. 2011 Spring;2(2):205–1.
17. Wluka AE, Lombard CB, Cicuttini FM. Tackling obesity in knee osteoarthritis. Nat Rev Rheumatol. 2013;9(4):225–35. https://doi.org/10.1038/nrrheum.2012.224.
18. Regnaux JP, Lefevre-Colau MM, Trinquart L, et al. High-intensity versus low-intensity physical activity or exercise in people with hip or knee osteoarthritis. Cochrane Database Syst Rev. 2015;(10):CD010203. https://doi.org/10.1002/14651858.CD010203.pub2.
19. da Costa BR, Reichenbach S, Keller N, et al. Effectiveness of non-steroidal anti-inflammatory drugs for the treatment of pain in knee and hip osteoarthritis: a network meta-analysis. Lancet. 2016;387(10033):2093–105.
20. Vickers AJ, Cronin AM, Maschino AC, et al. Acupuncture for chronic pain: individual patient data meta-analysis. Arch Intern Med. 2012;172(19):1444–53.

21. Hinman RS, McCrory P, Pirotta M, et al. Acupuncture for chronic knee pain: a randomized clinical trial. JAMA. 2014;312(13):1313–22.
22. Carr AJ, Robertsson O, Graves S, et al. Knee replacement. Lancet. 2012;379(9823):1331–40.
23. Nguyen C, Lefèvre-Colau MM, Poiraudeau S, Rannou F. Evidence and recommendations for use of intra-articular injections for knee osteoarthritis. Ann Phys Rehabil Med. 2016;59(3):184–9.
24. Xing D, Wang B, Zhang W, Yang Z, Hou Y, Chen Y, Lin J. Intra-articular platelet-rich plasma injections for knee osteoarthritis: an overview of systematic reviews and risk of bias considerations. Int J Rheum Dis. 2017;20(11):1612–30.
25. Lyon C, Spencer E, Spittler J, Desanto K. Clinical inquiries: how do hyaluronic acid and corticosteroid injections compare for knee OA relief? J Fam Pract. 2018;67(1):E13–4.
26. Bao X, Tan JW, Flyzik M, Ma XC, Liu H, Liu HY. Effect of therapeutic exercise on knee osteoarthritis after intra-articular injection of botulinum toxin type a, hyaluronate or saline: a randomized controlled trial. J Rehabil Med. 2018;50(6):534–41.
27. Mahowald ML, Singh JA, Dykstra D. Long term effects of intra-articular botulinum toxin A for refractory joint pain. Neurotox Res. 2006;9(2–3):179–88.
28. Choi W-J, Hwang S-J, Song J-G, et al. Radiofrequency treatment relieves chronic knee osteoarthritis pain: a double-blind randomized controlled trial. Pain. 2011;152:481–7.
29. El-Hakeim EH, Elawamy A, Kamel EZ, et al. Fluoroscopic guided radiofrequency of genicular nerves for pain alleviation in chronic knee osteoarthritis: a single-blind randomized controlled trial. Pain Physician. 2018;21:169–77.
30. Kim SY, Le PU, Kosharskyy B, et al. Is Genicular nerve radiofrequency ablation safe? A literature review and anatomical study. Pain Physician. 2016;19:E697–705.
31. Jamison DE, Cohen SP. Radiofrequency techniques to treat chronic knee pain: a comprehensive review of anatomy, effectiveness, treatment parameters, and patient selection. J Pain Res. 2018;11:1879–88.
32. McCormick ZL, Korn M, Reddy R, et al. Cooled radiofrequency ablation of the Genicular nerves for chronic pain due to knee osteoarthritis: six-month outcomes. Pain Med. 2017;18:1631–41.
33. McCormick ZL, Reddy R, Korn M, et al. A prospective randomized trial of prognostic Genicular nerve blocks to determine the predictive value for the outcome of cooled radiofrequency ablation for chronic knee pain due to osteoarthritis. Pain Med. 2018;19:1628–38.

A 55-Year-Old Man with Pain After Above Knee Amputation

29

E. B. Braun, A. Sack, J. M. Foster, T. M. Sowder, and T. W. Khan

Case Description

A 55-year-old male presents to the pain clinic with complaint of right lower extremity pain. The patient reports pain that began following trauma to the right lower extremity due to a motorcycle accident 3 months ago. After multiple surgeries failed, he was finally treated with above knee amputation. He was discharged to a rehab facility for gait training with a prosthetic leg. He was referred to the pain clinic for better pain control as it was interfering in his rehabilitation. He recalls having better pain control on oxycodone, but once he was weaned off it, he noticed constant pain in his leg. He characterized his pain as intermittently sharp and dull in the stump. At 1 month post amputation, he noticed that his missing limb felt shortened and painful. He described the pain as tingling and itching, worse with stress and weather changes. The patient noticed that over time pain character has changed. He could notice two distinct pains, ongoing moderate generalized stump pain that was intermittently sharp and dull and paresthesias and itching distal to the stump. He also had new-onset severe focal pain posterior to the mid incision. This pain was described as intermittent, sharp, and burning pain that radiated several centimeters. He was started on gabapentin and referred to the pain clinic for further pain management.

E. B. Braun (✉) · A. Sack · J. M. Foster
T. M. Sowder · T. W. Khan
Department of Anesthesiology, University of Kansas Medical Center, Kansas City, KS, USA
e-mail: ebraun@kumc.edu

What Is Your Preliminary Diagnosis?

Most likely, the patient is suffering from post-amputation pain. It is still important to take a detailed history and perform physical exam to rule out any infection, non-healing ulcers, or a bony spur causing lingering nociceptive pain. Post-amputation pain (PAP) includes residual limb pain (RLP, also known as stump pain) and phantom limb pain (PLP).

How Is the Diagnosis Confirmed?

Following amputation, most amputees still report feeling the missing limb and often describe these feelings as painful. Such experiences have been reported since the early sixteenth century, and the term "phantom limb" was used by Silas Weir Mitchell to describe the symptoms he observed in American Civil War soldiers [1]. Given that there are no tests to definitively diagnose phantom pain, the condition is primarily identified by history of traumatic or surgical amputation with ongoing painful sensations in the absent limb.

Physical exam and diagnostic procedures can support the diagnosis of PLP. Areas of sensitiv-

T. Malik (ed.), *Practical Chronic Pain Management*, https://doi.org/10.1007/978-3-030-46675-6_29

ity are identified by tapping on areas of known peripheral nerve distribution, which can illicit pain and/or paresthesias (Tinel's sign). Injection of local anesthetic in the region of the affected nerve may provide relief for the approximate duration of the local anesthetic, which can assist in establishing the diagnosis.

What Is the Pathophysiology of These Conditions?

Phantom pain is a chronic neuropathic pain condition. The exact underlying mechanism is unclear. The mechanism for RLP is thought to be an abnormal growth on damaged nerve endings (neuroma). Infection at the surgical site, poor wound healing, diabetes, or circulatory problems increase the likelihood of development of RLP [2]. There are several proposed mechanisms for PLP believed to be due to a combination of morphologic, physiologic, and chemical changes in the peripheral and central nervous systems.

Peripheral Mechanism

Typically, when axonal injury has occurred, inflammation and the release of pro-nociceptive factors, including cytokines, prostaglandins, and substance P, cause lowered thresholds of nociception and spontaneous discharge of nociceptive pathways [2]. Injured neurons exhibit upregulation of sodium channels, downregulation of potassium channels, altered expression of transduction molecules, and the development of non-functional connections between axons [3, 4]. Increased sympathetic discharge and circulating catecholamines may also lead to spontaneous pain [5]. In addition, the skin may manifest catecholamine sensitivity, and it has been suggested that skin temperature is inversely related to the intensity of phantom limb pain. [6]

Neuronal regeneration then begins, which can result in the formation of a neuroma at the proximal site of the nerve injury. Neuromas can generate spontaneous ectopic activity, have increased mechanical sensitivity, and increased catecholamine sensitivity. Neuromas have been implicated in the development of spontaneous and provoked pain [7].

Mechanical stimulation of neuromas can lead to enhanced RLP and PLP, reinforcing the role of peripheral mechanisms in PLP. [8] In addition, local anesthetic injected to the stump or in the region of a neuroma can reduce phantom pain, in the same way that surgical excision of a neuroma can reduce or eliminate phantom pain. [9, 10]

Dorsal root ganglion (DRG) cells also undergo significant changes after axonal transection and deafferentation resulting in loss and fibrosis of DRG cells [11]. Without inhibition, dorsal horn neurons have increased autonomous activity and ectopic neurochemical stimulation, resulting in the amplification of ectopic signals and increasing the likelihood of pain perception [7, 12, 13]. Frequently, as with other pain syndromes, PLP is exacerbated during times of emotional distress [14].

Spinal Mechanism

In addition to contributions from the peripheral nervous system, substantial evidence exists implicating a central component in the development of phantom limb pain. Central sensitization occurs when C fibers and A-delta afferents contribute to an increase in synaptic responsiveness of spinal cord neurons [15]. This process is mediated by the release of glutamate, substance P, and neurokinins, which increases activity in N-methyl-D-aspartate (NMDA) receptor-operated excitatory pathways [16]. These neurotransmitters decrease the threshold for activation of NMDA receptors and increase neuronal responsiveness [17]. Intrinsic spinal neurons and primary afferent nerve endings undergo downregulation of opioid receptors, decreasing the effectiveness of inhibitory pathways [18]. This may lead to spinal hyperexcitability in spinal cord segments adjacent to the deafferented regions, manifesting as pain in those regions.

Supraspinal Mechanism

Similar to the spinal reorganization theory, a phenomenon known as cortical reorganization is thought to occur in the brainstem, thalamus, and cerebral cortex [19]. Topographical mapping of the somatosensory cortex reveals a close association between the magnitude of PLP and specific alterations of somatosensory patterns [20]. An example of cortical reorganization is a patient experiencing pain in the affected extremity when touched on the cheek.

How Is This Problem Managed?

Phantom pain is quite difficult to manage. Management of PLP requires a multimodal approach that may include pharmacotherapy, injections, neuromodulation, surgical intervention, complementary and alternative therapies, and preventative treatments. Most therapies available for treatment of PLP are based on evidence for treatment of other neuropathic pain conditions.

Pharmacotherapy

It is important to use a stepwise approach when beginning pharmacotherapy, and the predominant pain type should influence the choice of medication. The World Health Organization Analgesic Ladder provides a useful guideline and recommends non-opioid analgesics (e.g., NSAIDs, acetaminophen) +/− an adjuvant as the initial intervention. In the setting of persistent or increasing pain, a weak opioid (e.g., tramadol, hydrocodone) can be added with continued optimization of non-opioid analgesics and adjuvants. Finally, a potent opioid (e.g., fentanyl, morphine) can be trialed in conjunction with non-opioid analgesics and adjuvants if pain persists or worsens. Each treatment progression should prompt an evaluation of medication regimen efficacy weighed against side effects as well as a consideration of interventional techniques. This consideration is especially important to minimize opioids due to their wide range of side effects and potential for abuse, tolerance, and dependence [21].

Anticonvulsant Agents

There is strong evidence for anticonvulsant therapy in the management of neuropathic pain in post-amputation patients [22].

Anticonvulsants treat neuropathic pain via several mechanisms. Anticonvulsants act both centrally and peripherally by inhibiting excitatory transmission via the NMDA receptor, as well as by antagonizing sodium channel conduction and enhancing inhibition through the GABA pathway. Gabapentin and pregabalin have similar tolerability and efficacy to antidepressants in the treatment of neuropathic pain [23].

Gabapentin causes inhibition of voltage-gated calcium channels in afferent neurons and acts as a central GABA agonist [24]. Several trials have shown the efficacy of gabapentin in the treatment of post-amputation PLP [25]. A common dosing strategy starts with 300 mg nightly and adds an additional daily dose every 7 days until the dose of 300 mg three times per day is reached. The typical maximally effective dose is 3600 mg per day and is usually well tolerated if gradual titration is performed [26]. Sedation, fatigue, nausea, and weight gain are the most common adverse effects. Temporarily suspending dose titration may minimize the chronicity of these adverse effects. Patients with chronic renal insufficiency require dose adjustment based on creatinine clearance to avoid supra-therapeutic blood levels of the medication.

Pregabalin (isobutyl-GABA) has similar mechanisms to gabapentin and may be more tolerable than gabapentin for some patients. No direct comparison of gabapentin and pregabalin has been published, but both have similar efficacy in the treatment of diabetic peripheral neuropathy and postherpetic neuralgia [27]. Small case studies have shown benefit of pregabalin in the treatment of PLP [28, 29].

Phenytoin, an older anticonvulsant, also suppresses ectopic neural discharges but does so through inhibition of voltage-gated sodium channels and suppression of glutamate release [30]. Phenytoin is considered an acceptable second-line agent in patients with neuropathic pain, but the paucity of evidence in the treatment of other neuropathic conditions combined with the need for serum monitoring noted adverse effects, and the introduction of newer, safer agents have decreased its use [31, 32].

Carbamazepine, a sodium channel blocker, has shown efficacy over placebo in treatment of neuropathic pain conditions including post-herpetic neuralgia and diabetic peripheral neuropathy and remarkable efficacy in the management of trigeminal neuralgia [30]. It has been shown to be beneficial for the treatment of lancinating-type PLP [33, 34]. During the initial period of therapy, adverse effects such as hyponatremia, aplastic anemia, and leukopenia may develop. Baseline hematologic and electrolyte lab values should be checked and periodically repeated throughout the treatment [30]. Oxcarbazepine, a carbamazepine analogue, may have fewer drug interactions and adverse effects than carbamazepine [32].

Antidepressants

Antidepressants are commonly used for treatment of RLP and PLP. These medications inhibit the reuptake of neurotransmitters such as dopamine, norepinephrine, and/or serotonin. The increased availability of these neurotransmitters decreases pain by enhancing descending spinal inhibitory pain pathways, which act to suppress pain. Treatment of depression may be an important secondary effect [31].

Tricyclic antidepressants (TCAs), such as amitriptyline and nortriptyline, have multiple mechanisms of action and have been used successfully for treatment of neuropathic pain. TCAs have the disadvantage of multiple potential adverse effects, such as anticholinergic effects, tachycardia, orthostatic hypotension, and blurred vision. Comorbid conditions and a high variability in an individual's response necessitate careful initiation and titration.

Selective serotonin reuptake inhibitors, such as fluoxetine and citalopram, are typically not as effective for the treatment of pain as are agents that also inhibit norepinephrine reuptake (SNRIs) [35, 36]. However, some case studies have shown fluoxetine to completely treat PLP [37]. SNRIs, such as duloxetine and venlafaxine, appear to have less adverse effects than TCAs. Venlafaxine and duloxetine have been shown to approach the efficacy of the TCA imipramine in treatment of neuropathic pain associated with painful polyneuropathy with fewer side effects and are among the most commonly recommended antidepressants in use today for neuropathic pain [36, 38, 39].

Both the provider and patient must exercise patience when initiating therapy with antidepressants. They are commonly discontinued too soon due to lack of effect prior to reaching therapeutic levels, or due to side effects that may resolve with more gradual titration [40]. Patients should be educated to monitor for common adverse effects such as somnolence, decreased salivation, hyperphagia, constipation, and urinary retention (Table 29.1) [30].

Interventional Techniques

Trigger Point Injections A trigger point is an isolated muscle spasm affecting a small area of muscle tissue. The spasming muscle can cut off its own blood supply leading to local metabolic crisis. Acute trauma or repetitive microtrauma may lead to the development of stress on muscle fibers and the formation of trigger points. Injections into the area relieve myofascial pain by decreasing muscular spasm, increasing range of motion, and improving blood circulation. The basic treatment principle is aimed at breaking the spasm-pain-spasm cycle in the muscles and eliminating the trigger point. Though the data is limited, trigger point injections have been reported to be helpful in PAP. One study of 21 patients found significant improvement of pain on the Visual Analogue Scale in most patients with post-amputation pain within 5 weeks [41]. Another study comparing botulinum toxin to a combination of lidocaine and methylprednisolone acetate found that both resulted in immediate improvement of RLP (not PLP) and pain tolerance, which lasted for 6 months in amputees who failed conventional treatments [42].

Lumbar Sympathetic Blocks The sympathetic division of the autonomic nervous system has been implicated in neuropathic pain and visceral pain. The lumbar sympathetic chain contains pre-

Table 29.1 Drugs and their properties

Drugs	Dosage and titration	Mechanism of action	Pharmacokinetics	Adverse effect	Monitoring
Anticonvulsants					
Gabapentin IR	Initial dose: 100–300 mg QHS up to TID Titration: ↑ dose 300–900 mg/day based on efficacy and tolerability over 2 weeks Max dose: 3600 mg/day	Antagonizes voltage-gated Ca^{2+}channels	Elimination: renal Dose reduction (max dose): CrCl 30–59 mL/min: 200–700 mg BID CrCl 15–30 mL/min: 200–700 mg/day	Edema, somnolence, dizziness, fatigue, weight gain	Serum creatinine
Pregabalin IR	Initial dose: 150 mg/day in 2–3 divided doses Titration: may ↑ to 300 mg/day within 1 week if tolerated; further ↑ to 600 mg/day after 2–3 weeks may be considered Max dose: 600 mg/day	Antagonizes voltage-gated Ca^{2+} channels (at alpha-2-delta subunit)	Elimination: renal Dose reduction (max dose): CrCl 30–60 mL/min: 300 mg/day CrCl 15–30 mL/min: 150 mg/day	Weight gain, fatigue, edema, somnolence, dizziness	Serum creatinine
Carbamazepine	Initial dose: 100 mg BID Titration: ↑ by up to 200 mg/day at weekly intervals Max dose: 1200 mg/day	Blocks Na^{+} and Ca^{2+}channels, modulates descending inhibition	Metabolism: hepatic Elimination: hepatic Consider dose reduction in hepatic impairment	Hepatotoxicity, diplopia, nystagmus, memory loss, drowsiness, nausea, GI upset	CBC, platelets, LFT, electrolytes, TSH
Oxcarbazepine IR	Initial dose: 300 mg/day Titration: ↑ after 3 days to 300 mg BID, then adjust dose in increments of 300 mg every 5 days Max dose: 1800 mg/day	Blocks Na^{+} channel	Metabolism: hepatic Elimination: hepatic and renal Dose reduction: CrCl <30 mL/min – initiate at 50% of the usual starting dose and titrate slowly	Hyponatremia, rash, sedation, GI upset, diplopia	LFT, electrolytes
Topiramate (50–600 mg/day)	Initial dose: 25 mg QHS Titration: ↑ 25 mg/day at weekly intervals Max dose: 100 mg/day divided into two doses	Na^{+} and Ca^{2+} channel blockade, GABA potentiation, glutamate blockage	Metabolism: hepatic Elimination: renal Dose reduction: CrCl <70 mL/min – reduce dose to 50% of usual dose and titrate slowly	Open angle glaucoma, nephrolithiasis (1–5%), dizziness, cognitive dysfunction, weight loss, paresthesias	Serum creatinine

(continued)

Table 29.1 (continued)

Drugs	Dosage and titration	Mechanism of action	Pharmacokinetics	Adverse effect	Monitoring
Serotonin norepinephrine reuptake inhibitors (SNRIs)					
Duloxetine	Initial dose: 30 mg/day Titration: ↑ to 60 mg/day after 1 week as tolerated Max dose: 60 mg/day (no additional benefit noted at 120 mg/day)	Selective reuptake inhibition of serotonin and norepinephrine	Metabolism: hepatic Elimination: renal and hepatic CrCl <30 mL/min: avoid use	Nausea, somnolence, constipation, dry mouth, dizziness, sweating, decreased appetite	
Venlafaxine ER	Initial dose: 37.5–75 mg/day Titration: ↑ by 75 mg weekly Max dose: 225 mg/day	Selective reuptake inhibition of serotonin and norepinephrine	Metabolism: hepatic Elimination: renal	Insomnia, sexual dysfunction, sweating, headache, anorexia, hypertension	
Tricyclic antidepressants (TCAs)					
Amitriptyline	Initial dose: 25–50 mg QHS Titration: ↑ as tolerated Max dose: 150 mg/day	Tricyclic antidepressant-inhibition of serotonin, norepinephrine, and dopamine	Metabolism: hepatic Elimination: hepatic and renal	Urinary retention, xerostomia, orthostasis, blurry vision, weight gain, constipation, sedation	Serum levels may need to be monitored at higher dosing levels or in those at higher risk of altered metabolism such as the elderly
Nortriptyline	Initial dose: 10–25 mg QHS Titration: ↑ as tolerated up to every 3 days Max dose: 150 mg/day	Tricyclic antidepressant-inhibition of serotonin, norepinephrine, and dopamine	Metabolism: hepatic Elimination: renal	Anxiety, urinary retention, orthostasis, weight gain, blurry vision, constipation, sedation, most side effects are less pronounced than with amitriptyline	Serum levels may need to be monitored at higher dosing levels
Imipramine	Initial dose: 50 mg/day in 1–2 doses Titration: ↑ gradually as tolerated Max dose: 150 mg/day	Tricyclic antidepressant-inhibition of serotonin, norepinephrine, and dopamine	Metabolism: hepatic Elimination: hepatic and renal	Dry mouth, tachycardia, orthostatic hypotension, and weight gain, constipation, urinary retention, blurred vision, and sexual dysfunction, most side effects are better tolerated than amitriptyline	

and post-ganglionic fibers to the pelvis and lower extremities and is located primarily at the anterolateral aspect of the L2-L4 vertebral bodies. Blockade of sympathetic ganglia with local anesthetic, neurolytic chemicals, neuroablative techniques, and intravenous regional techniques can be helpful in reducing post-amputation pain. In a small study of patients with post-amputation pain, treatment with a single lumbar sympathetic block resulted in reduction of both residual limb pain and phantom limb pain as well as perceived disability on the Pain Disability Index at 3 month follow-up in comparison to sham procedure [43]. For sympathetic blocks to support lasting improvement, they should be combined with concomitant physical and behavioral therapies. Neuromodulation Peripheral nerve stimulation (PNS) delivers an electrical current to a peripheral nerve via an array of electrodes placed adjacent to the nerve. This results in the sensation of paresthesias instead of pain. This technique can be especially useful when the pain is confined to the distribution of one or two peripheral nerves [44, 45]. Spinal cord stimulation (SCS) also uses electrical energy, but the electrodes are placed in the epidural space superficial to the dorsal columns and may provide coverage for a larger area of pain. A more recently developed neurostimulation technology involves stimulation of the dorsal root ganglion (DRG). The lead is placed through the epidural space close to the DRG receiving input from the painful area. This method may be effective in the treatment of complex regional pain syndrome (CRPS) and PLP, including in cases of failed conventional spinal cord stimulation [46, 47].

Surgical Intervention Stump revision or resection of distinct pathologic lesions such as neuromas and heterotopic ossification should be considered in patients whose pain is refractory to conservative treatments. Results of surgical revision for PAP have historically been mixed with some patients reporting short-term relief and eventual regrowth of neuroma [47–49]. More recent studies have shown promising results using surgical revision to treat both PLP [50] and RLP [51–53].

Behavioral, Complementary, and Alternative Therapies

Cognitive Behavioral Therapy Cognitive behavioral therapy (CBT) has long been a part of the multidisciplinary approach to the treatment of chronic pain conditions. While CBT has been reported to be helpful in treating neuropathic pain syndromes [54], there is a lack of data evaluating its efficacy in PAP. A small RCT found that combining CBT and mirror therapy did not have robust effects above those of general psychotherapeutic interventions [55].

Mirror Therapy Mirror therapy (MT) is a non-pharmacological treatment that involves placing a mirror adjacent to the intact limb to create the illusion that the amputated limb is present and can be moved without pain. MT is believed to treat PAP by influencing cortical reorganization. This is thought to occur because the brain prefers visual information over somatosensory feedback. A meta-analysis of the literature, including Medline, the Cochrane Database, and Embase identified 20 studies examining the efficacy of MT. MT was not recommended as a first-line treatment of PLP due to low-level evidence, but it was noted that high-level evidence exists for improvement in phantom limb movement [56].

Prevention Perioperative epidural catheter infusions with the goal of preventing development of chronic PAP have been studied extensively. The thought is that blocking nociceptive input after peripheral nerve injury might avoid long-term sensitization. A prospective study of 65 patients undergoing lower-limb amputation revealed median PAP at 6 month follow-up to be significantly improved if pain was optimized starting 48 hours pre-operatively with either epidural or parenteral analgesia [57].

What Is the Prognosis of This Condition?

Patients presenting with extremity injury due to trauma who require amputation have lower mortality rates compared with patients with peripheral artery disease. A retrospective review of 154 patients in the Veterans Affairs (VA) system after above knee amputation revealed overall survival of 78% at 1 year and 55% at 3 years [58]. Absence of vascular impairment of the residual limb and age less than 65 significantly improve the chances of autonomy in mobility as patients progress through rehabilitation post AKA [59].

What Is the Long-Term Outcome – Complete Cure or Recurrent/Chronic Persistent Problem?

RLP pain persists beyond 18 months in only approximately 15% of cases, and these patients are less likely to improve over time [60]. In contrast, a prospective study evaluating 58 patients who underwent limb amputation found that PLP persists after 2 years in 59% of patients [61]. A meta-analysis of the literature revealed a 66% return-to-work rate, with a high percentage of those subjects requiring a change in occupation [62].

Discussion

Prevalence

Post amputation pain is a highly prevalent disease state. Approximately 1.9 million amputees live in the United States, with worldwide projections expected to double by the year 2050 [63]. Vascular pathology accounts for 82% of limb loss, followed by trauma at 16.4% [64]. A study of 914 patients with limb loss found that up to 95% pateints suffer from some combination of PLP, RLP, or phantom sensations [65]. These sensations may be painless and range from vague sensations to an appreciation of full limb size and position. There is a wide variation in the reported incidence of phantom limb pain, possibly due to the lack of standardized definition and method of reporting the presence of pain [66].

Differential Diagnosis

While PAP is primarily a clinical diagnosis made through detailed history and physical exam, there are tests that can assist in ruling out certain causes. Ischemic injury must always be considered in patients presenting with PAP, as many amputees suffer from vascular insufficiency as their underlying etiology. Transcutaneous oxygen tension is indicative of ischemia if less than 20 mmHg at the level of the residual limb. Infections such as osteomyelitis can cause PAP and can be assessed with ESR, CRP, and WBC count. A neuroma can be diagnosed with a positive Tinel's sign as well as an improvement in pain following injection of local anesthetic. Prosthesis-related pain can result from changes in stump shape relative to the prosthetic mold and can cause skin breakdown. Pressure points and skin breakdown can also occur due to pathologic bone formation and/or heterotopic ossification. These types of anomalous bone formations can be evaluated with X-rays. Patients undergoing amputation have a higher prevalence of back pain compared to the general population [67]. Lumbar radiculopathy, facet arthropathy, sacroiliitis, and hip arthritis can present with referred pain and be mistaken for PAP [68]. Radiographic evaluation of these other anatomic regions with X-ray and MRI can help rule these out as causes of pain. PLP and CRPS should always be considered, but are difficult to test for [69].

Strength of Evidence for Different Treatment Modalities

The 2016 Cochrane Review on Pharmacologic interventions for treating PLP reveals an overall paucity of data on pharmacologic interventions. Conclusions from the review include favorable short-term analgesic efficacy for morphine, gabapentin, and ketamine with the caveat that the results were mostly based on small studies that varied considerably and lacked long-term efficacy and safety outcomes. Larger randomized controlled trials are needed to make stronger recommendations about which medications would be useful for clinical practice. There is more evidence available for treatment of the broader category of neuropathic pain [70]. In 2015, Finnerup et al. used the GRADE classification and found strong evidence for the use of gabapentin, gabapentin ER/enacarbil, pregabalin, SNRIs, and TCAs. There was weak evidence for capsaicin patches, lidocaine patches, tramadol, botulinum toxin A (subcutaneous), and strong opioids. The data was inconclusive

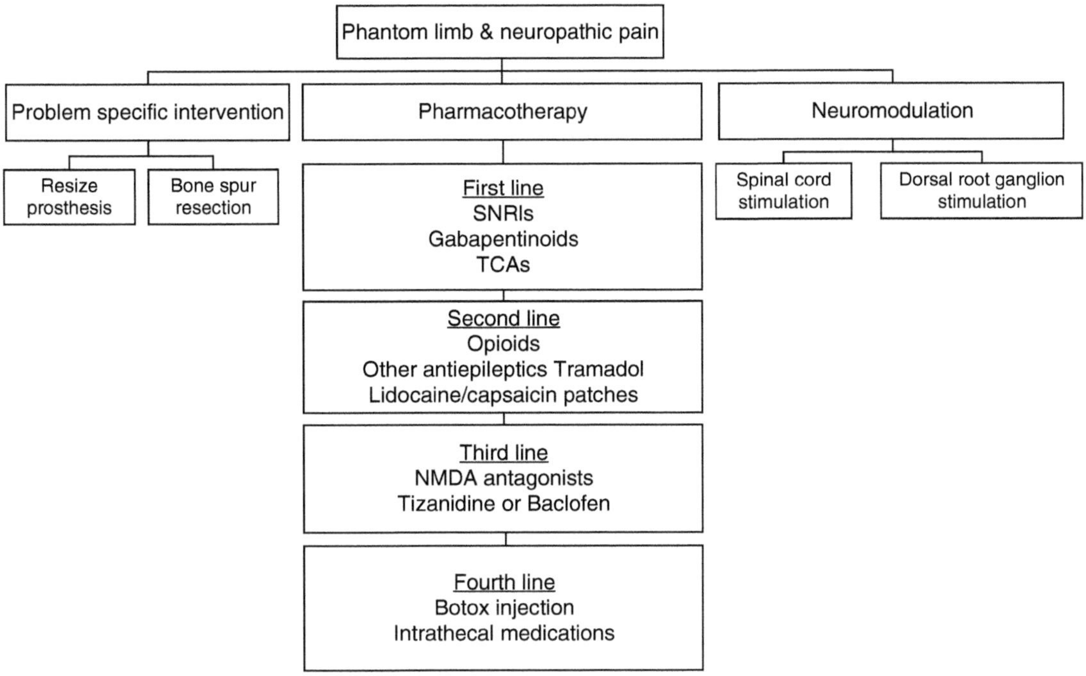

Fig. 29.1 Phantom limb pain treatment options

for combination therapy, capsaicin cream, carbamazepine, clonidine topical, lacosamide, lamotrigine, NMDA antagonists, oxcarbazepine, SSRI antidepressants, tapentadol, topiramate, and zonisamide. The evidence was weak for cannabinoids and valproate and strong for levetiracetam and mexiletine [71].

Evidence for newer treatment modalities such as neuromodulation is also lacking (Fig. 29.1). While there are not any randomized clinical trials, there are case reports of using PNS to successfully treat PAP. Spinal cord stimulation has been shown to be effective in many neuropathic pain states, and a comprehensive review of evidence for SCS implanted for the treatment of neuropathic pain and CRPS establishes a 1B+ level of evidence for perception of pain relief, reduction in pain scores, quality-of-life improvement, and patient satisfaction [72]. The evidence for its efficacy in the specific setting of PAP is less strong as the current data is primarily limited to small case series with variable criteria used to define a successful outcome. In a randomized controlled trial comparing SCS and DRG stimulation, DRG had a higher success rate at both 3 and 12 months [73]. Motor cortex stimulation in PAP is considered investigational by the Food and Drug Administration but has some promising initial studies. A meta-analysis of 155 patients who underwent motor cortex stimulation showed that 53% of patients with PLP were treated successfully [69, 74].

Future Directions or Clinical Trials in Progress

Monoclonal antibody–based therapeutics have shown efficacy in the treatment of inflammatory and oncologic conditions and could be useful in the treatment of PAP. In patients with rheumatoid arthritis, anti-interleukin-6 receptor monoclonal antibody shows promise in reducing disease activity and improving physical function per patient reports [75].

Genetic testing also appears to have a role in the treatment of pain conditions which should become more prevalent in the future. In the treatment of migraine headaches, 38 genetic variants have been identified and it is thought that establishing a polygenic risk score may lead to personalized treatment of migraine in identifying responders to specific drugs [76]. Pharmacogenomic testing revealed that some patients exhibit an allele which results in rapid metabolism of buprenorphine, necessitating higher dosing in the treatment of opioid use disorder [77]. Genetic testing could prove useful as a clinical decision support tool to assist with individualization in the pharmacologic treatment of PAP.

Conclusion/Summary

PAP occurs with a high prevalence and can be a challenge to treat. Multimodal therapy provides the most comprehensive approach to optimize analgesia and improve function. Much of the evidence supporting treatment of PAP is extrapolated from the literature for other neuropathic pain conditions. Further controlled studies that focus on the use of multimodal treatments and preventative measures could help to improve the management of this complex condition.

References

1. Nathanson M. Phantom limbs as reported by S. Weir Mitchell. Neurology. 1988;38(3):504–5.
2. Neil MJE. Pain after amputation. BJA Education. 2016;16(3):107–12.
3. Flor H, Nikolajsen L, Jensen TS. Phantom limb pain: a case of maladaptive CNS plasticity? Nat Rev Neurosci. 2006;7(11):873–81.
4. Devor M. Sodium channels and mechanisms of neuropathic pain. J Pain. 2006;Suppl 1:S3–S12.
5. Bartels K, Cohen SP, Raja SN. Postamputation pain. In: Benzon H, Raja SN, Fishman SM, Liu SS, Cohen SP, editors. Essentials of pain medicine. 3rd ed. Philadelphia: Elsevier Health; 2011. p. 365–9.
6. Sherman RA, Bruno GM. Concurrent variation of burning phantom limb and stump pain with near surface blood flow in the stump. Orthopedics. 1987;10:1395–402.
7. Devor M. In: Koltzenburg M, McMahon SB, editors. Wall and Melzack's textbook of pain. Amsterdam: Elsevier; 2005. p. 905–27.
8. Nyström B, Hagbarth KE. Microelectrode recordings from transected nerves in amputees with phantom limb pain. Neurosci Lett. 1981;27:211–6.
9. Chabal C, Jacobson L, Russell LC, et al. Pain responses to perineuromal injection of normal saline, gallamine, and lidocaine in humans. Pain. 1989;36:321–5.
10. Sehirlioglu A, Ozturk C, Yazicioglu K, et al. Painful neuroma requiring surgical excision after lower limb amputation caused by landmine explosions. Int Orthop. 2009;33:533–6.
11. Liss AG, af Ekenstam FW, Wiberg M. Loss of neurons in the dorsal root ganglia after transection of a peripheral sensory nerve. Scand J Plast Reconstr Surg Hand Surg. 1996;30:1–6.
12. Kajander KC, Wakisaka S, Bennett GJ. Spontaneous discharge originates in the dorsal root ganglion at the onset of a painful peripheral neuropathy in the rat. Neurosci Lett. 1992;138:225–8.
13. Chen Y, Michaelis M, Jänig W, Devor M. Adrenoreceptor subtype mediating sympathetic-sensory coupling in injured sensory neurons. J Neurophysiol. 1996;76:3721–30.
14. Woolf CJ. Dissecting out mechanisms responsible for peripheral neuropathic pain: implications for diagnosis and therapy. Life Sci. 2004;74:2605–1510.
15. Woolf CJ, Salter MW. In: Koltzenburg M, McMahon SB, editors. Wall and Melzack's textbook of pain. Amsterdam: Elsevier; 2005. p. 91–105.
16. Torsney C, MacDermott AB. Disinhibition opens the gate to pathological pain signaling in superficial neurokinin 1 receptor-expressing neurons in rat spinal cord. J Neurosci. 2006;26:1833–43.
17. Woolf CJ, Salter MW. Neuronal plasticity: increasing the gain in pain. Science. 2000;288:1765–9.
18. Wang S, et al. A rat model of unilateral hindpaw burn injury: slowly developing rightwards shift of the morphine dose-response curve. Pain. 2005;116:87–95.
19. Grusser SM, Winter C, Muhlnickel W, et al. The relationship of perceptual phenomena and cortical reorganization in upper extremity amputees. Neuroscience. 2001;102:263–72.
20. Flor H, et al. Phantom-limb pain as a perceptual correlate of cortical reorganization following arm amputation. Nature. 1995;375:482–4.
21. Manchikanti L, Kaye AM, Knezevic NN, et al. Responsible, safe and effective prescription of opioids for chronic non-cancer pain: American society of interventional pain physicians (ASIPP) guidelines. Pain Physician. 2017;20(2S):S3–S92.
22. Wiffen PJ, McQuay HJ, Edwards JE, Moore RA. Gabapentin for acute and chronic pain. Cochrane Database Syst Rev. 2005;(3):CD005452. https://doi.org/10.1002/14651858D005452.
23. Backonja MM. Use of anticonvulsants for treatment of neuropathic pain. Neurology. 2002;59:S14.
24. Sarantopoulos C, McCallum B, Kwok WM, et al. Gabapentin decreases membrane calcium currents in injured as well as in control mammalian primary afferent neurons. Reg Anesth Pain Med. 2002;27:47.

25. Bone M, Critchley P, Buggy DJ. Gabapentin in postamputation phantom limb pain: a randomized, double-blind, placebo-controlled, cross-over study. Reg Anesth Pain Med. 2002;27(5):481–6.
26. Backonja M, Glanzman RL. Gabapentin dosing for neuropathic pain: evidence from randomized, placebo-controlled clinical trials. Clin Ther. 2003;25:81.
27. Dworkin RH, Corbin AE, Young JP Jr, et al. Pregabalin for the treatment of postherpetic neuralgia: a randomized, placebo-controlled trial. Neurology. 2003;60:1274.
28. Spiegel DR, Lappinen E, Gottlieb M. A presumed case of phantom limb pain treated successfully with duloxetine and pregabalin. Gen Hosp Psychiatry. 2010;32(2):2285–7.
29. Wossner S, Weber K, Steinbeck A, Oberhauser M, Feuerecker M. Pregabalin as adjunct in a multimodal pain therapy after traumatic foot amputation – a case report of a 4-year-old girl. Scand J Pain. 2017;9(1):146–9.
30. Chen H, Lamer TJ, Rho RH, et al. Contemporary management of neuropathic pain for the primary care physician. Mayo Clin Proc. 2004;79:1533.
31. Sawynok J, Esser MJ, Reid AR. Antidepressants as analgesics: an overview of central and peripheral mechanisms of action. J Psychiatry Neurosci. 2001;26:21.
32. McLean MJ, Schmutz M, Wamil AW, et al. Oxcarbazepine: mechanisms of action. Epilepsia. 1994;35 Suppl 3:S5.
33. Elliott F, Little A, Milbrandt W. Carbamazepine for phantom-limb phenomena. N Engl J Med. 1976;295:678.
34. Patterson JF. Carbamazepine in the treatment of phantom limb pain. South Med J. 1988;81:1100–2.
35. Max MB, Lynch SA, Muir J, et al. Effects of desipramine, amitriptyline and fluoxetine on pain in diabetic neuropathy. N Engl J Med. 1992;326:1250.
36. Sindrup SH, Gram LF, Brosen K, et al. The selective serotonin reuptake inhibitor paroxetine is effective in the treatment of diabetic neuropathy symptoms. Pain. 1990;42:135.
37. Power-Smith P, Turkington D. Fluoxetine in phantom limb pain. Br J Psychiatry. 1993;163:105–6.
38. Sindrup SH, Bach FW, Madsen C, et al. Venlafaxine versus imipramine in painful polyneuropathy: a randomized, controlled trial. Neurology. 2003;60:284.
39. Dworkin RH, O'Connor AB, Backonia M, et al. Pharmacologic management of neuropathic pain: evidence-based recommendations. Pain. 2007;132:237.
40. McQuay HJ, Carroll D, Glynn CJ. Dose-response for analgesic effect of amitriptyline in chronic pain. Anaesthesia. 1993;48:281.
41. Reiestad F, Kulkarni J. Role of myofascial trigger points in post-amputation pain: causation and management. Prosthetics Orthot Int. 2013;37(2):120–3. https://doi.org/10.1177/0309364612447807. Epub 2012 Jun 20.
42. Wu H, et al. A prospective randomized double-blinded pilot study to examine the effect of botulinum toxin Type A injection versus lidocaine/depomedrol injection on residual and phantom limb pain. Clin J Pain. 2012;28(2). https://doi.org/10.1097/AJP.0b013e3182264fe9.
43. McCormick ZL, Hendrix A, Davanim D, Clay B, Kirsling A, Harden N. Lumbar sympathetic plexus block as a treatment for postamputation pain: methodology for a randomized controlled trial. Pain Med. 2018;19(12):2496–503.
44. Rauck RL, et al. Treatment of post-amputation pain with peripheral nerve stimulation. Neuromodulation. 2014;17(2):188–97.
45. Van Buyten JP, Smet I, Liem L, Russo M, Huygen F. Stimulation of the dorsal root ganglia for the management of complex regional pain syndrome: a prospective case series. Pain Pract. 2015;15:208–16.
46. Goebel A, Lewis S, Phyillip R, Sharma M. Dorsal root ganglion stimulation for complex regional pain syndrome (CRPS) recurrence after amputation for CRPS, and failure of conventional spinal cord stimulation. Pain Pract. 2018;18(1):104–8.
47. Sturm V, Kroger M, Penzholz H. Problems of peripheral nerve surgery in amputation stump pain and phantom limbs. Chirurg. 1975;46:389–91.
48. Dellon AL, Mackinnon SE. Treatment of the painful neuroma by neuroma resection and muscle implantation. Plast Reconstr Surg. 1986;77:427–38.
49. Burchiel KJ, Johans TJ, Ochoa J. The surgical treatment of painful traumatic neuromas. J Neurosurg. 1993;78:714–9.
50. Prantl L, Schreml S, Heine N, Eisenmann-Klein M, Angele P. Surgical treatment of chronic phantom limb sensation and limb pain after lower limb amputation. Plast Reconstr Surg. 2006;118:1562–72.
51. Potter BK, Burns TC, Lacap AP, Granville RR, Grajewski DA. Heterotopic ossification following traumatic and combat-related amputations: prevalence, risk factors, and preliminary results of excision. J Bone Joint Surg. 2007;89:476–85.
52. Ducic I, Mesbahi AN, Attinger CE, Graw K. The role of peripheral nerve surgery in the treatment of chronic pain associated with amputation stumps. Plast Reconstr Surg. 2008;121:908–14.
53. Poppler LH, Parikh RP, Bichanich MJ, Rebehn K, Bettlach CR, Mackinnon SE, Moore AM. Surgical interventions for the treatment of painful neuroma: a comparative meta-analysis. Pain. 2018;159(2):214–23. https://doi.org/10.1097/j.pain.0000000000001101.
54. Wetering EJVD, Lemmens KMM, Nieboer AP, Huijsman R. Cognitive and behavioral interventions for the management of chronic neuropathic pain in adults—a systematic review. Eur J Pain. 2010;14(7):670–81.
55. McQuaid J, Peterzell D, Rutledge T, Cone R, Nance P, Velez D, Coeshott R, Ortega J, Van Duyn M, Otilingam P, Atkinson J. Integrated Cognitive-Behavioral Therapy (CBT) and Mirror Visual Feedback (MVF)

for phantom limb pain: a randomized clinical trial. J Pain. 2014;15(4 Suppl):S108.
56. Barbin J, Seetha V, Casillas JM, Paysant J, Perennou D. The effects of mirror therapy on pain and motor control of phantom limb in amputees: a systemic review. Ann Phys Rehabil Med. 2016;59:270–5.
57. Karanikolas M, Aretha D, Tsolakis I, et al. Optimized perioperative analgesia reduces chronic phantom limb pain intensity, prevalence and frequency: a prospective, randomized, clinical trial. Anesthesiology. 2011;114(5):1144–54.
58. Nehler MR, Coll JR, Hiatt WR, et al. Functional outcome in a contemporary series of major lower extremity amputations. J Vasc Surg. 2003;38:7.
59. Traballesi M, Brunelli S, Pratesi L, Pulcini M, Angioni C, Paolucci S. Prognostic factors in rehabilitation of above knee amputees for vascular diseases. Disabil Rehabil. 1998;20(10):380–4.
60. De Mos M, Huygen FJPM, van der Hoeven-Borgman M, Dieleman JP, Stricker BHC, Sturkenboom MCJM. Outcome of the complex regional pain syndrome. Clin J Pain. 2009;25:590–7.
61. Jensen T, Krebs B, Nielson J, Rasmussen P. Immediate and long-term phantom limb pain in amputees: incidence, clinical characteristics and relationship to preamputation limb pain. Pain. 1985;21:267–78.
62. Burger H, Marinek C. Return to work after lower limb amputation. Disabil Rehabil. 2007;29(17):1323–9.
63. Ziegler-Graham K, MacKenzie EJ, Ephraim PL, Travison TG, Brookmeyer R. Estimating the prevalence of limb loss in the United States: 2005 to 2050. Arch Phys Med Rehabil. 2008;89(3):422–9.
64. Dillingham T, Pezzin L, MacKenzie EJ. Limb amputation and limb deficiencies: epidemiology and recent trends in the United States. South Med J. 2002;95:875–83.
65. Sherman RA, Sherman CJ. Prevalence and characteristics of chronic phantom limb pain among American veterans: results of a trial survey. Am J Phys Med. 1983;62(5):227–8.
66. Jensen T, Rasmussen P. Phantom pain and related phenomena after amputation. In: Wall P, Melzak R, editors. Textbook of pain. 2nd ed. Edinburgh: Churchill Livingstone; 1989. p. 159.
67. Smith DG, Ehde DM, Legro MW, et al. Phantom limb, residual limb, and back pain after lower extremity amputations. Clin Orthop Relat Res. 1999;361:29–38. [PubMed].
68. Cohen SP, Raja SN. Pathogenesis, diagnosis, and treatment of lumbar zygapophysial (facet) joint pain. Anesthesiology. 2007;106:591–614.
69. Hsu E, Cohen S. Postamputation pain:epidemiology, mechanisms, and treatment. J Pain Res. 2013;6:121–36.
70. Alviar MJM, Hale T, Lim-Dungca M. Pharmacologic interventions for treating phantom limb pain. Cochrane Database Syst Rev. 2016;(10):CD006380. https://doi.org/10.1002/14651858.CD006380.pub3.
71. Finnerup NB, et al. Pharmacotherapy for neuropathic pain in adults: systematic review, meta-analysis and updated NeuPSIG recommendations. Lancet Neurol. 2015;14(2):162–73. https://doi.org/10.1016/S1474-4422(14)70251-0.
72. Visnjevac O, Costandi S, Patel B, Azer G, Bolash R, Mekhail NA. A comprehensive outcome-specific review of spinal cord stimulation for complex regional pain syndrome. Pain Pract. 2017;17(4):533–45.
73. Deer TR, et al. Dorsal root ganglion stimulation yielded higher treatment success rate for complex regional pain syndrome and causalgia at 3 and 12 months: a randomized comparative trial. Pain. 2017;158(4):669–81.
74. Nguyen JP, Lefaucheur JP, Raoul S, et al. Motor cortex stimulation for the treatment of neuropathic pain. In: Krames ES, Peckham PH, Rezai AR, editors. Neuromodulation. 1st ed. Amsterdam: Elsevier Science; 2009. p. 515–26.
75. Strand V, Gossec L, Proudfoot CWJ, Chen CI, Reaney M, Guillonneau S, Kimura T, van Adelsberg J, Lin Y, Mangan EK, van Hoogstraten H, Burmester GR. Patient-reported outcomes from a randomized phase III trial of sarilumab monotherapy versus adalimumab monotherapy in patients with rheumatoid arthritis. Arthritis Res Ther. 2018;20(1):129.
76. Chalmer MA, Esserlind AL, Olesen J, Hansen TF. Polygenic risk score: use in migraine research. J Headache Pain. 2018;19(1):29.
77. Ettienne EB, Chapman E, Maneno M, Ofoegbu A, Wilson B, Settles-Reaves B, Clarke M, Dunston G, Rosenblatt K. Pharmacogenomics-guided policy in opioid use disorder (OUD) management: an ethnically diverse case-based approach. Addict Behav Rep. 2017;6:8–14.

A 45-Year-Old Patient with Chronic Sole Pain

30

Wyatt Kupperman and Tariq Malik

Case Description

This is a 45-year-old woman who presents to the pain clinic with complaint of long-standing left heel pain. She is an avid marathon runner, but left heel pain has prompted her to quit her last marathon and she is afraid to run marathon anymore. There was no inciting event. Pain started gradually and has been there for the last 1 year. Pain is worse in the morning and when standing after prolonged sitting. It also gets worse toward the end of the day. She has been managing her pain with over-the-counter pain killers. They help, but she is getting tired of taking them every day. She tried using different shoes and shoe insert but nothing has helped so far. She went to see her PCP who did some blood work and foot X-ray but saw nothing and referred her to the pain clinic. Foot examination is negative for any discoloration, swelling, or deformity but is significant for tenderness over the heel and some pain with dorsiflexion. Range of motion of the ankle and foot is unremarkable; her gait is normal too.

W. Kupperman
Neurological Institute, Cleveland Clinic, Cleveland, OH, USA

T. Malik (✉)
Department of Anesthesia and Critical Care, University of Chicago, Chicago, IL, USA
e-mail: TMuslim@dacc.uchicago.edu; tmalik@dacc.uchicago.edu

What Is Your Preliminary Diagnosis?

She has a chronic painful condition of her foot, which seems to get worse with weight bearing. There are no constitutional symptoms like fever, weight loss, swelling of the foot, or major trauma. She is tender over the insertion of plantar fascia in the heel and when the fascia is stretched with dorsiflexion. She is also a runner. This would suggest that she most likely has plantar fasciitis.

Heel pain can be from tear or rupture of ligaments or tendons but they tend to happen following major injury and often accompanied by swelling and discoloration. Calcaneus is prone to stress fracture from running and can be missed in plan X-ray imaging. Tumor of the bone both primary (Ewing sarcoma) and secondary (from lung, stomach, bladder, or endometrial) cannot be discounted. But long-standing history of pain with no other symptoms and negative foot X-ray make it an unlikely diagnosis. Calcaneal bone spur is often seen on X-ray in patients with heel pain. Though bone spur may cause pain, half the patients with bony spur never complain of heel pain. Thinning of heel pad can cause pain. Heel fat pad is a potent shock absorber, but after age 40, it starts deteriorating. Obesity and running can accelerate heel pad degeneration with age. Loss of fat pad cushion causes pain as heel experiences force equal to 110% of body weight during simple walking and up to 250% of body weight when running. Rheumatological diseases

T. Malik (ed.), *Practical Chronic Pain Management*, https://doi.org/10.1007/978-3-030-46675-6_30

(Ankylosing Spondylitis, Reiter's disease) can cause foot or heel pain but often it causes bilateral foot pain, and other joints of the body are also involved and often blood work is positive. Entrapment neuropathies (Tarsal Tunnel syndrome, Medial calcaneal neuropathy, Baxter's Neuropathy) can cause pain, but often there are accompanying symptoms of tingling and numbness.

How Is Diagnosis Confirmed?

Plantar fasciitis is a clinical diagnosis. Plantar fasciitis can generally be suspected from patient history and examination. It usually reveals a slow and gradual onset of discomfort along the inferior-medial heel [1–3]. It has been reported that pain can be present along the plantar fascia distally from the insertion point as well [4]. Discomfort is most appreciated after long periods of inactivity at the onset of action, i.e., in the morning after sleep with the first few steps [4, 5].

On physical examination, there may be acute tenderness along the plantar fascia insertion along the medial tuberosity of the calcaneus [5]. One should examine the plantar fascia superficially and with deep palpation, as well as in a relaxed state with toes flexed and stressed with toes extended [5].

The examiner should complete a motor, sensory, and postural assessment of the feet and proximal biomechanical chain. One may find tightness within the fascia network, and tightness of the heel chord [6–8]. Discomfort with reduced toe extension and diminished range in dorsiflexion may be appreciated [6–8]. Saban and Masharawi found that three office base tests (static single leg stance 30 seconds, 10 repetitions of a half squat, and 10 repetitions of heel rise may benefit diagnosis of plantar heel pain syndrome [9]. On gait assessment, if performed, there may be an antalgic gait, and/or the patient may show a preference to have the affected foot held in plantar flexion with attempts to avoid heel strike.

Utility of radiographs has been highly debated regarding the diagnostic benefit for plantar fasciitis [4].

In one study, Levy et al. found 59.5% of symptomatic patients with calcaneal spur and 46.5% with an Achilles spur. This did not lead to changes in management [10].

Findings of spurs on imaging continues to stir controversy, with Ahmad et al. finding no correlation between the size or shape with complaints [11].

The spurs that are found on imaging may simply represent other conditions of the foot potentially causing discomfort (Fig. 30.1) [12]. Subcalcaneal spurs can even be seen in patients who do not have symptoms of PF [13]. According to the American College of Foot and Ankle surgeons, advanced imaging is usually not required to make the diagnosis [4].

Ultrasound (US) investigation for diagnosis and treatment is gaining popularity for many musculoskeletal conditions. US investigation by Radwin et al. found it effective to assess fascial structure, but utility to be determined [14]. Fagan et al. found US of plantar fascia thickness to be superior than clinical diagnosis, though study is limited by sample size [15]. In another study, the sensitivity and specificity for diagnosing plantar fasciitis were found to be 80.9% and 85.7% using ultrasound investigation [16]. It has been further determined in a systematic retrospective review

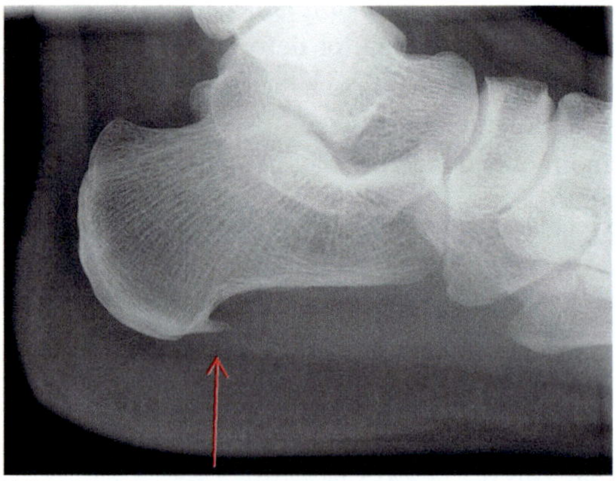

Fig. 30.1 Calcaneal spur. (From https://en.wikipedia.org/wiki/Plantar_fasciitis)

by Ali Mohseni-Bandpei et al. that US may be comparable with MRI in diagnosis [17]. If using US for fascial assessment, proximal thickness of more than 4 mm may be seen in PF [13].

Though PF may be picked up on clinical assessment, ultrasound investigation may be a helpful adjunct in the hand of a skilled practitioner. Further advanced imaging should be considered if there is concern for other pathologies depending on mechanism of injury that may be affecting the osseous and/or soft tissues of the foot, including tumor.

What Is the Pathophysiology of This Condition?

The disorder arises secondary to repetitive micro tears of the plantar fascia usually near the insertion point on the inferomedial calcaneus [18]. Multiple factors have been associated with this condition, mainly increased BMI, repetitive trauma, pes planus/cavus foot, aging, sedentary and active lifestyles [18].

Some do not believe this condition to be acute in nature and may reference "plantar fasciosis" as it is believed to be a chronic degenerative process in the active and even sedentary individual [13, 19].

The importance of the plantar fascia is for stabilization, particularly regarding the longitudinal arch between heal rise and toe off in the gait cycle [20]. During the heel rise phase of the gait cylce, the phalanges dorsi-flex which reciprocally tightens the plantar fascia, most notably on the medial aspect of the foot [20]. This causes an elevation of the longitudinal arch [20]. Due to the medial attachment site on the heel, one will see hindfoot inversion and an externally rotated tibia [21]. These accommodations aid in foot stabilization, and more effective toe-off [20, 21].

How Is This Problem Managed?

There are a variety of treatments that have been reported for plantar fasciitis with varying evidence and benefit. The goal for treatment like many musculoskeletal conditions is to treat early in a graduated manner if required. It has been shown that 90% of patients will improve with conservative measures [19, 22]. However, it may take many months for improvement of symptoms.

Conservative measures may be initiated including such things as rest, OTC pain medications, ice massage, and stretching exercises for a 6 week course [23, 24].

In a 2013 National Health and Wellness Survey (75,000), 650 respondents stated having plantar fasciitis symptoms in a month period [25]. Four hundred and sixty-six respondents reported using an OTC medication [25]. Still, according to Brotzman and Jasko, there is weak evidence to support NSAID use [23].

Stretching exercises have been focused on the plantar fascia and Achilles tendon. DiGiovanni et al. found plantar fascial stretching to improve symptoms significantly, up to 92% patient satisfaction in their prospective study [26]. If the patient continues to be symptomatic, a referral to a physical therapist may allow for a tailored program for the patient, to include education on eccentrically controlled exercises with a home exercise program and intrinsic foot techniques [27]. The physical therapist may further provide joint and soft tissues mobilization, which is a grade A recommendation by the American Physical Therapy Association [28].

Patients may further benefit from foot and ankle support. According to McPoil et al., prefabricated/custom foot orthoses provided improved function and improved pain for roughly 3 months [29]. Further, the American Physical Therapy Association (APTA) recommends orthosis for a short course, even up to 1 year. [28]. If patients can tolerate night splints with sleep, there is moderate evidence for symptoms lasting greater than 6 months, when the night splints are used for a duration of 1–3 months [28]. Night splints are recommended by the APTA especially for patients who consistently feel pain with the first step when walking in the morning [28].

Per Cochrane review, the orthosis type may not matter, but custom orthosis with a night splint may be effective [30].

Patients who continue to have discomfort after the above conservative measures have been explored, and may benefit from corticosteroid injection. This injection has been described using various duration of action corticosteroids, with either a blind technique or under ultrasound guidance. As an example, one may use a mixture of 2–3 ml of 0.25% bupivacaine and 40–80 mg methylprednisolone. Risk of injection is similar to other peripheral injections, including bleeding and infection. However, there is a risk of plantar fascial rupture and fat pad atrophy [31]. In a retrospective review by Chen, Wu, and Yu, including Cochrane trials, they concluded that a corticosteroid injection was more effective within the first month than a PRP injection [32]. But an injection of platelet-rich plasma was superior in VAS reduction at 6 months [32].

Botox, commonly used for cosmetic procedures and for spasticity management, has been investigated for the treatment of plantar fasciitis. Babcock et al.'s randomized controlled study determined improvement in symptoms and function at 3 and 8 weeks after treatment [33].

If the patient is still having significant difficulties, extracorporeal shockwave therapy has also been used for chronic plantar fasciitis, possibly after 6 months of symptoms with no benefit from multiple conservative measures. Kudo et al., in a double blind multi-center placebo-controlled trial, investigated ESWT on adult subjects with failure to conservative treatment for a minimum of 6 months. They found a statistical benefit in the treatment arm at 3 months compared to placebo [34]. This intervention, recommended by Ogden et al., may be worth considering prior to surgical intervention [35].

Surgery is reserved for refractory cases who failed to respond to 6–12 months of conservative management who continue with moderate to severe symptoms [5].

Complications of surgery are rare, but like with any other surgical interventions there is always a risk of developing wound infection and wound dehiscence [5]. Also there have been reports of further injury to the plantar fascia, loss of the medial arch, injury of lateral plantar nerve, and even CRPS [5].

Response to surgical intervention seems to be beneficial. According to Kadkia from DeLee and Drez's *Orthopedic Sports Medicine*, recurrence rate is roughly 10% following incomplete plantar fasciectomy [5]. Regarding the approach to surgery, if there is concern for nerve compression particularly of the first branch of lateral plantar nerve, open investigation may be warranted [36]. However, it has been seen with endoscopic investigation that one may return to activities up to 4 weeks earlier, (6 weeks vs. 10 weeks) [37]. Regardless of the approach, a total excision of the fascia is normally not performed, as this can lead to lateral column syndrome [38].

What Is the Prognosis of This Condition?

The prognosis for treatment of plantar fasciitis is quite good, with and overall cure/tolerance rate of 90% by following conservative measures [31]. However, patients will need encouragement, as in some cases it may take many months for symptom relief. It is a chronic degenerative disease and, once pain abates with treatment, requires life-long adjustment including life style modification like weight control and exercise routine to prevent it from recurrence or effecting the other foot.

Discussion

Approximately 10% in the United States will develop plantar fasciitis at some point in their life [39]. Incidence seems to be greatest among people between 40 and 60 years of age [40, 41]. About one million patients consult their physicians for plantar fasciitis management a year. Total cost of plantar fasciitis management is estimated at 300 million dollars a year. Plantar fascia is a broad fibrous aponeurosis that spans the plantar surface of the foot. It originates from the medial and anterior aspects of the calcaneus and inserts into the bases of proximal phalanges. It acts as a beam when the metatarsals are subjected to important bending forces (propulsion) and a truss when the foot absorbs forces of impact

Table 30.1 Differential diagnosis of plantar fasciitis

Calcaneal pain	Tumor Fracture Cysts
Entrapment syndromes	Tarsal tunnel syndrome Medial calcaneal nerve entrapment Baxter's nerve compression S1 radicular neuropathy
Inflammatory tendinopathy	Rheumatoid Spondyloarthritis Reiter's
Soft tissue pain	Heel fat pad atrophy Acute plantar fascia rupture Retrocalcaneal bursitis Achilles tendonitis

Table 30.2 Risk factors for developing plantar fasciitis

Anatomical	Leg-length discrepancy Foot arch abnormality Calf muscle tightness Overweight Loss of heel pad
Extrinsic	Overuse Poor footwear Improper training

expanded during landing and in the stance phase of gait. It is a common cause of foot pain in adults, worsening the patients' quality of life. It affects both sexes, either in professional or recreational athletes, and women are affected slightly more often than men. Many different healthcare providers (podiatrists, orthopedic surgeons, physical therapists, and chiropractors) are involved in the treatment of PF.

A number of different conditions can cause heel pain as discussed above but can be ruled out using history, physical examination, and lab work or imaging (Tables 30.1 and 30.2).

Plantar fasciitis can normally be diagnosed based solely on history and physical exam findings. Radiographs have been ordered for examination of osseous structures, but significance of spurs is highly debated [4]. US investigation is frequently used in the office based setting. It has been determined to have sensitivity and specificity of 80.9% and 85.7%, and comparable to MRI as previously stated [16, 17]. MRI has the added benefit to investigate for stress fracture/bone marrow reaction if suspected given history, mechanism of injury, and physical exam.

Conservative measures are very effective for treating plantar fasciitis. According to the American Physical Therapy Association, there is grade A evidence for specific stretching to the plantar fascia and gastrocnemius. Foot orthoses are recommended [28]. Further recommendation for night splints up to 3 months has been beneficial [28].

For continued symptoms despite above, corticosteroid injection has shown good short-term benefit, with PRP injection providing perhaps more sustained benefit [32]. Prior to surgery, it may be worthwhile to discuss a trial of extracorporeal shockwave therapy, even with varying opinions on the intervention [34, 35].

Surgery referral should be considered following failure of conservative modalities, and continued symptoms for a 6–12 month period.

More research should focus on interventions including PRP/stem cell, fat pad atrophy with silicone implantation, and botulinum toxin injection.

Conclusion

Plantar heel pain is a common chronic pain condition that transcends multiple medical specialties, including orthopedic surgery and primary care. Plantar fasciitis is the diagnosis in great majority of cases. However, other mechanical, rheumatologic, neurologic, and infectious causes exist; a comprehensive history and physical examination is pivotal to making the correct diagnosis. If there is no obvious etiology and pain is resistant to therapy, MRI, bone scan, and serological blood work is ordered. Mainstay of treatment is stretching of plantar fascia, NSAIDs, orthoses, and steroid injections. Operative intervention is only indicated after 6 months of failed conservative modalities.

References

1. Bordelon RL. Subcalcaneal pain: a method of evaluation and plan for treatment. Clin Orthop. 1983;177:49–53.
2. Bordelon RL. Subcalcaneal pain: present status, evaluation, and management. Instr Course Lect. 1984;33:283–7.

3. Bordelon RL. Surgical and conservative foot care. Slack: Thorofare; 1988.
4. Schneider HP, Baca JM, Carpenter BB, Dayton PD, Fleischer AE, Sachs BD. American College of Foot and Ankle Surgeons Clinical Consensus Statement: diagnosis and treatment of adult acquired Infracalcaneal heel pain. J Foot Ankle Surg. 2018;57(2):370–81.
5. Kadakia AR. Heel pain and plantar fasciitis: hindfoot conditions. In: DeLee & Drez's orthopaedic sports medicine. 4th ed. Philadelphia: Saunders; 2015. p. 1442–52.e1.
6. Buchbinder R. Plantar fasciitis. N Engl J Med. 2004;350:2159–66.
7. Thomas JL, Christensen JC, Kravitz SR, Mendicino RW, Schuberth JM, Vanore JV, Weil LS Sr, Zlotoff HJ, Bouché R, Baker J. The diagnosis and treatment of heel pain: a clinical practice guideline—Revision 2010. J Foot Ankle Surg. 2010;49:S1–S19.
8. Young CC, Rutherford DS, Niedfeldt MW. Treatment of plantar fasciitis. Am Fam Physician. 2001;63:467–74.
9. Saban B, Masharawi Y. Three single leg standing tests for clinical assessment of chronic plantar heel pain syndrome: static stance, half-squat and heel rise. Physiotherapy. 2017;103(2):237–44.
10. Levy JC, Mizel MS, Clifford PD, Temple HT. Value of radiographs in the initial evaluation of nontraumatic adult heel pain. Foot Ankle Int. 2006;27:427–30.
11. Ahmad J, Karim A, Daniel JN. Relationship and classification of plantar heel spurs in patients with plantar fasciitis. Foot Ankle Int. 2016;37:994–1000.
12. Moroney PJ, O'Neill BJ, Khan-Bhambro K, O'Flanagan SJ, Keogh P, Kenny PJ. The conundrum of calcaneal spurs: do they matter? Foot Ankle Spec. 2014;7:95–101.
13. Karabay N, Toros T, Hurel C. Ultrasonographic evaluation in plantar fasciitis. J Foot Ankle Surg. 2007;46:442–6; McMillan AM, Landorf KB, Barrett JT, Menz HB, Bird AR. Diagnostic imaging for chronic plantar heel pain: a systematic review and meta-analysis. J Foot Ankle Res. 2009;2:32.
14. Radwan A, Wyland M, Applequist L, Bolowsky E, Klingensmith H, Virag I. Ultrasonography, an effective tool in diagnosing plantar fasciitis: a systematic review of diagnostic trials. Int J Sports Phys Ther. 2016;11:663–71.
15. Fagan R, Cuddy V, Ashton J, Clarke M, French H. Validity of clinical assessment compared with plantar fascia thickness on ultrasound for plantar fasciitis: a cross-sectional study. Manual Therapy. 2016;25:e141.
16. Sabir N, Demirlenk S, Yagci B, Karabulut N, Cubukcu S. Clinical utility of sonography in diagnosing plantar fasciitis. J Ultrasound Med. 2005;24:1041–8.
17. Ali Mohseni-Bandpei M, Nakhaee M, Ebrahim Mousavi M, Shakourirad A, Reza Safari M, Vahab KR. Application of ultrasound in the assessment of plantar fascia in patients with plantar fasciitis: a systematic review. Ultrasound Med Biol. 2014;40(8):1737–54.
18. Reider B, Davies GJ, Provencher MT, undefined undefined undefined. Plantar fasciitis. In: Orthopaedic rehabilitation of the athlete: getting back in the game. Philadelphia: Elsevier/Saunders; 2015. p. 1511–30. https://www.clinicalkey.com/#!/content/book/3-s2.0-B9781455727803000421?scrollTo=%23hl0000446.
19. Thomas JL, Christensen JC, Kravitz SR, American College of Foot and Ankle Surgeons Heel Pain Committee, et al. The diagnosis and treatment of heel pain: a clinical practice guideline-revision 2010. J Foot Ankle Surg. 2010;49:S1–S19.
20. Haskell A, Mann R. Biomechanics of the foot and ankle. In: Mann's surgery of the foot and ankle. 9th ed. Philadelphia: Elsevier; 2014. p. 3–36. https://www.clinicalkey.com/#!/content/book/3-s2.0-B9780323072427000012?scrollTo=%23hl0000669.
21. Carlson RE, Fleming LL, Hutton WC. The biomechanical relationship between the tendoachilles, plantar fascia and metatarsophalangeal joint dorsiflexion angle. Foot Ankle Int. 2000;21:18–25.
22. Donley BG, Moore T, Sferra J, Gozdanovic J, Smith R. The efficacy of oral nonsteroidal anti-inflammatory medication (NSAID) in the treatment of plantar fasciitis a randomized, prospective, placebo-controlled study. Foot Ankle Int. 2007;28:20–3.
23. Giangarra CE, Manske RC, Brotzman BS, Jasko JJ. Inferior heel pain. In: Clinical orthopaedic rehabilitation: a team approach. 4th ed. Philadelphia: Elsevier; 2018. p. 281–289e.1.
24. Reider B, Davies GJ, Provencher MT. Plantar fasciitis. In: Orthopaedic rehabilitation of the athlete: getting back in the game. Philadelphia: Elsevier/Saunders; 2015. p. 1511–30.
25. Nahin RL. Prevalence and pharmaceutical treatment of plantar fasciitis in United States adults. J Pain. 2018;19:885.
26. Digiovanni BF, Nawoczenski DA, Malay DP, Graci PA, Williams TT, Wilding GE, Baumhauer JF. l: chronic plantar fasciitis. A prospective clinical trial with two-year follow-up. J Bone Joint Surg Am. 2006;88:1775–81.
27. Hyland MR, Webber-Gaffney A, Cohen L, Lichtman PT. Randomized controlled trial of calcaneal taping, sham taping, and plantar fascia stretching for the short-term management of plantar heel pain. J Orthop Sports Phys Ther. 2006;36:364–71.
28. Martin RL, Davenport TE, Reischl SF, McPoil TG, Matheson JW, Wukich DK, McDonough CM, American Physical Therapy Association. Heel pain-plantar fasciitis: revision 2014. J Orthop Sports Phys Ther. 2014;44(11):A1–33.
29. McPoil TG, Martin RL, Cornwall MW, Wukich DK, Irrgang JJ, Godgess JJ. Heel pain—plantar fasciitis: clinical practice guidelines linked to the International Classification of Function, Disability, and Health from the Orthopaedic Section of the American

Physical Therapy Association. J Orthop Sports Phys Ther. 2008;38:A1–A18.
30. Hawke F, Burns J, Radford JA, du Toit V. Custom-made foot orthoses for the treatment of foot pain. Cochrane Database Syst Rev. 2008;(undefined):CD006801.
31. Miller MD, Hart JA, MacKnight JM, Khoon Tan C, Molloy A. Plantar fasciitis. In: Essential orthopaedics. IV. Philadelphia: Saunders/Elsevier; 2010. p. 758–60.
32. Chen YJ, Yi-Cheng W, Tung-Yang Y. Platelet-rich plasma or autologous blood VS corticosteroids for treatment of plantar fasciitis: a meta-analysis. Arch Phys Med Rehabil. 2017;98(10):e136–7.
33. Babcock MS, Foster L, Pasquina P, Jabbari B. Treatment of pain attributed to plantar fasciitis with botulinum toxin A: a short-term, randomized, placebo-controlled, double-blind study. Am J Phys Med Rehabil. 2005;84:649–54.
34. Kudo P. Randomized, placebo-controlled, double-blind clinical trial evaluating the treatment of plantar fasciitis with an extracorporeal shockwave therapy (ESWT) device: a North American confirmatory study. J Orthop Res. 2006;24:115–23.
35. Ogden JA, Alvarez R, Levitt R, et al. Shock wave therapy for chronic proximal plantar fasciitis. Clin Orthop Relat Res. 2001;387:47–59.
36. Baxter DE, Pfeffer GB. Treatment of chronic heel pain by surgical release of the first branch of the lateral plantar nerve. Clin Orthop Relat Res. 1992;279:229–36.
37. Kinley S, Frascone S, Calderone D, et al. Endoscopic plantar fasciotomy versus traditional heel spur surgery: a prospective study. J Foot Ankle Surg. 1993;32:595–603.
38. Myerson M. Foot and ankle disorders, vol. 2. Baltimore: W.B Saunders; 2000.
39. Cole C, Seto C, Gazewood J. Plantar fasciitis: evidence-based review of diagnosis and therapy. Am Fam Physician. 2005;72:2237–42.
40. Riddle DL, Schappert SM. Volume of ambulatory care visits and patterns of care for patients diagnosed with plantar fasciitis: a national study of medical doctors. Foot Ankle Int. 2004;25:303–10.
41. Taunton JE, Ryan MB, Clement DB, McKenzie DC, Lloyd-Smith D. Plantar fasciitis: a retrospective analysis of 267 cases. Phys Ther Sport. 2002;3:57–65.

A 33-Year-Old Patient with Persistent Back Pain

31

Muhammad Zubair, Kenneth D. Candido, and Nebojsa Nick Knezevic

Case Description

A 33-year-old male with a past medical history of uveitis, psoriasis, and a recent surgical history of open inguinal hernia repair presented to the clinic for evaluation of chronic, dull, lower back, and bilateral hip pain, which started insidiously and which was aggravated with rest and alleviated by exercise. The pain was located in the bilateral sacroiliac (SI) joints and was non-radiating, not associated with numbness, tingling, and kept changing in sensation or with motor weakness. The patient reported a family history of similar problems. On examination, he was found to have bilateral SI joint tenderness with limited external rotation and abduction of the hips bilaterally.

On initial evaluation by the primary care physician (PCP), the patient was prescribed nonsteroidal anti-inflammatory drugs (NSAIDs) with minimal improvement, and after lumbar spine imaging demonstrated SI joint arthropathy, the patient was sent home and referred to the pain clinic for persistence of pain and suspicion of SI joint inflammation. After being evaluated in the pain clinic, the patient had an AP X-ray of the pelvis taken that was inconclusive. Subsequently, an MRI of the lower lumbar spine (as being the most symptomatic region) was performed, which demonstrated sacroiliitis.

M. Zubair
Department of Anesthesiology, Advocate Illinois Masonic Medical Center, Chicago, IL, USA
e-mail: muhammad.zubair@advocatehealth.com

K. D. Candido · N. N. Knezevic (✉)
Department of Anesthesiology, Advocate Illinois Masonic Medical Center, Chicago, IL, USA

Department of Anesthesiology, University of Illinois, Chicago, IL, USA

Department of Surgery, University of Illinois, Chicago, IL, USA

What Is Your Preliminary Diagnosis?

SI joint inflammation due to ankylosing spondylitis (AS).

How Is the Diagnosis Confirmed?

The diagnosis of this clinical condition can be confirmed in two steps: the first step involves a detailed history that identifies lower back pain (LBP) of >3 month's duration, age of onset before 45 years, AP radiograph of the pelvis that demonstrates sacroiliitis, and involvement of the SI joint. The second step involved in the diagnosis is taken into account in the patient population in whom imaging is inconclusive. Clinicians have looked at 11 pertinent clinical features (LBP, heel pain, improvement with NSAIDs, uveitis, dactylitis, elevated acute phase reactants such as ESR and CRP, psoriasis, alternating buttock pain, asymmetric arthritis,

T. Malik (ed.), *Practical Chronic Pain Management*, https://doi.org/10.1007/978-3-030-46675-6_31

and Inflamatory Bowel Disease -IBD) and presence of 4 out of the 11 features is required to confirm the diagnosis [1]. In the case described, the patient demonstrated both sacroiliitis on the pelvic AP film and uveitis, psoriasis, and improvement with NSAIDs.

What Is the Pathophysiology of This Condition?

Multiple factors have been implicated in the pathogenesis of ankylosing spondylitis. The factors include a genetic background and its interaction with target anatomic structures, gut microbes, and innate immune mechanisms. At the affected organs, *IL-17*, *IL-17A*, and TNF-alpha have been shown to play a significant role [2].

The most significant contribution comes from an *HLA-B27* gene. However, the presence of *HLA-B27* gene is not necessary for diagnosing the disease, as this disease is also present in patients without this gene.

Some of the significant challenges experienced by researchers are, but not limited to, the simultaneous bone formation and resorption extending to a pathological degree. The osteoblastic process eventually leads to syndesmophytes and, in extreme conditions, can cause rigidity of the vertebral column. Below are the three postulated mechanisms of pathogenesis.

Genetic Factors

HLA-B27 has been primarily implicated in the disease and has been shown to be present in 85–95% of people who are of a certain ethnicity as well as in 6% of the US population [3]. *HLA-B27* differs from other HLA1 molecules, and these differences could be responsible for its pathogenesis. The differences include the presence of an unpaired cysteine at residue 67 and this unique configuration allows the human leukocyte antigen (HLA) to form homodimers and oligomers of free chains. *HLA-B27*, as a massive loose chain, can exist as a dimer and is involved in AS pathogenesis. These dimers are located in the gut and joints and when presented to antigen-presenting cells (APCs) can augment IL-23 cells and ultimately produce IL-17 [4]. *HLA-B27* has also been involved in autophagy.

Non-HLA genes, though not many, may still provide the clue about AS. These non-MHC AS-causing genes can be grouped into several functional categories: *ERAP1* and *ERAP2*, *IL 23/17*, *TNF* gene family, T lymphocytes.

Proinflammatory Mediators

The roles of proinflammatory mediators have been highlighted in observational studies. COX, TNF, and IL17 are the targets of current therapy.

Role of the Gut Mucosa, IL-23, and Microbes

In patients with the presence of microscopic bowel lesions, the disease process begins within the gut where IL-23 receptor (IL-23R)-positive innate lymphoid cells (ILCs) that produce IL-17 (a proinflammatory cytokine) and IL-22, are activated by spondyloarthritides (SpA)-specific gut microbiota [5]. Activated ILCs migrate to the joint and regions where they begin an inflammatory process involving the TNF-alpha. The implicated IL-22 activates osteoclasts.

How Is the Problem Managed?

Taking the treatment of this clinical problem into consideration, it has been elucidated in the literature that the treatment of ankylosing spondylitis (AS) is extensive and is separated into medical, interventional, and surgical options.

Non-pharmacological Treatment

Non-pharmacological treatments of joint inflammation and sacroiliitis, resulting from the disease, are limited to patients with grade 1A. Physical therapy by trained individuals with the help of an exercise program should be started for individuals with the minimal disease and as an initial treatment. Exercises ranging from stretching to hydrotherapy help increase patients' ranges of motion.

Pharmacological Therapy

Pharmacological therapy involves either one or more of the following agents: NSAIDs, sulfasalazine, TNF-alpha inhibitors, and glucocorticoids. Indomethacin, as the most effective NSAID, is used with the usual dose of 25 mg twice or three times daily, and for the extended-release 75 mg once daily with a maximum one dose of 50 mg and maximum daily dose of 100 mg. The treatment can be used in increments of 25–50 mg per week.

Patients who have persistent, active, symptomatic AS should use continuous NSAIDs to control symptoms. This approach is in agreement with the 2010 Assessment of SpondyloArthritis International Society (ASAS)/European League Against Rheumatism (EULAR) recommendations [6]. Analgesics, including opioids, are rarely used and are preferable when side effects like renal failure, myocardial infarction, gastric ulcers, and vision and skin changes have to be avoided.

Retrospective studies have highlighted the role of low-dose steroids (5 mg daily) used for 1 week. Low-dose modified-release (MR) prednisone significantly reduced disease activity, fatigue, stiffness, and pain in steroid-naïve patients with SpA.

Pain management strategies for SI joint inflammation or sacroiliitis can be broadly grouped into the following:

1. Non-pharmacological, including exercise regimens with a trained therapist, for example, range of motion exercises and hydrotherapy
2. Pharmacological management with NSAIDs as highlighted above
3. Oral steroids
4. Disease-modifying agents like sulfasalazine
5. Sacroiliac joint injections

Role of SI Joint Injections in Sacroiliitis or Hip Pain due to AS

Ankylosing spondylitis in a patient can present as hip and bilateral lower back pain, and the pain experienced by the patient is due to inflammation and spondylitis of the SI joint. The treatment aimed at using SI joint injections has proven to be beneficial to many (Fig. 31.1) [7].

The SI joint is richly innervated and pain sensitive and has a significant amount of muscle insertions. A double diagnostic block of sacroiliac joints has been shown to reduce the false-positive favorable rates of single diag-

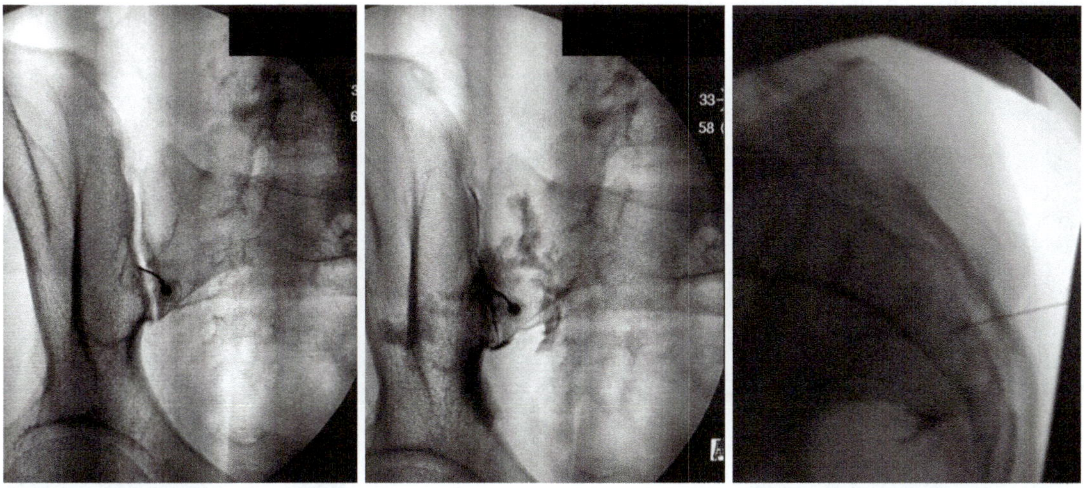

Fig. 31.1 Sacroiliac injection of corticosteroids

nostic blocks by some 20%. Recently, SI joint injections have proven to be beneficial in spondyloarthropathy [8].

A systematic review was performed to evaluate the utility of physical therapy for patients with ankylosing spondyloarthropathy, but the exact regimen and the type of exercise are still to be determined [9].

Role of Radiofrequency Ablation for SI Joint Inflammation

Radiofrequency ablation (RFA) offers a long-term effective pain control intervention when the side effects of repetitive steroid injections are undesirable and also as a long-term pain control measure for people not responsive to conventional pain control strategies (Fig. 31.2). Even though the sensory innervation of the SI joint is still under debate, a significant number of posterior sensory innervation is thought to be transmitted from S1, S2, and S3 dorsal rami via the lateral branches and medial branches from L4 and L5 dorsal rami [10]. The anterior portion of the joint is thought to be obtaining sensory innervation from the lumbosacral plexus [11]. There are schools of thought that believe some regions of SI joint are either devoid or receive innervation from obturator and gluteal nerves. There are three types of RFA: low-intensity RFA, cooled RFA, and pulsed RFA. There are no definitive techniques, as the understanding of the sensory innervation is still evolving. There are no set standards or guidelines for specific nerve roots targets. However, the three most common techniques, as highlighted in the literature, are three puncture technique (focused at the lateral upper quadrant of S1–S3 dorsal foramina and targeted to dorsal rami of L4, L5 and S1-S3 nerves) [12], strip lesion technique (continuous lesion pattern from L4–L5 dorsal rami to S1–S3 dorsal lateral foraminal aperture) [13], and leap frog technique (multiple probes close together to allow the production of consistent and large thermal lesion) [14]. Overall, RFA of the SI joint has been shown to be beneficial for SI joint inflammation.

What Is the Prognosis of This Condition?

Sacroiliitis due to ankylosing spondylitis seems to have a moderate to poor prognosis and is usually dependent upon the nature of the disease. For instance, in people with ankylosing spondylitis, the quality of the progression of this disease determines the overall prognosis. There is no complete cure and the treatment is symptomatic.

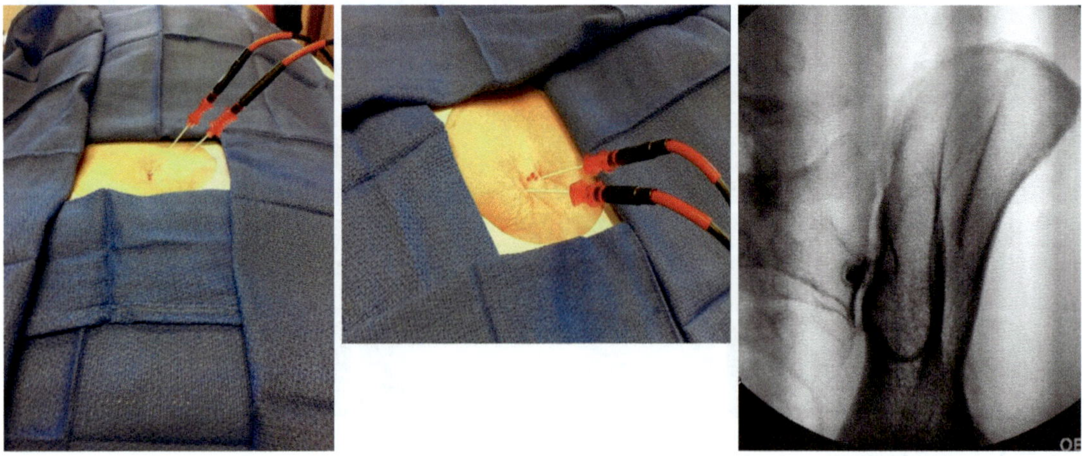

Fig. 31.2 Radiofrequency ablation of SIJ

Discussion

Prevalence

The prevalence of sacroiliac joint pain is estimated to range between 10% and 62% based on the setting; however, quite a number of analyzed studies suggest a point prevalence of around 25%, with a false-positive rate for uncontrolled blocks of approximately 20%. [15] Up to 10–25% of the pain in patients with persistent lower back pain below L5 is due to sacroiliac joint inflammation.

Lower back pain is a widespread clinical problem and accounts for a significant number of visits to healthcare providers. Lower back pain was found to have a point prevalence of 22–65% in a global review performed in 2000. The mean overall prevalence of lower back pain is around 38%. An analysis by the *Journal of the American Medical Association* highlighted that the annual cost from lower back and neck pain accounted for 87.6 billion dollars (US Spending on Personal Health Care and Public Health, 1996–2013).

Differential Diagnosis

In this review, we have described a 33-year-old male patient with ankylosing spondylitis who was referred to the pain clinic by his PCP for chronic lower back pain and sacroiliac inflammation. On evaluation, an MRI of the pelvis was performed, which implicated sacroiliitis as the cause of back pain.

There are multiple etiologies of lower back pain, ranging from lumbar radiculopathy to hip and lumbar spine syndrome, lumbar stenosis, facet arthropathy, sacroiliac joint inflammation, and arthropathy.

Lower back pain is a widespread clinical problem and is typically multifactorial. Some of the common differential diagnoses of lower back pain include lumbar radiculopathy, lumbar stenosis, sacroiliac joint inflammation, tumor of the spinal cord, and facet arthropathy.

Predictive Value of Different Clinical Features and Lab Testing/ Imaging

The presence of four out of the five features in patients with lower back pain (onset of back pain before the age of 40, insidious onset, improvement with exercise, no improvement with rest, and pain at night with improvement upon arising) has a sensitivity of 80% and specificity of 74% for an inflammatory cause of the back pain.

Imaging is important in the workup of patients with AS and axial SpA. Specific radiographic and MRI findings are a cornerstone in the diagnosis, and these modalities are also useful in monitoring the disease. CT is the conventional, but insensitive, gold standard method for the assessment of structural damage in spine and sacroiliac joints, whereas MRI can help in monitoring the disease progression [11].

Strength of Evidence for Different Treatment Modalities

Ankylosing spondylitis, primarily responsible for sacroiliitis evident in this patient, is a multifactorial disease with an interaction of the genetic component with gut microbes and immune modulation with IL-17 as a critical mediator. Understanding the pathogenesis of the disease also simplifies the treatment options. The treatment options can be divided into non-pharmacological and pharmacological treatments. Non-pharmacological treatments include physical therapy, such as scheduled and supervised physical therapy that was particularly shown to be superior to non-supervised physical training. A recently published Cochrane review was intended to demonstrate an exercise regime for the lower back pain resulting from ankylosing spondylitis. However, the authors were unable to formulate a specific exercise plan that would help the people with lower back pain. Pharmacological treatments include first-line drugs such as NSAIDs; however, TNF-alpha inhibitors and glucocorticoids have a distinct role in suppressing the inflammation.

One of the critical, interventional strategies that has helped with the sacroiliac joint inflammation from ankylosing spondylitis is sacroiliac joint steroid injection. These steroid injections have also helped in diagnosis while alleviating the sacroiliac joint pain and swelling. Though the evidence is not overwhelming, they seem to be helping with pain reduction and may be promising when used with pharmacological treatment. While taking into consideration the aforementioned strategies for sacroiliitis from ankylosing spondylitis, it is also imperative to adhere to and manage patients systematically in a stepwise approach based on practice guidelines established by the American College of Physician and the American Pain Society.

Seventy to eighty percent of patients with lower back pain have experienced relief, including improvement in stiffness, with NSAIDs [16]. Analgesics, including opioids, are rarely useful. Eighty percent of the patients with AS respond to treatment with one of the TNF antagonists, and roughly one-half get at least 50% improvement in a composite index, modified from the one adopted by the Ankylosing Spondylitis Assessment Group [17]. The role of sacroiliac joint injections has been shown to have moderate benefit; however, further studies are needed.

Joint clinical practice guidelines from the American College of Physicians and American Pain Society has included the following recommendations for the treatment of chronic lower back pain [18].

Clinicians should conduct a focused history and physical examination to help place patients with low back pain into one of three broad categories: nonspecific low back pain, back pain potentially associated with radiculopathy or spinal stenosis, and back pain possibly associated with another specific spinal cause. The history should include assessment of psychosocial risk factors, which predict the risk for chronic disabling back pain (strong recommendation, moderate-quality evidence).

Clinicians should not routinely obtain imaging or other diagnostic tests in patients with nonspecific low back pain (strong recommendation, moderate-quality evidence).

Clinicians should perform diagnostic imaging and testing for patients with low back pain when severe or progressive neurologic deficits are present or when harsh underlying conditions are suspected from history and physical examination (strong recommendation, moderate-quality evidence).

Clinicians should evaluate patients with persistent low back pain as well as patients with signs or symptoms of radiculopathy or spinal stenosis with magnetic resonance imaging (preferred) or computed tomography only if they are potential candidates for surgery or epidural steroid injection (for suspected radiculopathy) (strong recommendation, moderate-quality evidence).

Clinicians should provide patients with evidence-based information on low back pain concerning their expected course, advise patients to remain active, and provide information about useful self-care options (strong recommendation, moderate-quality evidence).

For patients with low back pain, clinicians should consider the use of medications with proven benefits in conjunction with back care and self-care information. Clinicians should assess the severity of baseline pain and functional deficits, along with potential benefits, risks, and relative lack of long-term efficacy and safety data before initiating therapy (strong recommendation, moderate-quality evidence). For most patients, first-line medication options are acetaminophen or nonsteroidal anti-inflammatory drugs.

For patients who do not improve with self-care options, clinicians should consider the addition of non-pharmacologic therapy with proven benefits: spinal manipulation for acute low back pain; intensive interdisciplinary rehabilitation, exercise therapy, acupuncture, massage therapy, spinal manipulation, yoga, cognitive-behavioral therapy, or progressive relaxation (weak recommendation, moderate-quality evidence) for chronic or subacute low back pain.

Future Directions or Clinical Trials in Progress

Future directions and clinical trials are underway to determine specific exercise regimens that are tailored to patients with sacroiliitis, as well as for immunotherapies targeting the mechanisms involved in inciting and progression of the disease.

Conclusion

In conclusion, there are multiple etiologies regarding lower back pain; however, for patient under 33 years of age in the presence of history of other immune-mediated diseases, the origin of the pain is likely due to sacroiliac joint disease of ankylosing spondylitis. The treatment options range from non-pharmacologic therapies such as exercise regimes and pharmacological options including NSAIDs, TNF-alpha inhibitors, and glucocorticoids. SI joint steroid injections have an important role in ameliorating pain and also for diagnostic purposes. Further studies are needed to further elaborate on SI joint steroid injections, tailored exercise regimes, and disease-modifying agents.

References

1. den Berg V, Hooge MD, Rudwaleit M, Sieper J, Gaalen FV, Reijnierse M, Landewé R, Huizinga T, van der Heijde D. ASAS modification of the Berlin algorithm for diagnosing axial spondyloarthritis: results from the SPondyloArthritis Caught Early (SPACE)-cohort and the Assessment of SpondyloArthritis international Society (ASAS)-cohort. Ann Rheum Dis. 2012;72(10):1646–53.
2. Raychaudhuri SP, Raychaudhuri SK. Mechanistic rationales for targeting interleukin-17A in spondyloarthritis. Arthritis Res Ther. 2017;19(1):51.
3. Schlosstein L, Terasaki PI, Bluestone R, Pearson CM. High association of an HL-A antigen, W27, with ankylosing spondylitis. N Engl J Med. 1973;288(14):704–6.
4. Ranganathan V, Gracey E, Brown MA, Inman RD, Haroon N. Pathogenesis of ankylosing spondylitis — recent advances and future directions. Nat Rev Rheumatol. 2017;13(6):359–67.
5. Praet LV, Bosch VFD, Mielants H, Elewaut D. Mucosal inflammsation in spondylarthritides: past, present, and future. Curr Rheumatol Rep. 2011;13(5):409–15.
6. Braun J, Van den Berg R, Baraliakos X, Boehm H, Burgos-Vargas R, Collantes-Estevez E, et al. Update of the ASAS/EULAR recommendations for the management of ankylosing spondylitis. Ann Rheum Dis. 2011;70:896–904.
7. Braun J, Bollow M, Seyrekbasan F, Häberle HJ, Eggens U, Mertz A, Distler A, Sieper J. Computed tomography guided corticosteroid injection of the sacroiliac joint in patients with spondylarthropathy with sacroiliitis: clinical outcome and follow-up by dynamic magnetic resonance imaging. J Rheumatol. 1996;23:659–64.
8. Levin JH. Prospective, double-blind, randomized placebo-controlled trials in interventional spine: what the highest quality literature tells us. Spine J. 2009;9:690–703.
9. Sharan D, Rajkumar JS. Physiotherapy for ankylosing spondylitis: systematic review and a proposed rehabilitation protocol. Curr Rheumatol Rev. 2017;13:121–5.
10. Dreyfuss P, Henning T, Malladi N, Goldstein B, Bogduk N. The ability of multi- site, multi-depth sacral lateral branch blocks to anesthetize the sacroiliac joint complex. Pain Med. 2009;10:679–88.
11. Foley BS, Buschbacher RM. Sacroiliac joint pain: anatomy, biomechanics, diagnosis, and treatment. Am J Phys Med Rehabil. 2006;85:997–1006.
12. Buijs EJ, Kamphuis ET, Groen GJ. Radiofrequency treatment of sacroiliac joint-related pain aimed at the first three sacral dorsal rami: a minimal approach. Pain Clinic. 2004;16:139–46.
13. Burnham RS, Yasui Y. An alternate method of radiofrequency neurotomy of the sacroiliac joint: a pilot study of the effect of pain, function, and satisfaction. Reg Anesth Pain Med. 2007;32:12–9.
14. Ferrante FM, King LF, Roche EA, et al. Radio frequency sacroiliac joint denervation for sacroiliac syndrome. Regl Anesth Pain Med. 2001;26:137–42.
15. Simopoulos TT, Manchikanti L, Singh V, Gupta S, Hameed H, Diwan S, Bollow M, Seyrekbasan F, Häberle HJ, Eggens U, Mertz A, Distler A, Sieper J. A systematic evaluation of prevalence and diagnostic accuracy of sacroiliac joint interventions. Pain Physician. 2012;15(3):E305–44.
16. Song IH, Poddubnyy DA, Rudwaleit M, Sieper J. Benefits and risks of ankylosing spondylitis treatment with nonsteroidal antiinflammatory drugs. Arthritis Rheum. 2008;58:929–38.
17. Anderson JJ, Baron G, van der Heijde D, Felson DT, Dougados M. Ankylosing spondylitis assessment group preliminary definition of short-term improvement in ankylosing spondylitis. Arthritis Rheum. 2001;44:1876–86.
18. Chou R, Qaseem A, Snow V, Casey D, Cross JT Jr, Shekelle P, Owens DK, Clinical Efficacy Assessment Subcommittee of the American College of Physicians, American College of Physicians, American Pain Society Low back Pain Guidelines Panel. Diagnosis and treatment of low back pain: a joint clinical practice guideline from the American College of Physicians and the American Pain Society. Ann Intern Med. 2007;147(7):478–91.

45-Year-Old Man with Leg Pain and Numbness

32

Robert Fuino and Waqar Waheed

Case Description

A 45-year-old man presents with a 5-day history of right leg pain. He describes the pain as acute in onset with constant numbness with overlying pins and needles burning involving his anterior shin. He has noticed that the toes on his right foot have been dragging on the floor, causing him to trip. One day prior to presentation, he developed similar but milder symptoms on his left leg. He denies history of low back pain, trauma, rashes, joint pain, constitutional symptoms, polydipsia, polyuria, or history of hepatitis. There is no history of prolonged kneeling, squatting, leg crossing, or prolonged immobility. He has no medical problems, takes no medications, and has no family history of neurologic problems. He does not use any tobacco, alcohol, or any illicit substances.

His general examination reveals intact peripheral pulses and no joint swelling nor decreased range of motion. His strength examination is notable for right foot weakness in dorsiflexion and eversion, with preserved strength of foot inversion, knee flexion and extension, and hip abduction. His sensory examination reveals diminished sensation over the anterolateral shin and dorsum of the foot, sparing high thigh or posterior lower leg. There are similar but milder examination findings on his left leg. There are no asymmetries in reflexes and his plantar responses are downgoing. He walks with a steppage quality to his gait on his left.

What Is Your Preliminary Diagnosis?

The differential diagnosis for unilateral leg pain is broad and can be divided into neurologic and non-neurological disorders. A thorough history and examination are essential to narrow down such a broad differential. A history needs to include the onset and progression of symptoms, location, presence of numbness or weakness, and aggravating or alleviating factors. Assessment of comorbid medical conditions such as diabetes, alcohol use, infections such as hepatitis, travel history, and family history of neuropathy are useful. The presence of rash, weight loss, and constitutional symptoms is also helpful. Non-neurologic disorders, such as bursitis, peripheral vascular disease, fibromyalgia,

The original version of this chapter was revised. The correction to this chapter can be found at https://doi.org/10.1007/978-3-030-46675-6_47

R. Fuino
Department of Neurology, University of Vermont Medical Center, Burlington, VT, USA

W. Waheed (✉)
Department of Neurosciences, University of Vermont Medical Center, Burlington, VT, USA
e-mail: waqar.waheed@uvmhealth.org

T. Malik (ed.), *Practical Chronic Pain Management*, https://doi.org/10.1007/978-3-030-46675-6_32

and other musculoskeletal causes, can be considered initially in this patient prior to the history. As this patient has signs suggestive of focal neuropathic pain, sensory loss, and asymmetric foot drop, the diagnosis appears most consistent with neurologic causes.

The next step in diagnosis involves the physical examination. A general examination, including examination of skin for rashes, joint examination, and presence of peripheral pulses, can also provide additional diagnostic clues. A focused neurologic examination is needed if a neurologic cause is suspected, including strength examination, sensory examination, deep tendon reflexes, and observation of gait.

Prior to examination, his differential diagnosis for a neurologic cause of leg pain and foot drop depended on the area of the nervous system involved. The absence of upper motor neuron signs (increased tone, hyper-reflexia, and upgoing plantar response), a sensory level, and bowel/bladder involvement suggests that the site of the lesion is at or distal to the anterior horn cell of the spinal cord. The presence of sensory symptoms excludes pure motor disorders such as motor neuron diseases, neuromuscular junction, or muscle disorders. The most probable site of disease is at the nerve roots, plexus, or peripheral nerves.

Atypical L5 radiculopathy could cause pain in this distribution, but it is classically associated with intermittent radiation and back pain. Disc herniation, spinal foraminal stenosis, mass lesions, infections (such as Lyme disease or tuberculosis), or inflammatory conditions, such as sarcoidosis, are potential considerations for a radiculopathy. Similarly, causes of a lumbosacral radiculoplexopathy were possible, such as structural lesions, diabetic amyotrophy, and nondiabetic lumbar radiculoplexopathy. However, absence of findings suggesting multiple nerve root involvement within the same limb, such as involvement of proximal muscles or calves, makes this less likely.

The motor examination narrows down the differential diagnosis considerably. It is important to perform a neurologic examination as to avoid unnecessary testing, interventional procedures, and even surgery [1]. Attention can be paid to his strength and sensory examination, particularly asymmetry in testing. The presence of weakness in foot dorsiflexion and ankle eversion indicates involvement of the peroneal nerve. However, preserved strength of ankle inversion, knee flexion, or hip abduction shows integrity of more proximal tibial, sciatic, and superior gluteal nerves, respectively. This examination is suggestive of a common peroneal nerve neuropathy, and the sensory examination is also consistent with this conclusion.

An approach to evaluating a patient with suspected polyneuropathy is demonstrated in Fig. 32.1. Characterizing the patient's symptoms can help diagnose and characterize different types of polyneuropathy, which can inform further testing to refine the differential diagnosis. One should first characterize whether the symptoms are sensory, motor, autonomic, or a combination of these. In addition, the pattern of involvement, onset, and progression of symptoms can suggest categories of causes of symptoms. Finally, as one would do for the evaluation of polyneuropathy, inquiring about red flags associated with atypical causes is necessary. These are also listed in Fig. 32.1 and include acute or subacute onset, relapsing or remitting course, marked asymmetric pattern of pain, concomitant cranial nerve deficits, and upper extremities being more severely affected than lower extremities. The presence of these could suggest immune-mediated, vasculitic, neoplastic, or paraneoplastic causes. The presence of these historical signs in a neuropathy, rather than a radiculopathy, should lead to prompt neurological referral and additional investigations, including electro-diagnostic testing and serology. Lumbar puncture, expanded serologic evaluation, and a potential nerve or muscle biopsy are possible additional considerations.

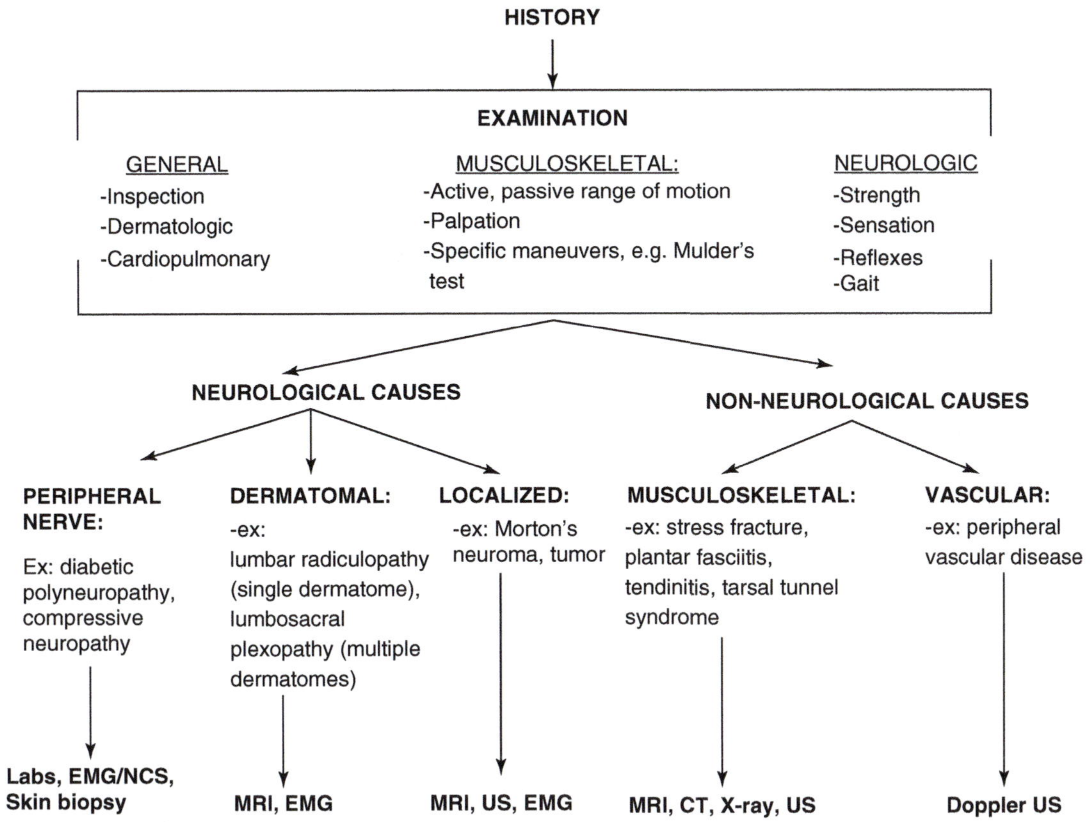

Fig. 32.1 Approach to polyneuropathy

This patient's history and examination is suggestive of asymmetric bilateral peroneal neuropathy, with features suggestive of an inflammatory cause such as mononeuritis multiplex. Further diagnostic testing will be needed to determine the cause. A list of diagnostic considerations for asymmetric or the beginning of a multifocal neuropathy is listed in Table 32.1.

How Is Diagnosis Confirmed?

The differential diagnosis based on this patient's history is confirmed by pertinent diagnostic testing. Imaging of the affected extremity, such as an MRI, is an option should a structural cause be suspected. Electro-diagnostic testing, including electromyography and nerve conduction studies with an experienced provider, is necessary to confirm and characterize the diagnosis of nerve pathology. It allows insight into the severity of the process and whether the process is primarily related to axon degeneration or peripheral demyelination. Findings of demyelination are not consistent with vasculitic neuropathy. This information further informs the likelihood of certain diagnoses, as well as prognosis and timing of treatment. Initial evaluation and selected additional labs to consider are listed in Table 32.2. Given the morbidity associated with systemic vasculitis, as well as its long-term treatment with immunosuppressant, nerve/muscle biopsy is important for definitive diagnosis

Table 32.1 Differential diagnosis of asymmetric or multifocal neuropathy [30, 31]

1. *Vascular/ischemic*	3. *Mechanical*
Vasculitis	Multiple injuries or burns
Primary systemic vasculitis	Entrapment syndromes
Microscopic polyangiitis	Wartenberg's migratory sensory neuritis
Polyarteritis nodosa	4. *Infections*
Granulomatosis without polyangiitis	Viral disease: HBV[a], HCV[a], HIV[a], VZV, CMV[a], WNV, HTLV-1[a]
Granulomatosis with polyangiitis	Lyme disease[a]
Eosinophilic granulomatosis with polyangiitis	Tuberculosis
Essential mixed cryoglobulinemia	Leprosy[a]
Vasculitis secondary to other connective tissue disorders	Other
Rheumatoid arthritis	5. *Neoplastic*[a]
Systemic lupus erythematosus	Direct infiltration
Sjogren's syndrome	Paraneoplastic syndromes
Systemic sclerosis	Tumor compression
Dermatomyositis	Primary AL amyloidosis
Mixed connective tissue disease	Intravascular large B-cell lymphoma
Hypocomplementemic urticarial vasculitis syndrome	Lymphomatoid granulomatosis
Non-systemic vasculitides	Acute leukemia
Non-systemic vasculitic neuropathy	6. *Genetic*
Diabetic radiculoplexus neuropathy	Charcot Marie Tooth variants
Localized cutaneous or neuropathic vasculitis	Krabbe disease
Sickle cell anemia	Tangier disease
Thrombophilic or hemophilic states	Porphyria
Idiopathic thrombocytopenic purpura	Hereditary neuropathy with liability to pressure palsies
Embolic causes	Mitochondrial disorders
Cholesterol emboli	Familial amyloid polyneuropathy
Atrial myxoma	7. *Drug-induced*[a]
Infective endocarditis	Antibiotics: penicillin, sulfonamides, minocycline
2. *Inflammation/Immune-mediated*	Interferon-alpha
Sarcoidosis[a]	TNF-alpha inhibitors
Behcet's disease[a]	Montelukast and leukotriene receptor antagonists
Guillain-Barre variants	Amphetamines
Multifocal motor neuropathy	Cocaine
Lewis-Sumner syndrome	Heroin
Inflammatory bowel disease[a]	Others
Other	

[a]Occasionally associated with vasculitis

in the evaluation of a suspected vasculitic neuropathy.

In this case, electro-diagnostic testing performed in the patient showed findings consistent with moderate-to-severe asymmetric bilateral axonal peroneal neuropathies, left worse than right, raising concern for a mononeuritis multiplex pattern. Initial workup showed normal hemoglobin A1c, elevated erythrocyte sedimentation rate and C-reactive protein, a negative antinuclear antibody, negative hepatitis B and C testing, negative rheumatologic markers, and otherwise unremarkable labs. A nerve biopsy was ultimately pursued, which demonstrated

Table 32.2 Laboratory and imaging evaluation when immune-mediated neuropathy is suspected [30, 31]

Routine	Second line
Complete metabolic panel (electrolytes, urea, creatinine, liver function tests)	Anti double-stranded DNA antibody, anti-Smith antibody, cyclic citrullinated peptide antibodies
Complete blood cell count (for anemia or eosinophilia)	Sinus X-ray
Serum protein electrophoresis	Chest CT
Urine protein electrophoresis	Anti-SSA/SSB, Schirmer test
Hemoglobin A1c or 2-hour glucose tolerance test	Angiotensin-converting enzyme level
Chest X-ray	Porphyria screen
Erythrocyte sedimentation rate, C-reactive protein	HIV, West Nile virus, Lyme disease, cytomegalovirus
Hepatitis B and C serologies	Lumbar puncture and CSF analysis
Antinuclear antibody, antineutrophil cytoplasmic antibody, rheumatoid factor	Paraneoplastic antibodies
Cryoglobulins, C3, C4	Imaging for malignancy

mononuclear inflammatory cells with associated fibrinoid necrosis of the vessel wall consistent with vasculitic neuropathy. After rheumatologic consultation, it was determined that there was no other organ involvement and he did not meet diagnostic criteria for polyarteritis nodosa or other systemic vasculitides. Therefore, his diagnosis was determined to be mononeuritis multiplex as a consequence of non-systemic vasculitic neuropathy.

What Is the Pathophysiology of This Condition?

The pathophysiologies of immune-mediated neuropathies are varied, as are those of the different vasculitides. Vasculitis as a disorder can be either systemic, affecting multiple organs, or localized to the nervous system. When neuropathy occurs in absence of a systemic vasculitis, this is referred to as non-systemic vasculitic neuropathy (NSVN). NSVN is the most commonly reported vasculitic neuropathy [2–4]. Systemic vasculitis can be a primary disorder, related to inflammation of small, medium, or large blood vessels. For example, neuropathy can affect 60–70% of patients with polyarteritis nodosa and eosinophilic granulomatosis with polyangiitis, whereas it can affect 40–50% of patients with microscopic polyangiitis [5]. In addition, vasculitis can be secondary as a result of infections, drugs, and cancers. No specific trigger can be found for some.

Primary vasculitic neuropathies represent a group of heterogeneous disorders, each with different mechanisms that may not be completely understood for each disease. For example, microscopic polyangiitis and non-systemic vasculitic neuropathy are caused by separate mechanisms involving anti-neutrophilic antibodies and complement pathways, respectively [6]. Whether immune complex deposition in vessel walls leads to an inflammatory cascade, or cell-mediated immunity by T-cell pathways leads to vessel wall injury, the final common pathway leads to ischemic injury of nerves. Damage of the vasa nevorum, particularly epineurial arteries, leads to ischemic injury and resultant degeneration of axons [7].

How Is This Problem Managed?

The primary focus of treatment in immune-mediated (including vasculitic) neuropathy is based on treating underlying inflammation. Treatment of other primary systemic vasculitides is used to guide treatment based on paucity of randomized clinical trials for NSVN. This often involves immunosuppressive agents such as glucocorticoids, cyclophosphamide, rituximab, azathioprine, and methotrexate. The approach to treatment, including in NSVN, involves two phases. First, remission-induction therapy is meant to stop inflammatory damage from continuing acutely to sub-acutely, usually with corticosteroids. This can be accomplished with monotherapy of prednisone 1 mg/kg daily with prolonged taper. Combination therapy with a second agent, such as azathioprine or mycophenolate mofetil, can also be used for additional effects seen later in the course on induction and remission. The choice of whether to use a second agent in the acute phase depends on the severity of disease. For example, less intense agents such as methotrexate or mycophenolate mofetil can be added for milder cases, and plasma exchange can be substituted in for severe cases [8].

After induction therapy, maintenance therapy involves continued treatment with these medications for at least 18–24 months with the aim of reducing the likelihood of clinical relapses. Escalation in the intensity of regimen (such as addition of plasma exchange, IVIG) is guided by the initial severity as mentioned previously, or also the response to less intense therapy. Treatment with maintenance immunosuppression with tapering corticosteroids and a second agent (azathioprine, methotrexate, mycophenolate mofetil, cyclophosphamide, etc.) is continued until remission has been achieved. If there is associated hepatitis B or C infection, treatment with antivirals is warranted, with timing of treatment determined on a case-by-case basis.

Multidisciplinary teamwork between neurology and rheumatology is important in vasculitic neuropathy. Management of immune-mediated neuropathy is focused on supportive care as well as its underlying cause. Physical and occupational therapy is helpful for recovery in presence of sensory and motor deficits. Management of analgesic treatment is warranted for pain associated with vasculitic neuropathy. Several medication classes are options for pain control, including anticonvulsants, tricyclic antidepressants (TCAs), serotonin-norepinephrine reuptake inhibitors (SNRIs), and opioids, which are to be discussed later in this chapter. It is important to note that symptomatic treatment of pain in these conditions is often not based on large, randomized controlled trials for each separate disease process resulting in neuropathy. Instead, symptomatic treatment of pain is often borrowed by successful treatments in studies dominated by more common neuropathic pain conditions such as painful diabetic neuropathy or post-herpetic neuralgia [9–11]. Please refer to prior chapters on diabetic neuropathy for further information.

As mentioned previously, the strength of evidence for treatment specific to NSVN is suboptimal. More importantly, it is worth noting that these trials for primary systemic vasculitides are often not focused on neuropathy or appropriate measurements of efficacy in neuropathy. Therefore, their efficacy is extrapolated for vasculitic neuropathy and cannot be definitively relied on [12]. Consultation with a rheumatologist or neurologist is warranted in immunosuppressant management.

In summary, treatments are often individualized based on disease process, severity, and patient factors. Either corticosteroid monotherapy or combination with another immunosuppressive agent is used in a higher dose induction phase, followed by tapering doses over a maintenance period. Urgent consultation for treatment regimens with rheumatology or neurology is warranted based on the organ systems involved.

What Is the Prognosis of This Condition?

The prognosis of a neuropathy depends on its cause and its mechanism. As a general principle, nerve injury resulting in axonal damage has a longer recovery time than damage from demyelination. As vasculitic neuropathy is axonal in nature, this underscores the need for prompt diagnosis and treatment to mitigate damage with prolonged consequences.

NSVN rarely spreads beyond the peripheral nervous system to other organs. The relapse rate is estimated to be 30% after treatment is started [13]. The prognosis is good in those who receive treatment. In a cohort study, approximately 13% of treated patients become asymptomatic, and 68% have mild or moderate symptoms while remaining independent and ambulatory [14]. Mortality is noted to be approximately 10% at 5 years [14]. Chronic pain is common and ranges from 37 to 60% of patients who are treated [14, 15].

Discussion

Prevalence

The epidemiology of NSVN is poorly studied, but it can be estimated based on studies of systemic vasculitides. The annual incidence of primary and secondary vasculitis was 140 cases per million people in a Spanish study. Primary systemic vasculitis represented 82 percent of these cases, [16] with the most common secondary vasculitis resulting from connective tissue disease. A separate Parisian study estimated the prevalence of individual primary systemic vasculitides, finding a range from 10 to 31 per 1,000,000 adults for each disease process [17]. For example, most common disease was polyarteritis nodosa, with prevalence of 30 per 1 million, followed by microscopic polyangiitis.

These studies do not account for the prevalence of neuropathy in these patients. Neuropathy is a common manifestation of some primary and secondary vasculitides. As an example, it occurs in approximately 74% of PAN patients, [18] most commonly resulting in a mononeuritis multiplex pattern. The most common vasculitic neuropathies include NSVN, microscopic polyangiitis, and polyarteritis nodosa [2]. It is not uncommon for painful asymmetric neuropathy to be a presenting symptom for these disorders and the majority of presentations of NSVN. [14]

Differential Diagnosis

The use of the history and physical is important to accurately determine whether symptoms are related to a polyneuropathy, mononeuropathy, radiculopathy, or other neurologic process. The differential for polyneuropathies and radiculopathies is beyond the scope of this chapter. A differential diagnosis for asymmetric or multifocal neuropathy is listed in Table 32.1.

Compressive or multifocal mass lesions or burns should not be missed on history or diagnostic testing. Non-compressive causes can result from inflammation, infection, degeneration, and infarction. A more detailed list of diagnostic considerations for asymmetric or multifocal neuropathies is listed in Table 32.1. Underlying diabetes, gammopathies, or alcoholism can result in asymmetric nerve dysfunction, but more classically causes a distal, symmetric polyneuropathy. Non-compressive causes can also result from inflammatory insults such systemic vasculitides. Primary vasculitic disorders associated with neuropathy include polyarteritis nodosa, microscopic polyangiitis, ANCA-associated vasculitis, among others. Systemic vasculitides can also result secondarily from connective tissues disease (such as rheumatoid arthritis or systemic lupus erythematosus), sarcoidosis, infections, drugs, or malignancy. Finally, non-systemic vasculitis of the peripheral nervous system is a syndrome with peripheral nerve vasculitis without clinical or laboratory evidence of another systemic vasculitis. Diabetic neuropathic injury, if asymmetric, classically results in an asymmetric radiculoplexus neuropathy, but it can rarely cause individual nerve injury. Once considered a separate entity, diabetic radiculoplexus neuropathy (also known as diabetic amyotrophy) is classified as a form of NSVN.

It is worth noting that an acute or subacute mononeuropathy can sometimes be the initial phase of mononeuritis multiplex, a syndrome that requires an expedited evaluation to reveal the underlying cause, many of which are listed in Table 32.1.

Predictive Value of Different Clinical Features (Both on History and Physical Exam) and Lab Testing/Imaging

Neuropathy secondary to vasculitis presents focally (over a peripheral nerve distribution) and painfully over an acute to subacute time period. There have been limited studies, often small case-control or retrospective cohort studies, which have addressed predictors of a vasculitic neuropathy. For example, pain is a particularly sensitive finding in vasculitic neuropathy, which occurs in 90% of patients [14]. Rapid onset, defined as symptom onset less than 1 month from biopsy, was poorly sensitive and 100 percent specific in one small retrospective study of 40 patients [19].

The most common pattern of involvement is classically mononeuritis multiplex (multiple mononeuropathies), but plexopathy and distal sensorimotor polyneuropathy can also occur. Asymmetry or multifocal involvement (either clinically or by electrodiagnostics) is common due to characteristic patchy involvement and is one of the more specific characteristics [20–22]. However, due to varying EMG definitions and small sample sizes, precise estimates of specificity are difficult to assess. In addition, as the neuropathy progresses and more nerves are affected, the overall pattern may look similar to a distal length-dependent polyneuropathy.

Just as clinical and electrophysiological data is not completely sensitive or specific to vasculitic neuropathy, laboratory data also has considerable overlap with other diagnoses. Elevated erythrocyte sedimentation rate and C-reactive protein were studied in two small studies and were at least sensitive for vasculitis, although they were not specific to this diagnosis [19, 23]. In addition, this does not distinguish between causes of vasculitic neuropathy, other neuropathic disorders that would result in elevated markers, and elevation due to other chronic conditions. No other laboratory or radiographic findings have been studied that have reliable predictive value for NSVN. There are additional clinical and laboratory data that, conversely, have low association with NSVN and systemic vasculitic neuropathy. These include demyelination, CSF pleocytosis, CSF protein >110 mg/dL, and pure motor symptoms [24].

Arguably the most important diagnostic test is the nerve and muscle biopsy. One cohort study of 70 combined superficial peroneal nerve (SPN) and peroneus brevis muscle (PBM) biopsies classified biopsy samples as positive, suspicious, or negative for vasculitic neuropathy. A positive SPN/PBM biopsy had 60% sensitivity for vasculitic neuropathy, while the group of positive or suspicious biopsies had a 86% sensitivity and 85% specificity [25]. The yield of sural nerve biopsy is less robust, [26] perhaps related to this nerve being less involved in vasculitic neuropathies. The combined nerve and muscle biopsy has also been questioned in terms of its yield over nerve biopsy alone [4, 25]. It is worth noting that these studies are not specific to NSVN and, therefore, the exact sensitivity for biopsy in NSVN can only be estimated imprecisely, some suggest approximately 50% [13].

While the sensitivity and specificity of biopsies are imprecise, the diagnosis of vasculitic neuropathy often relies upon the use of histopathologic data to establish high confidence in diagnosis according to the Brighton Collaboration group [27]. In the absence of a classic clinical presentation with either classic electrodiagnostic or clinical exam findings, a biopsy is essential for diagnosis.

Strength of Evidence for Different Treatment Modalities

As previously mentioned, the evidence for specific treatments for NSVN is largely based on data from treatment of systemic vasculitis, although studies did not have reliable outcome measures for neuropathy or pain. Therefore, it is difficult to accurately extrapolate the quality of evidence for vasculitis confined to the peripheral nervous system.

Regarding analgesic treatment, evidence for specific agents can be borrowed from trials in more common neuropathic pain conditions, such as diabetic neuropathy or post-herpetic neuralgia. These medications include SNRIs, TCAs, anticonvulsants, and consideration of opioid agents with consideration of risks and benefits. Discussion of the level of evidence supporting these agents can be found in a separate chapter on diabetic neuropathy.

As mentioned previously, treatment regimens for vasculitic neuropathy utilize corticosteroids with or without a second immunosuppressive agent, such as cyclophosphamide, rituximab, mycophenolate mofetil, or others. Specific regimens can be customized to each individual patient and disease process, which is beyond the scope of this chapter. Rheumatologic or neurologic consultation is warranted for creating treatment regimens.

Recognizing the heterogeneity of disease processes, treatment regimens, and strength of evidence surrounding each, in this case of NSVN, immunomodulatory treatment is unsurprisingly without strong evidence for specific regimen. A 2007 Cochrane review of immunosuppressive treatment of non-systemic vasculitic neuropathy found no adequate randomized controlled trials [28]. Two retrospective cohort studies have analyzed corticosteroid monotherapy versus corticosteroid plus second-line therapy [14, 29]. One study demonstrated that combination (cyclophosphamide plus steroid) therapy was more effective than corticosteroid monotherapy in achieving sustained improvement at 6 months in a cohort of 48 NSVN patients [14].

Future Directions or Clinical Trials in Progress

Future study is warranted on specific treatment regimens for specific vasculitic disease entities, although the prevalence of individual disorders makes design of studies challenging. Registries, such as one from the UK and Ireland Vasculitis Study group, can be useful in the study and understanding of these disorders and their treatments. Research continues to focus on the pathogenesis of NSVN as it compares to other organ vasculitides.

Conclusion/Summary

Non-systemic vasculitic neuropathy is an isolated vasculitis of the peripheral nervous system. It is the most common of the vasculitic neuropathies, which often results in asymmetric, painful sensorimotor deficits. History of asymmetry, rapid progression, or other red flags could suggest a vasculitic process, which could result in significant morbidity if left untreated. It is paramount to evaluate if an underlying systemic vasculitis is contributing to avoid damage to other organ systems.

Diagnosis is based on history and exam findings, supported by laboratory data, and often needs confirmation by nerve biopsy. The prognosis of vasculitic neuropathy depends on the underlying cause and chronic pain is common. Control of neuropathic pain is possible with the similar agents as other neuropathic pain (TCAs, anticonvulsants, SNRIs), with consideration of opioids in select cases. In addition, control of inflammation with corticosteroids and immunosuppressants is needed to prevent further progression, although the exact treatment regimen has not been rigorously studied in NSVN. Consultation with neurology or rheumatology is needed on an urgent basis. Further research is needed into optimal treatment regimens and mechanisms of injury.

References

1. Reife MD, Coulis CM. Peroneal neuropathy misdiagnosed as L5 radiculopathy: a case report. Chiropr Man Therap. 2013;21(1):12.
2. Collins MP, Periquet MI. Isolated vasculitis of the peripheral nervous system. Clin Exp Rheumatol. 2008;26(3):S118–30.
3. Kararizou E, Davaki P, Karandreas N, Davou R, Vassilopoulos D. Nonsystemic vasculitic neuropathy: a clinicopathological study of 22 cases. J Rheumatol. 2005;32(5):853–8.
4. Bennett DL, Groves M, Blake J, Holton JL, King RHM, Orrell RW, et al. The use of nerve and muscle biopsy in the diagnosis of vasculitis: a 5 year retrospective study. J Neurol Neurosurg Psychiatry. 2008;79(12):1376–81.
5. Collins MP, Arnold WD, Kissel JT. The neuropathies of vasculitis. Neurol Clin. 2013;31(2):557–95.
6. Takahashi M, Koike H, Ikeda S, Kawagashira Y, Iijima M, Hashizume A, et al. Distinct pathogenesis in nonsystemic vasculitic neuropathy and microscopic polyangiitis. Neurol Neuroimmunol Neuroinflamm. 2017;4(6):e407.
7. Morozumi S, Koike H, Tomita M, Kawagashira Y, Iijima M, Katsuno M, et al. Spatial distribution of nerve fiber pathology and vasculitis in microscopic polyangiitis-associated neuropathy. J Neuropathol Exp Neurol. 2011;70(5):340–8.
8. Ntatsaki E, Carruthers D, Chakravarty K, D'Cruz D, Harper L, Jayne D, et al. BSR and BHPR guideline for the management of adults with ANCA-associated vasculitis. Rheumatology (Oxford). 2014;53(12):2306–9.
9. Waldfogel JM, Nesbit SA, Dy SM, Sharma R, Zhang A, Wilson LM, et al. Pharmacotherapy for diabetic peripheral neuropathy pain and quality of life: a systematic review. Neurology. 2017;88(20):1958–67.
10. Bril V, England J, Franklin GM, Backonja M, Cohen J, Del Toro D, et al. Evidence-based guideline: treatment of painful diabetic neuropathy: report of the American Academy of Neurology, the American Association of Neuromuscular and Electrodiagnostic Medicine, and the American Academy of Physical Medicine and Rehabilitation. PM R. 2011;3(4):345–52, 52.e1–21.
11. Attal N, Cruccu G, Baron R, Haanpaa M, Hansson P, Jensen TS, et al. EFNS guidelines on the pharmacological treatment of neuropathic pain: 2010 revision. Eur J Neurol. 2010;17(9):1113–e88.
12. De Vita S, Quartuccio L, Fabris M. Rituximab in mixed cryoglobulinemia: increased experience and perspectives. Dig Liver Dis. 2007;39:S122–8.
13. Collins MP, Hadden RD. The nonsystemic vasculitic neuropathies. Nat Rev Neurol. 2017;13(5):302–16.
14. Collins MP, Periquet MI, Mendell JR, Sahenk Z, Nagaraja HN, Kissel JT. Nonsystemic vasculitic neuropathy: insights from a clinical cohort. Neurology. 2003;61(5):623–30.
15. Uceyler N, Geng A, Reiners K, Toyka KV, Sommer C. Non-systemic vasculitic neuropathy: single-center follow-up of 60 patients. J Neurol. 2015;262(9):2092–100.
16. Gonzalez-Gay MA, Garcia-Porrua C. Systemic vasculitis in adults in northwestern Spain, 1988-1997. Clinical and epidemiologic aspects. Medicine (Baltimore). 1999;78(5):292–308.
17. Mahr A, Guillevin L, Poissonnet M, Ayme S. Prevalences of polyarteritis nodosa, microscopic polyangiitis, Wegener's granulomatosis, and Churg-Strauss syndrome in a French urban multiethnic population in 2000: a capture-recapture estimate. Arthritis Rheum. 2004;51(1):92–9.
18. Pagnoux C, Seror R, Henegar C, Mahr A, Cohen P, Le Guern V, et al. Clinical features and outcomes in 348 patients with polyarteritis nodosa: a systematic retrospective study of patients diagnosed between 1963 and 2005 and entered into the French Vasculitis Study Group Database. Arthritis Rheum. 2010;62(2):616–26.
19. Terrier B, Lacroix C, Guillevin L, Hatron PY, Dhote R, Maillot F, et al. Diagnostic and prognostic relevance of neuromuscular biopsy in primary Sjogren's syndrome-related neuropathy. Arthritis Rheum. 2007;57(8):1520–9.
20. Zivkovic SA, Ascherman D, Lacomis D. Vasculitic neuropathy – electrodiagnostic findings and association with malignancies. Acta Neurol Scand. 2007;115(6):432–6.
21. Deprez M, de Groote CC, Gollogly L, Reznik M, Martin JJ. Clinical and neuropathological parameters affecting the diagnostic yield of nerve biopsy. Neuromuscul Disord. 2000;10(2):92–8.
22. Lindenlaub T, Sommer C. Cytokines in sural nerve biopsies from inflammatory and non-inflammatory neuropathies. Acta Neuropathol. 2003;105(6):593–602.
23. Vrancken AF, Notermans NC, Jansen GH, Wokke JH, Said G. Progressive idiopathic axonal neuropathy – a comparative clinical and histopathological study with vasculitic neuropathy. J Neurol. 2004;251(3):269–78.
24. Collins MP, Dyck PJ, Gronseth GS, Guillevin L, Hadden RD, Heuss D, et al. Peripheral nerve society guideline on the classification, diagnosis, investigation, and immunosuppressive therapy of non-systemic vasculitic neuropathy: executive summary. J Periph Nerv Syst. 2010;15(3):176–84.
25. Collins MP, Mendell JR, Periquet MI, Sahenk Z, Amato AA, Gronseth GS, et al. Superficial peroneal nerve/peroneus brevis muscle biopsy in vasculitic neuropathy. Neurology. 2000;55(5):636–43.
26. Rappaport WD, Valente J, Hunter GC, Rance NE, Lick S, Lewis T, et al. Clinical utilization and complications of sural nerve biopsy. Am J Surg. 1993;166(3):252–6.

27. Hadden RDM, Collins MP, Zivkovic SA, Hsieh ST, Bonetto C, Felicetti P, et al. Vasculitic peripheral neuropathy: case definition and guidelines for collection, analysis, and presentation of immunisation safety data. Vaccine. 2017;35(11):1567–78.
28. Vrancken AF, Hughes RA, Said G, Wokke JH, Notermans NC. Immunosuppressive treatment for non-systemic vasculitic neuropathy. Cochrane Database Syst Rev. 2007;(24):1.
29. Pollard JD, McLeod JG, Spies JM, Davies L. Vasculitis confined to peripheral nerves. Brain. 1996;119(5):1441–8.
30. Collins MP. The vasculitic neuropathies: an update. Curr Opin Neurol. 2012;25(5):573–85.
31. Gwathmey KG, Burns TM, Collins MP, Dyck PJ. Vasculitic neuropathies. Lancet Neurol. 2014;13(1):67–82.

A 65-Year-Old Man with Leg Pain While Walking

33

Mary Leemputte and Sophy C. Zheng

Case Description

A 65-year-old male nonsmoker with past medical history of scoliosis, diabetes type II, hypertension, hyperlipidemia, and depression/anxiety presents to the outpatient pain clinic with reports of left leg pain while walking.

He has been experiencing cramping pain in the buttocks, radiating down the lateral thigh to anterior shin on the left leg intermittently for the past year but significantly more frequently in the last 3 months. The symptoms are most pronounced on walking and ease up on resting. He feels his legs get heavy and crampy prompting him to sit and take a break. He has rare episodes of pain down his right leg as well. The patient was previously able to ambulate one to two miles without difficulties but now has difficulty completing two blocks before resting to relieve his symptoms. He reports occasional low back pain in the evening while he is lounging on the couch in addition to the leg pain. He previously had a left knee replacement with occasional residual knee pain and was told he has hip arthritis and had prior left knee replacement. He denies numbness or tingling. He also denies any fevers or chills, redness, skin changes, or wounds. No falls or trauma noted around onset of pain and no recent travels.

A systematic physical examination reveals a morbidly obese male who appears his stated age. He walks with a minimally hunched gait. On inspection, no skin changes, swelling, or warmth noted in either leg. Mild scoliosis can be seen on inspection. Sensation is subjectively decreased in the left lateral thigh and anterior shin. Strength is 4/5 in the left first toe compared to the right, otherwise equal. Patellar and Achilles reflexes are symmetric 2+ and dorsalis pedis and posterior tibial pulses are equal bilaterally. Pain is reproduced with extension and lateral bending to the left. Bilateral axial loading is positive. Palpation of sacroiliac joint, FABERS, and internal and external rotations of the hips are negative.

What Is Your Preliminary Diagnosis?

The patient's clinical presentation of leg pain with walking has a broad differential diagnosis that includes spine-related pathologies and vascular and musculoskeletal causes. Patient's symptom of crampy pain on walking is called intermittent claudication which could be vascular or neurogenic in origin. Vascular etiologies such as peripheral arterial disease should be considered,

M. Leemputte
Department of Anesthesiology, Northwestern University, Chicago, IL, USA
e-mail: mary.leemputte@northwestern.edu

S. C. Zheng (✉)
Department of Anesthesiology, Northwestern Memorial Hospital, Chicago, IL, USA
e-mail: sophy.zheng@nm.org

T. Malik (ed.), *Practical Chronic Pain Management*, https://doi.org/10.1007/978-3-030-46675-6_33

Table 33.1 Diagnosis for leg pain

	Neurogenic	Vascular
Pain	Neuropathic/nerve root based	Tissue/muscle ischemia
Distribution	Buttock/legs	Calf muscles
Relief	Flexion of lumbar spine	Rest
Diagnosis	MRI/CT	Angiography
Pulses	Normal	Weak/absent
Back pain	Yes (usually)	No (usually)

especially in an older individual with cardiovascular risk factors (Table 33.1). One would expect not only pain with walking but also often improvement of symptoms upon standing in such case. Physical exam findings may also include cool, shiny skin, distal extremity pallor on elevation, capillary refill, or nonhealing wounds [1]. Similarly, deep venous thrombosis should be suspected in a patient with unilateral lower extremity pain, especially if risk factors are present.

Musculoskeletal pathologies including hip or knee osteoarthritis, sacroiliitis, or stress fracture may also cause similar unilateral symptoms sometimes that are exacerbated by activities. Frequently, physical exam findings such as positive FABER's test and Ganslen's maneuver would help confirm diagnosis of sacroiliac disease, and hip pain is frequently worse with internal rotation of the hip. Less commonly, knee pain from range of causes including arthritis to ligamentous injuries on the left side may cause referred hip or lower leg pain, although tenderness is often maximum around the knee joint and rarely extends in dermatomal distribution. Diabetic neuropathy is possible in a patient with poorly controlled diabetes and with subjective sensory changes that follow a sock distribution from distal extremity upward, often bilaterally.

A few key features should promptly raise the suspicion of spinal stenosis. Of particular concern are age of the pateint (>50), his complain of leg heaviness with walking, worsening of leg symptoms significantly with back extension and radiation of pain/numbness or heaviness in a dermatomal distribution down the legs. On physical examination, his wide-based, hunched gait is also important, as it often decreases pain [2]. Broadly speaking, spinal stenosis may be central which results in bilateral symptoms, or foraminal in nature which may result in symptoms only on one side. All these clinical findings are suggestive but diagnostic of lumbar spinal stenosis, which still requires confirmation.

How Is the Diagnosis Confirmed?

The diagnosis of lumbar spinal stenosis requires evidence of anatomical reduction of the lumbar spinal canal as determined radiographically. However, studies indicate that up to 20% of asymptomatic patients have imaging consistent with the disease [1]. Many still rely on historical criteria published by Verbiest et al., in which relative spinal stenosis occurs with 10–12 mm and absolute stenosis less than 10 mm. In vitro and in situ studies by Schonstrom et al. have suggested that the diagnosis can be made with cross-sectional area of the dural sac. According to their criteria, stenosis above 70–80 mm^2 is unlikely to be symptomatic [2, 3]. The lateral recess when less than 4 mm in AP dimension is considered significant. In either case, the diagnosis can only be confirmed after radiographic reports have been correlated with clinical symptomatology.

MRI is often considered standard in confirming diagnosis (Fig. 33.1). It can not only evaluate stenosis but also rule out other causes like compression fracture, tumor, and infection. Also it can point out the etiology of stenosis like disc protrusion, facet joint hypertrophy or facet cyst causing lateral recess or foraminal stenosis, and extent of ligamentum flavum hypertrophy. This information is useful when planning for management. MRI provides superior soft tissue differentiation, including the nerve roots and disc versus bone material, and often demonstrates location of pathology. When MRI is contraindicated, CT may be used since it discriminates cortical bone from soft tissue, such as the ligamentum flavum [4]. Some reports indicate that the latter revealed smaller spinal canal areas [4]. With this in mind, MRI is often considered first line and would be appropriate for our patient.

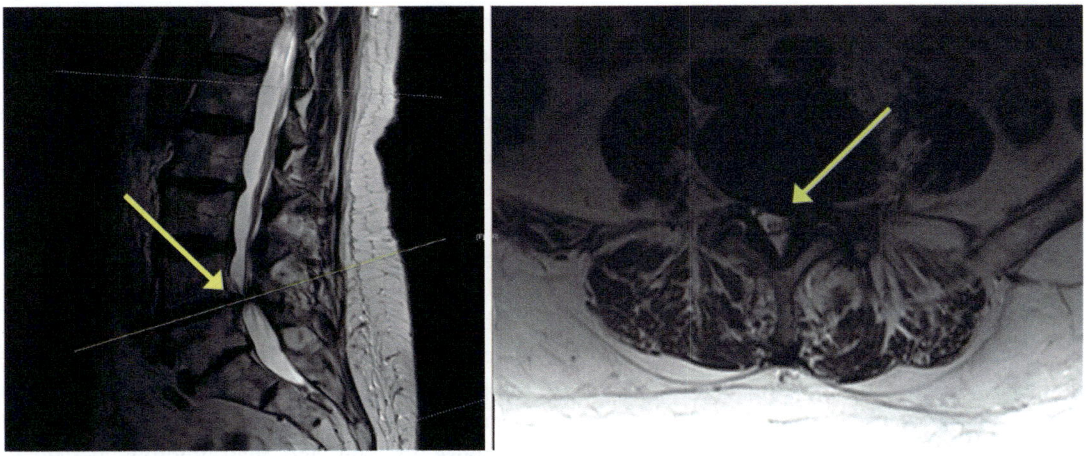

Fig. 33.1 Sagittal image on the left indicates spinal stenosis at L4–L5. Cross-sectional image on the right indicates that this stenosis is asymmetric to the left, and with combination of facet arthrosis, there is compression of the exiting left L5 nerve root consistent with the patient's symptoms

In cases for which the diagnosis is less clear, additional tests may be warranted. An A1c and a diabetic microfilament exam may be indicated to assess for diabetic neuropathy. Knee or hip osteoarthritis may be seen on X-ray, although patients may have both osteoarthritis and spinals stenosis simultaneously. Although in this case, physical examination was not fully consistent with PAD, ankle-brachial index may be performed with results <0.5 indicating critical ischemia [1]. The clinician may also consider Doppler ultrasonography if exam suggests deep venous thrombosis. New research has also assessed the utility of electromyography measurements in those with indeterminate radiographic findings. Some studies suggest an association between mid-zone stenosis and abnormal EMG, but correlation with clinical symptoms remains indeterminate [5].

What Is the Pathophysiology of This Condition?

Lumbar spinal stenosis is commonly explained on the basis of physical narrowing of the space around the nerves. This may explain some clinical features like worsening pain with extension and less pain with flexion, but not many other features. There is no correlation between the severity of stenosis on MRI and severity of symptoms. Many patients with severe stenosis of MRI are even asymptomatic. It has also been shown that the severity of stenosis on MRI does not even correlate with abnormal EMG findings. This lack of correlation between stenosis and clinical features explains lack of benefit in many patients after decompressive surgery.

MRI studies reveal venous dilatation proximal to stenosis pointing toward a physical component to the pathology. Some cadaveric studies reveal thickening of meninges around the nerve roots revealing an arachnoiditis-type pathology possibly from chronic compression; histopathological studies have revealed loss of axons and demyelination of large fibers in the involved nerve roots. There is suggestion of microcirculatory disturbance from endothelial dysfunction around the nerve roots, damaged blood–brain barrier, and poor CSF flow around the nerve roots, all contributing to poor health of nerve roots. The role of inflammatory mediators like IL-1 and tumor necrosis factor in mediating pain is also very likely as can be seen from good response to steroid injection in many cases.

Spinal stenosis is classified as primary, when it results from congenital pathology or postnatal abnormalities. More often etiology is secondary or acquired, as majority of the cases results from spinal degeneration or less commonly from infection, surgery, or trauma [3]. Of these, chronic degeneration represents the most typical cause and may occur at the level of the central canal, lateral recess, or foramina.

Central stenosis may result from hypertrophy of the ligamentum flavum caused by chronic mechanical stress. Studies suggest that fibrosis along the dorsal ligamentum flavum may be linked with transforming growth factor (TGF)-β released from endothelial cells, as well as interleukin (IL)-1β [3]. Decreased disc height may also cause anteroposterior or transversal loss of diameter, likewise resulting in central stenosis. Stenosis also occurs at the lateral recess due to degenerative changes, including facet joint hypertrophy with or without spondylolisthesis, vertebral endplate osteophytosis, and decreased disc height. Foraminal stenosis may result from both anteroposterior and vertical narrowing. The former results from disc space narrowing and extension of structures anterior to the facet joint capsule. Vertical stenosis is often due to vertebral endplate protrusion, lateral annulus fibrosis, or herniated discs compressing the nerve root along the superior pedicle. Of note, foraminal stenosis occurs most commonly at the L5 nerve root, as the L5-S1 foramen is smaller relative to root area [3]. While many patients exhibit generalized degeneration at multiple levels, those with central stenosis are more likely to exhibit bilateral radiculopathy as irritation and compression of both left and right dorsal nerve roots are impacted. Those with degeneration at the lateral recess or foramen experience greater compression unilaterally.

Unique in the presentation of spinal stenosis is a dynamic component in which positional changes may significantly alter anatomy. Central canal space may decrease with extension and with loading. Similarly, foraminal stenosis will increase 12% with flexion and up to 15% with extension [6]. These changes are important in that they reflect the dynamic clinical presentation, namely pain with extension and with standing.

How Is This Problem Managed?

Once appropriate imaging has been obtained, the physician should assess patient goals to facilitate appropriate treatment planning. The management of this condition is very personalized. Many patients have other comorbid conditions and many of them may not be mobile because of other issues. Most patients intuitively mange themselves by altering their activity, posture, and or using walking-assist devices to ambulate longer.

Physical therapy has been proposed for those with spinal stenosis, although few studies investigate its role as a sole intervention. Researchers suggest that it may protect against the further deconditioning that patients often experience in response to pain and may improve perceived recovery, although changes in pain or function are indeterminate [7].

In the SPORT study, subjects who received physical therapy along with other conservative therapies, in general, did well and were less likely to require surgery. The interventions are focused on improving range of motion, strengthening core and leg muscles, and posture training – all to stabilize lumbar spine and minimize lumbar lordosis. Improved activity may promote cardiovascular health and weight loss which is much more beneficial in the long run.

There is no proven effective pharmacological therapy. First-line options for those with moderate symptoms may include oral medications, physical therapy, and bracing. Neuropathic medications, NSAIDs, and muscle relaxants are often used. In patients with refractory symptoms, opioids may be added as adjunct as well [8]. However, as many patients are over 50–60 years old, these medications are not without risk. Gabapentin improved walking distance in one study that was unblended, results of which could not be reproduced. In a different retrospective study, gabapentin showed improvement in quality of life when patients were interviewed using QOL-5 questionnaire. In another observational study, pregabalin up to 150mg per day was given to 57 patients with leg pain more than 3. Of the 57 patients, 10 became pain free, 22 experienced pain to less than 2/10, and 15 reported pain was 3 or less. As a result, gabapentinoids are considered an essential part of conservative treatment. Studies in general suggest that they produce improved clinical outcomes compared with NSAIDs, including improved walking distance, recovery of sensory deficit, sleep, and improvement in pain scores [3, 9]. However, as with all conservative treatments, it is likely most beneficial in those with milder symptoms [10].

The use of epidural steroid injections for spinal stenosis has emerged as an important topic, as spinal stenosis accounts for up to 30% of all epidural steroid injections [11]. Delport et al. have reported improvements in pain scores in those receiving epidural steroids [3]. Further studies by Abdi et al. have indicated significant short-term relief defined as <6 weeks but variable long-term benefits [11]. Not surprisingly, there is no correlation between the severity of stenosis and response to steroid injection. Most studies and meta-analysis find short-term relief from steroid injection. A Cochrane review found no benefit of injection calcitonin in the epidural space.

Surgical decompression is considered a definite treatment when patient fails to respond to conservative interventions or is showing signs of nerve damage. Surgical interventions range from minimally invasive to open decompression with fusion. Unfortunately there are no guidelines on who will benefit from which type of surgery. In the 2016 Cochrane meta-analysis of surgical intervention versus non-surgical management, there was no clear benefit for surgery. The authors attributed this to lack of standardization in evaluation, patient selection, surgical management, and outcome reporting. The Spine Patient Outcome Research Trial (SPORT) revealed that, patients who opted for surgery had better pain control at year 2 but not much better functional status. The Main Lumbar Spine Study found that patients who predominantly have leg pain from spinal spinal stenosis tends to do better with surgical decompression compared to non-surgical interventions in the short-term.

Interestingly, spinal stenosis is a leading indication for spine surgery in older adults. Most commonly, the procedure involves a decompressive laminectomy with the goal of removing nerve root irritation with resulting success rates of 45–72% [12]. For those with multilevel pathology or malalignment of the vertebrae, some surgeons pursue concurrent fusion to avoid instability. The SPORT trial compared laminectomy to NSAIDS, exercise, and education. A small improvement in pain was seen at 2 years with surgical intervention [13]. Thus, these large studies show moderate improvement, but results vary based on outcome measured. In general, one-third of patients do not fare well after surgery, despite careful selection.

There are quite a few procedures on the market to target this condition, including a percutaneous or minimally invasive decompressive procedure. Their attraction stems from the fact that these can be done with minimal sedation and do not require post-procedure admission or rehab making them much cheaper and with much lower complication rates.

Minimally invasive lumbar decompression (MILD) is meant to decompress central spinal stenosis due to ligamentum flavum hypertrophy. It is an image-guided procedure, in which using a 5 mm cannula, ligament flavum is partially removed to improve central canal space. In a 2014 meta-analysis of available studies, Kreiner et al. found statistical improvement in Oswestery Disability Index (ODI) and Visual Analogue Score (VAS) after the treatment [14]. But they found these studies to be of low quality and heavily sponsored by industry. Per CMS insistence, the safety of the procedure was evaluated over a 2-year period. The data was published in 2018. It was found that patients followed over 2 year demonstrated no higher incidence of spinal instability and improvement in pain score and ODI was maintained for 2 years.

FDA has also approved interspinous process spacer as implantable device to treat spinal stenosis. Two such devices are X-STOP and Spurion. The devices work by introducing some kyphosis, limiting extension but permitting flexion of the lumbar spine. When compared to epidural steroid injection in 191 patients with mild to moderate symptoms, X-STOP provided long-term improvement. When compared to decompressive laminectomy, the devices have less complication, are cheaper, and have lower 90-day complications, but at 1 year have higher reoperation rates.

Neuromodulation therapy has also been proposed for nonsurgical candidates not responding to conservative therapy. In one study, 91 patients underwent spinal cord stimulation trial; among them, 60 patients responded with 50% improvement and 41 opted for permanent implant. They were followed up for a mean of 34.5 months (+/−22 months). Thirty-nine patients continued to show 50% or more pain relief.

What Is the Prognosis of This Condition?

The Spinal stenosis course is very variable. In an observational study where patients who refused surgery were followed for years, revealed a pattern of fluctuating symptoms with many patients showing improvement without any intervention. In another study with patients with neurogenic claudication and myelographically proven lumbar spinal stenosis, symptoms remained unchanged in 60% of the patients. The Maine Lumbar Spine Study also found that if a patient opts to delay surgery when indicated, he/she still gets equal benefit from it when he/she again opts for it. That is, delaying surgery does not cause any harm.

Research indicates approximately half of patients remain clinically stable, with one-fourth exhibiting improvement and one-fourth exhibiting worsening [6]. According to the North American Spine Society categorization, 30–50% of patients with mild to moderate symptoms experience a promising course [6]. However, the clinical outcomes of those who present with severe symptoms require further investigation.

Discussion

Lumbar spinal stenosis was first described by the Dutch surgeon Henk Verbiest in 1954. He in a series of seven patients ascribed symptoms of claudication to spinal stenosis. Spinal stenosis is a disease of old age, and with changing population, its incidence is bound to increase. Currently, more than 1 million physician office visits are due to lumbar spinal stenosis. About 89,000 laminectomies were performed for neurogenic claudication in 2009. Recent work has attempted to elucidate the prevalence of spinal stenosis. The Framingham Heart Study cohort revealed that only 20% of those under 40 years qualified for acquired stenosis compared 47.2% of those who were 60–69 years. Of note, those with a CT-derived absolute diagnosis were more likely to experience back pain [6].

The prevalence is higher in female compared to male. In age 70 or older, prevalence of spinal stenosis is 40–50% in females compared to 20–30% in males.

Patients with spinal stenosis represent an increasingly relevant cohort within the United States. Recently, the fastest growth in lumbar surgeries occurred in patients with spinal stenosis [1]. As discussed, some studies highlight the advantage of surgical intervention with focus on decompressive laminectomy over conservative treatment. As complex fusion procedures are performed on an aging population with growing medical comorbidities, further work is indicated to determine which patients best qualify for which procedures [1]. Thus, a thorough risk-benefit discussion weighing possible complications should be encouraged with each patient presenting clinically. The disease can cripple significant portion of older population. Even in those who seem to benefit from surgery, the effects tend to wear off with time. The benefit of repeat surgery is less clear and more complicated as older patients tend to have less favorable health for a more cumbersome repeat surgery.

Study of the predictive value of clinical symptoms has yielded results proposing high risk of diagnosis in those >60 years, symptoms for over 6 months, exacerbation with extension, exacerbation with standing, symptoms that occur with walking, and improvement with rest [15].

While no one treatment regimen has been consistently validated in long-term data, conservative regimens may be attempted for those with mild symptoms. Moderate to severe spinal stenosis is more likely to be symptomatic and represents the most common indication for epidural steroid injection [3]. Surgical treatments include decompressive laminectomy and spinal fusion. With the potential for protracted course and significant disability, spinal stenosis remains an important consideration for future investigation in an attempt to pair the appropriate patients with the most optimal interventions.

Conclusion/Summary

Spinal stenosis represents a dynamic decrease in the anatomic space afforded by the spinal canal, whether at the central canal, lateral recess, or foramina. Typically, this results from chronic degeneration of the spine and is seen in older individuals. Diagnosis includes radiographic evidence of such anatomic narrowing but is largely based on correlation with patient history and physical exam findings. Because the natural history of spinal stenosis may be difficult to predict, the physician should facilitate shared decision-making when assessing goals of treatment.

References

1. Bailey M, Griffin K, Scott D. Clinical assessment of patients with peripheral arterial disease. Semin Intervent Radiol. 2014;1:292–9.
2. Friedly J. Long-term effects of repeated injections of local anesthetic with or without corticosteroid for lumbar spinal stenosis: a randomized trial. Arch Phys Med Rehabil. 2017;98(8):1499–507.
3. Genevay S, Atlas S. Lumbar spinal stenosis. Best Pract Res Clin Rheumatol. 2010;24(2):253–65.
4. Eun S, Lee H, Lee S, Kim K, Liu W. MRI versus CT for the diagnosis of lumbar spinal stenosis. J Neuroradiol. 2012;39(2):104–9.
5. Kuittinen P, Sipola P, Aalto TJ, Määttä S, Parviainen A, Saari T, Sinikallio S, Savolainen S, Turunen V, Kröger H, Airaksinen O, Leinonen V. Correlation of lateral stenosis in MRI with symptoms, walking capacity and EMG findings in patients with surgically confirmed lateral lumbar spinal canal stenosis. BMC Musculoskelet Disord. 2014;15:241–2477.
6. Johnsson K, Rosen A. The natural course of lumbar spinal stenosis. Clin Orthop Relat Res. 1992;279(1):82–6.
7. Weinmeister K, Trentman T, Joseph J, Shinaman H, et al. Outcomes in 615 spinal stenosis patients treated with epidural steroids. Conference: 15th World-Federation-of-Societies-of Anaesthesiologists (WFSA) World. Argentina: La Rural, Predio Ferial de Buenos Aires; 2012. p. 25–30.
8. Koc Z, Ozcakir S, Sivrioglu K, Gurbet A, Kucukoglu S. Effectiveness of physical therapy and epidural steroid injections in lumbar spinal stenosis. Spine. 2009;34(10):985–9.
9. Ammendolia C, Stuber K, Tomkins-Lane C, Schneider M, Rampersaud Y, Furlan A, Kennedy C. What interventions improve walking ability in neurogenic claudication with lumbar spinal stenosis? A systematic review. Eur Spine J. 2014;10(14):3262–6.
10. Yaksi A, Ozgonenel L, Ozgonenel B. The efficiency of gabapentin therapy in patients with lumbar spinal stenosis. Spine. 2007;32(9):938–42.
11. Abdi S, Datta S, Lucas L. Role of epidural steroids in the management of chronic spinal pain: a systematic review of effectiveness and complications. Pain Physician. 2005;8(1):127–43.
12. Deyo R, Mirza S, Martin B, Kreuter W, Goodman D, Jarvik J. Trends, major medical complications, and charges associated with surgery for lumbar spinal stenosis in older adults. JAMA. 2010;303(13):1259–65.
13. Pearson A, Lurie J, Tsteson T, Zhao W, Abdu W, Weinstein J. Who should have surgery for spinal stenosis? treatment effect predictors in SPORT. Spine. 2012;37(21):1791–802.
14. Kreiner DS, MacVicar J, Duszynski B, Nampiaparampil DE. The mild® procedure: a systematic review of the current literature. Pain Med. 2014;15(2):196–205.
15. Konno S, Hayashino Y, Fukuhara S, Kikuchi S, Kaneda K, Seichi A, Chiba K, Satomia K, Nagata K, Kawai S. Development of a clinical diagnosis support tool to identify patients with lumbar spinal stenosis. Eur Spine J. 2007;16(11):1951–7.

34 Lower Back Pain in an Elderly Patient

Hassan Aboumerhi and Tariq Malik

Case Description

A 70-year-old man presents to your clinic with long-standing back pain that has got worse in the last 3 months after a hiking trip. He describes his pain as intense and achy that is partly relieved by resting, but worse with bending, twisting, and when standing from sitting position. . He denies any balance problem or fear of falling. The patient adds that his pain shoots down the both legs but not below the knees. He denies any weakness or abnormal sensation. The patient denies an inciting event or trauma. The patient also denies bowel or urinary incontinence. He had similar but much milder flare-ups in the past but they were all self-limited and responded to nonprescription medications. This time he has tried oral acetaminophen and ibuprofen, but has only been able to obtain minimal relief.

What Is Your Preliminary Diagnosis?

The patient has pain of long-standing duration. There is absence of any red flags, i.e., history of weight loss, fever, major trauma, immunosuppression, or neurodeficit in his history. These all suggest that his pain is most likely from a degenerative process. Also his pain is worse with certain movements that stress the low lumbar spine. The fact that it does not radiate down the leg means that there is no nerve root irritation. For a 70-year-old guy with low back pain (LBP), the most likely diagnosis is degenerative disc disease, facet arthropathy, and/or paravertebral muscle pain.

What Should We Look for in the Physical Examination of the Patient?

History is very suggestive that sensory motor examination is not affected at all. However, it should be objectively confirmed with physical examination. Focus would be on gait, balance, and range of motion of lumbar spine.

He has stable gait and good balance. He has good strength in his lower limb muscles and no evidence of muscle wasting. Straight leg raising test is negative; he has good range of lumbar flexion in his lumbar spine, but extension of lumbar spine is limited and more painful than flexion. Sensory examination is unremarkable. There is no paravertebral tenderness. In the absence of any tender muscles, the pain is most likely from either the facet disease or the degenerative discs.

H. Aboumerhi
Department of Anesthesiology, Northwestern University, Chicago, IL, USA

T. Malik (✉)
Department of Anesthesia and Critical Care, University of Chicago, Chicago, IL, USA
e-mail: TMuslim@dacc.uchicago.edu; tmalik@dacc.uchicago.edu

T. Malik (ed.), *Practical Chronic Pain Management*, https://doi.org/10.1007/978-3-030-46675-6_34

It is unlikely to be from sacroiliac joint as there is no history of trauma and pain is not unilateral; but no back pain disease process has any pathognomonic clinical features.

How Is Diagnosis Confirmed?

It is almost impossible to be certain of a diagnosis based on history and physical examination. Imaging is obtained to rule out infection, tumor, trauma, or inflammatory disorders, but rarely imaging confirms an etiology of a chronic pain disorder. Imaging can also evaluate the extent of degeneration as a marker of a disease process. In this patient, it is suspected that pain is either from lumbar degenerative disc disease or from facet arthropathy. MRI of the lumbar spine will be able to evaluate both apart from ruling any tumor process since that is always a possibility at advanced age like this patient. Computed tomogram can also be used if MRI is not possible. Xray of the lumbar spine is must if MRI or CT spine cannot be done for one reason or another in an elderly patient who has worsening of his chronic back pain or a new onset back pain to rule out a malignant process even though it is not as sensitive as the other two images mentioned above. Pain from facet disease is confirmed by performing medial nerve branch block at the suspected level. More than 75% pain relief after a properly done procedure confirms the pain source is from these joints. In the absence of significant pain relief (less than 50%), pain is most likely coming from the discs.

What Is the Pathophysiology of This Condition?

Facet joints are synovial joints. They can be potentially afflicted by all the diseases that can affect a synovial joint. The pathogenesis involves degradation of hyaline cartilage from overactive proteases (collagenases, stromelysins, and gelatinases) and the failure of the chondrocytes to repair the loss caused by the proteases. Inflammatory cells release pro-inflammatory chemicals and enzymes that either initiate or accelerate the process of cartilage degradation. The exposure of the underlying subchondral bone results in sclerosis, followed by reactive remodeling changes that lead to the formation of osteophytes. Facet arthropathy is quite often preceded by degenerative disc disease. Loss of disc height may alter the mechanics that trigger the osteoarthritic changes in the facet joints.

How Is This Problem Managed?

Once the diagnosis is established, it is important to find out the factors that potentiate the problem. The changes in the facet joint themselves are irreversible; hence, it is vital to focus on factors that can be modified. Comprehensive evaluation should include evalauting the biopsychosocial aspects of pain. The main goal is how to improve the pateint fucntional status instead of just focussing on the pain score. Treatments may be conservative, interventional, or operative.

In general, patient is advised to try over-the-counter pain medications. This patient has already tried that. In that case the next step is to refer him to a physical therapy session to improve his biomechanics along with strengthening of his core muscles. The purpose of physical therapy sessions is to improve endurance of his core muscles. Patient is informed that the improvement in pain takes time and there may be a temporary increase in pain for 1–2 weeks as he mobilizes his painful muscles. He is asked to come back for evaluation after 2 months.

He Comes Back in Months After Completing His Physical Therapy and Still Has Pain. What Is the Next Step?

On close questioning, he admits that pain has gone better after physical therapy. He is ambulating better and sleeping better, but still low back pain is holding him back. He cannot play golf effectively and is missing on social events with his friends. You suggest that since he has failed conservative therapy, he should undergo diagnostic facet block injections, and if he gets good relief, he should undergo radiofrequency ablation of the facet joints nerves. He agrees with the plan. He undergoes radiofrequency ablation procedure after a successful diagnostic block and is satisfied with the outcome.

What Is the Prognosis of This Condition?

This issue is generally age-related and its onset occurs exponentially more frequently in elderly patients. Its exact prognosis is unknown but since it is a degenerative disorder, once the joint develop the degenerative changes, the changes are irreversible. The pain from such joint is chronic, i.e, it would fluctuate but may not ever go away completely. The impact of pain on patients' functionality can be minimized with multimodal therapy by addressing any worsening factors such as physical, mental, or environmental. It is a chronic pain disorder and requires life-long effort on the part of patient and repeated denervation if needed.

Discussion

The facet joints have long been recognized as a source of low back pain since Goldthwaite first reported that the facet joints could be a significant source of back pain in 1911 [1]. Ghormley coined the term "facet syndrome," in 1933, describing a low pain with or without leg pain after a rotational injury [2]. Hirsch published the first account whereby the injection of l-z joints reproduced patients' back pain [3]. The prevalence rate of facet joint pain varies widely in the literature, ranging from less than 5% to more than 90%. The prevalence increases as the age of the populations studied increases.

The treatment of facet joint pain, like any other chronic pain condition, should consist of a multimodal approach comprising conservative therapy, medical management, procedural interventions, and, if indicated, psychotherapy [4, 5]. Conservative therapy is the first-line therapy and it usually involves myofascial manipulation along with non-opioid analgesics. No clinical studies have directly assessed the role of pharmacotherapy or non-interventional treatment for lumbar-facet mediated pain. Data is usually extrapolated from the several controlled studies evaluating conservative treatment for axial low back pain. Guided-exercise programs and yoga have shown to reduce pain and prevent relapses in patients with chronic axial low back pain. Chiropractic manipulation and acupuncture have also been shown in randomized trials to provide significant benefit in patients with chronic low back pain [6]. The data does not identify patients who will benefit the most from different treatments. Quite often patients need frequent visits and cost becomes an issue.

Nonsteroidal anti-inflammatory drugs and acetaminophen are the first-line drugs widely considered for the treatment of LBP, with little evidence to support one particular drug over another [7–9]. Adjuvants have also been shown to be effective in relieving LBP. Schintzer et al. reviewed published clinical trials evaluating pharmacotherapy in low back pain and found strong evidence for the use of antidepressants for chronic LBP and muscle relaxants in acute back pain [10]. Untreated psychopathology can adversely affect low back pain treatment outcomes. Features of depression, anxiety disorder, and substance abuse are quite prevalent in patients with chronic low back pain [11].

Weight loss is often advocated in these patients as being overweight contributes to degenerative disease and arthritis-related resultant pain.

Interventional treatment of facet-related pain begins with a diagnostic block. Diagnostic intraarticular or medial nerve branch block are considered the most reliable means to diagnose painful facets. Nerve block is in general preferred over intraarticular injection as leakage of injectate into the surrounding area has higher potential to give false-positive result. Injections are commonly performed on two different occasions due to high incidence of false positive with single injection. There are multiple reasons for the high incidence of false positive of these blocks. False-positive results can be minimized by judicious use of local anesthetic by numbing the needle track, avoiding use of opioids during the diagnostic procedure, positioning properly the needle tip lower on the groove to avoid epidural spread, and keeping the volume of diagnostic solution less than 0.5 ml. It's asserted that instead of selecting pateint who will benefit the most from radiofrequency ablation using diagnostic nerve blocks, performing the nerve ablation procedure on pateints using clinical criteria is economically more efficient. This may result in few patients getting the abltive procedure who will not benefit from it but oveall, skipping the diagnostic nerve block step is more cost effective.

The long-term relief of back pain, reported in uncontrolled studies, after intraarticular steroid injection is variable and ranges from 18% to 63% [12]. Relief has also been noticed after plain intraarticular LA alone as well as normal saline. In the controlled trials, the results were mixed. Studies using PET scan to evaluate facet joint disease found longer relief when steroids were injected as opposed to plain LA, indicating that in those subset of patients where inflammation is contributing to pain, steroid helps.

Radiofrequency denervation of medial nerve branch is an effective treatment for pain originating from the facet joints. A number of reviews on this subject have been done which may provide different level of evidence depending upon the studies included for analysis and also on the opinions of the reviewers [13–16]. In general, relief lasts from 6 months to 2 years with a median time of 10 months. Radiofrequency denervation lasts longer and is more reliable compared to pulsed radiofrequency technique and is backed by more robust clinical evidence. The technical aspects of radiofrequency merits close attention. Focus is on achieving a sizable lesion which requires proper needle gauge and proper needle alignment. Flouroscopic guidance is invaluable in proper needle placement. Sensory testing of reproducing pain at 0.5 V is not very reliable, but reproducing motor twitch of multifidis muscles is a useful sign for proper needle placement. Twitch presence is good enough response and obtaining twitch at low voltage is not necessary. The radiofrequency ablation procedure can be repeated in future if and when the pain comes back at 6 months or longer interval and subsequent denervation provides equally long and extent of pain relief.

The evidence for intraarticular steroid injection and radiofrequency ablation of medial branch of dorsal ramus is weak to moderate at best; and for pulsed radiofrequency of these nerves to treat facet joint pain is not there at all and is now not recommended.

Facet interventions are low-risk procedures. Risk of infection is always there but has not been reported. Metabolic effects of repeated steroid injections cannot be discounted but have not been reported. Few cases of post-dural puncture headache and intrathecal placement of local anesthetic have been reported after intraarticular injection. Numbness and/or dysesthesias after radiofrequency denervation are uncommon and tend to be transient and self-limiting [17–19]. Burns with radiofrequency procedures are possible and result from electrical faults, insulation breaks in the electrodes, or generator malfunction. The most common complication after facet joint radiofrequency is neuritis, with a reported incidence of less than 5%. Administration of corticosteroid (methylprednisolone) or pentoxifylline may reduce the incidence of post-procedure pain after radiofrequency denervation.

Surgery is occasionally performed to treat facet arthropathy, despite a lack of evidence supporting fusion for degenerative spinal disorders. One reason patients with facet joint pain might respond to arthrodesis is because during surgery, medial branch often gets destroyed during pedicle screw placement.

Conclusion/Summary

Low back pain is an issue that affects a majority of Americans at some point in their lives and will progressively become more relevant to all physicians as our population ages. Healthcare providers must recognize low back pain as chief complaint rather than a diagnosis. Pain originating from the facet joints is a recognized source of LBP. The facet joints become weak with age and changes in their orientation predispose them to injury from rotational and bending stresses. The three most caudal facet joints, L3–L4, L4–L5, and L5–S1, are exposed to the greatest strain and are thus more prone to inflammation, joint hypertrophy, and osteophyte formation. Osteoarthritis of the facet joints is seen commonly in association with degenerative disc disease. There are no pathognomonic findings in history and/or physical examination that are diagnostic for lumbar facet syndrome. The pain patterns arising from the lumbar facet joints at different levels overlap considerably. Along with axial low back pain, pain from diseased lower facet joints is associated with referred pain to the buttock, thigh, groin, and even to leg, whereas that referred from the upper lumbar facet joints extends into the flank, hip, groin, and lateral thigh. Reports on the correlation between CT and MRI evidence of facet arthropathy and the response to diagnostic lumbar facet blocks are conflicting. Medial branch blocks have diagnostic, therapeutic, and prognostic values. In properly selected patients, intraarticular steroid injections and radiofrequency denervation are good treatment options even if conservative interventions have failed. The results of surgical therapies including arthrodesis for facet arthropathy are discouraging.

References

1. Goldthwait JE. The lumbosacral articulation: an explanation of many cases of lumbago, sciatica and paraplegia. Boston Med Surg J. 1911;164:365–72. [Google Scholar]
2. Ghormley RK. Low back pain with special reference to the articular facets, with presentation of an operative procedure. JAMA. 1933;101:773.
3. Hirsch D, Inglemark B, Miller M. The anatomical basis for low back pain. Acta Orthoscan. 1963;33:1–17.
4. .Qaseem A, Wilt TJ, McLean RM, Forciea MA. Noninvasive treatments for acute, subacute, and chronic low back pain: a clinical practice guideline from the American College of Physicians. Ann Intern Med. 2017;166(7):514–30. Clinical Guidelines.
5. .De Leon-Casasola. American College of Physicians clinical practice guidelines for non-invasive treatments for scute, subacute, and chronic low back pain. ASRA. https://www.asra.com/news/141/american-college-of-physicians-clinical. 21 Feb 2017.
6. Kerr DP, Walsh DM, Baxter D. Acupuncture in the management of chronic low back pain: a blinded randomized controlled trial. Clin J Pain. 2003;19:364–70.
7. Zerbini C, Ozturk ZE, Grifka J, Maini M, Nilganuwong S, Morales R, Hupli M, Shivaprakash M, Giezek H. Efficacy of etoricoxib 60 mg/day and diclofenac 150 mg/day in reduction of pain and disability in patients with chronic low back pain: results of a 4-week, multinational, randomized, double-blind study. Curr Med Res Opin. 2005;21:2037–49.
8. Videman T, Osterman K. Double-blind parallel study of piroxicam *versus* indomethacin in the treatment of low back pain. Ann Clin Res. 1984;16:156–60.
9. Mens JM. The use of medication in low back pain. Best Pract Res Clin Rheumatol. 2005;19:609–21.
10. Schnitzer TJ, Ferraro A, Hunsche E, Kong SX. A comprehensive review of clinical trials on the efficacy and safety of drugs for the treatment of low back pain. J Pain Symptom Manag. 2004;28:72–9.
11. Polatin PB, Kinney RK, Gatchel RJ, Lillo E, Mayer TG. Psychiatric illness and chronic low-back pain: the mind and the spine-which goes first? Spine. 1993;18:66–71.
12. Bogduk N. A narrative review of intra-articular corticosteroid injections for low back pain. Pain Med. 2005;6:287–96.
13. Slipman CW, Bhat AL, Gilchrist RV, Isaac Z, Chou L, Lenrow DA. A critical review of the evidence for the use of zygapophysial injections and radiofrequency denervation in the treatment of low back pain. Spine J. 2003;3:310–6.
14. Schofferman J, Kine G. Effectiveness of repeated radiofrequency neurotomy for lumbar facet pain. Spine. 2004;29:2471–3.
15. Mikeladze G, Espinal R, Finnegan R, Routon J, Martin D. Pulsed radiofrequency application in treatment of chronic zygapophyseal joint pain. Spine J. 2003;3(5):360–2.
16. Dreyfuss P, Halbrook B, Pauza K, Joshi A, McLarty J, Bogduk N. Efficacy and validity of radiofrequency neurotomy for chronic lumbar zygapophysial joint pain. Spine. 2000;25:1270–7.
17. Kornick C, Kramarich SS, Lamer TJ, Sitzman BT. Complications of lumbar facet radiofrequency denervation. Spine. 2004;29:1352–4.
18. Bogduk N, Holmes S. Controlled zygapophysial joint blocks: the travesty of cost-effectiveness. Pain Med. 2000;1:24–34.
19. Cohen SP, Hurley RW, Christo PJ, Winkley J, Mohiuddin MM, Stojanovic MP. Clinical predictors of success and failure for lumbar facet radiofrequency denervation. Clin J Pain. 2007;23:45–52.

A 55-Year-Old Woman with Chronic Gluteal Pain

35

Hassan Aboumerhi and Tariq Malik

Case Description

A 55-year-old female presents to your clinic with 5 months of persistent right-sided gluteal pain. She describes her pain as constantly aching, especially during activity. The pain is worst on transitioning from sitting to standing and when climbing stairs. Meanwhile, it is alleviated by resting seated or lying down. Acetaminophen and non-steroidal anti-inflammatory drugs (NSAIDs) originally provided relief, but they have become less effective. The pain originates in her right upper buttocks and radiates down to her right posterior thigh. She denies any weakness, numbness, or paresthesia. The patient denies an inciting event or trauma. The patient also denies bowel or urinary incontinence. Of note, the patient has a history of Crohn's disease.

Physical exam reveals tenderness over the deep back muscles on the right side. She also has tenderness along the right side of the sacrum and in the buttock area. The patient exhibits strong, symmetrical strength throughout her lower extremities with normal sensitivity to pinprick. Her gait is stable and she has problem walking in the room.

What Is Your Preliminary Diagnosis?

The key aspects of any diagnostic process are to localize pain inciting point (pain generator) and the pathological process causing or sustaining it. Gluteal pain has a multitude of etiologies. Gluteal pain can be mechanical in nature from musculoskeletal tissue or visceral in nature being referred from the tissues inside the pelvis. It is important to consider ischemic disease, especially in a patient with a history of coronary artery disease, carotid artery disease, or cerebrovascular disease. Patients with peripheral artery disease experience vascular claudication characterized by progressive pain with activity that is relieved with rest.

The patient points to her gluteal region as the site of pain; pain could come from any underlying structure namely muscles or joints or it could be a referred pain. Pain is associated with movement, making it more likely musculoskeletal in origin. Pain is insidious in onset without any traumatic event and there is no sign of any systemic illness, even though she has Crohn's disease. It is unlikely to be a referred pain as she has reproducible tenderness in the gluteal area and no sign or symptom of nerve compression or irritation as she has no motor weakness or presence of numbness or

H. Aboumerhi
Department of Anesthesiology, Northwestern University, Chicago, IL, USA
e-mail: hassan.aboumerhi@northwestern.edu

T. Malik (✉)
Department of Anesthesia and Critical Care University of Chicago, Chicago, IL, USA
e-mail: tmalik@dacc.uchicago.edu; TMuslim@dacc.uchicago.edu

T. Malik (ed.), *Practical Chronic Pain Management*, https://doi.org/10.1007/978-3-030-46675-6_35

paresthesia. This makes it most likely either a sacroiliac joint issue or gluteal muscle issue, something like piriformis dysfunction.

Gluteal muscle strain can present with pain and tenderness. This is usually due to strenuous overactivity and has a more acute presentation and resolution. Piriformis syndrome involves spasm of the piriformis muscle with impingement on the sciatic nerve. This pain can be reproduced by palpating a band-like piriformis muscle and performing Patrick's test (extension, abduction, external rotation of the ipsilateral hip). Spinal stenosis can present with gluteal pain that is worse with spinal extension and relieved by flexion.

This patient most likely has either sacroiliitis or piriformis dysfunction. Sacroiliitis is a disease-associated inflammation of the sacroiliac (SI) joint. This inflammatory process may be due to a number of causes including osteoarthritic degeneration, spondyloarthropathy related to inflammatory bowel disease, pregnancy, trauma, cancer, and infection. Sacroiliitis generally presents with lower back or gluteal pain that may or may not radiate down the lower extremity. This pain is reproducible with palpation of the sacroiliac joint or any maneuver that stresses the joint. Piriformis muscle dysfunction is usually from direct trauma or repeated micro-trauma, leg length discrepancy, obesity, pregnancy, and lumbar hyperlordosis. Pain in the buttock area that gets aggravated with sitting, tenderness to palpation pain on physcial examination manuvers that stretch the piriformis muscle are very suggestive of piriformis pain syndrome.

How Is Diagnosis Confirmed?

History and physical examination are suggestive but not diagnostic. Physical examination of patient encompassing stretching of target point is quite helpful. It has been shown that tests evaluating sacroiliac joints may be positive in about 20% of asymptomatic subjects. The sensitivity and specificity of various tests are variable. The sensitivity and the specificity of these various physical examination manuvers have been reported to be in low 20s to high 80s. The best use of these tests is that they entertain SI joint dysfunction in the differential diagnosis. Cibulka found that if three out of four commonly used SI joint tests are positive, then the sensitivity and specificity of the combined tests are 0.82 and 0.88, respectively, with positive predictive value of 0.86 and negative predictive value of 0.84.

Sacroiliitis is a clinical diagnosis based on symptoms in correlation with physical exam. Examination should reveal pain in the lower back and buttocks reproduced with palpation of the SI joint. Sacroiliitis can be confirmed with a diagnostic block and can be quantified by imaging. There is level III evidence for single diagnostic block with local anesthetic providing 75% pain relief and level II evidence for double diagnostic block providing 70% pain relief [1]. Technetium bone scintigraphy can localize the disease. Meanwhile, computed tomography (CT) or magnetic resonance imaging (MRI) can characterize the anatomy and degree of pathology [2].

What Is the Pathophysiology of This Condition?

Pain is either from trauma/injury or from inflammation. This causes damage or disruption of number of structure. It can cause capsular disruption, ligamentous injury, myofascial pain, hypermobility, microfracture, chondromalacia, and inflammation. Persistent nociception can lead to central sensitization contributing to creation of a chronic pain state. Intraarticular pathology is usually from age-related arthritis or spondyloarthropathies causing inflammatory processes in the SI joint. Extracapsular pain usually comes from ligamentous. This is more likely the case in age-related painful SI joints. Intraarticular structure tends to be more painful in younger patients, as in this population the etiology tends to be injury from a major trauma or a sytemic or local disease process causing intense inflammation. The distinction may be useful as the ablation of lateral branches of posterior division tends to be more effective when pain is extracapsular in origin. Trauma, infection, and tumor invasion may also propagate sacroiliitis when involving the SI joint.

In the parturient, the SI joint widens and stretches with the growing uterus. This factor combined with the added weight of the pregnancy may inflame the SI joint to result in sacroiliitis.

How Is This Problem Managed?

Sacroiliitis, most often caused by degeneration of the SI joint, can be approached via conservative and invasive measures. Most cases can be treated without surgery. Initial treatment includes proper rest and physical therapy to exercise the joint and strengthen supporting muscle. Superficial heat and ice can be applied over the painful area to soothe and decrease inflammation. Oral NSAIDs can be taken at safe doses as needed to treat inflammation and, along with acetaminophen, decrease pain. In the acute phase, ibuprofen 600–800 mg PO three times a day as needed is not unreasonable. Patients with a history of or at risk of gastric ulcer or renal disease should take a reduced dose to avoid exacerbation of these diseases. Acetaminophen can be taken as 1000 mg three times a day as needed. Patients with liver disease may need a reduced dose to avoid toxicity and overdose.

If conservative medical management is not sufficient in treating sacroiliitis, interventional procedures may help. Under fluoroscopic guidance, pain physicians may inject a combination of local anesthetic and steroid into the SI joint to directly decrease inflammation.

Risks of joint injection are very small, but include those generic to interventional therapy including bleeding, infection, and nerve damage. Generally speaking, patients who are coagulopathic or on chronic anticoagulation are at higher risk of developing a bleeding complication. Injecting through an infected area such as cellulitis may spread infection, just as injecting through tumor can seed cancer cells. Targeting the SI joint itself leaves nerve damage highly unlikely as the needle does not traverse major nerve tissue. The SI joint normally cannot hold more than 3 cc of volume and so a common anesthetic injection mixture is 2 cc of 0.25% bupivacaine with 40 mg triamcinolone. The steroid dose may be adjusted in a patient undergoing multiple injections in the same day or if they are at risk of hyperglycemia as with uncontrolled diabetes.

Other forms of interventional therapy include cooled radiofrequency ablation, conventional radiofrequency ablation, and botulinum toxin injection with varying degrees of reported success. The surgical option include fusion of the joint either via open approach or percutaneoulsy. However, it is reserved for pateints who are refractory to conservative and interventional therapies. These patients can undergo minimally invasive SI joint fusion for stabilization and increased weight-bearing [3].

What Is the Prognosis of This Condition?

As most cases of sacroiliac joint pain are due to age-related degeneration, many persist lifelong. Goal therapy is to make pain as tolerable as possible to ensure quality of life and proper functionality. Several Cochrane systematic reviews have shown that there is level III–IV evidence that intraarticular steroid injections provide pain relief with notably more success in the short term. There is level II–IV evidence for the efficacy of radiofrequency ablations, but patients who pass diagnostic blocks are much more likely to respond to this intervention [4, 5].

Discussion

Gluteal pain is a persistent issue in the American population. The etiology, however, is wide and varied. Patients may present with gluteal pain in the acute or chronic setting. A physician's differential diagnosis must be broad to address the multitude of possible causes and also as not to miss more critical cases.

One of the more morbid reasons for gluteal pain is peripheral vascular disease (PVD). Nonradicular gluteal pain with activity that predictably resolves with rest is a classic presentation of vascular claudication consistent with aorto-iliac occlusive disease. This disease is progressive and may be limb- or life- threatening. The American Heart Association estimates PVD prevalence at close to 12% [6]. According to the American College of Cardiology, PVD risk factors include age, smoking, diabetes, and known ischemic disease such as coronary, renal, or cerebrovascular disease. Treatment of PVD includes lifestyle changes such as diet, smoking cessation, and exercise. Management of diabetes and hypertension is crucial. Many of these patients require aggressive antiplatelet therapy. Patients refractive to this treatment require revascularization via fluoroscopic interventions or bypass surgery. PVD patients should be referred to a specialist such as a vascular surgeon for proper management [7].

The more common etiologies of gluteal pain seen by the pain physician are musculoskeletal or neuraxial in nature. Musculoskeletal pain includes myofascial pain syndromes such as that of the gluteus maximus. This happens as a result of strain or overuse and can make sitting or rising from the seated position more strenuous. Myofascial pain syndrome is a clinical diagnosis verified by the reproducibility of pain on palpation of trigger points in the muscle. Treatment includes oral acetaminophen and NSAIDs as well as physical therapy. Stretching and strength training improve coordination and flexibility, which results in greater range of motion [8]. These patients may also benefit from massage therapy or even trigger point injections. In fact, dry needling has been shown to provide similar pain relief to physiotherapy [9]. Posture evaluation and ergonomic lifestyle changes can prevent myofascial pain occurrence or worsening.

Piriformis syndrome involves spasm of the piriformis muscle with impingement on the sciatic nerve. Prevalence is estimated at 6.25% of patients with low back and buttock pain [10]. Common causes include trauma or repeated piriformis muscle stress [11]. These patients may exhibit gluteal pain that coincides with sciatica, increase in pain with prolonged sitting position, tenderness over the sciatic notch, and pain on manuvers that stretch the muscles. Patrick's test can be used to reproduce the patient's symptoms. The piriformis muscle can be palpated deep in the buttock over the greater sciatic notch where it runs from the greater sciatic notch through the sacral foramen to the greater trochanter. Patients with piriformis syndrome may have a very tender muscle that feels cord-like. Diagnosis is clinical, but EMG, CT, and MRI may show some sort of pathology that would corroborate piriformis muscle dysfunction. EMG would show a delay in H-reflex while CT and MRI would show muscle thickening.

As with general myofascial pain, piriformis syndrome can be prevented with ergonomics. Avoiding sitting on provocative or hard surfaces may be imperative in preventing the development or progression of this issue in at-risk patients. Treatment is also similar in that stretching and strengthening exercises may prevent or improve symptoms. These exercises include hip adductor and abductor strengthening [12]. Acetaminophen and NSAIDs are helpful in controlling day-to-day pain. Transcutaneous electrical nerve stimulation (TENS) and massage therapy may also treat piriformis syndrome. TENS is explained by the gate theory of pain according to which stimulation of large diameter A-beta fibers via a pulsed electrical current inhibits nociceptive fibers in the dorsal horn of the spinal cord. A-beta cutaneous mechanoreceptors inhibit signaling through A-delta and C pain fibers, thereby closing a "gate."

If conservative therapy fails, interventional therapy such as via steroid or botulinum toxin injection may treat persistent piriformis syndrome. These injections are classically performed under CT or fluoroscopic guidance, but studies have shown ultrasound guidance, which avoids radiation exposure, is more accessible, the ultrasound-guided injections are just as safe and effective when done by trained providers [13]. In extreme cases, which are rare, surgical release of the muscle may be warranted [14]. In this scenario, immobilization or release of the muscle is compensated for by the surrounding musculature.

Gluteal pain derived from the neuraxiom can be either radicular or referred pain. Spinal stenosis can result in radiculopathy that manifests in gluteal pain, bilateral or one-sided. This disease is a clinical diagnosis defined as neurogenic claudication with or without back pain or lower extremity pain worsened by lumbar spinal extension. Spinal stenosis can be confirmed with CT or MRI. CT imaging elucidates bony structures. MRI better identifies nerve and soft tissue with 75–90% sensitivity and > 75% specificity [15, 16].

Lumbosacral spinal stenosis may also yield referred gluteal pain as can joint dysfunctions such as lumbosacral facet arthropathy and sacroiliitis. The pain pattern is quite overlapping and diagnostic blocks clinch the diagnosis for facet joint-based pain syndrome. Sacroiliitis affects 15–30% of individuals with chronic, non-radicular back pain [17]. SI joint is a complex joint and the largest joint of the spine. It is primarily for stability and its structure allows for very little rotation and sliding movement. Its innervation is complex and accounts for its variable pain pattern. A number of physical examination maneuvers have been described for eliciting pain from SI joint which only point toward the joint but are not diagnostic. Injection is the only way to diagnose pain form SI joint. Injection using only landmark are not recommended, as failure to place needle accurately in the joint is quite high (failure rate of 80%). Ultrasound is reliable if individual is not obese and space can be accurately visualized; the only limitation is skill and experience of the operator. Flouroscopic guidance is quite invaluable in placing the needle. The solution is injected intraarticularly during the joint injection; however there is a case to be made that part of the soultion should be injected just outside the capsule of the joint as extra-articular ligaments are also source of pain. Borowsky showed that combination injection may be more effective than intraarticular injection alone.

As with many of these osteoarthritic degenerative processes mediated by inflammation, initial treatment includes proper rest and physical therapy to exercise the affected joint and strengthen the supporting muscle. Patients may benefit from heat or ice therapy as well as oral NSAIDs and acetaminophen.

Patients who do not respond well to conservative treatment may undergo interventional procedures. These therapies include joint injections under fluoroscopic guidance that place a combination of local anesthetic and possibly steroid. Pain relief is both therapeutic and diagnostic in identifying the cause of the patient's complaints. The limitation of steroid-based injection is recurrence of pain in few months. The duration of relief reported has been from 1 month to almost a year. Most of the studies were uncontrolled and some included repeat injections. Patients who respond well to joint injections may be candidates for radiofrequency ablation, which can provide more lasting relief. The reported percentage of patients achieving significant long-lasting pain relief (> 50% pain improvement lasting 6 or more months) after the ablation procedure is quite variable but is around 50%–60%. The SI joint is hard to denervate as the nerve supply and nerve location are variable. Various strategies employed to get as many nerve ablated as possible include multiple lesions, multipronged needles, longer lesion time, and cooled RF. Using such extensive burn technique has reportedly led to much higher incidence of post-procedure neuritis. Current RF technique does not address the pain emanating from the ventral aspect of the joint and failure to identify such patients will lead to failure of the treatment. Cohn el al found that older patient, opioid use, higher pre-procedural pain score, and pain radiation below the knee are risk factors for failure of RF treatment [17]. Meanwhile, surgery such as sacroiliac joint fusion remains a last resort. The surgery is based on the principle of fusion. It can be done using minimally invasive approach.

There is ongoing research to explore the various causes of gluteal pain and their treatments. Radial shock wave and acupuncture carry potential in myofascial pain and piriformis syndrome. Research in spinal stenosis is examining new surgical techniques as well as reviewing various rehabilitative strategies for non-operative management. In sacroiliac dysfunction and facet arthropathy, ongoing studies are examining new surgical strategies as well as radiofrequency ablation efficacies. Beyond that, the utility of hyaluronic acid and stem cell therapy is becoming more apparent. With these exciting projects, patients will have more avenues for success in controlling their gluteal pain [18].

Conclusion/Summary

Gluteal pain is a common complaint reported to primary care providers, emergency medicine providers, and specialists alike. It is a more common musculoskeletal problem in the athlete or those with daily work or activities that predispose them to developing myofascial issues. Other patients develop gluteal pain progressively with age-related disease in their spine or its articulating joints. From a pain perspective, it is important to rule out critical medical etiologies such as vascular claudication, which may warrant a vascular surgeon's evaluation. Gluteal pain is a complaint with a variety of etiologies, each with their own work-up and treatment. Pain specialists must perform a thorough examination when consulting these patients and consider a complete clinical picture before considering what imaging may corroborate the suspected diagnosis. Various physical examination tests employed to identify SI joint as source of pain are suggestive, but not diagnostic; only a controlled diagnostic injection can identify the SI joint as source of pain. Best long-term pain relief is obtained when the underlying source causing SI joint pain is fixed. Steroid injection (intra- or peri-articular) tends to provide short-term relief, so should be used in conjunction with physical therapy. RF of lateral branches is effective in properly selected patients but quality of evidence is intermediate. With these strategies, a care provider can assess the suffering patient and begin treating their pain in a safe and efficient manner.

References

1. Simopoulos TT, Manchikanti L, Gupta S, Aydin SM, Kim CH, Solanki D, Nampiaparampil DE, Singh V, Staats PS, Hirsch JA. Systematic review of the diagnostic accuracy and therapeutic effectiveness of sacroiliac joint interventions. Pain Physician. 2015;18(5):E713–56.
2. Slobodin G, Rimar D, Boulman N, Kaly L, Rozenbaum M, Rosner I, Odeh M. Acute Sacroiliitis. Clin Rheumatol. 2016;35(4):851–6.
3. Kancherla V, McGowan S, Audley B, Sokunbi GO, Puccio ST. Early outcomes following percutaneous sacroiliac joint fusion. Spine J. 2015;15(10):255.
4. Hansen HC, McKenzie-Brown AM, Cohen SP, Swicegood JR, Colson JD, Manchikanti L. Sacroiliac joint interventions: a systematic review. Pain Physician. 2007;10(1):165–84.
5. McKenzie-Brown AM, Shah RV, Sehgal N, Everett CR. A systematic review of sacroiliac joint interventions. Pain Physician. 2005;8(1):115–25.
6. Kalbaugh CA, Kucharska-Newton A, Wruck L, Lund JL, Selvin E, Matsushita K, Bengtson LGS, Heiss G, Loehr L. Peripheral artery disease prevalence and incidence estimated from both outpatient and inpatient settings among medicare fee-for-service beneficiaries in the atherosclerosis risk in communities (ARIC) study. J Am Heart Assoc. 2017;6:e003796.
7. Rooke TW, Hirsch AT, Misra S, Sidawy AN, Beckman JA, Findeiss L, Golzarian J, Gornik HL, Jaff MR, Moneta GL, Olin JW, Stanley JC, White CJ, White JV, Zierler RE, American College of Cardiology Foundation Task, Force; American Heart Association Task, Force. Management of patients with peripheral artery disease (compilation of 2005 and 2011 ACCF/AHA Guideline Recommendations): a report of the American College of Cardiology Foundation/ American Heart Association Task Force on Practice Guidelines. J Am Coll Cardiol. 2013;61(14):1555–70.
8. Starlanyl DJ, Copeland ME. Fibromyalgia & chronic myofascial pain: a survival manual. 2nd ed. Oakland: New Harbinger Publications; 2001.
9. Rayegani SM, Bayat M, Bahrami MH, Raeissadat SA, Kargozar E. Comparison of dry needling and physiotherapy in treatment of myofascial pain syndrome. Clin Rheumatol. 2014;33(6):859–64.
10. Singh US, Meena RK, Singh CAK, Singh AKJ, Singh AM, Langshong R. Prevalence of piriformis syndrome among the cases of low back/buttock pain with sciatica: a prospective study. J Med Soc. 2013;27(2):94–9.
11. Jawish RM, Assoum HA, Khamis CF. Anatomical, clinical and electrical observations in piriformis syndrome. J Orthop Surg Res. 2010;5:3.
12. Boyajian-O'Neill LA, McClain RL, Coleman MK, Thomas PP. Diagnosis and management of piriformis syndrome: an osteopathic approach. J Am Osteopath Assoc. 2008;108(11):657–64.
13. Fabregat G, Rosello M, Asensio-Samper JM, Villanueva-Perez VL, Martinez-Sanjuan V, De Andres

J, Eichenberger U. Computer-tomographic verification of ultrasound-guided piriformis muscle injection: a feasibility study. Pain Physician. 2014;17(6):507–13.
14. Filler AG, Haynes J, Jordan SE, Prager J, Villablanca JP, Farahani K, McBride DQ, Tsuruda JS, Morisoli B, Batzdorf U, Johnson JP. Sciatica of nondisc origin and piriformis syndrome: diagnosis by magnetic resonance neurography and interventional magnetic resonance imaging with outcome study of resulting treatment. J Neurosurg Spine. 2005;2(2):99–115.
15. Starling A, Hernandez F, Hoxworth JM, Trentman T, Halker R, Vargas BB, Hastriter E, Dodick D. Sensitivity of MRI of the spine compared with CT myelography in orthostatic headache with CSF leak. Neurology. 2013;81(20):1789–92.
16. Wassenaar M, van Rijn RM, van Tulder MW, et al. Magnetic resonance imaging for diagnosing lumbar spinal pathology in adult patients with low back pain or sciatica: a diagnostic systematic review. Eur Spine J. 2012;21:220–7.
17. Cohen SP, Chen Y, Neufeld NJ. Sacroiliac joint pain: a comprehensive review of epidemiology, diagnosis and treatment. Expert Rev Neurother. 2014;13(1):99–116.
18. Low back pain. NIH U.S. National Library of Medicine. https://www.clinicaltrials.gov. 13 Jun 2018.

A 75-Year-Old Woman with Mid-thoracic Pain (Compression Fracture)

36

Jonathan K. Song and Tariq Malik

Case Description

A 75-year-old Caucasian woman comes to your office complaining of mid-thoracic back pain. Past medical history includes osteoporosis, hypertension, congestive heart failure (CHF), history of smoking, and hyperthyroidism. Patient has had frequent hospitalizations over the past 2 years for hypotension and acute CHF exacerbation. Patient has had functional decline after each hospitalization, with intermittent mid back pain that has progressively gotten worse. Patient completed 2 weeks of rehabilitation after the most recent hospitalization with little improvement in her functionality. While at home, she had an incident where she slipped while getting up from her commode and abruptly sat back down onto the commode, causing excruciating back pain. She is here today to discuss workup and treatment options.

J. K. Song
Department of Physical Medicine and Rehabilitation, Schwab Rehabilitation Hospital/University of Chicago, Chicago, IL, USA
e-mail: jonathan.song@sinai.org

T. Malik (✉)
Department of Anesthesia and Critical Care University of Chicago, Chicago, IL, USA
e-mail: tmalik@dacc.uchicago.edu; TMuslim@dacc.uchicago.edu

What Is Your Preliminary Diagnosis?

Vertebral Compression Fracture (VCF)

Vertebral compression fractures are common in older adults and are usually caused by age-related osteoporosis. This is an elderly female with multiple comorbidities that affect bone mass and can disrupt bone integrity. A non-traumatic fall acutely exacerbated an already weakened spinal structure that caused an acute fracture. This patient has many risk factors for osteoporosis, including race (Caucasian), female gender, advanced age, risk for falls, tobacco abuse, and hypothyroidism. The decrease in bone strength directly correlates with an increased chance of bone fractures. Osteoporotic compression fractures often occur at the T7-T8 and T12-L1 junction, resulting in pain, limited activity, and overall decline in functionality [1].

What Is the Pathophysiology of This Condition?

As a growing child and adolescent, there is rapid linear skeletal growth. Old bone is removed by osteoclasts and new bone is formed by osteoblasts. Structural integrity of bones is maintained by this process of bone remodeling. Lifestyle factors, such as diet and exercise, as well as genetics determine peak bone mass. Most people reach peak bone mass between 25 and 30 years of age,

T. Malik (ed.), *Practical Chronic Pain Management*, https://doi.org/10.1007/978-3-030-46675-6_36

while people slowly start to lose bone mass at 40 years old [2].

Osteoporosis is a condition that describes the loss of calcium in bones, causing thinning of the bone. Bone density of the spine is positively correlated with a number of factors, both modifiable and non-modifiable factors. Uncontrolled risk factors include being over 50 years old, female, menopause, and family history. Controllable risk factors include smoking, drinking too much alcohol, inactive lifestyle, and calcium and vitamin D deficiency [3].

VCFs are the hallmark of osteoporosis and directly correlate with the strength and integrity of bone, although infection, neoplasm, and trauma can also cause VCFs. Postmenopausal women have the greatest risk of VCFs due to hormonal changes that directly affect the microarchitecture of bone. Estrogen deficiency is associated with increased bone resorption, leading to an increased number of osteoclasts (both enhanced production and decreased apoptosis of osteoclasts) [4].

Acute fractures occur in patients when the weight on the bone exceeds its tolerable capacity to hold the load. A small event or activity, such as sneezing, lifting an object, or navigating stairs can cause a VCF in those with severe osteoporosis. 30% of compression fractures even occur while in bed [5]. More force and trauma are needed to create a fracture for those with less severe osteoporosis.

A trademark of VCFs is an anterior wedge fracture on imaging, caused by a combination of flexion and axial compression loading force on the anterior part of the vertebral body. This results in height loss and, as the anterior vertebrae fuse together in a bent forward position, a kyphotic deformity forms. The majority of the damage is usually sustained by the anterior vertebral column and rarely involves neurological complications [6].

Overtime, multiple fractures can occur, further causing loss of height, and, in effect, causes a shortening of paraspinal muscles that produces pain from muscle fatigue that can persist despite fracture healing.

How Is the Diagnosis Confirmed?

A thorough history and physical is always the initial starting point; however, diagnosis must be confirmed with spinal imaging. Evaluating the patient's comorbidities, inciting events leading to injury, structural exam, and range of motion are all important to help develop a differential diagnosis. About 1 in 3 vertebral fractures are diagnosed as many patients regard their back pain as arthritis or a normal effect of aging [1]. Tenderness to palpation over the area of fracture, increased kyphosis, and decreased spinal mobility are common presentations. Neurological deficits are not as common in anterior vertebral compression fractures and do not usually involve retropulsion of bone fragments into the vertebral canal. Pain is usually intensified with walking or standing.

Plain frontal and lateral radiographs of the spine should be obtained for initial assessment. They are low cost and allow for a quick screening for possible vertebral fractures. Anterior wedging, vertebral collapse, and endplate irregularity are more common findings while posterior wedging is a less common finding that may be suggestive of an underlying lesion (Table 36.1) [7]. Indicators of vertebral disruption on radiographs include loss of vertebral height, disruption of anterior and posterior vertebral body lines, and increased interpedicular and interspinous space that is >7 mm. Wedge fractures are the most common and account for greater than 50% of all VCFs.

Table 36.1 Vertebral compression fracture radiograph findings

Radiograph findings for VCF	% of the time	Description of lesion
Wedge VCF	50	Compression of anterior segment of vertebral body
Biconcave	17	Involve only the middle portion of the vertebral body
Crush compression fractures	13	The entire anterior column, anterior and posterior margins have collapsed
Complex fractures	20	

From Black et al. [7], with permission

X-rays can also be helpful in tracking post-traumatic kyphotic angulation to assess fracture progression (Fig. 36.1). A plain radiograph may be all that is needed for the majority of compression fractures. A major disadvantage to plain radiographs, however, is its lack of ability to assess ligamentous injuries [8].

Most patients will not require an MRI or CT scan to confirm diagnosis, although it is appropriate when further diagnostic evaluation is needed to further evaluate results from X-rays and labs. Computed tomography (CT) gives the best bony anatomy imaging, but also has greater expense and irradiation to the patient than plain radiographs. CTs can help determine the level of instability in an anterior wedge compression fracture and is more appropriate when assessing complex fractures to measure the degree of vertebral involvement.

Magnetic resonance imaging (MRI) is not usually needed. Circumstances in which an MRI would be obtained in a VCF are when there is a neurological deficit or there are concerns for an underlying infectious or malignant process. MRIs can also accurately assess the age of the compression fracture (increased T2 signal from water in the vertebral body) [9].

Without a history of trauma, a vertebral compression fracture is usually diagnostic for underlying osteoporosis. A dual-energy X-ray absorptiometry (DEXA) scan can be obtained to assess overall bone density. Approximately 50% of patients with vertebral fractures have osteoporosis (T score < 2.5), while roughly 40% have osteopenia (T score − 1 to −2.5) [10]. DEXA scans can be used to predict future fracture risk based on bone density quality.

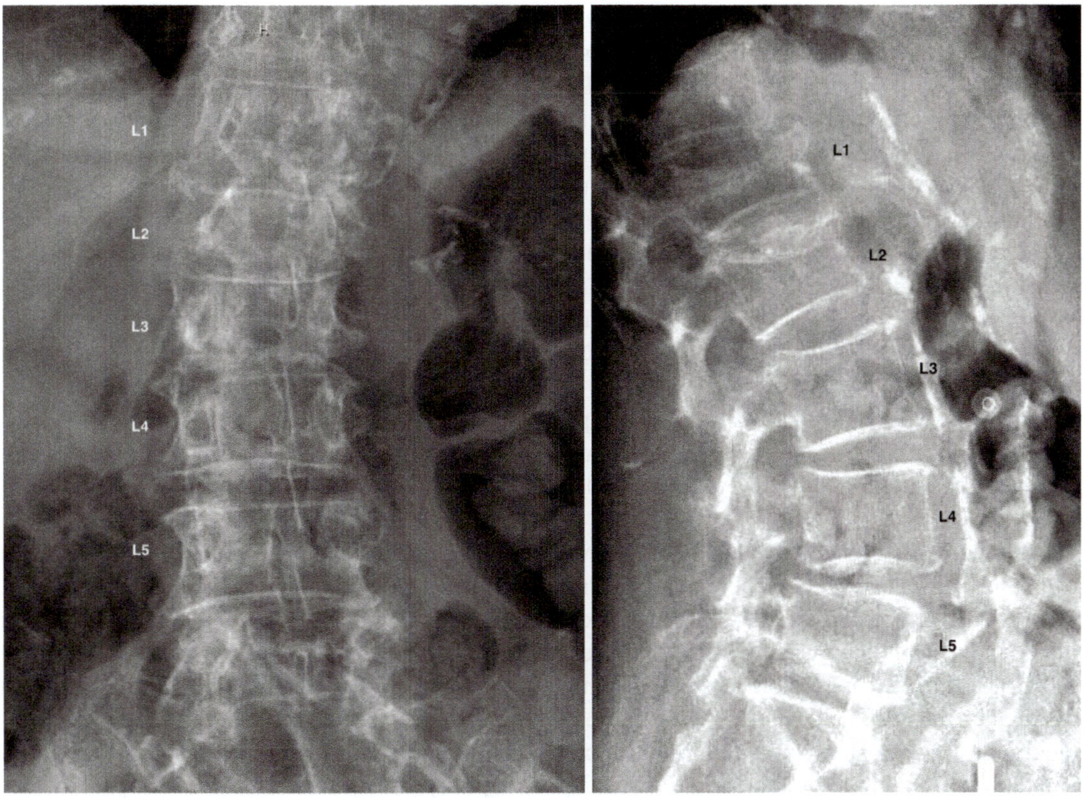

Fig. 36.1 Lumbar spine X-ray. Description: Moderate compression deformity of L1 vertebral body superior endplate and age-indeterminate mild compression deformity of L2 vertebral body superior endplate. Mild dextroconvex curvature of lumbar spine. Grade 1 anterolisthesis of L3 on L4, L4 on L5, and L5 on S1

How Is This Problem Managed?

Vertebral compression fracture ranges from benign, asymptomatic, incidental findings to debilitating and agonizing sources of pain. Initial management includes pain control and activity modification. Anterior vertebral compression fractures are traditionally considered benign and can heal without complications, while middle and/or posterior involvement in the compression fracture are unstable in quality and may require prompter surgical intervention [11]. Complete bed rest should be avoided if possible, as it can accelerate bone loss and cardiopulmonary deconditioning [12].

First-line oral analgesics for acute pain include acetaminophen (500 to 1000 mg four times a day), naproxen (220 to 500 mg twice a day), ibuprofen (200 to 800 mg every 8 hours), and topical/transdermal lidocaine [1]. Acetaminophen side effects include hepatotoxicity, thrombocytopenia, and acute renal tubular necrosis. Nonsteroidal anti-inflammatory drugs (NSAIDs) inhibit platelets and, as such, can cause possible bleeding, gastrointestinal damage, and renal injury. NSAIDs can also interfere with fracture healing due to COX-2 inhibition, so the lowest effective dose should be used for the shortest duration. Topical lidocaine side effects include skin irritation (dermatitis), edema, and urticaria.

A two- to four-week course of calcitonin can be used for mild to moderate pain with little to no improvement with oral analgesics (200 IU per day intranasal). There are some trials that suggest intranasal calcitonin may reduce pain at modest levels [13].

Although pain from VCF typically improves over the course of a few weeks, narcotics are often needed temporarily to help encourage continued movement and prevent complete bed rest. If pain is still uncontrollable despite first-line treatments, the lowest effective dose of oral opioids with or without a combination with acetaminophen should be initiated. In cases of extreme, debilitating pain, hospitalization and IV narcotics may be needed.

There are many side effects and risks with use of opioids (i.e., hydrocodone, hydromorphone, oxycodone), including addiction, constipation, delirium, respiratory depression, and cognitive impairment. Tramadol is both an opioid pain medication and acts as a serotonin-norepinephrine reuptake inhibitor (SNRI). Caution should be taken when giving tramadol for patients on serotonin reuptake inhibitor medications so as to avoid causing serotonin syndrome. Serotonin syndrome is a potentially life-threatening syndrome caused by an overload of serotonin in the system that can potentially cause mental status change, autonomic hyperactivity (hyperthermia, hypertension), and neuromuscular hyperactivity (rigidity) [14].

Exercise is very beneficial in patients with osteoporosis. Improving strength (back extensors especially) can help increase bone density and reduce the risk of a vertebral fracture. There are mixed recommendations with the use of back braces but are still used. While some studies report improved pain, posture, and strength [15], others suggest no improvement in disability scores and deemed non-effective [16].

At least 3–6 weeks should be given to trial and exhaust non-surgical options. If pain is persistent after 6 weeks, medical management can be continued or vertebral augmentation can be considered. Medical management should be continued if there was some improvement in pain or if the patient can tolerate therapies. Vertebral augmentation may be appropriate for patients with inadequate symptomatic relief, continued decline in functionality, or inability to tolerate medications (i.e., opioid side effects). Recommendations remain controversial for the indications of vertebral augmentation procedures. Vertebroplasty and kyphoplasty are procedures involving a percutaneous injection of cement into the fracture vertebra. Optimal timing, effectiveness, and indications are still unclear and controversial. In 2010, the American Academy of Orthopaedic Surgeons recommended against vertebroplasty in neurological intact patients with vertebral compression fractures [17]. Other studies show vertebroplasty was more effective in pain relief, functionality, and overall quality of life compared to conservative care treatments [18]. The National Institute for Health and Clinical Excellence (NICE) recommended vertebra augmentation as possibilities for osteoporotic spinal compression fractures with severe, ongoing pain despite pain treatment [19]. Even though kyphoplasties are performed more frequently, vertebroplasty may be more preferred for patients with endplate fractures since they are easier to perform and are also less expensive. Surgical complications include cement leakage into the spinal canal resulting in neurologic deficits, such as radiculopathy or spinal cord compression [9].

Current controversy regarding vertebral augmentation techniques revolve around when to intervene after a compression fracture is diagnosed. Optimum time to intervention is unknown. In general if patient has failed few weeks of conservative therapy and is not ambulating enough, then this injection therapy should be employed. The focus should be on ambulation and not pain. Waiting too long may defeat the purpose of interventional therapy. It should be stressed that the augmentation therapy works best when the fracture has not healed (as seen by presence of edema on MRI and read by radiologist as acute or subacute fracture) and the pain is truly coming from the fracture and limiting ambulation. It has been a concern that the fracture by causing loss of height stresses the posterior elements of the spine, i.e., facet joint, and it's the joint that are the pain generator and not the fracture itself. In such case it is not a bad idea to do diagnostic medial branch block, which if helpful will spare the patient a more invasive and fruitless procedure especially if the fracture is more than 6 months old and MRI findings non-diagnostic.

A trial of conservative, non-operative treatments should be initiated and exhausted before surgery is considered, unless there is imaging evidence of instability, uncontrollable pain, or neurological deficits.

What Is the Prognosis of This Condition? What Is the Long-Term Outcome – Complete Cure, Recurrent, or Chronic Persistent Problem?

Severity of fracture deformation is the most significant factor in predicting severity and longevity of symptoms after a low energy vertebral compression. Most patients can make a full recovery or at least some improvement after 6–12 weeks and can return to normal exercise after the fracture has healed [1]. The more severe the deformed fracture, the more disabling and functional deterioration is seen during the first post fracture year [20].

Incidence of new fractures is similar regardless of conservative therapy versus surgical therapy, due to ongoing osteoporosis and not the type of treatment therapy. The largest improvements can be seen between the initial visit and 3 month follow-up; after the 3 month mark, outcome measures tend to level out or deteriorate [21]. Approximately 20% of patients with a history of osteoporotic VCF will experience a new vertebral fracture within a year depending on the severity of the previous fracture [22]. Compared to non-operative patients, kyphoplasty patients had a 34% greater life expectancy than vertebroplasty patients [23].

Discussion

Prevalence

1. Osteoporosis causing vertebral fractures are common, causing approximately 700,000 out of 1.5million osteoporotic fractures a year in the United States alone. This is likely an under-estimate due to the number of compression fractures that go undiagnosed, with only a third of vertebral fractures formally diagnosed [24].
2. Prevalence estimates range from 10% to 15% for women 50–59 years old to 50% for women greater than 80 years old [25].
3. Approximately 30% of post-menopausal white women in the United States have osteoporosis, 16% of the lumbar spine. Vertebral fractures are more common in Caucasian females and less common among men, African-American, and Asian women.
4. Although most commonly found in osteoporotic patients (DEXA T score ≤ 2.5), vertebral fractures occur up to 18% in women older than 60 with low bone mass (T score > 2.5 but < -1.4).

5. More than a third of post-menopausal women who do not meet criteria for osteoporosis suffer from vertebral fractures [26].
6. The lifetime risk for fragility fractures in Caucasian females greater than 50 years old is approximately 40% [27].

Differential Diagnosis

Back pain differential: Back strain, acute disc herniation, osteoarthritis, spinal stenosis, spondylolisthesis, acute fracture.

Causes of low bone mass: Osteoporosis, osteomalacia, hyperparathyroidism, metastatic cancer, granulomatous disease, sarcoidosis.

Predictive Value of Different Clinical Features (Both on History and Physical Exam), and Lab Testing/Imaging

Physical Exam Tests

Closed fist percussion sign: Patient stands in front of a mirror so practitioner can gauge reaction. Using firm, closed fist percussion along entire length of spine; + test when complains of sharp, sudden, fracture pain. Sn 87.5, Sn 90 [28]

Supine sign: Laying supine, with only one pillow; + when unable to lay supine d/t severe pain in spine. Sn 81.25, Sp 93.33 [24].

Plain Radiographs

- Plain x-ray technique diagnose compression fractures in patients only 55%–65% of the time (emergency department experince) [29, 30].
- Multinational study of 2000 postmenopausal women with osteoporosis reported a false negative rate of Osteoporotic VFs from 27–45% [31].

Plain radiographs make it difficult to interpret the underlying cause of an atraumatic vertebral compression fracture, making it difficult to distinguish between osteoporosis, metastatic lesion, or other primary bone neoplasm. Generally, plain radiographs have no problem showing diagnostic evidence for moderate to severe vertebral fractures, with a diagnostic rate of 87 [32], yet may underestimate the amount of trauma the spine has endured by possibly missing other lesions (i.e., hairline fractures, non-displaced fractures) [33].

Computed tomography is useful for more detailed evaluation of bone structure and level of cortical bone destruction. CT scans have a higher sensitivity and specificity in evaluating spine injuries when compared with plain film radiographs [33].

Magnetic resonance imaging is the most helpful radiological modality in distinguishing between metastatic versus osteoporosis causing compression fractures. MRIs have the highest sensitivity (99), specificity (98.7), and diagnostic rate (98) compared to plain radiographs and CT scans [32]

Strength of Evidence for Different Treatment Modalities

While there is statistically significant data in favor of use of NSAIDs for effectiveness, there was a trade-off in significantly increased side effects. COX-2 NSAIDs have statistically significant fewer side effects than traditional NSAIDs while having strong evidence as being just as effective as NSAIDs for acute low back pain [34].

The American Academy of Neurology states there is significant effectiveness in short-term use of opioids for pain relief but no significant evidence in longer-term maintenance of pain without suffering serious side effects [35]. The American Association of Family Physicians has published their recommendations as well. [36]

With regards to surgery, there is ongoing debate on the effectiveness of surgery. In 2009, McGirt et al. [37] published a 20-year review of vertebral augmentation and found:

- Level I evidence – vertebroplasty has superior pain control over medical management in the first 2 weeks
- Level II-III evidence – within first 3 months, superior outcomes in analgesic use in disability and general health

- Level II-III evidence – kyphoplasty improved daily activity, physical function, and pain control at 6 months compared to medical management.

It should be noted; however, the studies were favorable for tumor-related fractures.

The larger VERTOS II trial found sustained evidence of significant differences at the 1-year follow-up mark with continued pain relief from the vertebroplasty group [38].

In 2009, the *New England Journal of Medicine* discussed how there was no difference in pain control of functionality between vertebroplasty and sham procedure group, and suggested vertebroplasty benefits in prior trials were secondary to placebo effect [39].

Future Directions or Clinical Trials in Progress

There have been improvements made to minimize the risk of complications from kyphoplasty, such as vesselplasty, an inflatable balloon left in the patient and filled with cement. Kyphoplasty with Sky Bone Expander has shown promising results, improving Cobb's angle, alleviating pain, and improving quality of life in a relatively short time period [40].

Cortoss is a bioactive, injective composite made up of highly cross-linked resins and bioactive glass fibers that can decrease subsequent fractures but restores more physiologic load transfer through the vertebra [41].

Conclusion/Summary

Compression fracture is a symptoms and not a disease. The most common underlying disease process leading to this problem is osteoporosis, one of the most prevalent disease listed by World Health Organization among the top 10 diseases that affect human race the most worldwide. The prevalence of osteoporosis is bound to increase as the whole world is aging. The best treatment of treating compression fracture is preventing development of osteoporosis and then treating it if it happens. This requires extensive education on the part of heath care providers as the solution is simple. The current conundrum is lack of high level evidence in when to intervene if compression fracture happens. This is due to lack of knowledge of the prognosis of the fracture in general. In addition, there is no good evidence how best to treat the pain from the fracture. In general, there is no need to intervene if pain is not affecting quality of life and interventions should be focused on treating the underlying disease. If the pain is truly debilitating, then vertebral augmentation is truly affective in restoring quality of life in the short term. The literature is still not clear, when is the best time to intervene. Presence of edema on MRI is often used as a marker that the vertebral fracture may still benefit from augmentation, but this is not always the case. Current guidelines suggest that conservative therapy should be tried for few weeks before augmentation should be considered. The issue of resorting height has not been found beneficial clinically in any trial even though it is the catch phrase of various device manufacturing companies.

References

1. Calvert M. Vertebral compression fractures in the elderly. Am Fam Physician. 2004;69(1):111–6. https://www.aafp.org/afp/2004/0101/p111.html
2. Healthy bones at every age – OrthoInfo - AAOS. Clavicle Fracture (Broken Collarbone) – OrthoInfo – AAOS. https://orthoinfo.aaos.org/en/staying-healthy/healthy-bones-at-every-age/.
3. Are you at risk? National Osteoporosis Foundation. https://www.nof.org/preventing-fractures/general-facts/bone-basics/are-you-at-risk/ (accessed June 29, 2018).
4. Manolagas SC. Birth and death of bone cells: basic regulatory mechanisms and implications for the pathogenesis and treatment of osteoporosis. Endocr Rev. 2000;21:115–37. https://doi.org/10.1210/er.21.2.115.
5. Patel U, Skingle S, Campbell GA, Crisp AJ, Boyle IT. Clinical profile of acute vertebral compression fractures in osteoporosis. Rheumatology. 1991;30:418–21. https://doi.org/10.1093/rheumatology/30.6.418.
6. Rockwood CA Jr, Green DP. Rockwood and green's fractures in adults, vol. 2. 4th ed. Philadelphia: Lippincott-Raven; 1996. p. 1544–5.

7. Black DM, Arden NK, Palermo L, Pearson J, Cummings SR. Prevalent vertebral deformities predict hip fractures and new vertebral deformities but not wrist fractures. J Bone Miner Res. 1999;14:821–8. https://doi.org/10.1359/jbmr.1999.14.5.821.
8. Epstein O, Ludwig S, Gelb D, Poelstra K, O'Brien J. Comparison of computed tomography and plain radiography in assessing traumatic spinal deformity. J Spinal Disord Tech. 2009;22(3):197–201. DOI. https://doi.org/10.1097/BSD.0b013e31817e6fa8.
9. Alexandru D. Evaluation and management of vertebral compression fractures. Perm J. 2012;16:46–51. https://doi.org/10.7812/tpp/12-037.
10. Unnanuntana A, Gladnic B, Donnely E, Lane J. The assessment of fracture risk. J Bone Joint Surg. 2010 Mar;92(3):743–53. https://doi.org/10.2106/JBJS.I.00919.
11. Kim DH, Vaccaro AR. Osteoporotic compression fractures of the spine: current options and considerations for treatment. Spine J. 2006;6:479–87.
12. Parry SM, Puthucheary ZA. The impact of extended bed rest on the musculoskeletal system in the critical care environment. Extrem Physiol Med. 2015. https://extremephysiolmed.biomedcentral.com/articles/10.1186/s13728-015-0036-7. Accessed 29 June 2018);4:16.
13. Knopp JA, Diner BM, Blitz M, Lyritis GP, Rowe BH. Calcitonin for treating acute pain of osteoporotic vertebral compression fractures: a systematic review of randomized, controlled trials. Osteoporos Int. 2005;16:1281–90.
14. Gayle JA, Abadie JV, Kaye AM, Kaye AD. Serotonin syndrome. Essentials of pharmacology for anesthesia, pain medicine, and critical care 2014:797–807. https://doi.org/10.1007/978-1-4614-8948-1_49.
15. Pfeifer M, Begerow B, Minne HW. Effects of a new spinal orthosis on posture, trunk strength, and quality of life in women with postmenopausal osteoporosis. Am J Phys Med Rehabil. 2004;83:177–86. https://doi.org/10.1097/01.phm.0000113403.16617.93.
16. Sinaki M, Itoi E, Wahner H, Wollan P, Gelzcer R, Mullan B, et al. Stronger back muscles reduce the incidence of vertebral fractures: a prospective 10 year follow-up of postmenopausal women. Bone. 2002;30:836–41. https://doi.org/10.1016/s8756-3282(02)00739-1.
17. AAOS guideline on the treatment of osteoporotic spinal compression fractures: summary of recommendations. https://www.aaos.org/research/guidelines/scfsummary.pdf
18. Anderson PA, Froyshteter AB, Tontz WL. Meta-analysis of vertebral augmentation compared with conservative treatment for osteoporotic spinal fractures. J Bone Miner Res. 2013;28:372–82. https://doi.org/10.1002/jbmr.1762.
19. National Institute for Healthy and Clinical Excellence. Percutaneous vertebroplasty and percutaneous balloon kyphoplasty for treating osteoporotic vertebral compression fractures. https://www.nice.org.uk/guidance/ta279/documents/vertebral-fractures-vertebroplasty-and-kyphoplasty-final-appraisal-determination-document2.
20. Suzuki N, Ogikubo O, Hansson T. The prognosis for pain, disability, activities of daily living and quality of life after an acute osteoporotic vertebral body fracture: its relation to fracture level, type of fracture and grade of fracture deformation. Eur Spine J. 2008a;18(1):77–88. https://doi.org/10.1007/s00586-008-0847-y.
21. Suzuki N, Ogikubo O, Hansson T. The course of the acute vertebral body fragility fracture: its effect on pain, disability and quality of life during 12 months. Eur Spine J. 2008b;17(10):1380–90. https://doi.org/10.1007/s00586-008-0753-3.
22. Klotzbuecher CM, Ross PD, Landsman PB, Abbott TA, Berger M. Patients with prior fractures have an increased risk of future fractures: a summary of the literature and statistical synthesis. J Bone Mineral Res. 2010;15(4):721–39. https://doi.org/10.1359/jbmr.2000.15.4.721.
23. Edidin AA, Ong KL, Lau E, Kurtz SM. Life expectancy following diagnosis of a vertebral compression fracture. Osteoporos Int. 2012;24(2):451–8. https://doi.org/10.1007/s00198-012-1965-2.
24. Ensrud KE, Schousboe JT. Clinical practice. Vertebral fractures. N Engl J Med. 2011a;364(17):1634–42.
25. Cauley JA, Palermo L, Vogt M, Ensrud KE, Ewing S, Hochberg M, et al. Prevalent vertebral fractures in Black women and white women. J Bone Miner Res. 2008;23:1458–67. https://doi.org/10.1359/jbmr.080411.
26. Ensrud KE, Schousboe JT. Vertebral Fractures. N Engl J Med. 2011b;364:1634–42. https://doi.org/10.1056/nejmcp1009697.
27. Melton LJ. Who has osteoporosis? A conflict between clinical and public health perspectives. J Bone Mineral Res. 2000;15(12):2309–14. https://doi.org/10.1359/jbmr.2000.15.12.2309.
28. Langdon J, Way A, Heaton S, Bernard J, Molloy S. Vertebral compression fractures – new clinical signs to aid diagnosis. Ann R Coll Surg Engl. 2010;92:163–6. https://doi.org/10.1308/003588410x12518836440162.
29. Kim N, Rowe BH, Raymond G, Jen H, Colman I, Jackson SA, et al. Underreporting of vertebral fractures on routine chest radiography. Am J Roentgenol. 2004;182:297–300. https://doi.org/10.2214/ajr.182.2.1820297.
30. Majumdar SR, Kim N, Colman I, Chahal AM, Raymond G, Jen H, et al. Incidental vertebral fractures discovered with chest radiography in the emergency department. Arch Intern Med. 2005;165:905. https://doi.org/10.1001/archinte.165.8.905.
31. Delmas PD, Langerijt LVD, Watts NB, Eastell R, Genant H, Grauer A, et al. Underdiagnosis of vertebral fractures is a worldwide problem: the IMPACT study. J Bone Miner Res. 2004;20:557–63. https://doi.org/10.1359/jbmr.041214.
32. Sung JK, Jee WH, Jung JY, Choi M, Lee SY, Kim YH, et al. Differentiation of acute osteoporotic and malignant compression fractures of the spine: use of

additive qualitative and quantitative axial diffusion-weighted MR imaging to conventional MR imaging at 3.0 T. Adv Pediatr. 2014. https://www.ncbi.nlm.nih.gov/pubmed/24484060. Accessed 29 June 2018.
33. Parizel PM, Zijden TVD, Gaudino S, Spaepen M, Voormolen MHJ, Venstermans C, et al. Trauma of the spine and spinal cord: imaging strategies. Eur Spine J. 2009;19:8–17. https://doi.org/10.1007/s00586-009-1123-5.
34. Tulder MV, Scholten R, Koes B, Deyo R. Non-steroidal anti-inflammatory drugs for low-back pain. Cochrane Database Syst Rev 2000. doi:https://doi.org/10.1002/14651858.cd000396.
35. Franklin GM. Opioids for chronic noncancer pain: a position paper of the American Academy of Neurology. Neurology. 2014;83:1277–84. https://doi.org/10.1212/wnl.0000000000000839.
36. McCarthy J, Davis A. Diagnosis and management of vertebral compression fractures. Am Fam Physician. 2016. https://www.aafp.org/afp/2016/0701/p44.html#afp20160701p44-b19. Accessed 29 June 2018.
37. Wong MM. Vertebral compression fractures: a review of current management and multimodal therapy. J Multidiscip Healthc. 2013;6:205. https://doi.org/10.2147/jmdh.s31659.
38. Klazen CA, Lohle PN, de Vries J, et al. Vertebroplasty versus conservative treatment in acute osteoporotic vertebral compression fractures (Vertos II): an open-label randomised trial. Lancet. 2010;376(9746):1085–92. Epub 2010 Aug 9. The Spine Journal 2011;11:88–. https://doi.org/10.1016/j.spinee.2010.11.011.
39. A randomized trial of vertebroplasty for osteoporotic spinal fractures | NEJM. New Eng J Med. https://www.nejm.org/doi/full/10.1056/NEJMoa0900563. Accessed 29 June 2018.
40. Xiong J, Dang Y, Jiang BG, Fu ZG, Zhang DY. Treatment of osteoporotic compression fracture of thoracic/lumbar vertebrae by kyphoplasty with SKY bone expander system. 2010;3:270–4. Retrieved from https://www.ncbi.nlm.nih.gov/pubmed/20880451.
41. Gilula L, Persenaire M. Subsequent fractures post–vertebral augmentation: analysis of a prospective randomized trial in osteoporotic vertebral compression fractures. Am J Neuroradiol. 2012;34(1):221–7. https://doi.org/10.3174/ajnr.a3156.

Piriformis Syndrome

37

Nicholas Kirch and Maunak V. Rana

Case Description

A 45-year-old man presents to pain clinic with 6 month history of right-sided buttock pain. He describes that pain as sharp and stabbing present deep in the buttock, radiating down the leg into the heel. The pain increases after 30 min of sitting, prompting him to stand up or shift his weight to the left buttock, making hard to work during the day. Walking and lying down is least uncomfortable while bending and lifting things makes the pain worse. The patient describes a tingling sensation that occurs, whether seated or standing. He has been to physical therapy, which has not been of benefit, and he has tried rest, NSAIDs and OTC topical analgesic medications without benefit. On examination, his gait is antalgic. He has distinct tenderness to deep palpation over the gluteal muscles. Internal and external rotation of his hip is painful. Lumbar spine range of motion is within normal limits. Neuro examination is intact, and he has a negative straight leg raise test on examination.

What Is Your Preliminary Diagnosis?

The patient has a vague radicular pain with no sign of nerve compression. His neuro examination is unremarkable. There is no finding on lumbar spine physical examination. There is pain on rotation of the hip joint which requires close scrutiny of hip joint as a cause of his pain. The list of potential structures as source of pain for such kind of presentation would include sacroiliac joint, ischial or greater trochanter bursas, lumbar disc disease, lumbar facet joint, lumbosacral radiculopathies, and piriformis/gluteal muscles [1–5].

Sacroiliac joint tends to cause pain in the low back, rarely radiate below the knee, and tends to ease up with sitting. Lumbar disc pain does get worse with sitting, but pain localization tends to be over the spine, with limitation of lumbar range of motion due to pain. Facet joint pain is usually ipsilateral, gets better with sitting, and tends to occur in older patients unless due to injury. Hip joint pain does not tend to get worse with sitting, though pain with hip joint rotation can point toward the hip joint as a source of problem [6]. Considering the overall clinical features of the pain symptom constellation, it looks most likely piriformis syndrome.

N. Kirch · M. V. Rana (✉)
Department of Anesthesiology and Critical Care, University of Chicago, Chicago, IL, USA
e-mail: nkirch@dacc.uchicago.edu; mrana@dacc.uchicago.edu

T. Malik (ed.), *Practical Chronic Pain Management*, https://doi.org/10.1007/978-3-030-46675-6_37

How Is the Diagnosis Confirmed?

Piriformis syndrome is a diagnosis of exclusion. The diagnosis is confirmed when a patient demonstrate certain clinical features in the absence of other pathologies as confirmed by chemical testing or imaging. Clinical feature have not been validated; pain relief after piriformis muscle injection is considered as the most diagnostic test.

Patients will describe deep buttock pain that may or may not radiate down the leg, which improves with movement and worsens by sitting/standing for even short periods of time (10–15 min) (Table 37.1). This pain may be associated with difficulty walking due to antalgic gait or foot drop, weakness of the ipsilateral lower extremity, numbness in the ipsilateral foot, or even contralateral SI pain. As these symptoms are similar to a variety of other causes of lower back, hip, and lower extremity pain, physical exam isolating the piriformis muscle is critical in differentiating it as the primary diagnosis.

In a systematic review of more than 50 case studies of piriformis syndrome, the most common presenting symptoms were buttock pain, external tenderness over the greater sciatic notch, and aggravation of the pain through sitting.

On physical exam, a patient will have point tenderness over the piriformis muscle, especially over the attachment points at the greater trochanter (Table 37.2) [5]. There may be tenderness extending to the SI joint as well. In the supine position, a relaxed patient would show ipsilateral foot external rotation, referred to as *a positive piriformis sign∗*. In the setting of chronic piriformis syndrome, surrounding neurovascular and muscular tissues can be impacted, leading to sacral plexus neuropathies as well as ipsilateral weakness of gluteus muscles, adductor magnus, quadratus femoris, and obturator externus muscles, further confounding the diagnosis. Sacral anterior rotation is often seen in piriformis syndrome, which can result in a shortening of the ipsilateral leg as well as compensatory lumbar vertebral counter-rotation, which can cause confounding lower lumbar/thoracic pain and decreased range of motion.

As there is no single test that is specific to piriformis syndrome, a variety tests frequently used to aid in the diagnosis include Freiberg, Pace, FABER, FAIR, and Beatty tests [2–4]. In the *Freiberg* test, the patient is placed in a supine or prone position, the extended hip is passively internally rotated (Table 37.3). A positive test will elicit pain in the sciatic notch. The *Pace* test is performed with the patient in the seated position with patient abducting the legs, leading to a contraction of the piriformis muscle and a resulting deep buttock pain. The *FABER* (flexion, abduction, external rotation of the hip) will result in back and deep buttock pain, as will the *FAIR* (flexion, adduction and internal rotation of the hip), reproducing the patients sciatic pain. In the Beatty test, the patient is placed in the lateral decubitus position with the painful side up. The leg on the painful side is flexed and the knee is placed on the examining table. The patient is asked to lift and hold the knee. A positive finding yields deep buttock pain [7]. Even with multiple positive physical exam tests, it can still be difficult to discern the etiology of pain and isolate the pain to the piriformis muscle. In certain instances, EMG, CT, MR, and ultrasonography have been used to further differentiate the cause. MRI or CT

Table 37.1 Symptoms of piriformis syndrome

1. Point tenderness in buttocks
2. Pain radiating down back of leg
3. Tingling down back of leg
4. Pain improves with ambulation
5. Antalgic gait

Table 37.2 Diagnostic signs of piriformis syndrome (many of below will not be met, mostly diagnosis of exclusion)

1. Pain with palpation over piriformis muscle
2. Positive Freiberg test
3. Positive pace
4. Positive FABER test
5. Positive FAIR test
6. Negative MRI spine

Table 37.3 Freiberg's criteria

Tenderness at the sciatic notch
Positive Lasègue sign
Improvement with nonsurgical treatment

of the piriformis muscle have shown both atrophy and hypertrophy of the muscle, so assessing the size of the muscle on imaging does not refute or confirm anything. The imaging of spine or pelvis is more helpful in ruling out other pathologies. Neurophysiologic testing can distinguish piriformis syndrome from disc herniation based on which muscle groups show abnormalities, with disc herniation causing nerve impingement showing abnormalities in muscles proximal to the piriformis muscle, while in piriformis syndrome the abnormalities would be distal to it [8]. Some people use delay or loss of H-reflex in the peroneal or tibial nerve as a very important diagnostic information. The delay is more pronounced in the peroneal distribution. Increase in the delay of H-reflex or its loss when the test is repeated with leg in FAIR position will confirm the entrapment of the nerve at the piriformis muscle level. CT and MR studies can show hypertrophy of the piriformis muscle or anomalous course of sciatic nerve either above or splitting through the piriformis muscle, which are known risk factors for developing this syndrome [9, 10, 11]. Radiographic studies can additionally be used to rule out alternative causes of pain. Ultrasound can also be used to assess for hypertrophy of piriformis muscle as well as anatomic variations of sciatic nerve course.

What Is the Pathophysiology of This Condition?

In order to understand how the piriformis muscle can result in sciatic nerve irritation and pain, a basic understanding of the neuroanatomy as well as rare variations in the sciatic nerve course is critical. There are two types of piriformis syndrome, primary and secondary. The primary form results from anatomic variations of the piriformis muscle in relation to the sciatic nerve. The piriformis muscle functions to work at the hip joint, acting as an abductor, flexor, and external rotator of the joint. Anatomically, the muscle spans the anterior aspect of the sacrum to the greater trochanter, with the sciatic nerve exiting the greater sciatic foramen deep along the inferior surface of the piriformis muscle (Fig. 37.1). In as much as 22% of the population, the sciatic nerve pierces the piriformis muscle, splits the piriformis muscle, or both, predisposing these individuals to piriformis syndrome [12]. Secondary piriformis syndrome results from macro-/microtrauma resulting in ischemic mass effect or local inflammation of the sciatic nerve. This version of piriformis syndrome is most often caused by macrotrauma or direct trauma to soft tissue and the piriformis muscle, resulting in soft tissue inflammation and muscle spasm. This creates an impingement point as the sciatic nerve courses under the muscle. Microtrauma can be caused by repetitive use of the piriformis muscle, seen in long distance runners, or by direct compression, seen in people

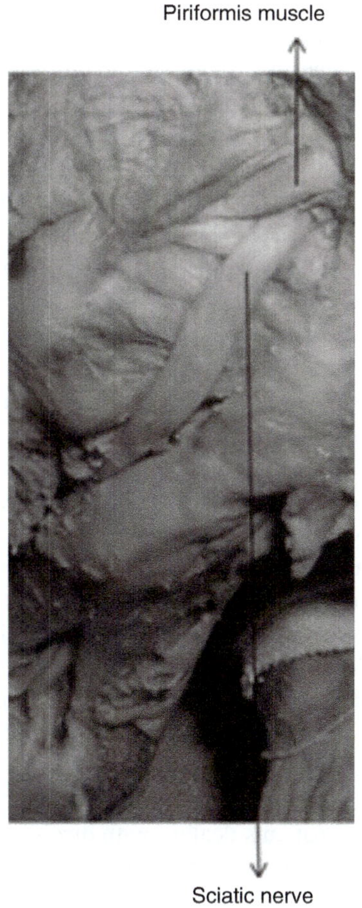

Fig. 37.1 Standard course of sciatic nerve inferior to the body of the piriformis muscle. (From Sulak et al. [22], with permission)

chronically sitting on hard surfaces, like taxi drivers or patients who sit on large wallets [7].

How Is This Problem Managed?

Initial treatment of piriformis syndrome includes rest, analgesics, and physical therapy. Pharmacotherapy includes NSAIDs, acetaminophen, muscle relaxants, gabapentin, and opiates. Initial therapies should be chosen based on symptoms and titrated to effect.

In patients refractory to conservative management, more invasive approaches should be considered. Diagnostic and therapeutic injections have been shown to be effective. While injections under fluoroscopy have been done, ultrasound-guided injections of the piriformis muscle have been shown to be superior in multiple studies.

Local anesthetic and steroid injections were evaluated in an approach correlating anatomical dissection with a combined fluoroscopic-nerve stimulator technique to demonstrate efficacy of therapy [4]. Other authors have studied the use of ultrasound as a combination modality to gauge feasibility and outcome [13, 14, 15]. One group compared the accuracy of fluoroscopically guided versus ultrasound piriformis injections in a cadaveric study, demonstrating a higher success rate in the ultrasound guided approach than in the X-ray guided group.

In addition to technique, the efficacy of different injectate has been debated with local anesthetic versus combination local and steroid preparations [16]. The addition of corticosteroid did not confer additional benefit. The limitations of the study include volume administration (5 mL) and the use of a singular steroid (betamethazone). No comparison was made with a different class of steroid, dexamethasone for example, in this evaluation.

Muscle relaxants are also a possible treatment option for patients dealing with discomfort from piriformis syndrome. Common routes include oral agents and also the use of botulinum toxin injections. A case report highlights the use of botulinum toxin A in a patient with chronic pain due to spasms [17]. Another study, a prospective single site trial, evaluated the effect of botulinum toxin using CT guidance [18]. Physical modalities including TENS, massage, and soft tissue mobilization have also demonstrated efficacy for the treatment [19].

What Is the Prognosis of This Condition?

The prognosis of the condition is unknown as most patients get better by themselves [20, 21]. Only recalcitrant cases come to seek medical help. It's suspected that a piriformis flare-up pain resolves over few weeks in general. It's more important to find the underlying factors that are causing piriformis muscle to act up, i.e., improve sitting posture, gait balance training, and fix leg length discrepancy or any anatomical factors that need surgical correction so that it does not happen again. Proper diagnosis and directed treatment can lead to improvement in symptoms and benefit for patients with piriformis syndrome.

Discussion

Prevalence

The lifetime prevalence of sciatica in the general population has been reported between 12% and 27% with an annual prevalence of between 2.2% and 19.5% [1]. Piriformis syndrome, compression of the sciatic nerve by the piriformis muscle, is a relatively rare cause of sciatica and is estimated to account for 0.6–8% of all cases of sciatica

With annual incidence of 40 million new cases of back pain, the annual incidence of piriformis syndrome would then be around 2 million cases. Prevalence rates variability is most likely due to alterations in diagnostic criteria used to diagnose piriformis syndrome.

Differential Diagnosis

The differential diagnosis of this syndrome includes lumbago, lumbar radiculopathy, ischial bursitis, and cluneal neuralgia. The possibilities can be eliminated with a thorough history and physical examination of the patient. Lumbago would be limited primarily to axial low back pain, with piriformis presenting as buttock and posterior thigh and leg pain. Piriformis syndrome is often confused with lumbar radiculopathy; however, in the absence of disk pathology on imaging (CT or MRI), piriformis is more likely. Additionally, physical examination findings such as palpation over the piriformis muscle, provocative tests, along with the history of pressure on the piriformis muscle (such as when seated) leading to radicular-type symptoms, lead to piriformis as a diagnosis. Ischial bursitis, while in the general gluteal region, is primarily diagnosed with palpation over the ischio-gluteal bursa. Cluneal neuralgia is the irritation of the cluneal nerves over the buttock and would not be expected to lead to radicular symptoms.

Predictive Value of Different Clinical Features and Lab Testing/Imaging

The predictive values of physical exam tests have not been validated. A FAIR and FABER tests have a reported sensitivity of 0.78 and specificity of 0.80. Pace test (seated stretch test) has sensitivity of 0.53 and a specificity of 0.90, while the Lasegue's test (straight leg raise) has a sensitivity of 0.15 and specificity of 0.95. The combination of the Pace test with other tests that actively stretch piriformis muscles has shown a sensitivity of 0.91 and specificity of 0.80 for the endoscopic finding of sciatic nerve entrapment. Hence, the diagnosis of piriformis syndrome is best achieved with a combination of the history, physical examination, and diagnostic studies.

Laboratory testing including EMG testing may be performed. Usually EMG test is normal in patients with piriformis syndrome. The test is usually done to exclude other conditions. If positive, it reveals slowing of conduction velocity and or amplitude of action potentials. The degree of slowing correlates with the duration of the pathology. Fishman et al. evaluated the H-reflex of 918 patients [8]. The test was done with their leg FAIR position. He found that a delay in the H-reflex greater than 3 SD had a sensitivity of 0.88 and specificity of 0.83 for the diagnosis of piriformis syndrome. Patients who have prolonged H-reflex in the FAIR position tend to improve significantly (improvement >50%) with conservative therapy. Needle EMG of piriformis muscle tends to be normal till the very end; presence of denervation sign may be present but unlikely and a sign of severe compression. MRI of the piriformis muscle may be equivocal, but the absence of degenerative disk disease can exclude discal pathology from the differential diagnosis of piriformis syndrome. Piriformis muscle asymmetry on MRI is looked for but has not diagnostic value. MRI neurography is a little more promising. MRI of the sciatic nerve when visualized using STIR sequence may show signs of nerve irritation or edema. Hyperintensity of sciatic nerve has been seen in 86–94% patients. The MRI finding of piriformis muscle asymmetry and ipsilateral sciatic nerve hyperintensity at the sciatic notch had a specificity of 0.93 and sensitivity of 0.64 for predicting good to excellent outcome from piriformis muscle release surgery. Additionally, Ultrasound imaging of the region may demonstrate nerve entrapment and possibly muscular trauma. Increase in size of the sciatic nerve is a sign of nerve swelling at the piriformis level, but more work is needed to make the test more useful.

Strength of Evidence for Different Treatment Modalities

Rest, analgesics, and stretching exercises all have a role in the treatment of this entity. Around half the patients respond to conservative therapy. Additionally, interventional options may hasten recovery from this syndrome. Landmark technique is not reliable at all. Some sort of imaging to guide injection is almost mandatory for accuracy reason. As described above, fluoroscopic guidance was traditionally used for treatment. With the advent of ultrasound-guided intervention for this entity, a robust and dynamic modality allows for direct visualization of target and treatment delivery. In one study, MRI-guided local anesthetic injection into the piriformis muscle in patients with piriformis syndrome gave complete relief to 15% of patients with no recurrence of pain, another 8% needed a repeat injection for complete relief, 37% had 2–4 months of relief with a subsequent recurrence despite repeat injection, 24% had less than 2 weeks of relief with subsequent recurrence, and 16% had no relief at all. There is no proof that addition of steroid to local anesthetic adds any benefit. In a double-blind, randomized, placebo-controlled trial, botulinum toxin was found to be superior to a combination of lidocaine and steroid as well as normal saline placebo for pain relief in patients with piriformis syndrome. When combined with physical therapy, injection of botulinum has shown to improve symptoms in resistant cases. When looking at more invasive treatments, including nerve blocks, steroid injections, and botox injections, there is a paucity of randomized controlled trials on injectate type for this pain condition. Surgical intervention often involves tenotomy of the piriformis muscle tendon and sciatic nerve decompression.

Future Directions or Clinical Trials in Progress

Greater use of ultrasound guidance for diagnosis and tracking of therapy is a direction of interest for pain providers. Identifying the etiology of piriformis syndrome, whether an isolated phenomenon, or the fruition of concomitant lumbago, or lumbar radiculopathy would allow providers to identify, stratify and intervene with therapy early on in the development of this entity. Early diagnosis is crucial in treating this process as intervening sooner with treatment modalities would improve treatment outcomes with less potential nerve damage.

Conclusion/Summary

Piriformis syndrome is a clinical entity that requires a pain provider to synthesize history, exam, and diagnostic tools to give a diagnosis. While a clinical diagnosis leads to treatment, precision can lead to improved outcomes. The use of combination of diagnostic tests, instead of relying on one, on physical exam allows practitioners to exclude confounding entities. The advent of ultrasound guidance for injections as well as for diagnostic purposes has led to an improvement in outcomes. Debate continues to exist as to the most effective mixture for injection to calm the musculature and underlying sciatic nerve. Future controlled trials should evaluate choice of injectate and speed and persistence of clinical result. What is not debatable, however, is the requirement for a multi-disciplinary approach, including pharmacology, interventional treatments, and physical modalities, to improve pain and numbness related to the piriformis syndrome.

References

1. Cass SP. Piriformis syndrome: a cause of nondiscogenic sciatica. Curr Sports Med Rep. 2015;14(1):41–4. https://doi.org/10.1249/JSR.0000000000000110. PMID 25574881.
2. Hopayian K, Danielyan A. Four symptoms define the piriformis syndrome: an updated systematic review of its clinical features. Eur J Orthop Surg Traumatol. 2017;28:155–64. https://doi.org/10.1007/s00590-017-2031-8. PMID 28836092.
3. Smoll NR. Variations of the piriformis and sciatic nerve with clinical consequence: a review. Clin Anat. 2010;23(1):8–17. https://doi.org/10.1002/ca.20893. PMID 19998490.
4. Benzon HT, Katz JA, Benzon HA, Iqbal MS. Piriformis syndrome: anatomic considerations, a new injection technique, and a review of the literature. Anesthesiology. 2003;98(6):1442–8. https://doi.org/10.1097/00000542-200306000-00022. PMID 12766656
5. Jawish RM, Assoum HA, Khamis CF. Anatomical, clinical and electrical observations in piriformis syndrome. J Orthop Surg Res. 2010;5:3. https://doi.org/10.1186/1749-799X-5-3. PMC 2828977 . PMID 20180984.
6. Hayek SM, Shah BJ, Desai MJ, Chelimsky TC. Pain medicine: an interdisciplinary case-based approach. Oxford: Oxford University Press; 2015. p. 240. ISBN 978-0-19-939081-6.
7. Boyajian-O'Neill LA, McClain RL, Coleman MK, Thomas PP. Diagnosis and management of piriformis syndrome: an osteopathic approach. J Am Osteopath Assoc. 2008;108:657–64.
8. Fishman L, Allen NW, Rosner B. Electrophysiologically Identified Piriformis Syndrome is successfully treated with Incobotulinum toxin A and Physical Therapy. Muscle Nerve. 2016;56:258–63. https://doi.org/10.1002/mus.25504.

9. Ro TH, Edmonds L. Diagnosis and management of piriformis syndrome: a rare anatomic variant analyzed by magnetic resonance imaging. J Clin Imaging Sci. 2018;8:6.
10. Rossi P, Cardinali P, Serrao M, Parisi L, Bianco F, De Bac S. Magnetic resonance imaging findings in piriformis syndrome: a case report. Arch Phys Med Rehabil. 2001;82(4):519–21.
11. Al-Al-Shaikh MF, Paratte B, Kastler B, Vidal C, Aubry S. An MRI evaluation of changes in piriformis muscle morphology induced by botulinum toxin injections in the treatment of piriformis syndrome. Diagn Interv Imaging. 2015;96(1):37–43.
12. Brooks JBB, Silva CAC, Soares SA, Kai MR, Cabral RH, Fragoso YD. Anatomical variations of the sciatic nerve in a Group of Brazilian Cadavers. Rev Dor Sao Paulo. 2011;12(4):332–6.
13. Huerto APS, Yeo SN, Ho KY. Piriformis muscle injection using ultrasonography and motor stimulation-report of a technique. Pain Physician. 2007;10:687–90.
14. Finnoff JT, Hurdle MFB, Smith J. Accuracy of ultrasound-guided versus fluoroscopically guided contrast-controlled piriformis injections. J Ultrasound Med. 2008;27(8):1157–63. Accessed online: https://doi.org/10.7863/jum.2008.27.8.1157.
15. Smith J, Hurdle MF, Locketz AJ, Wisniewski SJ. Ultrasound-guided piriformis injection: technique description and verification. Arch Phys Med Rehabil. 2006;87(12):1664–7.
16. Misirlioglu TO, Akgun K, Palamar D, Erden MG, Erbilir T. Effectiveness of local anesthetic and corticosteroid injections: a double-blinded randomized controlled study. Pain Physician. 2015;18:163–71.
17. Santamato A, Micello MF, Valeno G, Beatrice R, Cinone N, Baricich A, Picelli A, Panza F, Logroscino G, Fiore P, Ranieri M. Ultrasound-guided injection of botulinum toxin type a for piriformis muscle syndrome: a case report and review of the literature. Toxins (Basel). 2005;7(8):3045–56.
18. Yoon SJ, Ho J, Kang HY, Lee SH, Kim KI, Shin WG, Oh JM. Low-Dose botulinum toxin type A for the treatment of refractory piriformis syndrome. Pharmacotherapy. 2007;27(5):657–65.
19. Tonley JC, Yun SM, Kochevar RJ, Dye JA, Farrokhi S, Powers CM. Treatment of an individual with piriformis syndrome focusing on hip muscle strengthening and movement reeducation: a case report. J Orthop Sports Phys Ther. 2010;40(2):103–11.
20. Jeong HS, Lee GY, Lee EG, Joe EG, Lee JW, Kang HS. Long-term assessment of clinical outcomes of ultrasound-guided steroid injections in patients with piriformis syndrome. Ultrasonography. 2015;34(3):206–10.
21. Kean Chen C, Nizar AJ. Prevalence of piriformis syndrome in chronic low back pain patients. A clinical diagnosis with modified FAIR test.
22. Sulak O, Sakalli B, Ozguner G, Kastamoni Y. Anatomical relation between sciatic nerve and piriformis muscle and its birfurcation level during fetal period in human. Surg Radiol Anat. 2014;36(3):265–72.

A 25-Year-Old Cyclist with Persistent Perineal Pain

38

David H. Kim, Arjun Ramesh, and Adam C. Young

Case Presentation

A 25-year-old professional male cyclist notes an increasing dull ache in the perineum. His pain symptoms radiate to the penis and are exacerbated by long-distance cycling. Several weeks after his symptoms begin, he notices painful urination and perineal pain following intercourse. He is otherwise healthy. Prior to visiting your pain clinic, he was treated empirically for possible urinary tract infection or prostatitis by his primary care physician. Following a course of antibiotics, negative urinalysis, negative sexually transmitted disease panel, he was referred to a neurologist. Initial MRI of the lumbar and sacral spine is negative for central or foraminal stenosis. He was started on anti-inflammatory medications with moderate reduction in pain but ongoing symptoms were exacerbated by cycling activities and sitting. He admits the only alleviating factors are resting from cycling, changing to a wider saddle, massages, standing, laying down, or sitting on the toilet. He denies frank loss of bowel or bladder control but does note increased diminished sensation and increased straining during bowel movements and a mild degree of erectile dysfunction and genital sensitivity to light touch. He presents to your pain clinic for further evaluation and treatment.

What Is Your Preliminary Diagnosis?

The patient pain is distributed in the perineum and has mechanical component to it as it gets worse with sitting. There is associated visceral dysfunction affecting bladder and penile area. His medical work up is negative and he showed no response to antibiotics. He demonstrates increased sensitivity (allodynia) in the distribution of pudendal nerve. This along with relief of pain when sitting on the toilet and worsening pain with cycling and difficulty moving bowel suggest pudendal nerve dysfunction. The pudendal nerve dysfunction often results from entrapment, but direct damage from a trauma, surgery, infection, or any other medical condition causing demyelination can also do this. Pudendal neuralgia diagnosis requires high level of suspicion as there are no obvious signs or symptoms.

D. H. Kim
Department of Anesthesiology and Pain Medicine, Kansas University Medical Center, Kansas City, KS, USA

A. Ramesh
Department of Anesthesiology, Rush University, Chicago, IL, USA

A. C. Young (✉)
Department of Anesthesiology and Pain Management, Illinois Bone & Joint Institute, Morton Grove, IL, USA
e-mail: Adam_Young@Rush.Edu

T. Malik (ed.), *Practical Chronic Pain Management*, https://doi.org/10.1007/978-3-030-46675-6_38

How Is the Condition Diagnosed?

Pudendal neuralgia is a clinical diagnosis. Like many other chronic pain conditions, it is a diagnosis of exclusion. A patient with clinical feature suggestive of pudendal neuralgia can have confirmatory diagnosis if the pudendal nerve block provides complete relief. There are no specific tests for pudendal neuralgia. Imaging study like MRI or CT helps in excluding other pathologies. Neurophysiology tests such as pudendal nerve terminal motor latency (PNTML) test and electromyography (EMG) may serve as complementary diagnostic measures. However, these electrophysiologic findings are not specific for patients with pudendal neuralgia can be abnormal in other conditions and explain their limitation in female after child birth. PNTML is done by sending a signal along the pudendal nerve and the time it takes for a muscle to contract. PNTML test can pick a demyelination process but cannot detect axon loss. It cannot detect any sensory nerve damage. The test would be normal if only sensory fibers are affected. A latency longer than 2.2 ms is considered abnormal. PNTML relies on the largest, fastest conducting nerves. EMG and single-fiber EMG with fiber density measurements are better able to evaluate neuropathy compared with latency tests, but these tests are more cumbersome and even too painful for a patient already in pain.

How Do You Manage This Condition?

If the precipitating factors are well defined, they can be avoided. Physical therapy is first line of intervention. Patient would need referral to place who specialize in pelvic floor exercises. This may entail manual techniques to relax the muscles, improve range of motion, posture training, strengthening pelvic, back, and hip muscles. Membrane stabilizers (Lyrica), muscle relaxers (flexeril, baclofen), and tricyclic antidepressants (amitriptyline) have also been tried. Pudendal nerve block is performed both for diagnostic and therapeutic reasons. A number of approaches and medications have been used with variable success in different reports. Pain relief up to few months has been described. In few cases where there is a strong suspicion of nerve entrapment, surgical decompression is done when everything else has failed.

Discussion

Pudendal neuralgia is a rare and painful condition along the distribution of the pudendal nerve with varied clinical presentations. Pudendal neuralgia is classically described as a sharp or burning pain in the perineum with extension to the genitals, including both the scrotum and penis in males and the vulva, vagina, and clitoris in females. Associated symptoms include dyspareunia, dysuria, urinary frequency and/or urgency, decreased rectal sensation during defecation, and allodynia or hyperpathia of the perineum or genitals [1]. Clinical signs associated with pudendal neuralgia include exacerbation when sitting or cycling and alleviation with standing, laying down, sitting on a toilet seat. The diagnosis of this condition is often delayed due to shared characteristics with other pain etiologies with average diagnosis from symptom onset of 2–10 years [2].

The varied presentation of pudendal neuralgia is secondary to the anatomical course of pudendal nerve with three main branches and the fact that it is a mixed sensory-motor nerve. The nerve is derived from S2-S4 ventral roots and courses along the greater sciatic notch, piriformis muscle, sacrospinous ligament, sacrotuberous ligament, lesser sciatic foramen, and Alcock's canal. The three terminal branches are the inferior rectal nerve, the perineal nerve, and the dorsal nerve of the penis and clitoris. The inferior rectal nerve controls the external anal sphincter, sensation of the distal anal canal below the pectinate line, and perianal sensation. The perineal nerve has both a motor component innervating perineal muscles within the urogenital triangle – superficial transverse perineal muscle, bulbospongiosus, ischiocavernosus, sphincter urethra, but also provides sensation from the scrotum or labia. The dorsal nerve provides genital sensation from the penis and clitoris. Several anatomic entrapment areas have been previously characterized: (1) exit of the greater sciatic notch associated with the piriformis muscle; (2) ischial spine associated with the sacrotuberous ligament; (3) obturator internus muscle at entrance of the pudendal or Alcock canal; and (4) entrapment of distal terminal branches [2].

Although classically described in the cyclist population, pudendal neuralgia is also associated with obstetrical complications, urologic surgery, pelvic fractures, pelvic radiation, and infectious complications. During vaginal delivery, the pudendal nerve may suffer mechanical compression or stretch injury. Vaginal sling procedures for urinary incontinence have also been associated with scarring initiated by mesh, suture, or trocar placement with likely entrapment [3, 4]. Sacrospinous ligament fixation for treatment of vaginal vault prolapse may similarly cause entrapment of the pudendal nerve [3, 5]. Patients who have suffered pelvic or hip fractures can have subsequent direct transection or stretch/compression injuries to the pudendal nerve [6, 7]. Scarring or adhesions as a result of pelvic radiation may be associated with entrapment [8]. Infectious etiologies are also possible as post-herpetic pudendal neuralgia has also been described [9].

Differential Diagnosis

The differential diagnosis for chronic pelvic and perineal pain is broad. As no definitive test exists for this condition, the proper diagnosis depends on history and physical examination along with exclusion of other diagnoses. Other etiologies of chronic pelvic and perineal pain include the following:

- Sciatica (or lumbosacral radiculopathy)
- Piriformis syndrome
- Coccycodynia
- Ischial bursitis
- Tarlov cyst
- Sacral central stenosis
- Sacral foraminal stenosis
- Interstitial cystitis
- Abacterial chronic prostatitis
- Prostatodynia
- Idiopathic proctalgia
- Vulvodynia
- Vaginismus/pelvic floor myalgia
- Endometriosis
- Hemorrhoids
- Proctalgia fugax
- Levator ani syndrome
- Persistent genital arousal disorder
- Chronic pelvic pain syndrome

Confirming the Diagnosis

The diagnostic dilemma of pudendal neuralgia as with many other chronic pelvic pain conditions is that no specific and definitive diagnostic testing exists. A careful history and physical examination guiding subsequent diagnostic testing with either laboratory testing or imaging studies is necessary to rule out other diagnoses. Diagnostic criteria (Nantes Criteria) for pudendal have been refined and validated [10] (Table 38.1). Essential criteria include the following: (1) pain in the territory of the pudendal nerve: from the anus to the penis or clitoris, (2) pain is predominantly experienced while sitting, (3) the pain does not wake the patient at night, (4) pain with no objective sensory impairment, and (5) pain relieved by diagnostic pudendal nerve block. It should be noted that neurophysiology findings are complementary or supportive and no mention is made of imaging modalities. The diagnosis is primarily a clinical one, guided by history.

Testing for lack of pain upon palpation, allodynia, hyperpathia in other nerve distributions such as the cluneal, ilioinguinal, iliohypogastric nerves along with testing for lack of objective sensory impairment may support a diagnosis of pudendal neuralgia (Table 38.2). Given overlapping sensory innervation in the perineum and genital area from the iliohypogastric, ilioinguinal, genitofemoral, posterior femoral cutaneous, and cluneal nerves, an isolated sensory deficit would be more consistent with a radiculopathy or plexopathy [11]. Palpation of the greater or lesser sciatic notch and the obturator internus may reproduce symptoms and point out areas of

Table 38.1 Nantes diagnostic criteria for pudendal neuralgia

Essential diagnostic criteria	Complementary diagnostic criteria	Exclusion criteria	Associated signs not excluding the diagnosis
Pain in the territory of the pudendal nerve: from the anus to the penis or clitoris	Burning, shooting, stabbing pain, numbness	Exclusively coccygeal, gluteal, pubic, or hypogastric pain	Buttock pain on sitting
Pain is predominantly experienced while siting	Allodynia or hyperpathia	Pruritis	Referred sciatic pain
The pain does not wake the patient at night	Rectal or vaginal foreign body sensation (sympathalgia)	Exclusively paroxysmal pain	Pain referred to the medial aspect of the thigh
Pain with no objective sensory impairment	Worsening of pain during the day	Imaging abnormalities able to account for the pain	Suprapubic pain
Pain relieved by diagnostic pudendal nerve block	Predominantly unilateral pain		Urinary frequency and/or pain on a full bladder
	Pain triggered by defecation		Pain occurring after ejaculation
	Presence of exquisite tenderness on palpation of the ischial spine		Dyspareunia and/or pain after sexual intercourse
	Clinical neurophysiology findings in men or nulliparous women		Erectile dysfunction
			Normal clinical neurophysiology

From Labat et al. [10], with permission

Table 38.2 Diagnostic tests for pudendal neuralgia

Physical features	Tenderness around ischial spine
Nerve block	Relief with nerve block at the ischial spine
Ultrasound	Thickening of nerve may be visible
MRI	May reveal source of nerve entrapment, rule out other pathologies
Angiography	AV pathologies causing nerve compression
Pelvic X-ray	Fracture along the nerve route
Electrophysiology	Conduction delay

possible nerve entrapment [3, 12]. Tenderness on palpation of the ischial spine during rectal or vaginal examination, particularly when unilateral, supports a diagnosis of pudendal neuralgia [3, 11]. In addition, patients may favor one side to sit on during clinical evaluation [3]. No clinical sign or physical examination finding has been shown to be both sensitive and/or specific.

Neurophysiology testing may focus on pudendal nerve terminal motor latencies or electromyography [13]. However, this testing is not specific to pudendal neuralgia and may not be a sensitive measure with poor correlation to clinical symptoms such as fecal incontinence or physiologic changes such as perineal descent, which was theorized to initiate pudendal nerve injury [14]. It should be noted that as the pudendal nerve is a mixed nerve, any branch may be affected; neurophysiologic testing of the pudendal nerve terminal motor latencies or electromyography does not address pain or sensory manifestations of pudendal neuralgia. At present MR neurography is considered a relatively new and unvalidated technique to diagnose pudendal neuralgia.

Treatment

Behavioral modification is an important modality when treating pudendal neuralgia. In one study of 64 patients with pudendal neuralgia symptoms, behavioral modification by sitting on pads along with medication therapy resulted in pain relief in all patients, albeit with mild to moderate symptom relief [15]. Other behavioral modifications more specific to cyclists may include halting cycling activity to decrease inflammation, stretching exercises, wider or softer seats, cycling in a more upright position, or intermittently relieving pressure by standing up while riding [12, 16, 17].

Physical therapy, specifically active release technique, has been described in a case report with good results in an ironman triathlete [12]. For patients suffering from pudendal myalgia, optimal therapy may be achieved by a physical therapist specializing in pelvic floor dysfunction. Techniques that have been described include basic palpation, posture optimization, range of motion, and strength exercises to myofascial and trigger point release, which may include transvaginal or transrectal approaches. Based on this, protocols have been developed that utilized myofascial trigger points and relaxation therapy in the treatment of pelvic pain in general. However, no specific large-scale trials utilizing physical therapy have been performed for the specific diagnosis of pudendal neuralgia. Although biofeedback has been applied for the diagnosis of pudendal neuralgia, this treatment modality is utilized typically as an adjunct therapy along with behavioral modification and physical therapy [18].

Medication classes that are historically utilized in the treatment of pudendal neuralgia included tricyclic antidepressants, NSAIDS, gabapentinoids, opioids, and muscle relaxants [3, 19]. Recommended dosing for pregabalin is 75 mg twice per day with up-titration as tolerated. Although oral muscle relaxants are readily available, a variety locally delivered muscle relaxants have been described. Vaginal valium, diazepam, or baclofen suppositories are commonly used in the obstetrics and gynecologic population [3, 20]. Rectal belladonna and opium suppositories twice per day have also been used for local muscle relaxant and pain relief effects [18]. Perineal 8% capsaicin patches have recently been utilized for a variety of chronic pelvic and perineal pain syndromes with one study demonstrating a response rate of 24% in a pelvic pain population with "very much improved" or "much improved" with an overall improvement of 58% and 3.4 score reduction on NRS scales [21].

Pudendal nerve blockade can be accomplished with various imaging modalities although duration relief has been limited. A recent study demonstrated long-term relief in 2 of 29 patients with the diagnosis of pudendal neuralgia confirmed by initial response to pudendal nerve blockade [22]. And a larger scale retrospective study of 95 patients utilizing CT-guided dual pudendal nerve blockade both at the ischial spine and pudendal canal demonstrated an efficacy rate at 6 month follow-up of 25.2% with self-reported improvement of 60% [23]. The addition of corticosteroids to the nerve block does not appear to confer additional analgesia [24]. The evidence for pudendal nerve radiofrequency ablation appears to be more promising. One case series demonstrated mean reduction in VAS scores from 9.0 down to 1.9 at 1 year post-procedure [13].

Neuromodulation has been successfully utilized for refractory cases of pudendal neuralgia. Spinal cord stimulation of the conus medullaris in a case series of 27 patients had a response rate of 74% and estimated improvement of 55.5% over an average follow-up time of 29 months [25]. In that study, the majority of spinal cord stimulator systems at the permanent implant phase was single column and placed with the termination of last stimulator plot just below the level of the conus medullaris as determined by MRI of the spinal cord pre-implant. More recently, dorsal root ganglion stimulation has been utilized for refractory chronic pelvic pain. In a small case series of 7 patients with severe chronic pelvic pain, some of whom had failed dorsal column spinal cord stimulation, bilateral L1 and S2 dorsal root ganglion trial leads were utilized with significant relief in all patients [26]. Average VAS pain score was 7.6 pre-trial and 1.6 post-trial. Sacral stimulation utilizing lead placement at bilateral S3 and S4 foramina has been shown in a case report to have significant pain relief with 10/10 NRS pre-stimulator to 2/10 NRS post-stimulator over a 4 year follow-up period with significant improved function such as the ability to resume horseback riding and significant reduction in opioid medication [27]. Peripheral nerve stimulation of the pudendal nerve at the ischio-rectal fossa has been described with complete to significant pain relief in 16 out of 19 patients following lead placement [28].

Surgical decompression has been historically effective in approximately 75% of patients. In one of the earliest larger case series of pudendal nerve decompression, a success rate of 70% was reported in a population of 170 patients [29]. A more recent prospective study of 200 patients resulted in sustained 50–100% improvement in 87% of patients over a 12 month follow-up period [2]. A randomized controlled trial comparing surgical versus non-surgical treatment of pudendal neuralgia revealed a significantly greater percentage of patients reporting improvement at 3 month follow-up, 50% versus 6.2%. This trial also replicated prior larger case series in that 71.4% of patients in the surgical group reported improvement at 12 month follow-up [30]. Non-response has been hypothesized to be secondary to chronic nerve injury via crush, stretch, or transection injury rather than secondary to an anatomic entrapment.

Conclusion

Pudendal neuralgia is a painful condition affecting the nerve distribution of the pudendal nerve that is quite common in certain population and often underdiagnosed or mistreated. The Nantes criteria are quite useful in helping to make the diagnosis of this confusing condition. There is no definite treatment for this condition like many other chronic pain conditions since pathophysiology is still poorly understood. More research is needed to clarify the optimal diagnostic and treatment methods for this condition.

References

1. Robert R, Labat JJ, Riant T, et al. The pudendal nerve: clinical and therapeutic morphogenesis, anatomy, and physiopathology. Neurochirurgie. 2009;55(4–5):463–9.
2. Filler AG. Diagnosis and treatment of pudendal nerve entrapment syndrome subtypes: imaging, injections, and minimal access surgery. Neurosurg Focus. 2009;26(2):E9.
3. Khoder W, Hale D. Pudendal Neuralgia. Obstet Gynecol Clin N Am. 2014;41(3):443–52.
4. Fisher HW, Lotze PM. Nerve injury locations during retropubic sling procedures. Int Urogynecol J. 2011;22(4):439–41.
5. Alevizon SJ, Finan MA. Sacrospinous colpopexy: management of postoperative pudendal nerve entrapment. Obstet Gynecol. 1996;88(4 Pt 2):713–5.
6. Lyon T, Koval KJ, Kummer F, Zuckerman JD. Pudendal nerve palsy induced by fracture table. Orthop Rev. 1993;22(5):521–5.
7. Báča V, Báčová T, Grill R, et al. Pudendal nerve in pelvic bone fractures. Injury. 2013;44(7):952–6.
8. Elahi F, Callahan D, Greenlee J, Dann TL. Pudendal entrapment neuropathy: a rare complication of pelvic radiation therapy. Pain Physician. 2013;16(6):E793–7.
9. Howard EJ. Postherpetic pudendal neuralgia. JAMA. 1985;253(15):2196.
10. Labat JJ, Riant T, Robert R, et al. Diagnostic criteria for pudendal neuralgia by pudendal nerve entrapment (Nantes criteria). Neurourol Urodyn. 2008;27(4):306–10.
11. Ploteau S, Cardaillac C, Perrouin-Verbe MA, et al. Pudendal neuralgia due to pudendal nerve entrapment: warning signs observed in two cases and review of the literature. Pain Physician. 2016;19(3):E449–54.
12. Durante JA, MacIntyre IG. Pudendal nerve entrapment in an Ironman athlete: a case report. J Can Chiropr Assoc. 2010;54(4):276–81.
13. Masala S, Calabria E, Cuzzolino A, et al. CT-guided percutaneous pulse-dose radiofrequency for pudendal neuralgia. Cardiovasc Intervent Radiol. 2014;37(2):476–81.
14. Lefaucheur JP, Labat JJ, Amarenco G, et al. What is the place of electroneuromyogrpahic studies in the diagnosis and management of pudendal neuralgia related to entrapment syndrome? Neurophysiol Clin. 2007;37(4):223–8.
15. Benson JT, Griffis K. Pudendal neuralgia, a severe pain syndrome. Am J Obstet Gynecol. 2005;192(5):1663–8.
16. Carpes FP, Dagnese F, Kleinpaul JF, et al. Effects of workload on seat pressure while cycling with two different saddles. J Sex Med. 2009;6(10):2728–35.
17. Gemery JM, Nangia AK, Mamourian AC, Reid SK. Digital three-dimensional modelling of the male pelvis and bicycle seats: impact of riderposition and seat design on potential penile hypoxia and erectile dysfunction. BJU Int. 2007;99(1):135–40.
18. Hibner M, Desai N, Robertson LJ, Nour M. Pudendal neuralgia. J Minim Invasive Gynecol. 2010;17(2):148–53.
19. Pereira A, Pérez-Medina T, Rodríguez-Tapia A, et al. Chronic perineal pain: analyses of prognostic factors in pudendal neuralgia. Clin J Pain. 2014;30(7):577–82.
20. Elkins N, Hunt J, Scott KM. Neurogenic Pelvic Pain. Phys Med Rehabil Clin N Am. 2017;28(3):551–69.
21. Levesque A, Riant T, Labat JJ, Ploteau S. Use of high-concentration capsaicin patch for the treatment of

pelvic pain: observational study of 60 inpatients. Pain Physician. 2017;20(1):E161–7.
22. Mamlouk MD, vanSonnenberg E, Dehkharghani S. CT-guided nerve block for pudendal neuralgia: diagnostic and therapeutic implications. AJR Am J Roentgenol. 2014;203(1):196–200.
23. Kastler A, Puget J, Tiberghien F, et al. Dual site pudendal nerve infiltration: more than just a diagnostic test? Pain Physician. 2018;21(1):83–90.
24. Labat JJ, Riant T, Lassaux A, et al. Adding corticosteroids to the pudendal nerve block for pudendal neuralgia: a randomized, double-blind, controlled trial. BJOG. 2017;124(2):251–60.
25. Buffenoir K, Rioult B, Hamel O, et al. Spinal cord stimulation of the conus medullaris for refractory pudendal neuralgia: a prospective study of 27 consecutive cases. Neurourol Urodyn. 2015;34(2):177–82.
26. Hunter CW, Yang A. Dorsal root ganglion stimulation for chronic pelvic pain: a case series and technical report on a novel lead configuration. Neuromodulation. 2019;22(1):87–95.
27. Valovska A, Peccora CD, Philip CN, et al. Sacral neuromodulation as a treatment for pudendal neuralgia. Pain Physician. 2014;17(5):E645–50.
28. Peters KM, Killinger KA, Jaeger C, Chen C. Pilot study exploring chronic pudendal neuromodulation as a treatment option for pain associated with pudendal neuralgia. Low Urin Tract Symptoms. 2015;7(3):138–42.
29. Robert R, Prat-Pradal D, Labat JJ, et al. Anatomic basis of chronic perineal pain: role of the pudendal nerve. Surg Radiol Anat. 1998;20(2):93–8.
30. Robert R, Labat JJ, Bensignor M, et al. Decompression and transposition of the pudendal nerve in pudendal neuralgia: a randomized controlled trial and long-term evaluation. Eur Urol. 2005;47(3):403–8.

A 55-Year-Old Patient with Recurrent Pain After Back Surgery

39

Thomas Zouki, Kenneth D. Candido, and Nebojsa Nick Knezevic

Case Description

A 55-year-old man with a history of 10 years of progressive low back pain (LBP) radiating in the left lower extremity, which proved refractory to conservative treatment, was evaluated. The pain was insidious in onset, progressed to an 8/10 on a visual assessment numerical rating scale (VAS) score at its worst, and was poorly controlled with ibuprofen, gabapentin, hydrocodone/acetaminophen, and epidural steroid injections (ESI). He experienced "mild relief" with physical therapy but the benefits were only transient. He worked as a mechanic and, although he did not have any motor deficit from his condition, he experienced a substantially reduced quality of life and functional status due to the pain he perceived, to a point where he even would have to regularly miss days of work. He had MRI evidence of an L4-L5 disc herniation, spinal canal stenosis, and degenerative changes of the lumbar spine (Fig. 39.1). He lives alone and his medical problems are acid reflux for which he takes omeprazole, mild depression for which he takes amitriptyline and he is mildly obese with a BMI of 34. After consultation with a neurosurgeon, a decision was made to undergo an L4-L5 discectomy with accompanied L4 and L5 laminectomies. The surgery was uncomplicated but after only 2 months post-operatively, the patient presented to our pain clinic with complaints of recurrent back pain that he then considered to be potentially more aggravating than what it was at baseline.

What Is Your Preliminary Diagnosis?

There is no precise or well-accepted definition of failed back surgery syndrome (FBSS). In general, specialists agree that it is a term used to identify "the surgical end-stage after one or several interventions on the lumbar neuroaxis indicated to relieve lower back pain, radicular pain or the combination of both, without effect" [1]. In other words, "when the outcome of lumbar spinal surgery does not meet the pre-surgical expectations of the patient and surgeon" [2]. It does not mean failure to obtain total pain relief or return to total normal function since, for some spinal conditions, it is clear that complete pain relief is not realistic.

The case presented in this chapter is a typical case of FBSS, involving a patient who had significantly reduced quality of life due to his spine

T. Zouki
Department of Anesthesiology, Texas Tech University Health Sciences Center, Lubbock, TX, USA

K. D. Candido · N. N. Knezevic (✉)
Department of Anesthesiology, Advocate Illinois Masonic Medical Center, Chicago, IL, USA

Department of Anesthesiology, University of Illinois, Chicago, IL, USA

Department of Surgery, University of Illinois, Chicago, IL, USA

T. Malik (ed.), *Practical Chronic Pain Management*, https://doi.org/10.1007/978-3-030-46675-6_39

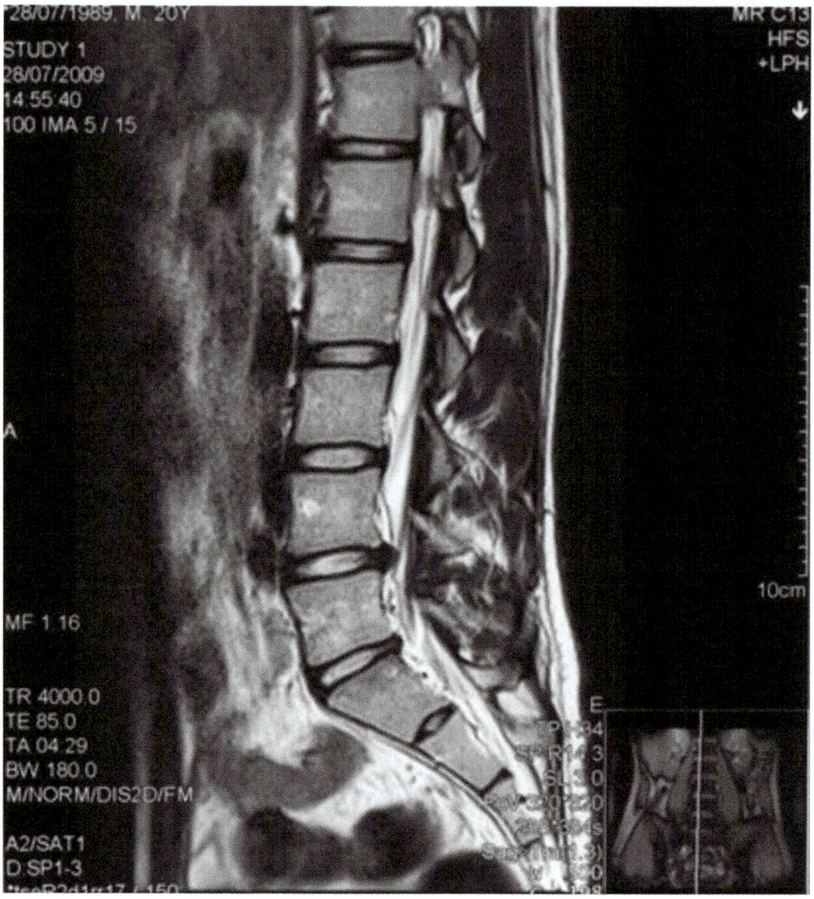

Fig. 39.1 T2-weighted sagittal lumbar MRI showing significant disc bulging at L4-L5 leading to spinal canal stenosis at the associated level

condition and also had MRI evidence of discogenic disease. After undergoing surgery, the patient did not show signs of improvement and, according to him, felt worse than before undergoing surgery. But the diagnosis of FBSS itself is very broad, and the exact etiology of the disease must be worked up to know the exact cause of FBSS. Improved knowledge of the root of the condition leads to better choice for course of treatment. Studies done on patients with FBSS identified that common causes included patients who had lateral canal stenosis post-op, central canal stenosis, recurrent or residual disc herniation, arachnoiditis or epidural fibrosis. Less common causes included nerve injury during surgery (leading to neuropathic pain), chronic mechanical pain, painful segment (disc) above or below the operated segment, pseudoarthritis, foreign body, and surgery performed at the wrong level. When a clinician is faced with a patient who presents to him/her with suspected FBSS, a careful assessment must be undertaken and all possible causes must be considered. A careful history and physical examination as well as the use of the appropriate investigation tools available to the clinician are imperative.

How is the Diagnosis Confirmed?

History

A careful history should include a thorough psychosocial well-being assessment since poor psychosocial status prior to surgery has a strong correlation with poor surgical outcome [3]. The presence of Workers' Compensation claims as well as disability claims should be taken into account. A detailed pain history with pre-operative and post-operative comparison is crucial to determine the likely source of pain. A temporal relationship between the pain following the surgery undertaken to address the underlying condition should be established. Pain that appears shortly after surgery is most likely due to pre-operative and intra-operative factors (see Discussion). If the patient complains of a pain that is more "radicular" in origin, then the source is more likely to be due to inadequate decompression, foraminal stenosis, epidural fibrosis, recurrent disc herniation, or residual disk or fragment. Post-op new onset leg pain is suggestive of an instrumentation issue such as a pedicle screw compressing an exiting nerve root [4, 5]. On the other hand, pain that is predominantly in the lower back is more suggestive of sources such as sacroiliac joint (SIJ), myofascial issues, facet joint dysfunction, or discogenic causes. Careful evaluation to rule out any red flags should not be dismissed. Other rare causes such as abscesses, hematomas, abdominal or pelvic inflammatory diseases, thoracic or abdominal aortic aneurysms, and malignancies should be kept in mind. Signs and symptoms such as early onset of back pain that is different than pre-op, new onset neurological deficit such as bowel and bladder paralysis, and weight loss should further prompt rapid investigation and treatment. The presence of night pain with or without weight loss should also be considered a cause for concern. A thorough documentation of previous treatment should also be undertaken.

Physical Examination

Even a thorough physical examination does not necessarily "rule in" the etiology of post-op back pain, but it can be helpful in "ruling out" serious pathologies. Examination of vital signs as well as abdominal, pelvic, and vascular system is important, especially if one or more of the "red flags" mentioned earlier are present. Functional examination during patient visits, including assessment of posture, gait, need of assistance such as a cane or wheelchair, ability to sit straight, and ability to undress, should all be observed and documented during the patient's visit. The patient's spine should be visibly inspected; surgical scars and vertebral alignment need to be assessed. Palpation of the lumbar spine to elicit areas of tenderness, step-offs, and indentations suggestive of spondylolisthesis is also important. Furthermore, assessing the patient's spinal range of motion with pain elicited on motion is necessary. Laying the patient down and performing a "straight leg raise test" can help identify patients with spinal stenosis, in which case the pain increases with hyperextension of the spine and is reduced when leaning forward. Focal or global muscular involvement can be evaluated by assessing each of the patient's muscle groups against resistance and comparing that to the contralateral side. Sensation is also tested bilaterally and, if affected, dermatomal or peripheral nerve distribution patterns should be assessed. Provocative testing for the integrity and functional stability of the SIJ should also be performed.

Investigations

The findings on history and physical examination should dictate the choice of investigational tools. When feasible, it is always preferable to compare post-operative results with those obtained pre-operatively. Tools for assessing the functional capacity such as the Oswestry low back pain disability index (ODI) or the EuroQuol 5D (EQ-5D) as well as simple pain assessment tools such as Numerical Rating Scales (NRS) for leg and back pain are necessary to support the diagnosis of FBSS. Plain radiographs can be used to assess the vertebral alignment as well as to detect significant degenerative changes. Lateral "extension/flexion" radiographs have been shown to be superior to MRI in detecting a spondylolisthesis [6]. However, these images will not provide any additional information regarding the involvement of soft tissue pathology such as neural impingement [7]. It is also not used as a reasonable tool in the evaluation of spinal stenosis. The gold standard in the evaluation of FBSS is MRI. Gadolinium-enhanced MRI is useful to differentiate from recurrent or residual disc herniation versus post-operative epidural fibrosis (scar tissue in the epidural space). The presence of enhancement of gadolinium-MRI may indicate the presence of infection. MRI is also the gold standard to evaluate stenosis in the lateral recess and neural foramens, discitis, and pseudomeningocele [7, 8].

Spinal endoscopy is a reliable tool used in the evaluation of epidural fibrosis. In those for whom MRI is contraindicated (pacemaker, cerebral aneurysm clip) or in whom the presence of surgical hardware produces significant artifacts on scanning, computed tomography (CT) myelogram is recommended in lieu of MRI. The CT-myelogram is useful in demonstrating compression of neural structures by bony elements [4]. Laboratory tests measuring markers of infection (white cell count, erythrocyte sedimentation rate, C reactive protein) can be considered if infection is suspected based upon history and physical examination. Electrodiagnostic studies may assist in distinguishing focal neural involvements such as peripheral neuropathy.

What Is the Pathophysiology of This Condition?

As discussed earlier, FBSS is not a precise diagnosis with a clear-cut cause and with associated symptoms. Rather, it is a constellation of etiologies and symptoms that all lead to a surgical outcome below the expectations of the patient and/or surgeon. The pathophysiology of the condition depends on the etiology, which can be divided into pre-operative, intra-operative, and post-operative factors [9].

Pre-operative Factors

As mentioned above, the patient's previous functional, socio-economic, and psychosocial statuses are important pre-surgical indicators of post-surgical success. A large study performed by Carragee et al. showed that psychosocial risk factors are stronger predictors of post-op disability than are structural abnormalities [3]. In this case, our patient suffered from depression, a psychological factor that has been found to be associated with poorer outcomes. Another relevant pre-operative factor is the amount of previous spine surgeries that the patient underwent. Repeated surgeries lead to repetitive insults to soft tissue structures as well as structural alterations in the spine and its contents and are associated with a reduced success rate [9].

Surgical Factors

Back surgery is very delicate and unforgiving; a surgical error or even routine perioperative bleeding into the spinal canal can lead not only to worsening pain of the same anatomic distribution as originally identified but also to a new source of pain. The bony spine is the main contributor to the human posture; a lumbar fusion can lead to the loss of the normal lumbar curve, putting excessive stress on the sacroiliac joints (SIJ), ultimately leading to SIJ pain. The use of instrumentation in a restricted space that is available to the surgeon generates a high risk of neural impingement.

Inappropriate surgery selection should always be considered in the event of FBSS. The most commonly reported error during spine surgery is the decompression of the wrong level [4]. The incidence of wrong level surgery is discovered following surgery in approximately 2.1–2.7%, while the incidence of unrecognized incorrect level of operation at the time of surgery is 0.57–0.72% [10–13]. Another common selection mistake is performing surgery on the basis of imaging solely; for example, performance of a discectomy on a patient with axial type of pain who could be better served with a more conservative approach such as a medial branch used to address facet joint mediated pain. Single-level decompression in a patient with spinal stenosis at multiple levels is unlikely to achieve the desired effects. On the other hand, FBSS stems from the inability to achieve the surgical goals because of an elevated level of surgical difficulty such as ligamentous hypertrophy or far lateral disc herniation.

Post-surgical Factors

Just like any other surgery, the risk of post-op bleeding and infection must be taken into consideration and identified as soon as possible given these complications can rapidly lead to permanent neurological deficiency and even death [14]. Inadvertent meningeal tear can cause pseudomeningocele and lead to post-dural puncture headache, wound swelling, and focal neurological symptoms. Prolonged and aggressive nerve root retraction leads to a condition known as "battered root syndrome" and can cause persistent radicular pain. Persistent inflammation of the arachnoid matter, known as arachnoiditis, results in chronic nerve root irritation and ultimately produces spine and lower limb pain.

A condition known as "fusion disease" originates from myofascial pain. The dissection and prolonged retraction of the paraspinal muscles results in denervation and atrophy of the musculature [15–17]. Furthermore, damage to the paraspinal muscles can lead to postural changes post-op. The patients will typically compensate with hyperextension of the thoracolumbar spine, which will further exacerbate back pain in the long term [18]. Recurrent disc herniation at the site of surgery (or at an adjacent segment due to altered load distribution) is known to occur in up to 15% of patients following discectomy. Epidural fibrosis is one of the biggest contributors to FBSS (up to 20–36% of FBSS patients). The condition stems from epidural scarring that occurs following spine surgery and, subsequently, causes tethering of nerve roots. Perineural fibrosis may interfere with cerebrospinal fluid mediated nutrition, resulting in hypersensitivity of the affected nerve roots. Additionally, fibrosis can interfere with adequate blood supply of the nerve roots. Lastly, the changes in weight distribution carried by the axial spine following back surgery may lead to a new instability. This can accelerate pre-existing disc degeneration of adjacent segments due to changes in biomechanics of the spine, a condition known as transition syndrome, which is thought to occur in up to 36% of patients [18–20]. Although a discectomy may initially relieve pain, it can ultimately reduce the height of the interspace and cause the involved facet joints to compress the exiting nerve root, which leads to pain. The latter is known as "vertical stenosis."

How Is the Problem Managed?

According to experts, the management options for FBSS consist mostly of physical therapy, pharmacotherapy, psychotherapy (such as cognitive behavioral therapy), injections, repeated surgery, and neuromodulation. There is, unfortunately, no miracle solution, and the probability of success of each respective management will be discussed later.

Conservative Management

The first step in the management of FBSS is a trial of conservative management with physical therapy and pharmacotherapy. Physical therapy should aim at improving the patient's core strength and spinal range of motion. There is no level I study evidence to support physical therapy or exercise, but there is a strong level II evidence that supports this approach [21]. Pharmacotherapy should initially start with the use of non-steroidal anti-inflammatory agents (NSAIDs) and/or acetaminophen, although both have shown weak evidence to support their effectiveness. The use of opioids is now, more than ever, controversial and is recommended as the last line of defense for intractable pain. The use of opioids has been shown to increase pain scores, risks of addiction, incur physiological and psychological dependence, and even lead to death. With the use of opioids on the decline, anticonvulsants such as gabapentin and pregabalin have gained immense popularity and have shown a certain level of effectiveness; there is at least one level I study to support their use [21]. As mentioned earlier, cognitive behavioral therapy has shown to reduce pain score in a certain patient population.

Interventional Pain Procedures

Epidural steroid injections (ESI) are the most commonly performed procedures employed in pain clinics, and FBSS is one of the most common indications for their use. Evidence has shown that ESI can prevent repeated surgery needs in the short term and furthermore that ESI is a useful tool in treating radicular type of pain from FBSS. Level I evidence shows that caudal ESI were similar or less expensive than reoperation, manipulation, and medical management [21]. As mentioned above, scar formation in the epidural space is very likely to occur and may be a source of pain for the FBSS patient. Furthermore, these scars create septations that can interfere with adequate spread of medications injected during ESI. Lysis of these adhesions is theoretically possible by delivering a hypertonic solution with a mixture of local anesthetics, x-ray contrast agents, and glucocorticosteroids (Racz procedure). There is level I evidence to support the Racz lysis procedure. Lysis of adhesion can also be done by means of epiduroscopy, but the level of evidence is II or III for this modality (Fig. 39.2). Another frequently performed procedure with proven success is radiofrequency ablation (RFA) of targeted structures (Fig. 39.3). The first step consists of blocking the targeted nerve(s) and observing the patient's responses; if the block is deemed successful (>80% reduction of pain, even transiently), then the patients are candidates for RFA. The most common locations where RFA is performed are medial branches and SIJ.

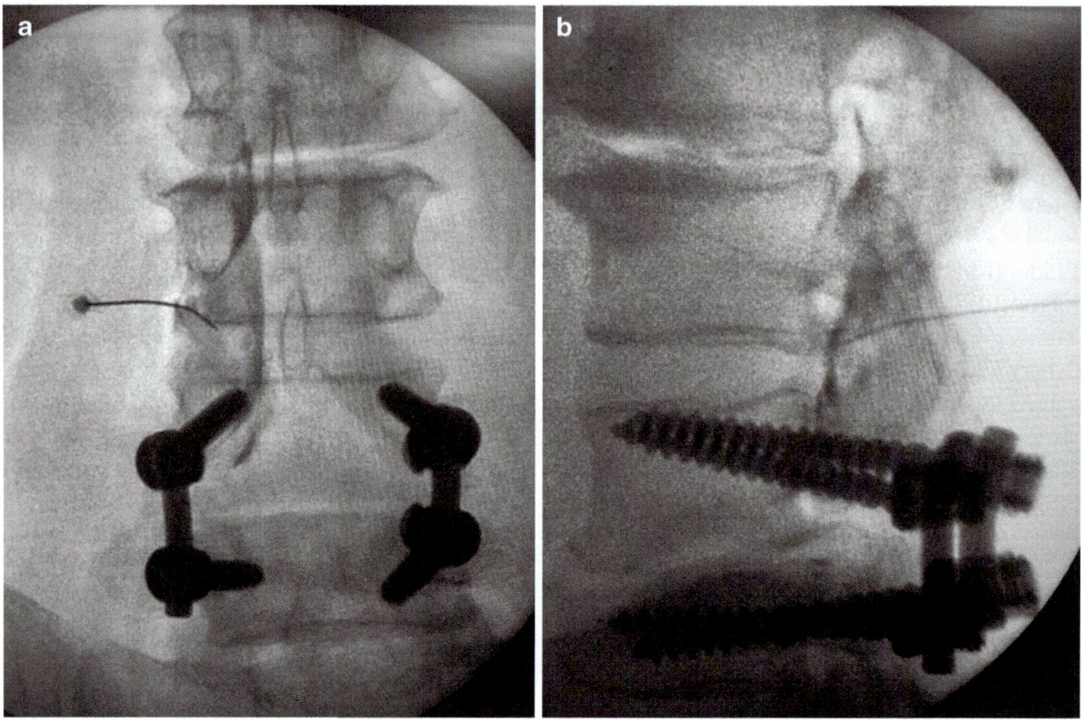

Fig. 39.2 Transforaminal epidural steroid injection in a patient with failed back surgery syndrome under fluoroscopic guidance. (**a**) Anteroposterior view. (**b**) Lateral view

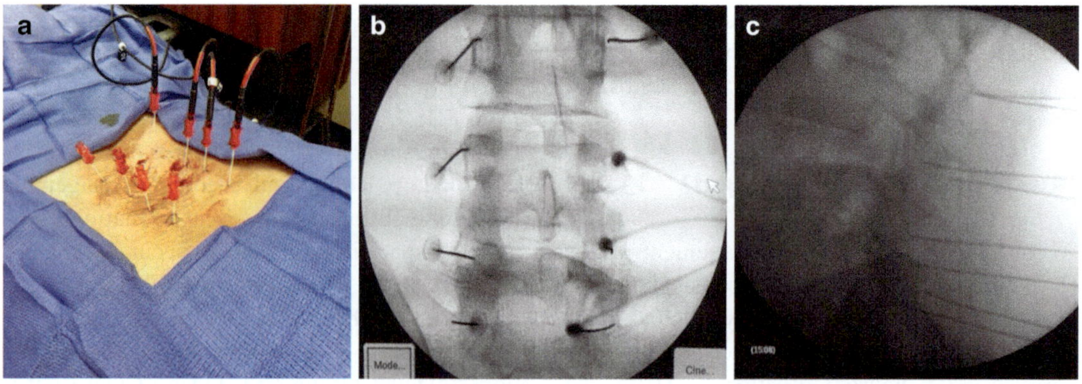

Fig. 39.3 (**a**–**c**) Radiofrequency ablation in a patient with failed back surgery syndrome under fluoroscopic guidance

Repeat Spine Surgery

Few indications exist for repeat spine surgery, and these include progressive neurological deficit, spinal instability, and removal of an improperly placed pedicle screw. There is no good level of evidence to support revision surgery and, overall, the success rate of such procedure is known to be very low and also leads to additional scarring and fibrosis in the epidural space. Studies have demonstrated that success rate for repeat surgery is no more than 30%, 15%, and 5% of the patients who experience a successful outcome after the second, third, and fourth surgeries, respectively [22].

Neuromodulation

Spinal cord stimulation has shown to be a treatment modality with tremendous potential. Its proposed mechanism of action consists of utilizing the "gate theory of pain control" (Wall and Melzack) at the spinal level to block the transmission of pain, thereby replacing it with a more favorable sensation. There is also a belief that a supraspinal component of pain relief exists, along with descending inhibitory pathway and inhibiting pain facilitation [23]. Evidence exists showing improved outcomes with SCS compared to conventional medical management for pain that is predominantly neuropathic. SCS is also superior to surgical management for pain that is predominantly radicular in nature. The PRECISE trial showed that SCS is more cost-effective than conservative medical management. There is a level I evidence to support that SCS is more effective than repeat surgery for a subpopulation with FBSS. There is also a level I evidence to support that SCS is more effective than conservative medical management in reducing pain, is more cost-effective, and offers better quality of life to FBSS patients [21].

What Is the Prognosis of This Condition?

The prognosis of the condition depends on the cause of FBSS and the decision to treat it or not to treat it. Furthermore, the treatment modality chosen will also impact the prognosis of the condition. Careful consideration of the type of therapy most appropriate for the treatment of FBSS is dependent on the etiology of the pain. The fact of the matter is that up to 40% of patients undergoing back surgery will fall under the heading of FBSS in the future. These patients will most likely live with some degree of chronic pain their entire lives, and the best options for these patients are options that modulate their pain.

Although there is strong level II evidence to suggest that exercise, physical therapy, and behavioral modification techniques are useful, there is no level I evidence to suggest these treatments are superior, one to the other. Anticonvulsants and antidepressants are frequently recommended for FBSS with a neuropathic pain component, despite inconclusive evidence for their efficacy [21]. The different interventional and surgical options were discussed earlier and all represent ways to intervene in order to manage FBSS.

Discussion

Prevalence

Chronic LBP is highly prevalent in our society and has an exceptional cost associated with it. The point prevalence of LBP is estimated to be about 11.9%, and the 1-month prevalence is estimated to be 23.2% [1]. In the United States, an estimated 149 million workdays are lost every year because of low back pain [2], with total costs estimated to be US $ 100 to 200 billion a year, of which two thirds are due to lost wages and lower productivity. With the increasing prevalence of LBP comes an increasing number of back surgeries. Between 1998 and 2008 in the United States alone, the number of lumbar fusion surgeries increased from 77,682 to 210,407. In the same time period, the number of laminectomies increased from 92,390 to 107,790 [24]. We discussed earlier that FBSS could be interpreted as "when the outcome of lumbar spinal surgery does not meet the pre-surgical expectations of the patient and surgeon." Compared to other developed countries such as Canada, Finland, and Australia, the rate of spine surgery is about double in the United States. When compared to the United Kingdom, it is about five times more common. In the United States, the failure rate of lumbar spine surgery is estimated to be between 10% and 40%, and with the increasing number of spine surgeries performed, the prevalence of FBSS is also increasing [25, 26]. These statistics incorporate the different kinds of procedures that can be performed on the spine (i.e., discectomy, lumbar decompression, etc.) as well as the different sources of pain that cause FBSS.

Differential Diagnosis

As discussed earlier, there is a wide range of etiologies that can lead to FBSS, and it also important to keep in mind that pain is a subjective sensation (Table 39.1).

Predictive Value of Different Clinical Features and Lab Testing/Imaging

A thorough evaluation of the patient with suspected FBSS is important and should include a good temporal history of the patients' pain, physical examination, labs, and imaging. Early onset of pain can be an indication that the surgery was performed inadequately or at the wrong level. Early onset is also a sign that a surgical screw could be misplaced. Radicular type of pain is most likely due to epidural fibrosis, foraminal stenosis, inadequate decompression, recurrent disc herniation, or residual disc or fragment. New onset of leg pain that is different from pre-op pain is most likely due to an instrumentation issue [4]. Pain in the lower back is suggestive of SIJ disease, myofascial pain, or discogenic causes. Pain in the central spine in response to repetitive movement is representative of discogenic pain.

Table 39.1 Differential diagnosis of postsurgical back pain

Malingering (litigation involvement or workers compensation)
Patient psychological factors (depression, hypochondriac, etc.)
Poor surgical selection (inadequate level operated on or discectomy performed while medial branch block would have been better option)
Poor surgical technique (inadequate decompression, misplaced screw)
Surgical complication (infection, nerve injury, hematoma)
Vertical stenosis (new spinal instability)
Myofascial pain development
Epidural fibrosis
New level disc herniation (secondary to altered biomechanics of the spine)
Recurrent disc herniation of same level
Spondylolisthesis (secondary to altered biomechanics of the spine)

Strength of Evidence for Different Treatment Modalities

Although no consistent physical exam exists to rule in FBSS, it is still strongly recommended to perform a thorough physical examination and to rule out any serious complications (see physical exam above). MRI is the gold standard radiological exam in the setting of FBSS. Nerve root enhancement on post-operative MRI has a strong correlation with recurrent or residual symptoms, with a positive predictive value (PPV) of 83.7%. In the presence of both nerve root thickening and recurrent disc herniation, the correlation is even stronger. Nerve root enhancement combined with nerve root thickening generates a PPV of 87.7%, and if recurrent disc herniation is also identified, the PPV is increased to 94.1%. Although epidural fibrosis is expected after spinal surgery, extensive epidural fibrosis is associated with a 3.2 times increased chance of experiencing recurrent radicular pain [27].

Future Directions or Clinical Trials in Progress

The strongest level of evidence that exists presently for the treatment of FBSS is use of neuromodulation. There is level I evidence suggesting that the use of SCS for the long-term treatment of FBSS, specifically at high frequency (10 kHz), is efficacious. SCS is superior to reoperation and conventional medical management. Studies show that SCS remains underutilized for the treatment of FBSS and therefore represents an avenue that should be considered as an early remedy for this condition. Newer studies have shown that burst stimulation SCS offers superior pain coverage and also offers better quality of life than does use of conventional SCS or placebo. Burst stimulation waveforms lead to further pain reduction than tonic stimulation. SCS has also been demonstrated to be more cost-effective than repeat surgery [28].

Conclusion

This case report involved a patient who underwent spine surgery but, unfortunately, did not get the expected benefit out of it. It represents a case of FBSS. With the volume of spine surgeries increasing and the ratio of failed surgery being the same over multiple decades, the yearly incidence of FBSS is therefore on the rise. Since response to back pain is subjective and multifactorial, better patient investigation and selection prior to undertaking surgery as well as employment of appropriate surgical procedure selection represent pre-operative areas that have substantial room for improvement. It is important to keep in mind that when FBSS is diagnosed, the pain is often multifactorial and the management necessitates a multi-disciplinary approach. One cannot overlook the social, psychological, and financial factors that are involved in the patient's medical situation. Care should be focused on maximizing the patient's functional status as much as possible. The initial approach should always be conservative medical management including physical therapy, with or without psychotherapy, and non-opioid analgesics, such as NSAIDs and acetaminophen. But there is now strong evidence to support the early use of SCS and epidural adhesiolysis. There are currently large-scale clinical trials in place to assess different methods of neuromodulation for the treatment of FBSS.

References

1. Follett KA, Dirks BA. Etiology and evaluation of the failed back surgery syndrome. Neurosurg Q. 1993;3(1):40–59.
2. Waguespack A, Schofferman J, Slosar P, Reynolds J. Etiology of long-term failures of lumbar spine surgery. Pain Med. 2002;3(1):18–22.
3. Carragee EJ, Alamin TF, Miller JL, Carragee JM. Discographic, MRI, and psychosocial determinants of low back pain disability and remission: a prospective study in subjects with benign persistent back pain. Spine J. 2005;5:24–35.
4. Guyer RD, Patterson M, Ohnmeiss DD. Failed back surgery syndrome: diagnostic evaluation. J Am Acad Orthop Surg. 2006;14(9):534–43.
5. Hazard RG. Failed back surgery syndrome: surgical and nonsurgical approaches. Clin Orthop Relat Res. 2006;443:228–32.
6. Kizilkilic O, Yalchin O, Sen O, et al. The role of standing flexion-extension radiographs for spondylolisthesis following single level disc surgery. Neurol Res. 2007;29:540–3.
7. van JWM G, Parizel PM, Jinkins JR. Review article: MRI of the postoperative, lumbar spine. Neuroradiology. 2002;44:723–9.
8. Phillips FM, Cunningham B. Managing chronic pain of spinal origin after lumbar surgery. The role of decompressive surgery. Spine. 2002;27:2547–53.
9. Fritsch EW, Heisel J, Rupp S. The failed back surgery syndrome: reasons, intraoperative findings, and long-terms results: a report of 182 operative treatments. Spine. 1996;21:626–33.
10. Eie N, Solgaard T, Kleppe H. The knee-elbow position in lumbar disc surgery: a review of complications. Spine. 1983;8:897–900.
11. McCulloch JA. Complications (adverse effects). In: McCulloch JA, editor. Principles of microsurgery for lumbar disc disease. New York: Raven Press; 1989. p. 225–38.
12. Williams RW. Microlumbar discectomy: a conservative surgical approach to the virgin herniated lumbar disc. Spine. 1978;3:175–82.
13. Ruggieri F, Specchia L, Sabalt S, et al. Lumbar disc herniation: diagnosis, surgical treatment, recurrence. J Orthop Traumatol. 1988;14:15–22.
14. Chan CW, Peng P. Failed back surgery syndrome. Pain Med. 2011;12(4):577–606.
15. Kahanovitz N, Viola K, Gallagher M. Long-term strength assessment of postoperative discectomy patients. Spine. 1989;14:402–3.
16. Kawaguchi Y, Matsui H, Tsuji H. Back muscle injury after posterior lumbar spine surgery. Part 2: histologic and histochemical analyses in humans. Spine. 1994;19:2598–602.
17. Kawaguchi Y, Matsui H, Tsuji H. Back muscle injury after posterior lumbar spine surgery: a histologic and enzymatic analysis. Spine. 1996;21:941–4.

18. Onesti ST. Failed back syndrome. Neurologist. 2004;10:259–64.
19. Carroll SE, Wiesel SW. Neurological complications and lumbar laminectomy. A standardized approach to the multiply-operated lumbar spine. Clin Orthop Relat Res. 1992;284:14–23.
20. Kumar MN, Baklanov A, Chopin D. Correlation between sagittal plane changes and adjacent segmental degeneration following lumbar spine fusion. Eur Spine J. 2001;10:314–9.
21. Amirdelfan K, Webster L, Poree L, Sukul V, Mcroberts P. Treatment options for failed back surgery syndrome patients with refractory chronic pain: an evidence based approach. Spine (Phila Pa 1976). 2017;42(14):S41–52.
22. Nachemson AL. Evaluation of results in lumbar spine surgery. Acta Orthop Scand Suppl. 1993;251:130–3.
23. Guan Y. Spinal cord stimulation: neurophysiological and neurochemical mechanisms of action. Curr Pain Headache Rep. 2012;16:217–25.
24. Rajaee SS, Bae HW, Kanim LE, Delamarter RB. Spinal fusion in the United States: analysis of trends from 1998 to 2008. Spine. 2012;37(1):67–76.
25. North RB, Kidd DH, Zahurak M, et al. Spinal cord stimulation for chronic, intractable pain: experience over two decades. Neurosurgery. 1993;32:384–94.
26. Wilkinson HA. The failed back syndrome: etiology and therapy. Philadelphia: Harper & Row; 1991.
27. Lee YS, Choi ES, Song CJ. Symptomatic nerve root changes on contrast-enhanced MR imaging after surgery for lumbar disk herniation. AJNR Am J Neuroradiol. 2009;30:1062–7.
28. Linderoth B, Foreman RD. Conventional and novel spinal stimulation algorithms: hypothetical mechanisms of action and comments on outcomes. Neuromodulation. 2017;20(6):525–33.

A 55-Year-Old Diabetic Woman with Feet Pain

40

Robert Fuino, Rup Tandan, and Waqar Waheed

Case Description

A 55-year-old woman presents with 8 months history of gradually progressive pain in her feet. The pain is a constant burning with associated pins and needles involving all of the toes. There is no low back pain, trauma, difficulty with balance, foot swelling or discoloration, or particular aggravating or alleviating factors. Her medical problems include obesity, type 2 diabetes mellitus, and hypertension. Her medications include metformin and hydrochlorothiazide. She has been drinking two glasses of wine per day for over 20 years. Her general and musculoskeletal examinations demonstrate normal appearance of the feet with no deformity or point tenderness, negative Tinel's sign at the tarsal tunnels, negative Mulder's sign, and intact peripheral pulses. The neurologic examination is notable for diminished sensation to touch, pinprick, vibration in the feet circumferentially up to the mid-foot, as well as diminished ankle reflexes bilaterally.

R. Fuino · R. Tandan
Department of Neurology, University of Vermont Medical Center, Burlington, VT, USA

W. Waheed (✉)
Department of Neurosciences, University of Vermont Medical Center, Burlington, VT, USA
e-mail: Waqar.Waheed@uvmhealth.org

What Is Your Preliminary Diagnosis?

The diagnosis of any medical disorder is based upon the combination of history, examination findings, and confirmation with pertinent investigations. The differential diagnosis of foot pain is broad and can be divided into neurological and non-neurological disorders, as seen in Fig. 40.1.

Musculoskeletal causes of foot pain are varied and there are some features that are more suggestive of this group of diagnoses. Specifically, localizing pain to the forefoot, mid-foot, and rear-foot tailors the differential diagnosis considerably. Conditions common to the rear foot include plantar fasciitis, tarsal tunnel syndrome, and Achilles tendon pain, among others. Mid-foot pain can result from bony, tendinous, and rheumatologic causes (gout, rheumatoid arthritis), as well as neuropathic Charcot disease of the foot. Features suggestive of musculoskeletal causes of foot pain, besides pain location, include recent foot injuries, changes in weight or activity level, or improvement with shoe removal. Nocturnal pain can be seen in neurologic and non-neurologic diagnoses, such as severe arthritis, stress fractures, tumors, and DPN. Color changes in feet, along with claudication history, may be indicative of vascular basis of the patient's presentation. During examination, while evaluating both neurological and non-neurological disorders, it is important to expose the patient's lower legs and feet to inspect the legs and

T. Malik (ed.), *Practical Chronic Pain Management*, https://doi.org/10.1007/978-3-030-46675-6_40

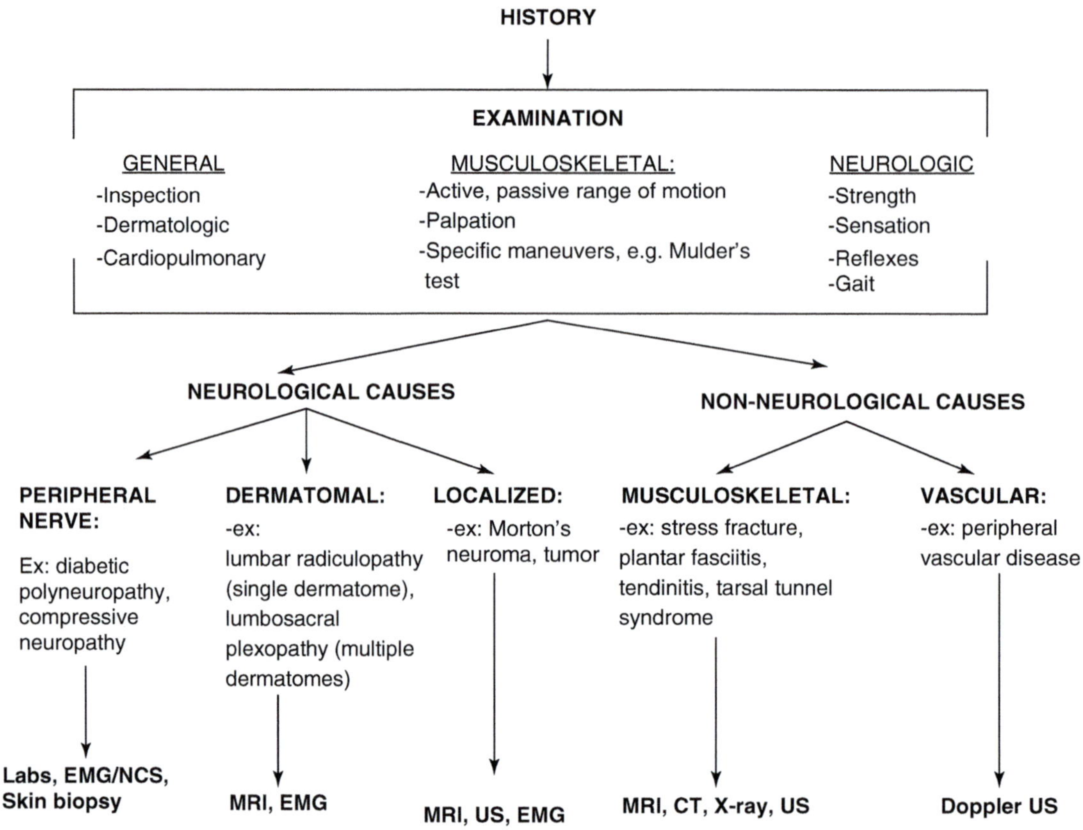

Fig. 40.1 History and examination of foot pain, including focused diagnoses and diagnostic considerations

interdigital spaces. The presence of skin changes, such as hair loss or ulcers, can indicate peripheral vascular disease. Pallor, cyanosis, edema, or erythema can indicate vascular, cardiac, rheumatologic, or infectious contributions to pain. Foot deformity, such as high or flat arches, can indicate neuropathic or diabetic insults, such as Charcot arthropathy. Additional maneuvers, such as Tinel's sign for tarsal tunnel syndrome or Mulder's test for Morton's neuroma, as well palpation of the feet to elicit tenderness, should also be performed. Tinel's sign is positive if electrical shooting pain along the sensory innervation of the posterior tibial nerve is elicited by tapping along the posterior aspect of the medial malleolus. Mulder's test is performed by applying pressure with the index and thumb on the dorsal and plantar aspect of the painful inter-metatarsal space in question. With palpation of the feet, the forefoot is compressed with the opposite hand by squeezing the adjacent metatarsal heads together; a palpable click or pain radiating into the affected toes indicates a positive test.

Assessment of comorbid medical conditions is important. One should ask questions about diabetes, alcohol intake, diet, signs or symptoms of hypothyroidism, infections such as hepatitis, travel history, and family history of similar problems, as these can provide diagnostic clues. A focused neurologic examination includes large fiber (i.e., light touch, position, and vibration) and small fiber (i.e., temperature and pinprick) sensory testing, deep tendon reflexes, strength examination, Romberg test, and observation of gait. Patients with neuropathy can have reduced sensation and reflexes, a positive Romberg sign, or a steppage quality to their gait. Muscle weakness and its symmetry should be noted. The presence of upper motor neuron signs, a sensory level or bowel, and bladder involvement all suggest a process occurring in either the spinal cord, brainstem, or brain itself and warrant urgent evaluation should there be no prior diagnosis to explain these findings. Neurologic disorders can be further divided into patterns suggestive of polyneuropathy (such as stocking and glove distribution of deficits), lumbar radiculopathy or lumbosacral plexus lesions (based upon the presence of back pain with radiation in a dermatomal distribution), mono-neuropathies, or focal structural causes (deficits involving individual nerves or its branches, such as tarsal tunnel syndrome due to tibial nerve entrapment).

In this case, considering the patient's history of chronic symmetrical burning pain involving the forefeet, examination findings of stocking-type sensory loss, ankle hypo-reflexia and absent musculoskeletal/vascular findings, the most likely preliminary diagnosis is of a polyneuropathy, likely caused by diabetes and contributed by alcohol. The absence of a family history, as well as of musculoskeletal deformities such as high arched feet or hammer toes, suggests that a hereditary neuropathy (such as Charcot Marie tooth disease) is an unlikely cause.

How Is the Diagnosis Confirmed?

The suspected diagnosis based upon the clinical evaluation is confirmed by pertinent diagnostic testing. Non-neurologic disorders can be assessed, when appropriate, using vascular or radiological studies based on the suspected diagnosis. Electromyography, nerve conduction studies, or imaging can be used, depending on the suspected neurologic diagnoses, for further confirmation. Of note, normal electro-diagnostic testing does not rule out the presence of a small fiber neuropathy, which requires skin biopsy to evaluate the density of un-myelinated nerve fibers (intraepidermal nerve fiber density) to support the diagnosis of a small fiber neuropathy. Further investigations into underlying causes can be made after these initial assessments.

Electro-diagnostic testing performed in this patient showed findings consistent with the presence of a moderately severe length-dependent axonal sensorimotor neuropathy. Work up for common causes of a symmetrical length-dependent polyneuropathy, besides an elevated hemoglobin A1c of 9.1%, was negative (including serum protein electrophoresis, TSH, and vitamin B12 level).

What Is the Pathophysiology of This Condition?

The pathophysiology of DPN is not well understood. It is evident that impaired glycemic control contributes to neuropathy. High quality evidence suggests that glucose control can prevent the development of clinical neuropathy in type 1 diabetic patients and trends towards reducing the incidence of neuropathy in type 2 diabetic patients [1]. Excess intracellular glucose can increase glycolysis and secondary generalization of reactive oxygen species (ROS) [2]. In addition, increased glucose transport can cause oxidative stress and inflammatory injury through separate pathways beyond the scope of this discussion [3]. Advanced glycation end products (AGEs) are also generated, resulting in binding to corresponding receptors (RAGEs) and the initiation of inflammatory signal cascades and increased production of ROS [4]. Dyslipidemia, common in diabetics, has also been implicated in increased oxidative stress [5]. Finally, as insulin has been shown to have neurotropic effects [6], insulin deficiency or resistance has been implicated in the pathogenesis of DPN [7].

How Is This Problem Managed?

Management of DPN is based on a combination of simultaneous risk factor modification, pain control, and avoidance of disease complications. All patients with severe DPN should be advised to routinely check their feet to identify occult injury or the development of ulcers. Blood glucose control is necessary to prevent progression of the neuropathy. Lifestyle modification counseling and medications to control blood glucose are warranted. Specific medication regimens to use for glycemic control are beyond the scope of this chapter.

Several medication classes are options for pain control, and it is worth noting that pain is one of the primary reasons for which patients with DPN seek care [8]. These are listed in Table 40.1, including starting doses and ranges, side effects, and supporting evidence. A 2017 systematic review of 57 eligible studies of pain reduction therapies in DPN found that, among others, duloxetine, venlafaxine, tricyclic antidepressants, pregabalin, oxcarbazepine, and tramadol were more effective than placebo [9].

Pregabalin and gabapentin are both neuronal-type calcium channel alpha^2-delta subunit antagonists. Analysis of 15 randomized controlled trials (RCTs) demonstrated that pregabalin had a mild beneficial effect on pain reduction when compared to placebo [9], consistent with prior systematic reviews [10]. Gabapentin has also been studied in painful DPN; although not all studies showed efficacy [9, 11], the American Academy of Neurology (AAN) and the European Federation of Neurological Societies (EFNS) still classify this agent as effective, and it is commonly used in clinical practice.

In addition, antidepressant agents have been well studied in painful DPN. Tricyclic antidepressants (TCAs) have demonstrated efficacy according to a two meta-analyses [12, 13], although a specific agent is not recommended on the basis of these studies. As amitriptyline has a higher level of evidence for efficacy [14], doses of 25–100 mg a day have been recommended. Initiation with a bedtime dose of 25 mg, with gradual titration, is recommended. Nortriptyline and desipramine are also utilized, but they have lower quality evidence supporting their use.

Serotonin-norepinephrine reuptake inhibitors (SNRIs), namely duloxetine and venlafaxine, are also potential treatment options. These agents are well studied and are found to produce significant pain reduction in trials and systematic reviews [9, 15]. Evidence for venlafaxine is less compelling, as a 2015 systematic review of six RCTs concluded that trials either showed no significant benefit or were at high risk of bias [16]. However, venlafaxine is still commonly used for DPN neuropathic pain in clinical practice. Patients should be advised to take duloxetine on a full stomach; transient GI discomfort may be associated with dose increases.

The use of opioids is another potential treatment option, although evidence is more inconsistent and of lesser quality [9, 17]. A 2017 systematic review found tramadol to have a moderate standardized mean difference in pain rating, suggesting benefit, as compared to placebo [9]. A careful discussion of the risks and benefits of these agents is necessary due to the enhanced risks of tolerance, dependence, addiction, and misuse.

Sodium valproate is classified as ineffective or with discrepant results by the EFNS but is classified as effective by the AAN. Oxcarbazepine may have some efficacy in neuropathic pain reduction [9], but due to discrepancies between study results, both the AAN and EFNS classify oxcarbazepine, lamotrigine, and lacosamide as ineffective and do not recommend their use [18].

Additional agents studied in painful DPN include topical capsaicin, isosorbide dinitrate spray, botulinum toxin injections, oral alpha lipoic acid, and lidocaine patches. Of these, Waldfogel et al.'s systematic review only identify botulinum toxin injections as effective, although only on the basis of two trials involving 60 patients [9]. Alpha lipoic acid is an antioxidant that is believed to reduce oxidative stress in painful DPN. One RCT in 181 diabetic patients showed that daily doses of 600–1800 mg of alpha lipoic acid mildly reduced burning pain (51% reduction in drug group vs. 32% reduction in placebo group [19].

The approach to pharmacologic management of diabetic neuropathic pain is addressed in several treatment algorithms [20, 21]. All recommend pregabalin, gabapentin, duloxetine, venlafaxine, and tricyclic antidepressants as first-line agents. These agents should be initiated, and the dose gradually increased, until the maximum tolerated dose before switching to another first-line agent. If partial efficacy from one drug is seen, or several agents do not show an acceptable benefit when used as monotherapy, a combination of first-line drugs from different classes can be

Table 40.1 Medication classes for pain control

	Society guidelines			Dose recommendations		Side effects	
	AAN[a] [15]	EFNS [b] [20]	Standardized mean difference in pain scale vs. placebo[c] [9]	Start daily dose	Recommended daily dose [15]	Common	Serious
Anticonvulsants							
Pregabalin	A	A	−0.34 [−0.50 to −0.18]	50 mg BID	300–600 mg	Dizziness, somnolence, peripheral edema, weight gain	Tolerance, dependence, discontinuation syndrome
Gabapentin	B	A	−0.73 [−1.54 to 0.09	900 mg	Up to 3200 mg	Dizziness, somnolence, peripheral edema, weight gain	Increased suicidal thoughts, tolerance, dependence, discontinuation syndrome
Oxcarbazepine	B[a]	A/B	−0.45 [−0.68 to −0.21]	600 mg	300–600 mg	Nausea, rash, hyponatremia, dizziness	SJS/TEN, hypersensitivity reactions, agranulocytosis, leukopenia, pancytopenia
Valproate	B	A/B	N/A	500 mg	500–1200 mg	Weight gain, nausea, vomiting, bruising, tremors, dizziness	Agranulocytosis, hepatic failure, SJS/TEN, dermatitis, pancreatitis, aplastic anemia
Antidepressants							
Tricyclic antidepressants (amitriptyline)	B	A	−0.78 [−1.24 to −0.33]	25 mg	25–100 mg	Somnolence, dry mouth, anticholinergic effects	Urinary retention
Duloxetine	B	A	−1.33 [−1.82 to −0.86]	60 mg	60–120 mg	Nausea, constipation, decreased appetite, somnolence	Rare cases of hepatotoxicity, withdrawal
Venlafaxine	B	A	−1.53 [−2.41 to −0.65]	75 mg	75–225 mg	Nausea, constipation, decreased appetite, somnolence	
Opioid agents							
Opioids (oxycodone)	B	A	−0.58 [−1.53 to 0.36]	Patient specific	Mean 37 mg/d, max 120 mg/d (oxycodone)	Sedation, constipation, tolerance, dependency	Dependency, risk of misuse, and diversion
Atypical opioids (tramadol)	B	A	−0.68 [−0.80 to −0.56]	Patient specific	210 mg (tramadol)	Sedation, constipation, tolerance, dependency, risk of misuse	Dependency, lowers seizure threshold, not recommended with serotonergic medications
Dextromethorphan	B	B	−0.28 [−1.49 to 0.92]	400 mg	400 mg	Sedation, constipation, tolerance, dependency, risk of misuse	

(continued)

Table 40.1 (continued)

	Society guidelines			Dose recommendations		Side effects	
	AAN[a] [15]	EFNS [b] [20]	Standardized mean difference in pain scale vs. placebo[c] [9]	Start daily dose	Recommended daily dose [15]	Common	Serious
Other agents							
Topical capsaicin 0.075% four times daily	B	A/B	−0.46 [−0.95 to 0.03]	N/A	N/A	Localized pain or erythema	Avoid on broken skin or wounds, hypersensitivity reactions
Botulinum toxin		B	Range: −0.79 to −0.96	N/A	N/A	Numbness, dysesthesias	Weakness of injected muscles
Isosorbide dinitrate spray	B	A	X	N/A	N/A	Local effects, headaches	Palpitations, fainting, avoid in patients with cardiac conditions and heart failure

Not consistently well recommended: lidocaine patches, lamotrigine, lacosamide

aAAN guidelines classify agents as A ("established as effective"), B ("probably effective"), or C ("possibly effective")

bEFNS has designations, from A to C, based on the quality of evidence supporting a given agent. A separate classification of A/B notes that the drug is either classified as ineffective or with discrepant results in studies

c95% confidence interval or a credible interval determined by investigators is in brackets. Standardized mean differences classified effect sizes into small (<0.5), moderate (0.5 to 0.8), and large (>0.8). Ineffective medications by this measure are listed in red tried. If TCAs, SNRIs, and anticonvulsants fail as monotherapy or combination therapy, tramadol or opioids can be trialed with careful consideration of the long-term side effect profile. The choice of specific agents should be made after consideration of the patient's medical comorbidities, use of other concomitant medications, addiction potential, cost, and tolerance in mind.

Role of Non-pharmacological Therapies

Quite often patient with diabetic neuropathy are offered or suggested nonpharmacological treatments. Most recently these treatments were reviewed by Amato et al. in 2018 [23]. Only those interventions evaluated in a randomized controlled trial were evaluated. Twenty-three trials were included. Alpha-lipoic acid and frequency-modulated electromagnetic stimulation were found to be more effective than control in the short term but not the long term while electrical stimulation was not effective for pain. Spinal cord stimulation was more effective than usual care for pain but strength of evidence was low. Evidence for cognitive behavioral therapy and acupuncture was insufficient; no exercise or physical therapy trials met inclusion criteria. No interventions reported sufficient evidence on quality of life. Frank Huygen et al. [24] reviewed evidence for interventional pain procedures for various chronic pain conditions; they found that evidence for performing lumbar sympathetic block was weak and for spinal cord stimulation moderate implying that the outcome in clinical practice may not match the results reported in the literature.

What Is the Prognosis of This Condition?

DPN is most often a persistent condition that often worsens over time. Spontaneous remissions are possible if the condition is triggered by short duration of diabetes, during diabetic ketoacidosis, or with significant weight loss [22]. Long-term improvement in pain and function can be achieved with medical management, according to some observational studies. In one study of 43 patients medically managed for painful DPN from Canadian tertiary pain centers, at 12 months 51.2% of patients had functional improvement, 37.2% of patients had more than 30% pain reduction, and 30.2% achieved both [25]. Control of other potential contributors to neuropathy is necessary to prevent continued progression of the disease.

Discussion

Prevalence

DPN is the most common cause of peripheral neuropathy. The prevalence is estimated at 2% of the general population, based on smaller studies [26, 27], and about 30% of patients with diabetes [28]. Peripheral neuropathic pain caused by peripheral neuropathy is estimated to occur in from 16.2 to 26.4% of diabetic patients [29, 30].

Differential Diagnosis

Polyneuropathies can be broadly divided into hereditary or acquired categories. Hereditary neuropathies frequently are long standing, insidious in onset, and positive sensory components (e.g., neuropathic pain) are often absent. Musculoskeletal deformities and a positive family history would also be supportive of a diagnosis of hereditary polyneuropathies. The most common pattern of involvement in an acquired polyneuropathy is of a length-dependent axonal polyneuropathy, seen most commonly with diabetes. In this pattern, neuropathic symptoms start in the feet gradually and by the time involvement reaches the mid-shin, the finger tips are also involved, creating the so-called glove and stocking-type of sensory loss. In one case series of 103 patients with diabetic sensory polyneuropathy, potential additional or alternative causes were identified in 53% [30]. The most common causes of peripheral neuropathy include diabetes, hypothyroidism, vitamin deficiencies (B12, B6, B1), monoclonal gammopathies, and effects of alcohol overuse. Therefore, screening for these disorders is recommended in patients with diabetic polyneuropathy.

While evaluating a patient with polyneuropathy, one should look for red flags associated with atypical causes, which often require urgent treatment to prevent further progression. Red flags include acute or subacute onset, relapsing or remitting course, marked asymmetric painful pattern, concomitant cranial nerve deficits, and lack of length dependence (upper extremities earlier and more severely affected than lower extremities). These red flags suggest the possibility of immune-mediated, vasculitic, infectious, neoplastic, or paraneoplastic etiologies. Prompt neurological referral and consideration of additional investigations, besides electro-diagnostic testing, in this group include lumbar puncture, expanded serologic evaluation, and potentially nerve and/or muscle biopsy.

Predictive Value of Different Clinical Features (Both on History and Physical Exam), and Lab Testing/Imaging

The diagnosis of peripheral neuropathy related to diabetes is complicated by the varying presentations it can have; these include varying tempo of onset and/or progression, symmetry, and distribution of involvement (proximal or distal). As the most common presentation is a symmetric, distal, sensorimotor polyneuropathy, this is the presentation referred to in most studies.

If typical features of a length-dependent neuropathy (i.e., involvement distal > proximal, feet earlier and greater than hands) are identified in diabetic patients, further evaluation with serology is indicated as described previously here. Other potential treatable causes of symmetric peripheral neuropathy should be identified and treated as previously mentioned. Neurology consultation can be considered for patients who have inconclusive serologic testing.

When compared to electro-diagnostic testing, a combination of clinical and examination findings are useful in the diagnosis of DPN. The sensitivity and specificity of the 10 g monofilament sensory test and vibration testing were studied in a 2001 analysis [31]. The presence of risk factors for neuropathy increased both the sensitivity and specificity of each, regardless of the results of each test. For the vibration test, a 128-Hz tuning fork was applied to the bony prominence of the first toe. Vibration was extinguished twice on each first toe, for a total of four potential responses. The presence of risk factors and a cut-off threshold equal to three or more incorrect responses demonstrated a sensitivity of 86% and specificity of 83% for the diagnosis of DPN. Similarly, the monofilament test utilized four stimuli just distal to the nail bed on each great toe for a total of eight potential responses. Three or more incorrect responses, with the presence of risk factors for neuropathy, were determined to have a sensitivity of 83% and a specificity of 73%. However, neither of these tests is able to discriminate between neuropathy due to diabetes or other modifiable causes, listed previously.

Symptoms alone can have poor diagnostic accuracy in DPN. Screening tests, such as those recommended by the San Antonio consensus conference [32], Toronto criteria [33], and others will incorporate a combination of neuropathic symptoms, diminished ankle reflexes, decreased distal sensations, and abnormal nerve conduction studies in the diagnostic process. For example, the Toronto criteria classify "probable diabetic sensory polyneuropathy" in patients with two of three of the following: neuropathic symptoms, decreased distal sensation, or decreased/absent ankle reflexes. The diagnosis of confirmed clinical DPN is based on the presence of signs and symptoms with an abnormal nerve conduction study. Specific criteria are not always used in practice but might have value for research studies.

Electromyography and nerve conduction studies should be performed for confirmation of the diagnosis. This allows one to confirm the acuity, nerve fiber type (motor, sensory, or both), pathophysiology (axonal loss versus demyelination), and distribution (focal, multifocal) of findings. As an example, metabolic/toxic or idiopathic neuropathies manifest primarily with axonal injury, while immune-mediated and inherited neuropathies can be either axonal or demyelinating. In addition, patients with previously mentioned atypical features for DPN (e.g., rapid progression, asymmetry, etc.) warrant both electro-diagnostic testing and a neurology consultation. Normal electro-diagnostic testing does not rule out small nerve fiber involvement in diabetes, but this is atypical for DPN.

Strength of Evidence for Different Treatment Modalities

Based on high quality evidence, a 2012 Cochrane systematic review concluded that improved glycemic control is effective in preventing the development of clinical neuropathy and reducing examination and electro-diagnostic abnormalities in patients with type 1 diabetes mellitus. In type 2 diabetes mellitus, there was a reduction in the incidence of clinical neuropathy with glucose control, but this was not statistically significant [34]. It did, however, reduce nerve conduction and vibration abnormalities.

Pharmacologic treatment modalities for painful DPN are previously mentioned. The AAN and EFNS both provide guidelines on various agents for neuropathic pain in diabetes, based on the strength of evidence. These are listed in Table 40.1.

Future Directions or Clinical Trials in Progress

Clinical trials for various experimental therapeutic agents are currently ongoing. Small studies with limited sample sizes have shown efficacy for percutaneous electrical nerve stimulation [35], but this technique is not commonly available in clinical practice. Spinal cord stimulation has also been studied in a small, open-label international trial, which reported a sustained positive effect at 24 months [36, 37], but further studies are needed before this invasive approach is recommended.

Conclusion/Summary

DPN is an often painful condition resulting from nerve damage due to oxidative stress consequent upon poor glycemic control. It has varying presentations and is among the most common causes of neuropathy. Most frequently, patients present with a progressive, length-dependent, distal sensory loss. History of neuropathic symptoms, including neuropathic pain, diminished ankle reflexes, and diminished distal vibratory sensation, is an important clinical diagnostic clue. Specific criteria for the diagnosis of DPN, including the Toronto criteria, have been described. They utilize these clinical findings, and use results nerve conduction testing, to confirm the diagnosis. This condition is rarely reversible and glucose control is necessary to prevent progression. Control of neuropathic pain is possible with either mono-therapy or combination therapy of anticonvulsants, tricyclic antidepressants, and SNRIs. Opioids have been utilized in prior studies but evidence is considered to be of low quality. This class also carries significant risk of long-term dependence and addiction, and each patient should be counseled accordingly. There are no interventions, at this time, that have high quality evidence showing pain reduction in this condition. Further research into disease pathogenesis and identification of novel therapeutic agents will further change how this disorder is treated.

References

1. Callaghan BC, Little AA, Feldman EL, Hughes RA. Enhanced glucose control for preventing and treating diabetic neuropathy. Cochrane Database Syst Rev. 2012;6:CD007543.
2. Vincent AM, Russell JW, Low P, Feldman EL. Oxidative stress in the pathogenesis of diabetic neuropathy. Endocri Rev. 2004;25(4):612–28.

3. Vincent AM, Callaghan BC, Al S, Feldman EL. Diabetic neuropathy: cellular mechanisms as therapeutic targets. Nat Rev Neurol. 2011;7(10):573–83.
4. Vincent AM, Perrone L, Sullivan KA, Backus C, Sastry AM, Lastoskie C, et al. Receptor for advanced glycation end products activation injures primary sensory neurons via oxidative stress. Endocrinology. 2007;148(2):548–58.
5. Padilla A, Descorbeth M, Al A, Payne K, De Leon M. Hyperglycemia magnifies Schwann cell dysfunction and cell death triggered by PA-induced lipotoxicity. Brain Res. 2011;1370:64–79.
6. Toth C, Brussee V, Martinez JA, McDonald D, Cunningham FA, Zochodne DW. Rescue and regeneration of injured peripheral nerve axons by intrathecal insulin. Neuroscience. 2006;139(2):429–49.
7. Kim B, Feldman EL. Insulin resistance in the nervous system. Trends Endocrinol Metab. 2012;23(3):133–41.
8. Vinik AI. Clinical practice. Diabetic sensory and motor neuropathy. N Engl J Med. 2016;374(15):1455–64.
9. Waldfogel JM, Nesbit SA, Dy SM, Sharma R, Zhang A, Wilson LM, et al. Pharmacotherapy for diabetic peripheral neuropathy pain and quality of life: a systematic review. Neurology. 2017;88(20):1958–67.
10. Freeman R, Durso-Decruz E, Emir B. Efficacy, safety, and tolerability of pregabalin treatment for painful diabetic peripheral neuropathy: findings from seven randomized, controlled trials across a range of doses. Diabetes Care. 2008;31(7):1448–54.
11. Vedula SS, Bero L, Scherer RW, Dickersin K. Outcome reporting in industry-sponsored trials of gabapentin for off-label use. N Engl J Med. 2009;361(20):1963–71.
12. Saarto T, Wiffen PJ. Antidepressants for neuropathic pain. Cochrane Database Syst Rev. 2007;4:CD005454.
13. Sindrup SH, Otto M, Finnerup NB, Jensen TS. Antidepressants in the treatment of neuropathic pain. Basic Clin Pharmacol Toxicol. 2005;96(6):399–409.
14. Max MB, Culnane M, Schafer SC, Gracely RH, Walther DJ, Smoller B, et al. Amitriptyline relieves diabetic neuropathy pain in patients with normal or depressed mood. Neurology. 1987;37(4):589–96.
15. Bril V, England J, Franklin GM, Backonja M, Cohen J, Del Toro D, et al. Evidence-based guideline: treatment of painful diabetic neuropathy: report of the American Academy of Neurology, the American Association of Neuromuscular and Electrodiagnostic Medicine, and the American Academy of Physical Medicine and Rehabilitation. PM R. 2011;3(4):345–52, 52.e1–21.
16. Gallagher HC, Gallagher RM, Butler M, Buggy DJ, Henman MC. Venlafaxine for neuropathic pain in adults. Cochrane Database Syst Rev. 2015;8:CD011091.
17. Gaskell H, Derry S, Stannard C, Moore RA. Oxycodone for neuropathic pain in adults. Cochrane Database Syst Rev. 2016;7:CD010692.
18. Callaghan BC, Cheng HT, Stables CL, Al S, Feldman EL. Diabetic neuropathy: clinical manifestations and current treatments. Lancet Neurol. 2012;11(6):521–34.
19. Ziegler D, Ametov A, Barinov A, Dyck PJ, Gurieva I, Low PA, et al. Oral treatment with alpha-lipoic acid improves symptomatic diabetic polyneuropathy: the SYDNEY 2 trial. Diabetes Care. 2006;29(11):2365–70.
20. Attal N, Cruccu G, Baron R, Haanpaa M, Hansson P, Jensen TS, et al. EFNS guidelines on the pharmacological treatment of neuropathic pain: 2010 revision. Eur J Neurol. 2010;17(9):1113–e88.
21. Dworkin RH, O'Connor AB, Audette J, Baron R, Gourlay GK, Haanpää MI, et al. Recommendations for the pharmacological management of neuropathic pain: an overview and literature update. Mayo Clin Proc. 2010;85(3 Suppl):S3–14.
22. Effect of intensive diabetes treatment on nerve conduction in the Diabetes Control and Complications Trial. Ann Neurol. 1995;38(6):869–80.
23. Amato S, Sharma R, Waldfogel JM, Zhang A, Bennett WL, Yeh HC, et al. Non-pharmacologic treatments for symptoms of diabetic peripheral neuropathy: a systematic review. Curr Med Res Opin. 2018 Aug;17:1–11.
24. Huygen F, Kallewaard JW, Tulder M, Boxem M, Vissers K, Kleef M, Zundert JV. Evidence-based interventional pain medicine according to clinical diagnoses: update, vol. 19; 2018. p. 664. https://doi.org/10.1111/papr.12786.
25. Mai L, Clark A, Gordon A, Lynch M, Morley-Forster P, Nathan H, et al. Long-term outcomes in the management of painful diabetic neuropathy. Can J Neurol Sci. 2017;44(4):337–42.
26. Bharucha NE, Bharucha AE, Bharucha EP. Prevalence of peripheral neuropathy in the Parsi community of Bombay. Neurology. 1991;41(8):1315–7.
27. Savettieri G, Rocca WA, Salemi G, Meneghini F, Grigoletto F, Morgante L, et al. Prevalence of diabetic neuropathy with somatic symptoms: a door-to-door survey in two Sicilian municipalities. Sicilian Neuro-Epidemiologic Study (SNES) Group. Neurology. 1993;43(6):1115–20.
28. Maser RE, Steenkiste AR, Dorman JS, Nielsen VK, Bass EB, Manjoo Q, et al. Epidemiological correlates of diabetic neuropathy. Report from Pittsburgh Epidemiology of Diabetes Complications Study. Diabetes. 1989;38(11):1456–61.
29. Daousi C, MacFarlane IA, Woodward A, Nurmikko TJ, Bundred PE, Benbow SJ. Chronic painful peripheral neuropathy in an urban community: a controlled comparison of people with and without diabetes. Diabet Med. 2004;21(9):976–82.
30. Davies M, Brophy S, Williams R, Taylor A. The prevalence, severity, and impact of painful diabetic peripheral neuropathy in type 2 diabetes. Diabetes Care. 2006;29(7):1518–22.
31. Olaleye D, Perkins BA, Bril V. Evaluation of three screening tests and a risk assessment model for diag-

nosing peripheral neuropathy in the diabetes clinic. Diabetes Res Clin Pract. 2001;54(2):115–28.
32. Consensus statement: Report and recommendations of the San Antonio conference on diabetic neuropathy. American Diabetes Association American Academy of Neurology. Diabetes Care. 1988;11(7):59207.
33. Dyck PJ, Albers JW, Andersen H, Arezzo JC, Biessels GJ, Bril V, et al. Diabetic polyneuropathies: update on research definition, diagnostic criteria and estimation of severity. Diabetes Metab Res Rev. 2011;27(7):620–8.
34. Callaghan BC, Little AA, Feldman EL, Hughes RA. Enhanced glucose control for preventing and treating diabetic neuropathy. 2012;6:CD007543.
35. Hamza MA, White PF, Craig WF, Ghoname ES, Ahmed HE, Proctor TJ, et al. Percutaneous electrical nerve stimulation: a novel analgesic therapy for diabetic neuropathic pain. Diabetes Care. 2000;23(3):365–70.
36. de Vos CC, Meier K, Zaalberg PB, Nijhuis HJ, Duyvendak W, Vesper J, et al. Spinal cord stimulation in patients with painful diabetic neuropathy: a multicentre randomized clinical trial. Pain. 2014;155(11):2426–31.
37. van Beek M, Slangen R, Schaper NC, Faber CG, Joosten EA, Dirksen CD, et al. Sustained treatment effect of spinal cord stimulation in painful diabetic peripheral neuropathy: 24-month follow-up of a prospective two-center randomized controlled trial. Diabetes Care. 2015;38(9):e132–4.

A 35-Year-Old Woman with Whole Body Pain: Fibromyalgia

41

Lynn R. Kohan and Xiaoying Zhu

Case Description

A 35-year-old woman presented to the pain management clinic as an initial visit. She stated that she has had ongoing fatigue and that her whole body hurts, especially her muscles and joints. She rated the pain a 7/10 on the numeric rating scale (NRS). She described the pain as achy in nature. She also complained of numbness and tingling in her arms and legs. She was unable to participate in activities with her children because of the pain. Nothing helped the pain. It was worse with prolonged activity. She was taking ibuprofen 600 mg by mouth about 2–3 times a day and Tylenol 500 mg as needed. In addition, she reported that she had not been sleeping well. Her symptoms began about 2 years ago but had steadily been getting worse. She presented asking what can be done about her pain.

Physical examination revealed normal vital signs. She was a moderately obese woman who appeared slightly anxious. She was tender to palpation in her bilateral trapezius, rhomboids, cervical paraspinal, latissimus dorsi, lumbar paraspinal, and gluteal musculature. The patient was given the widespread pain index (WPI) and symptom severity scale (SSS) questionnaire. She reported pain in 5 out of 5 quadrants in addition to indicating the following symptoms as moderate problems: fatigue, trouble concentrating, and waking up tired. Furthermore, she reported headaches and feelings of depression (Fig. 41.1). She was started on a course of duloxetine and given instructions to titrate up to 60 mg daily. In addition, she was offered an appointment with the pain psychologist and provided with a prescription for aqua-therapy. The patient returned 8 weeks later reporting mild improvement in her symptoms; however, secondary to delays obtaining appointments with physical therapy and pain psychology, she had just started those therapies. No changes were made to her regimen, and she was instructed to return to the clinic in 8 weeks. Upon return, she reported participating in both physical and psychological therapies and noted some additional improvement in her pain. She stated however that her function was still limited and was hoping for further improvements in her overall symptoms. She was started on a course of pregabalin at 75 mg twice a day (bid) and instructed to increase to 150 mg bid over 1 week. The patient returned at her follow-up appointment stating that she had been exercising regularly, using the techniques learned in pain psychology, and had been taking her duloxetine and pregabalin

L. R. Kohan (✉) · X. Zhu
Department of Anesthesiology, University of Virginia Health System, Charlottesville, VA, USA
e-mail: LRK9G@hscmail.mcc.virginia.edu

T. Malik (ed.), *Practical Chronic Pain Management*, https://doi.org/10.1007/978-3-030-46675-6_41

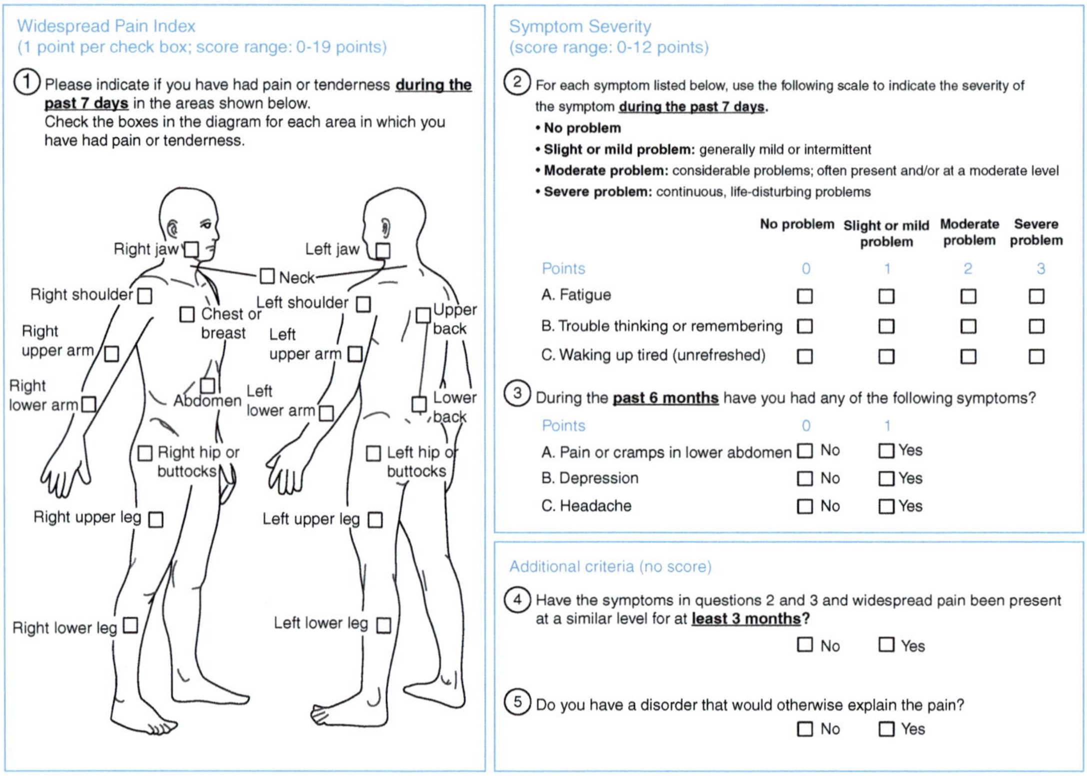

Fig. 41.1 Widespread pain index and symptom severity scale. (From Woolf [57], with permission)

without side effects. She reported overall improvement in her widespread pain, function, headaches, anxiety, and depression and was overall pleased.

What Is the Preliminary Diagnosis?

The primary diagnosis is fibromyalgia (FM) or chronic widespread pain syndrome. FM generally consists of a constellation of chronic syndromes including widespread pain, fatigue, stiffness, and insomnia [1]. The pain is mostly present in the musculoskeletal system and soft tissues. In addition, patients often report numerous associated symptoms such as altered mentation ("fibro-fog"), headaches, irritable bowel, anxiety, and depression. Given the lack of objective criteria, the American College of Rheumatology (ACR) has developed several diagnostic criteria since 1990 to better guide physicians to an appropriate diagnosis.

How Is the Diagnosis Confirmed?

The American College of Rheumatology first developed diagnostic criteria in 1990 in hope of providing improved guidance to physicians in diagnosing FM.

1990 Criteria

At that time there were two requirements for FM to be diagnosed: widespread pain (defined as axial pain in the upper and lower halves of the body) for at least 3 months; and 11 ≥ of 18 specific tender points identified on palpation [2]. Skill was required to locate the tender points and gradually press with 4 kg per square meter of pressure (Table 41.1).

The two greatest flaws with the 1990 criteria were the ability and/or confidence of practitioners to perform the tender point exam correctly and the fact that associated symptoms were

Table 41.1 The American College of Rheumatology 1990 criteria for the classification of fibromyalgia

1. History of Widespread Pain *Definition.*Pain is considered widespread when all of the following are present: pain in the right side of the body, pain above the waist, and pain below the waist. In addition, axial skeletal pain (cervical spine or anterior chest or thoracic spine or low back) must be present. In this definition, shoulder and buttock pain is considered as pain for each involved side. "Low back" pain is considered lower segment pain.
2. Pain in 11 of 18 tender sites on digital palpation *Definition.*Pain, on digital palpation, must be present in at least 11 of the following tender point sites: *Occiput:* bilateral, at suboccipital muscle insertions. *Low cervical:* bilateral, at the suboccipital muscle insertions. *Trapezius:* bilateral, at the midpoint of the upper border. *Supraspinatus:* bilateral, at origins, above the scapula spine near the medial border. *Second rib:* bilateral, at the second costochondral junctions, just lateral to the junction of the upper surfaces. *Lateral epicondyle:* bilateral, 2 cm distal to the epicondyles. *Gluteal:* bilateral, in upper outer quadrants of buttocks in anterior fold of muscle. *Greater trochanter:* bilateral, posterior to the trochanteric prominence. *Knee:* bilateral, at the medial fat pad proximal to the joint line. Digital palpation should be performed with an approximate force of 4 kg. For a tender point to be considered "positive," the subject must state that the palpation was painful. "Tender" is not considered painful.
For classification purposes, patients will be said to have fibromyalgia if both criteria are satisfied. Widespread pain must have been present for at least 3 months. The presence of a second clinical disorder does not exclude the diagnosis of fibromyalgia.

From Wolfe et al. [2], with permission

largely neglected. While the 1990 criteria were widely utilized, it became apparent that the majority of physicians were either not performing the tender point examination or performing it incorrectly [3–5]. The criteria were revised in 2010 to address these issues.

2010 ACR Criteria

The 2010 criteria were developed to offer clinicians a more practical method to diagnose FM. The tender point examination was eliminated, widespread pain was better quantified, and attention was drawn to associated symptoms of FM. The criteria involved two components that were scored: widespread pain index (WPI) which identified 19 painful regions on the body and the symptom severity scale which assessed for FM-associated symptoms [6]. The combination of scores was used to see whether the criteria were met. A medical evaluation was required and other disorders that could cause similar symptoms had to be ruled out (Table 41.2).

The criteria underwent slight revision in 2011 for research purposes which allowed a diagnosis to be determined solely based on patient self-report/questionnaire.

The criteria were once again revised in 2016 in order to better define widespread pain and to eliminate the exclusion criteria for other coexisting conditions [6].

2016 ACR Criteria

The most recent update seeks to better define widespread pain by identifying generalized pain in four of five body regions that have lasted for at least 3 months [6]. It also includes symptoms such as fatigue, cognitive issues, dizziness, numbness and tingling, nausea, chest pain, tinnitus, dry eyes, and easy bruising [6]. It also acknowledged that FM can coexist with other diseases [6] (Table 41.3).

A clinician should first start with a history and physical examination and use the diagnostic criteria to aid in questioning the patient. The physical examination should be complete but can focus

Table 41.2 American College of Rheumatology fibromyalgia diagnostic criteria (2010 Alternate)

Criteria	
A patient satisfies diagnostic criteria for fibromyalgia if the following three conditions are met:	
1. Widespread pain index (WPI) ≥ 7 and symptom severity scale score ≥ 5 or WPI and SS scale score ≥ 9.	
2. Symptoms have been present at a similar level for at least 3 months.	
3. The patient does not have a disorder that would otherwise explain the pain.	
Ascertainment	
1. *WPI:* note the number areas in which the patient has had pain over the last week. In how many areas has the patient had pain? Score will be between 0 and 19.	
Shoulder girdle, left	Hip (buttock, trochanter), left
Shoulder girdle, right	Hip (buttock, trochanter), right
Upper arm, left	Upper leg, left
Upper arm, right	Upper leg, right
Lower arm, left	Lower leg, left
Lower arm, right	Lower leg, right
Jaw, left	Upper back
Jaw, right	Lower back
Chest	Neck
Abdomen	
2. *SS scale score:*	
Fatigue	
Waking unrefreshed	
Cognitive symptoms	
For each of the three symptoms above, indicate the level of severity over the past week using the following scale:	
0 = No problem	
1 = Slight or mild problems, generally mild or intermittent	
2 = Moderate, considerable problems, often present and/or at a moderate level	
3 = Severe: pervasive, continuous, life-disturbing problems	
Considering somatic symptoms in general, indicate whether the patient has[a]:	
0 = No symptoms	
1 = Few symptoms	
2 = A moderate number of symptoms	
3 = A great deal of symptoms	
The SS scale score is the sum of the severity of the three symptoms (fatigue, waking unrefreshed, cognitive symptoms) plus the extent (severity) of somatic symptoms in general. The final score is between 0 and 12.	

From Wolfe [58], with permission

[a]Somatic symptoms that might be considered: muscle pain, irritable bowel syndrome, fatigue/tiredness, thinking or remembering problem, muscle weakness, headache, pain/cramps in the abdomen, numbness/tingling, dizziness, insomnia, depression, constipation, pain in the upper abdomen, nausea, nervousness, chest pain, blurred vision, fever, diarrhea, dry mouth, itching, wheezing, Raynaud's phenomenon, hives/welts, ringing in ears, vomiting, heartburn, oral ulcers, loss of/change in taste, seizures, dry eyes, shortness of breath, loss of appetite, rash, sun sensitivity, hearing difficulties, easy bruising, hair loss, frequent urination, painful urination, and bladder spasms

on the most symptomatic areas. There are no laboratory tests required in the diagnosis, but one can obtain certain tests such as basic chemistries, complete blood count, and thyroid tests if indicated. Based on the assessment of the patient, the diagnostic criteria can be scored to confirm the diagnosis of FM.

What Is the Pathophysiology of the Condition?

The exact pathophysiology of FM is unknown [7, 8]. There is no known specific triggering event; however, many physical or emotional stressors may worsen the condition [9]. It was traditionally thought that the disorder was secondary to mus-

Table 41.3 American College of Rheumatology 2016 Fibromyalgia Diagnostic Criteria

Criteria

A patient satisfies modified 2016 fibromyalgia criteria if the following 3 conditions are met:

(1) Widespread pain index (WPI) ≥ 7 and symptom severity scale (SSS) score ≥ 5 or WPI of 4–6 and SSS score ≥ 9

(2) Generalized pain, defined as pain in at least four of five regions, must be present. Jaw, chest, and abdominal pain are not included in generalized pain definition.

(3) Symptoms have been generally present for at least 3 months.

(4) A diagnosis of fibromyalgia is valid irrespective of other diagnoses. A diagnosis of fibromyalgia does not exclude the presence of other clinically important illnesses.

Ascertainment

WPI: note the number of areas in which the patient has had pain over the last week. In how many areas has the patient had pain? Score will be between 0 and 19

Left upper region (Region 1)
Jaw, left[a]
Shoulder girdle, left
Upper arm, left
Lower arm, left

Right upper region (Region 2)
Jaw, right[a]
Shoulder girdle, right
Upper arm, right
Lower arm, right

Left lower region (Region 3)
Hip (buttock, trochanter), left
Upper leg, left
Lower leg, left

Right lower region (Region 4)
Hip (buttock, trochanter), right
Upper leg, right
Lower leg, right

Axial region (Region 5)
Neck
Upper back
Lower back
Chest
Abdomen

2. Symptom severity scale (SSS) score
Fatigue
Waking unrefreshed
Cognitive symptoms

For each of the three symptoms above, indicate the level of severity over the past week using the following scale:
0 = No problem
1 = Slight or mild problems, generally mild or intermittent
2 = Moderate, considerable problems, often present and/or at a moderate level
3 = Severe: pervasive, continuous, life-disturbing problems

The symptom severity scale (SSS) score: it is the sum of the severity scores of the three symptoms (fatigue, waking unrefreshed, and cognitive symptoms) (0–9) plus the sum (0–3) of the number of the following symptoms the patient has been bothered by that occurred during the previous 6 months:
(1) Headaches (0–1)
(2) Pain or cramps in lower abdomen (0–1)
(3) Depression (0–1)

The final symptom severity score is between 0 and 12

The fibromyalgia severity (FS) scale is the sum of the WPI and SSS

The FS scale is also known as the polysymptomatic distress (PSD) scale.

From Wolfe et al. [6], with permission
[a]Not included in generalized pain definition

cle pathology; however, this idea has been refuted. It is now thought that any muscle pathology present is actually secondary to pain and inactivity and not a primary process [7].

Currently the most established pathophysiological mechanism for FM is thought to be central sensitization. Common symptoms of central sensitization such as hyperalgesia and allodynia are common in patients with FM. Patients with FM seem to be more sensitive to a variety of stimuli including heat, cold, and electrical stimulation [10], as well as auditory and visual stimuli suggesting a global central processing issue not just a pain processing issue [11].

Aside from genetic and psychological factors, use of functional magnetic resonance imaging has increased our understanding of chronic pain. Numerous studies have reported increased activation of pain processing networks in patients with FM compared to healthy controls in response to nociceptive stimuli [12–14]. There is also evidence that FM patients exhibit reduced activation or connectivity within the pain inhibitory network [15]. Furthermore, studies suggest a possibility of cross-talk between various sensory modalities as evidenced by increased insular activity evoked by aversive visual stimuli in patients with FM as compared to healthy controls [16]. Additional studies suggest that hyperconnectivity between the insular cortex (IC) to other parts of the brain processing network as well as networks involved in self-awareness and self-monitoring make the brain susceptible to increased pain perception and the development of a chronic pain state [17].

Use of proton magnetic resonance spectroscopy has also led to a better understanding of FM. This non-invasive modality can quantify concentrations of different metabolites such as glutamate and γ-aminobutyric acid (GABA). A study by Napadow suggests that increases in the excitatory neurotransmitters glutamate/glutamine or decreases in inhibitory neurotransmitters such as GABA in the IC can contribute to heightened pain [18].

Furthermore, it has been found that a polymorphism in the catechol-*O*-methyltransferase (COMT) enzyme may be associated with a predisposition to FM. COMT breaks down catecholamines such as dopamine and norepinephrine in addition to endorphins. This genetic defect has been associated with chronic pain and depression and is now thought to be linked to FM [19]. It is also interesting to note that endogenous opioid levels are actually increased in patients with FM. Researchers found through use of positron emission tomography (PET) that mu-opioid receptor binding potential was decreased in patients with FM. This finding may explain why patients with FM do not respond to opioids [20].

How Is the Problem Managed?

Treatment of FM is directed at reducing or ameliorating symptoms of the disease including chronic widespread pain, fatigue, insomnia, and cognitive dysfunction [21]. A step-wise approach should be taken (Table 41.4).

Patient education and collaboration with the patient to prioritize individual goals are paramount in the treatment of FM. An integrated approach encompassing continued patient education, pharmacologic treatments, and non-pharmacologic therapies is often necessary (Fig. 41.2).

Education

Education should focus on highlighting the importance of adherence to the treatment plan. The patient should be advised that treatment involves a slow and steady process for both physical therapy components as well as pharmacological treatments. Adhering to a starting low and going slow regimen will limit the risk for adverse effects and will lead to better efficacy.

Pharmacological Treatment

In regard to pharmacological treatments, three medications have been approved by the Food and Drug Administration (FDA) in the United States for the treatment of FM (pregabalin, duloxetine, and milnacipran) [22]. Patients and their families should be informed that while medications cannot cure FM, they may help to alleviate symptoms and improve function. Other medications such as tricyclic antidepressants (TCAs) (amitriptyline), medications with tricyclic properties

Table 41.4 Stepwise treatment of fibromyalgia

Step 1:
Confirm the patient's diagnosis.
Evaluate the patient for symptom variety, severity of symptoms, and level of function
Evaluate the patient for any comorbidities such as medical or psychiatric disease (sleep apnea, osteoarthritis, depression, or anxiety)
Evaluate level of fitness, and identify and psychological stressors or barriers to treatment
Review treatment options with the patient
Step 2:
Make treatment recommendations based on the results of the individual patient evaluation
A medication trial should be initiated in patients with moderate to severe pain
Patients with or without depression and anxiety: a trial of a selective serotonin and norepinephrine reuptake inhibitor should be started (do not use as sole medication in patients with history of bipolar disorder
Sleep disturbance or anxiety present: trial of alpha 2 delta ligand
If patient has partial response to SNRI or alpha 2 delta ligand monotherapies: trial of combination of these medications
If no response to monotherapy or combination therapy mentioned above—may try TCA, or combination of SSRI with TCA (monitor for serontonin syndrome) or SSRI with alpha 2 delta ligand
Provide adjunct treatments for comorbidities as warranted—for example, NSAIDS for OA, CPAP for sleep apnea
Step 3:
Initiate CBT for patients with comorbid psychosocial stressors, of problems with coping or functioning
Prescribe exercise according to patients fitness level—with a goal of 30–60 min at least 2–3 times per week
Encourage the patient to participate in supervised or group exercise

Modified from Arnold [23], with permission

(cyclobenzaprine, tramadol), and gabapentin are also frequently used in treatment. While these medications are not specifically approved by the FDA, they are often utilized as they are more affordable to patients than the FDA-approved medications. Selecting the appropriate medication should be tailored to the patient's individual needs based on a review of any comorbidities, such as sleep disturbance, fatigue, anxiety, and depression [21]. Patients may need a combination of medications to best treat all of their symptoms. Medications used should be started low and increased over time. It is also important to avoid medications that might result in drug-drug interactions. For example, if a patient is already on a selective serotonin re-uptake inhibitor that is working well to control his/her depression or anxiety, it may be better to avoid medications that also increase serotonin levels. In contrast, if a patient is exhibiting symptoms of depression/anxiety and is not on a medication to help control these symptoms, selecting a medication such as duloxetine or milnacipran may be beneficial. Table 41.5 provides a summary of treatment options that are available.

Non-pharmacological Therapies

Non-pharmacological therapies such as physical therapy, sleep hygiene, and cognitive behavioral therapy should be initiated at the beginning of treatment. In regard to exercise, aerobic activity appears to be the most beneficial. One should advise starting with low intensity activities and increase over time. An example would be to start with low impact walking or swimming for a short period of time and then increasing to a goal of 30–60 min at least 2–3 times per week [23].

What Is the Prognosis of This Condition?

FM is a chronic life-long illness for which there is no single identifiable cure. While medications are an important part of the treatment, research shows that patients treated with a multidisciplinary approach including medications, physical therapy, cognitive behavioral therapy, and self-

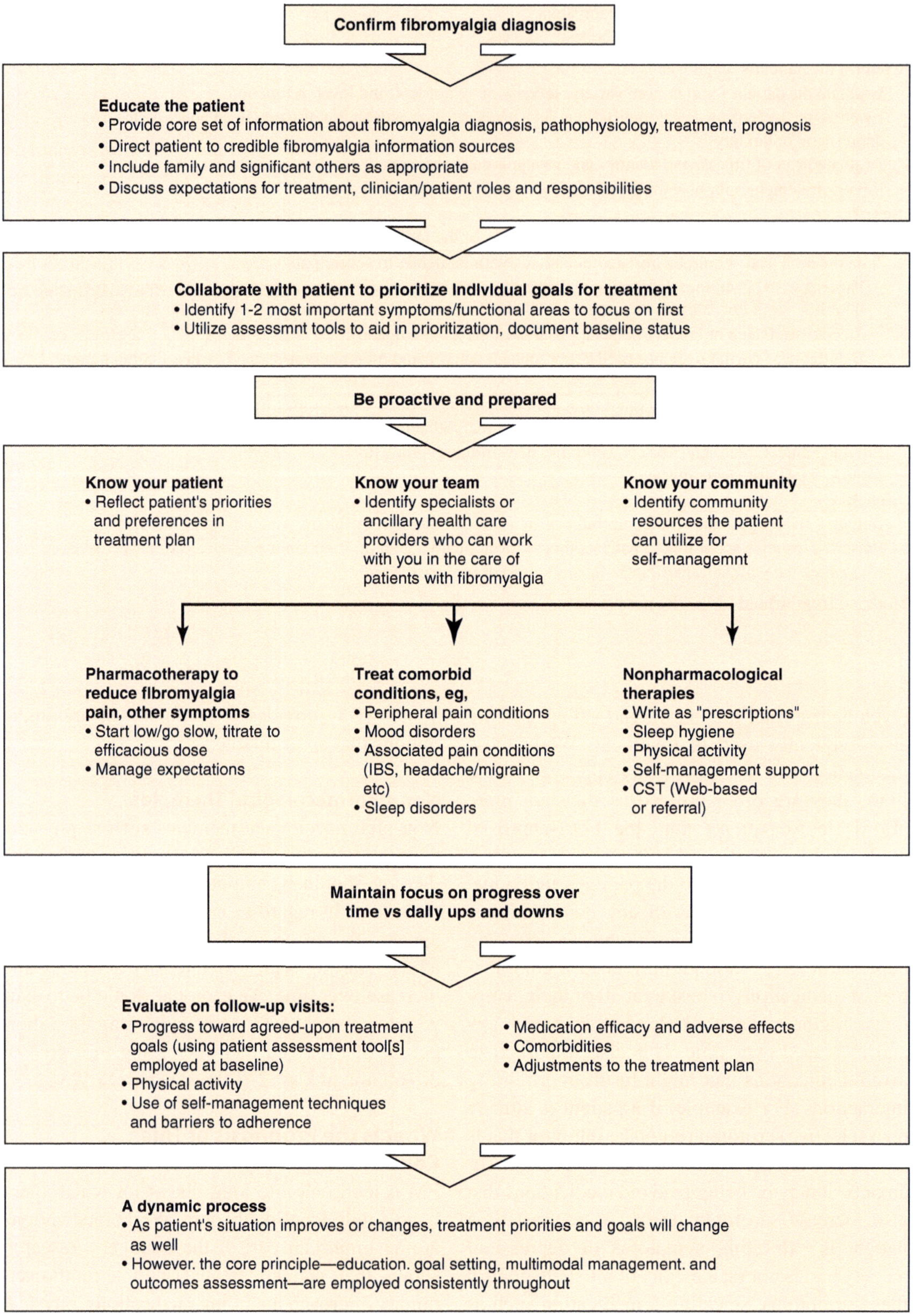

Fig. 41.2 Core principles for an integrated approach for fibromyalgia treatment. CBT cognitive behavioral therapy, IBS irritable bowel syndrome. (From Arnold et al. [22], with permission)

Table 41.5 Summary of treatment regimens for pharmacological and non-pharmacological therapies used in multimodal management of patients with fibromyalgia[a]

Therapy	Representative treatment regimen	Outcomes[b]
Pharmacotherapy		
Pregabalin	Start at 75 mg BID and up-titrate to 300–450 mg/d (150–225 mg twice a day)[c]	Significant reduction in pain (11-point NRS) Improvement in other subjective ratings of fibromyalgia symptoms (PGIC; FIQ total score) vs. placebo Most common AEs[b]: dizziness, somnolence, dry mouth, edema, blurred vision, weight gain, abnormal thinking (primarily difficulty with concentration/attention)[c] Discontinuation from clinical trials of fibromyalgia due to AEs: 19% for patients treated with pregabalin (150–600 mg/d) vs. 10% for placebo[c] AEs most often leading to discontinuation of pregabalin: dizziness (6%) and somnolence (3%)[c]
Duloxetine (SNRI)	Start at 30 mg/d and up-titrate to 60 mg once daily[d]	Significant reduction in pain (BPI and pain interference) Improvement in other subjective ratings of fibromyalgia symptoms (PGIC; FIQ total score) vs placebo Most common AEs[b]: nausea, dry mouth, somnolence, fatigue, constipation, decreased appetite, hyperhidrosis[d] Discontinuation from clinical trials of fibromyalgia due to AEs: 18.7% for patients treated with duloxetine (60–120 mg/d) vs. 10.8% for placebo[d] AEs most commonly leading to discontinuation of duloxetine: nausea (2.1%), somnolence (1.2%), and fatigue (1.1%)[d]
Milnacipran (SNRI)	Start at 12.5 mg/d and up-titrate to 50 mg twice a day[e]	Significant reduction in pain (VAS) and in composite responder rate Significant improvement in other subjective ratings of fibromyalgia symptoms (PGIC, SF-36 domains; FIQ total score) vs. placebo Most common AEs[b]: nausea, headache, constipation, dizziness, insomnia, hot flush, hyperhidrosis, vomiting, palpitations, increased heart rate, dry mouth, hypertension[e] Discontinuation from clinical trials of fibromyalgia due to AEs: 23% and 26% for patients treated with milnacipran (100 and 200 mg/d), respectively, vs. 12% for placebo[e] AEs most commonly leading to discontinuation of milnacipran: nausea (6%), palpitations (3%), and headache (2%)[e]
Non-pharmacological		
Education	Provide core information about fibromyalgia diagnosis, physiology, treatment, prognosis, importance of exercise, sleep. Manage expectations	Varied degrees of improvement in patient symptoms and/or functions through education (often in combination with CBT and/or exercise programs)
Physical activity	Start low, go slow; e.g., walk 10 min/d, build to 30–60 min of low or moderate activity up to 2–3 times/wk	Improvement in physical function and HRQoL and symptoms of fibromyalgia, including pain, depressed mood, and fatigue

(continued)

Table 41.5 (continued)

Therapy	Representative treatment regimen	Outcomes[b]
CBT/Web-based CBT	CFIDS and Fibromyalgia Self-Help (www.cfidsselfhelp.org; www.treatcfsfm.org) Arthritis Foundation's Fibromyalgia Self-Help Course Online self-help courses, tools, books, and CDs face-to-face CBT counseling	Improved knowledge about fibromyalgia and how to cope with pain Significant improvement in physical (pain, fatigue, and functional disability) and psychological (negative mood and anxiety) functioning and in impact of fibromyalgia in patients treated with CBT combined with exercise vs. no CBT
Sleep hygiene	Make sleep routine a priority. Optimize relaxing sleep environment. Provide advice on diet and exercise: avoid nighttime stimulants (e.g., coffee); exercise during the day; hide clock	Improving sleep hygiene can increase favorable outcomes on measures of pain (BPI) and mental well-being (SF-36)

From Arnold et al. [22]

[a]*AE* adverse event, *BPI* Brief Pain Inventory, *CBT* cognitive behavioral therapy, *CFIDS* chronic fatigue and immune dysfunction syndrome, *FIQ* Fibromyalgia Impact Questionnaire, *HRQoL* health-related quality of life, *NRS* numerical rating scale, *PGIC* Patient Global Impression of Change, *SF* short form, *SNRI* serotonin and norepinephrine reuptake inhibitor, *VAS* visual analog scale

[b]Safety is based on the most frequently occurring adverse reactions (≥5% and twice placebo for pregabalin[c] and duloxetine[d] or ≥ 5% and greater than placebo for milnacipran[e])

[c]For further detail, see prescribing information: http://labeling.pfizer.com/ShowLabeling.aspx?id=561

[d]For further detail, see prescribing information: http://pi.lilly.com/us/cymbalta-pi.pdf

[e]For further detail, see prescribing information: http://www.frx.com/pi/Savella_pi.pdf

management have better outcomes than those who do not engage in this approach. Patients should expect their symptoms to wax and wane over time. Overall signs of a better prognosis include increased sense of control over one's pain, the belief that one is not disabled, and that pain is not a sign of damage. In addition, those that seek help from others, exercise more, have less guarding during physical examination, and utilize good pacing activities do better. Efficacy of treatment is quite limited without improvements in physical and psychological stressors. The incidence of disability is high in patients with FM. Approximately 10–30% of FM patients experience work-related disability. This rate is three times greater than disability rates among patients with other types of widespread pain [24].

Discussion

Prevalence

Chronic pain is a serious health problem that affects about 15% of the population in Western countries [25–27]. FM, a centralized pain disorder, affects approximately 2–4% of the population and affects about five million Americans [28, 29]. It is more common in females than in males by a ratio of about 7–9:1. It most often affects patients around mid-life. Additionally, the prevalence of FM in women rises sharply in middle age to a peak of 7.4% in the 70–79 year-old age group before declining [28]. The prevalence among men also peaks in the 70–79-year-old age group but was only found to be slightly higher than 1% [28]. The prevalence of FM is higher among first-degree relatives which may suggest a genetic component to the disease [30, 31].

Differential Diagnosis

The differential diagnosis for FM is extensive as many different conditions present with pain and fatigue [21]. The differential diagnosis includes central pain syndromes, rheumatological conditions, myopathies, systemic connective tissue diseases, as well as endocrine disorders. Rheumatological diseases can also present with diffuse pain and fatigue; however, there are

Table 41.6 Differential diagnosis of fibromyalgia

Condition	Distinguishing features from fibromyalgia
Rheumatoid arthritis	Joint swelling, deformities, elevated erythrocyte sedimentation rate (ESR), C-reactive protein
Systemic lupus erythematosus	Rash, multisystemic inflammation, elevated ESR, antinuclear antibody
Myositis, myopathies	Weakness, elevated muscle enzymes
Ankylosing spondylitis	Back, neck immobility, elevated ESR, abnormal X-rays
Hypothyroidism	Abnormal thyroid function tests
Neuropathies	Weakness, loss of sensation, abnormal electromyography, nerve conduction studies

From Goldenberg [32], with permission

characteristics that help them to be distinguished from FM (Table 41.6).

Serological tests are usually not required. Physical exam findings can distinguish between diseases such as rheumatoid arthritis which presents with multiple joint swelling and systemic lupus erythematosus which presents with a facial rash and/or multi-systemic inflammation. These findings do not occur in FM. Polymyalgia rheumatic (PMR) may also present with similar features to FM; however, patients with PMR tend to be older at onset and present more often with generalized stiffness. The majority of patients with PMR will have an elevated sedimentation rate or C-reactive protein while those with FM will not.

Myopathies can also be distinguished from FM by history and physical examination as well as laboratory testing. Myositis and myopathies tend to cause muscle weakness while FM does not. Patients with FM also have normal muscle enzyme tests and normal muscle biopsies unlike in myopathies. Muscle biopsies are not recommended in the workup of FM.

Endocrine diseases such as hypothyroidism can be difficult to differentiate from FM as both conditions can cause generalized aches, fatigue, and sleep disorders. Thyroid function is normal in patients with FM unless they have co-existing disease, and thus it is reasonable to obtain thyroid function tests in the workup of FM [32]. In addition, non-icteric hepatitis may also present with myalgia and fatigue, and thus obtaining liver function tests as well as creatinine phosphokinase levels during initial presentation is reasonable [32].

Finally, somatic disorders can also mimic FM.

Predictive Value of Different Clinical Features

The different diagnostic criteria resulted in different specificity and sensitivities. Using the 1990 ACR criteria, widespread pain (axial plus upper and lower segment plus left- and right-sided pain) was found in 97.6% of all patients with FM and in 69.1% of all control patients. The combination of widespread pain and mild or greater tenderness in ≥11 of 18 tender point sites yielded a sensitivity of 88.4% and a specificity of 81.1% [2]. Using the 2010 ACR criteria, a symptom severity scale score of 6 identified patients satisfying the diagnostic criteria in 92.3% of cases [33]. Analysis of the 2010 criteria shows sensitivities of 90.2% and specificities of 89.5%, respectively [21].

Strength of Evidence for Different Treatment Modalities

In general, non-pharmacological treatments such as exercise and psychoeducational approaches have been shown to have the greatest efficacy in the treatment of FM [34]. These modalities should be tailored to the individual patient. The number of medications used for the treatment of FM has increased substantially over the last decade; however, only three drugs have been approved by the US FDA for the treatment of pain in FM: pregabalin, duloxetine, and milnacipran [17]. Amitriptyline, a non-selective 5-hydroxytryptamine and norepinephrine reuptake inhibitor, however, is the best-studied drug in the treatment of FM. It has been found to be efficacious in studies and is often considered a first-line medication [35]; however, the evidence supporting its use is of low quality as the studies conducted have been small and of short duration [36]. Duloxetine has marginal benefit in FM with a number needed to treat (NNT) of 8 and a number needed to harm (NNH) of 18 [37]. The European League Against Rheumatism as well as the Canadian Pain Society recommend a dose of 60 mg per day; however, the dose and duration of therapy is typically guided by patient response and side effects. Duloxetine at 20-30 mg per day has not been found to be efficacious, and there was no increase in efficacy when comparing 60–120 mg [37]. Milnacipran has high quality evidence that shows moderate effectiveness. It has an NNT for at least 30% decrease in pain of 11 and a NNH of 14 [38].

Antiepileptics are also often used in FM as they can help target the elevated levels of glutamate and substance P. Pregabalin and gabapentin are structurally similar to neurotransmitter GABA, but do not have activity on GABA receptors. They bind to voltage-gated calcium channels in the central nervous system exerting their analgesic effect [39]. Crofford et al. in 2005 performed an 8-week, double-blind, randomized controlled trial of over 500 patients with FM. They found that patients had >50% improvement in pain with 450 mg of pregabalin per day. In addition, improvements were also shown in sleep quality, fatigue, and health-related quality of life [40]. A Cochrane review showed a daily dose of 600 mg of pregabalin was no better than 450 mg/day for any outcome measures [41]. High quality evidence shows that the NNT for pregabalin is 12 with an NNH of 13 [42]. Pregabalin may also show a small benefit for sleep [42]. A Cochrane review on gabapentin, however, concluded, based on only very low quality evidence, that there is insufficient evidence to either support or refute the suggestion that gabapentin decreases pain in FM [43].

A recent Cochrane review concluded that there was no good quality evidence with regards to the superiority of selective serotonin reuptake inhibitors compared to placebo in treating pain, fatigue, and sleep problems in patients with FM [44]. Opioids are generally contraindicated in the treatment of FM because of their lack of clinical efficacy and increased risk of opioid induced hyperalgesia [45]. Cyclobenzaprine is a centrally acting muscle relaxant that is structurally similar to TCAs. Patients treated with this medication were three times more likely to report improvement overall; however, 85% of patients experienced side effects [46]. A recent Cochrane review did not conclude that NSAIDs were efficacious in the treatment of FM [47]. There has not been any direct evidence regarding the use of acetaminophen for the treatment of FM although it has been used in combination with tramadol with some efficacy [48].

In regards to physical exercise, a recent Cochrane review found that when compared to control, moderate quality evidence suggests that aerobic exercise improves health-related quality of life and low quality evidence suggests an improvement in pain intensity and physical function [49]. In addition, a recent meta-analysis concluded that aerobic exercise and muscle strengthening are the most effective way to decrease pain and improve global well-being in patients with FM and that both stretching and aerobic exercise improved health-related quality of life. Furthermore, exercise produced the largest beneficial effect on depression symptoms [50].

Future Directions or Clinical Trials in Progress

There has been increasing interest in cannabinoids to treat pain secondary to their analgesic properties as well as sleep promoting effects [51]; however, a recent Cochrane review did not demonstrate efficacy in the treatment of FM [52]. More studies are needed to better determine efficacy in the treatment of FM. In addition, there is emerging evidence that low dose naltrexone may be beneficial in treating FM [53]. Naltrexone may promote analgesia by attenuating the inflammatory process [54]. This mechanism of action is distinct from naltrexone's inhibition of neuronal opioid receptors and may instead involve antagonism of immune cell receptors such as microglial in the central nervous system [55]. Further research is necessary. A meta-analysis on repetitive transcranial magnetic stimulation concluded benefit for FM that was separate from depression at 1 month of therapy. This therapy is currently approved for depression but not for FM [56].

Summary/Conclusion

FM is a prevalent disease that significantly impacts patient's lives. It presents with widespread pain in multiple body regions for more than 3 months in addition to symptoms such as fatigue, difficulty concentrating, depression, and anxiety. The diagnosis can be made based on the ACR 2016 guidelines. While there is no known cure for FM, patients can improve through use of a multimodal treatment plan. More research is needed to better develop treatment options for this disease.

References

1. Smythe HA, Moldofsky H. Two contributions to understanding of the "fibrositis" syndrome. Bull Rheum Dis. 1977–1978;28(1):928–31.
2. Wolfe F, Smythe HA, Yunus MB, Bennett RM, Bombardier C, Goldenberg DL, et al. The American College of Rheumatology 1990 criteria for the classification of fibromyalgia. Report of the Multicenter Criteria Committee. Arthritis Rheum. 1990;33:160–72.
3. Fitzcharles MA, Boulos P. Inaccuracy in the diagnosis of fibromyalgia syndrome: analysis of referrals. Rheumatology (Oxford). 2003;42(2):263–7.
4. Bennett RM. Clinical manifestations and diagnosis of fibromyalgia. Rheum Dis Clin N Am. 2009;35(2):215–32.
5. Mease P. Fibromyalgia syndrome: review of clinical presentation, pathogenesis, outcomemeasures, and treatment. J Rheumatol Suppl 2005;75:6–21. Review. Erratum in: J Rheumatol Suppl. 2005;32(10):2063.
6. Wolfe F, Clauw D, Fitzcharles MA, Goldenberg D, Hauser W, Katz R, Russel A, Russel I, Walitt B. 2016 revisions to the 2010/2011 fibromyalgia diagnostic criteria. Semin Arthritis Rheum. 2016;46(3):319–29.
7. Sarzi-Puttini P, Atzeni F, Mease PJ. Chronic widespread pain: from the peripheral to central evolution. Best Pract Res Clin Rheumatol. 2011;25(2):133–9.
8. Schmidt-Wilcke T, Clauw DJ. Fibromyalgia: from pathophysiology to therapy. Nat Rev Rheumatol. 2011;7(9):518.
9. Goldenberg DL. Do infections trigger fibromyalgia? Arthritis Rheum. 1993;36:1489.
10. Petzke F, Clauw DJ, Ambrose K, Khine A, Gracely RH. Increased pain sensitivity in fibromyalgia: effects of stimulus type and mode of presentation. Pain. 2003;105(3):403–13.
11. Geisser ME, Glass JM, Rajcevska LD, Clauw DJ, Williams DA, Kileny PR, et al. A psychophysical study of auditory and pressure sensitivity in patients with fibromyalgia and healthy controls. J Pain. 2008;9(5):417–22.
12. Gracely RH, Petzke F, Wolf JM, Clauw DJ. Functional magnetic resonance imaging evidence of augmented central pain processing in fibromyalgia. Arthritiis Rheum. 2002;46:1333–43.
13. Giesecke T, Gracely R, Grant MA, Nachemson A, Petzke F, Williams D, Clauw D. Evidence of augmented central pain processing in idiopathic low back pain. Arthritis Rheum. 2004;50:613–23.
14. Cook DB, Lange G, Ciccone DS, Liu WC, Steffener J, Natelson BH. Functinal imaging of pain in patients with primary fibromyalgia. J Rheumatol. 2004;31:364–78.
15. Jensen KB, Loitoile R, Kosek E, Petzke F, Carville S, Fransson P, Marcus H, Williams SCR, Choy E, Mainguy Y, et al. Patients with fibromyalgia display less functional connectivity in the brain's pain inhibitory network. Mol Pain. 2012;8:32.
16. Harte SE, Ichesco E, Hampson JP, Peltier SJ, Schmidt-Wilcke T, Clauw DJ, Harris RE. Pharmacologic attenuation of cross-modal sensory augmentation within the chronic pain insula. Pain. 2016;157:1933.
17. Schmidt-Wilke T, Diers M. New insights into the pathophysiology and treatment of fibromyalgia. Biomedicine. 2017;5(22):E22.
18. Napadow V, Harris RE. What has functional connectivity and chemical neuroimaging in fibromyalgia taught us about the mechanisms and management of "centralized" pain? Arthritis Res Ther. 2014;16:425.
19. Gürsoy S, Erdal E, Herken H, Madenci E, Alaşehirli B, Erdal N. Significance of catechol-O-methyltransferase gene polymorphism in fibromyalgia syndrome. Rheumatol Int. 2003;23(3):104–7.
20. Harris RE, Clauw DJ, Scott DJ, McLean SA, Gracely RH, Zubieta JK. Decreased central mu-opioid receptor availability in fibromyalgia. J Neurosci. 2007;27(37):10000–6.
21. Clauw DJ. Fibromyalgia: a clinical review. JAMA. 2014;311:1547–55.
22. Arnold L, Clauw D, Dunegan J, Turk D. A framework for fibromyalgia management for primary care providers. Mayo Clinic Proc. 2012;87(5):488–96.
23. Arnold LM. Biology and therapy of fibromyalgia. New therapies in fibromyalgia. Arthritis Res Ther. 2006;8:212.
24. White KP, Speechley M, Harth M, Ostbye T. Comparing self-reported function and work disability in 100 community cases of fibromyalgia syndrome versus controls in London, Ontario: the London Fibromyalgia Epidemiology Study. Arthritis Rheum. 1999;42(1):76–83.

25. Blyth FM, March LM, Brnabic AJM, Jorm LR, Williamson M, Cousins MJ. Chronic pain in Australia: a prevalence study. Pain. 2001;89:127–34.
26. Harker, J.; Reid, K.J.; Bekkering, G.E.; Kellen, E.; Malgorzata, M.; Riemsma, R.; Worthy, G.; Misso, K.; Kleijnen, J. Epidemiology of chronic pain in Denmark and Sweden. Pain Res. Treat 2012; Art ID 371248:1–30.
27. Manchikanti L, Singh V, Datta S, Cohen SP, Hirsch J. A comprehensive review of epidemiology, scope, and impact of spinal pain. Pain Physician. 2009;12:E35–70.
28. Wolfe F, Ross K, Anderson J, Russell IJ, Hebert L. The prevalence and characteristics of fibromyalgia in the general population. Arthritis Rheumatol. 1995;38:19–28.
29. Assumpção A, Cavalcante A, Capela C, Al E. Prevalence of fibromyalgia in a low socioeconomic status population. BMC Musculoskelet Disord. 2009;10:64–70.
30. Baskila D, Neumann I. Fibromyalgia syndrome (FM) and nonarticular tenderness in relatives of patients with FM. J Rheumatol. 1997;24(5):941–0.
31. Chen J, Mckenzie-Brown AM. The epidemiology and prevalence of fibromyalgia syndrome. In: Lawson E, Wallace M, editors. Fibromyalgia: clinical guidelines and treatments. Switzerland: Springer Publishing; 2015.. Chapter 1.
32. Goldenberg D. Diagnosis and differential diagnosis of fibromyalgia. Am J Med. 2009;122(12):S14–21.
33. Wolfe F, Clauw DJ, Fitzcharles MA, Goldenberg DL, Katz RS, Mease P, Russell AS, Winfield JB, Yunus MB. Ther American college of rheumatology preliminary criteria for fibromyalgia and measurement of symptoms severity. Arthritis Care Res. 2010;62(5):600–10.
34. Macfarlane GJ, Kronisch C, Dean LE, Atzeni F, Häuser W, Fluß E, et al. EULAR revised recommendations for the management of fibromyalgia. Ann Rheum Dis. 2017;76:318–28.
35. Rico-Villademoros F, Slim M, Calandre EP. Amitriptyline for the treatment of fibromyalgia: a comprehensive review. Expert Rev Neurother. 2015;15:1123–50.
36. Kwiatek R. Treatment of fibromyalgia. Aust Prescr. 2017;40:179–83.
37. Lunn MP, Hughes RA, Wiffen PJ. Duloxetine for treating painful neuropathy, chronic pain or fibromyalgia. Cochrane Database Syst Rev. 2014;1:CD007115.
38. Cording M, Derry S, Phillips T, Moore RA, Wiffen PJ. Milnacipran for pain in fibromyalgia in adults. Cochrane Database Syst Rev. 2015;10:CD008244.
39. Taylor CP. Mechanisms of analgesia by gabapentin and pregabalin—Calcium channel α2-Δ [cavα2-Δ] ligands. Pain. 2009;142:13–6.
40. Crofford LJ, Rowbotham MC, Mease PJ, Russell IJ, Dworkin RH, Corbin AE, Young JP Jr, LaMoreaux LK, Martin SA, Sharma U. Pregabalin for the treatment of fibromyalgia syndrome: results of a randomized, double-blind, placebo-controlled trial. Arthritis Rheum. 2005;52:1264–73.
41. Moore RA, Straube S, Wiffen PJ, Derry S, McQuay HJ. Pregabalin for acute and chronic pain in adults. Cochrane Database Syst Rev. 2009;
42. Üçeyler N, Sommer C, Walitt B, Häuser W. Anticonvulsants for fibromyalgia. Cochrane Database Syst Rev. 2013;10:CD010782.
43. Cooper TE, Derry S, Wiffen PJ, Moore RA. Gabapentin for fibromyalgia in adults. Cochrane Database Syst Rev. 2017;(1):CD012188.
44. Walitt B, Urrútia G, Nishishinya MB, Cantrell SE, Häuser W. Selective serotonin reuptake inhibitors for fibromyalgia syndrome. Cochrane Database Syst Rev. 2015;6
45. Littlejohn GO, Guymer EK, Ngian GS. Is there a role for opioids in the treatment of fibromyalgia? Pain Manag. 2016;6:347–55.
46. Kia S, Choy E. Update on treatment guidelines in fibromyalgia syndrome with focus on pharmacology. Biomedicine. 2017;5(2):20.
47. Derry S, Wiffen PJ, Häuser W, Mücke M, Tölle TR, Bell RF, Moore RA. Oral nonsteroidal anti-inflammatory drugs for fibromyalgia in adults. Cochrane Lib. 2016; https://doi.org/10.1002/14651858.CD012332.
48. Bennett RM, Kamin M, Karim R, Rosenthal N. Tramadol and acetaminophen combination tablets in the treatment of fibromyalgia pain: a double-blind, randomized, placebo-controlled study. Am J Med. 2003;114:537–45.
49. Bidonde J, Busch A, Schachter C, Overend T, Kim S, et al. Aerobic exercise training for adults with fibromyalgia. Cochrane Database Syst Rev. 2017;(6):CD012700.
50. Sosa-Reina MD, Nunez-Nagy S, Gallego-Izquierdo T, Pecos-Martin D, Monserrat J, Alvarez-Mon M. Effectiveness of therapeutic exercise in fibromyalagia syndrome: a systematic review and meta-analysis of randomized clinical trials. Hindawi Biomed Research International. 2017; Art ID 2356346:1–14.
51. Hauser W, Walitt B, Fitzcharles MA, Sommer C. Review of pharmacological therapies in fibromyalgia syndrome. Arthritis Res Ther. 2014;16:201.
52. Walitt B, Klose P, Fitzcharles MA, et al. Cannabinoids for fibromyalgia. Cochrane Database Syst Rev. 2016;7:CD011694.
53. Younger J, Noor N, McCue R, Mackey S. Low-dose naltrexone for the treatment of fibromyalgia: findings of a small, randomized, double-blind, placebo-controlled, counterbalanced, crossover trial assessing daily pain levels. Arthritis Rheumatol. 2013;65(2):529–38.
54. Hutchinson MR, Zhang Y, Brown K, Coats BD, Shridhar M, Sholar PW, et al. Non-stereoselective reversal of neuropathic pain by naloxone and naltrexone: involvement of toll-like receptor 4 (TLR4). Eur J Neurosci. 2008;28:20–9.

55. Mattioli TA, Miline B, Cahill CM. Ultra-low dose naltrexone attenuates chronic morphine-induced gliosis in rats. Mol Pain. 2010;6:22.
56. Knijink LM, Dussan-Sarria JA, Rozisky JR, et al. Repetitive transcranial magnetic stimulation for fibromyalgia: a systematic review and meta-analysis. Pain Pract. 2016;16(3):294–304.
57. Woolf C. Central sensitization: implications for the diagnosis and treatment of pain. 2011;152(S3):S2–15.
58. Wolfe F, et al. The American College of Rheumatology preliminary diagnostic criteria for fibromyalgia and measurement of symptom severity. Arthritis Care Res. 2010;62(5):600–10.

A Puzzling Case of Increasing Pain After Chronic Opioid Therapy

42

Tariq Malik and Naveed Mameghani

Case Description

One of your longtime patients in your busy Family Medicine clinic comes to see you for a follow-up visit. The patient is a 55-year-old male with chronic low back pain. He has been on chronic opioid therapy for his back pain for several months now. When you first prescribed him opioids, his pain greatly improved and the patient was extremely satisfied. During his last two visits, he was complaining of worsening back pain so you increased the opioid dose on both occasions. Today he mentions that neither dose increase helped him, and in fact he feels that his pain is higher in intensity now. He also says that the pain is no longer localized to his low back, but it is now diffuse and all over his body. He even feels that things that should not be painful now cause him a great deal of pain, and they did not cause him pain before opioid therapy was started. He states he is in 11 out of 10 pain and begs you to "fix" him.

What Is Your Preliminary Diagnosis?

The patient is complaining of increasing pain in his back and over his body despite opioid intake. The dose has been increased twice in recent past with no analgesic improvement. It's important to rule out other reasons that may cause worsening pain. In the absence of any obvious cause, the clinical features are suggestive of tolerance or opioid-induced hyperalgesia. Since the patient is also complaining of pain at new sites and pain all over his body, it's more consistent with the diagnosis of opioid-induced hyperalgesia.

How Is Your Diagnosis Confirmed?

Opioid-induced hyperalgesia (OIH) is a clinical diagnosis. OIH is suspected in the context of worsening pain when patient is being treated with opioids. This is especially true if the pain of the patient seems worse than prior to initiation of opioid therapy in the absence of disease progression. This condition, when not immediately realized, often is confused with opioid tolerance and leads to increase in opioid doses which in turn further intensify pain. Tolerance also presents as loss of analgesia in a patient who has been chronically exposed to opioids. The two differ in two aspects. Patient develops tolerance complains of worsening pain for which he is being treated with opioids. In addition, increase in opioid dose will improve pain. This is in contrast to OIH, where patient not only complain of worsening pain at the original site but also develops pain at other sites, behaving like a being in a state of diffuse

T. Malik (✉) · N. Mameghani
Department of Anesthesia and Critical Care, University of Chicago, Chicago, IL, USA
e-mail: TMuslim@dacc.uchicago.edu; tmalik@dacc.uchicago.edu

T. Malik (ed.), *Practical Chronic Pain Management*, https://doi.org/10.1007/978-3-030-46675-6_42

hyperalgesia. Often patient cannot explain the pain clearly, and physician often treats this with increase in the opioid dose, which makes the pain worse. In research studies, OIH is often diagnosed with lowering in threshold to mechanical, chemical, or thermal painful stimuli using QST, but there is no accepted standardized definition of diagnosing OIH using these parameters, and OIH is still a diagnosis of exclusion and clinical suspicion.

In the end, OIH is diagnosed when lowering opioid dose in a person being treated with opioids improves pain when other causes have been excluded. Tolerance is a separate entity but can also lead to providers increasing opioid dosages, and thus, it can be difficult to differentiate between the two [1, 2]. Tolerance is the loss of drug potency, meaning a higher opioid dose is needed to achieve the same effect of the prior "baseline" dose. Tolerance is due to the desensitization of antinociceptive pathways to opioids while opioid-induced hyperalgesia is due to the sensitization of pronociceptive pathways [3]. Increased opioid doses may overcome tolerance but will further worsen opioid-induced hyperalgesia [3–5]. With OIH, pain is often worse than the original pain and not well defined in location or quality [1]. Pain in a state of tolerance tends to stay in the original location and has a similar quality to the initial pain [1]. In patients with OIH, reduction or cessation of opioid doses can actually improve pain [1, 6]. These two conditions often coexist with each other but not necessarily are always equal causal factors in the increased pain experienced by the patient.

Clinical Features of OIH

1. Increase in pain over time
2. Spreading of pain to other locations than the initial painful site
3. Lower threshold for pain to various stimuli (such as heat, mechanical pressure, and touch)
4. Exclude
   (a) Opioid withdrawal
   (b) Evidence of underlying disease progression
   (c) Exclude opioid tolerance

What Is the Pathophysiology of This Condition?

Its pathophysiology is poorly understood. Different mechanism has been proposed. Many factors are involved in the development of OIH. The development is influenced by gender, genetic make-up, dose, duration, and type of opioid exposure. Different mechanism has been proposed: (1) peripheral nerve sensitization; (2) augmented descending facilitation; (3) enhanced excitatory neurotransmitter release, production, or poor clearance; (4) second-order neuron sensitization to excitatory neurotransmitters. The changes are due to the neuroplastic property of neural transmission. In general mu-receptor persistent activation causes changes in the receptor structure and alters the attached G-protein and/or other proteins downstream that cause development of tolerance or OIH. NMDA glutamate receptor over-activation is commonly seen in cases with tolerance of OIH. Chronic mu-opioid exposure has been shown to cause overexpression of this receptor, which then causes activation of numerous intracellular enzymes and changes in mu-receptor that leads to receptor loss, deactivation, and over-activity of excitatory receptors (Table 42.1).

OIH can be seen when large doses of opioids are given over a prolonged time or even when given for a short duration. Acute administration of opioids can lead to reduction of pain for a few hours, but this is followed by a reduction of the pain threshold [3] for several hours to days. Use of long-acting opioids in the postoperative period can mask this effect. OIH can be reversible but will often require long periods without any opioid therapy [6]. The dose/effect curve with OIH is shifted down (analgesic effect is reduced over time with a given opioid dose and an increase in dose will not lead to improvement) [7]. This is in contrast to tolerance which the curve is shifted to the right (higher dose is needed to achieve the same effect as before) [7, 8]. With tolerance, G protein receptors are not able to reduce cyclic AMP and therefore not able to decrease the inward current of calcium and sodium. Furthermore, with tolerance membrane receptors

Table 42.1 Cellular mechanisms implicated in tolerance and hyperalgesia

(a) μ Opioid based
Increased cyclic adenosine monophosphate and protein kinase A
Protein kinase C
C-Jun N-terminal kinase
β-arrestin-2
Src kinase
(b) Transcriptional
cAMP response element-binding protein
Mammalian target of rapamycin complex
(c) Pronociceptive ion channels
NMNDA receptors
Transient receptor potential vanilloid channel
(d) Microglia
Toll-like receptor 4
P2X4 and P2X7 purinergic receptors
Src kinase
Brain-derived neurotrophic factor

are reduced in number by internalization. Again, OIH involves sensitization and tolerance involves desensitization. The pathophysiology of OIH is complex and not fully understood. OIH is associated with a changed pain threshold which is the point where a noxious stimulus is felt as pain along with pain tolerance which is the point that a noxious stimulus becomes intolerable [3]. Instead there are increases in NMDA receptors [2, 3, 9], increased excitatory neurotransmitters [1, 10], reduced inhibitory neurotransmitters, activation of COX in the spinal cord, second messengers, and both central and peripheral sensitization. The main mechanism seems to increase glutamate release in the dorsal horn of the spinal cord and increase NMDA receptor response due to protein kinase C (PKC) [7]. NMDA receptors are activated by opioids leading to calcium influx and central sensitization. This increased calcium can lead to increased PKC activity, phosphorylation, and thereby inactivation of opioid receptors and increased nitric oxide synthase. OIH has also been shown to be linked to increased levels of cholecystokinin, substance P [3], the calcitonin gene receptor polypeptide (CGRP) [3, 9, 11], and nociceptin – these peptides all have anti opioid properties [12]. One study in mice determined that sustained opioid therapy induces a neurokinin (NK-1) receptor-mediated hyperalgesia [3, 9, 13] along with increased spinal substance P. The hyperalgesia was reversed by an NK-1 receptor antagonist (L-732,138) and was not seen in NK-1 knockout mice [13]. This study argues that these mechanisms are similar to those seen in inflammatory pain states [13]. Further study of the role of the NK-1 receptor and the clinical effect of its antagonism could help find another avenue to treat OIH. Another study found similar results with the TRPV1 receptor (transient receptor potential vanilloid, a molecular sensor of noxious heat) and also found that antagonism of the receptor (with AMG 0347) or knockout mice leads to avoidance of hyperalgesia [14, 15]. Furthermore, descending facilitation of nociception from the rostroventral medulla also plays a role in OIH [3, 16]. This descending facilitation increases the endogenous opioid peptide dynorphin which is a paradoxically pronociceptive kappa opioid receptor agonist which modulates transmission using non-opioid receptor processes [7]. This leads to naloxone-insensitive pronociception due to increased neuronal field size and increased NMDA receptor sensitivity, thereby leading to increased glutamate [10, 17] (excitatory neurotransmitter), calcium, and cytokines. Microglia are also implicated in OIH as they are activated in response to opioid use and cause release of pro-inflammatory cytokines (e.g., tumor necrosis factor, interleukin 1 and 6), nitric oxide, matrix metalloproteases, and excitatory amino acids. All these agents increase excitatory neuronal transmission and downregulate GABA receptors [3]. These pro-inflammatory markers could potentially be used as biomarkers of microglial activation and therefore OIH.

How Is This Problem Managed?

OIH seems to be a complex issue. Different targets have been identified to reverse or stop the development of OIH. After identifying the problem, best option is to wean down the dose of opioid totally if possible. If not other drugs are tried as adjunct in an attempt to minimize the total dose of opioids.

1. NDAIDS
2. Tylenol
3. Gabapentin/Lyrica
4. IV lidocaine
5. Ketamine
6. Magnesium
7. Steroids
8. Clonidine
9. Dexmedetomidine
10. Opioid rotation, especially methadone and buprenorphine

NMDA receptor antagonists have been shown to reduce or prevent OIH as these receptors are upregulated by use of opioids [7, 16, 18]. A bolus of ketamine (NMDA antagonist) of 0.5 milligrams/kilogram with induction followed by a ketamine infusion of 5 micrograms/kilogram/minute reduces postoperative pain scores and opioid usage, as well as helps to prevent remifentanil-induced hyperalgesia [19]. Side effects of ketamine include increased intracranial pressure, psychomimetic reactions, increased secretions, and myocardial stimulation or depression. Methadone also has NMDA receptor antagonist properties, and other opioids can be switched to methadone when OIH is suspected [3, 18]. Side effects include QTc prolongation, respiratory depression, sedation, addiction, and constipation. Buprenorphine (partial mu and ORL-1 receptor agonist and kappa-delta antagonist, 4 mg every 6 h and 2 mg every 4 h as needed) has different G protein interactions than other opioids and has been shown to be helpful in treatment of OIH and pain that is not responsive to other opioids [2, 3, 18, 20]. The ORL-1 receptor is pronociceptive at supraspinal sites but antinociceptive in the dorsal horn [20]. Its activation can reduce hyperalgesia and neuropathic pain by downregulating calcium channels [20]. Propofol has been proposed as another agent to combat OIH due to its GABA agonism. It has delayed hyperalgesia caused by remifentanil in studies [given over 30 min to a target effect site concentration (concentration of drug at the site of its biological activity, e.g., bound to receptors) of 1.5 micrograms/milliliter] although once propofol was discontinued an increase in hyperalgesia was seen [21]. Side effects of propofol include pain on injection, respiratory depression, myocardial depression, and decreased systemic vascular resistance. COX 2 inhibitors have also been shown to reduce OIH by both blocking NMDA receptors and increasing glutamate reuptake in the dorsal horn of the spinal cord. Forty milligrams of parecoxib IV (COX 2 selective NSAID) was shown to reduce remifentanil-induced hyperalgesia if given prior to remifentanil [18]. If given at the same time as remifentanil, the benefit was not apparent [18]. Side effects include cardiovascular thrombotic events including myocardial infarction and stoke and gastrointestinal ulceration with bleeding. Clonidine 2 micrograms/kilogram has also been observed to have the same reduction on remifentanil-induced hyperalgesia [18, 19]. Side effects include hypotension, sedation, and rebound hypertension if used chronically and abruptly discontinued. Propranolol (nonselective Beta adrenergic agonist with side effects of bradycardia and hypotension) has been shown to reduce hyperalgesia in healthy volunteers who had remifentanil infusion. The beta adrenergic receptor has been linked to OIH in genetic studies, so it may be a useful agent but further research is needed [3]. Opioid sparing or opioid rotation (changing the opioid used, especially to longer acting opioids) are techniques used to combat OIH [4, 12, 22]. Low dose opioid antagonists can also help with this issue. Lastly, usage of multimodal analgesia helps to avoid or treat OIH [19, 20]. This entails the use of different analgesic medications with separate mechanisms of action in order to achieve a synergistic effect. This includes regional anesthesia and rescue blocks [19, 20], Acetaminophen (CNS COX activity inhibition with side effects of liver toxicity at high doses), NSAIDs [19, 20] (COX inhibitors with side effects of gastrointestinal bleeding and renal dysfunction), gabapentinoids [19] (such as gabapentin up to 600 mg TID or pregabalin up to 150 mg TID if tolerated, reduces calcium currents, and has a side effect of sedation), topical lidocaine, and patches [19] (sodium channel blocker, side effect of local anesthetic systemic toxicity if toxic levels reached which is unlikely with topicals and patches), along with other agents listed above. Unfortunately clinical guidelines for this condition are lacking, and there is no unanimous way of diagnosis or treatment. Progress needs to be made in these fronts.

Treatment of OIH

- Lower or discontinue the current opioid
- Opioid rotation (methadone, buprenorphine)
- Add acetaminophen and/or NSAIDs
- NMDA receptor antagonist
- Adjuvant therapies such as antidepressants, antiepileptics
- Regional/local anesthesia

What Is the Prognosis of This Condition?

While OIH can be "cured," it does have the tendency to resurface in patients who have experienced it in the past. It is thought that at least one opioid-free period is needed to reverse OIH, although there is no agreed-upon timeframe, and each patient is unique in this regard [1, 9, 23, 24]. The higher the chronic opioid dose the patient is on, the less successful their outcomes will be and the more expensive their medical care will be [25]. On admission to a comprehensive pain rehabilitation program, patients taking low or high dose opioids reported significantly higher instances of pain and depression when compared to their counterparts who underwent opioid withdrawal and stayed off opioids [26]. In studies, animals who have recovered from OIH went on to express recurrent hyperalgesia if given a single dose of either opioid agonist or antagonist [12]. This shows that animals that have recovered from OIH still remain sensitive to the hyperalgesic opioid effect. It also shows that the sensitization was likely being countered by an opposing endogenous opioid system since even administration of an opioid antagonist caused OIH to resurface. OIH resolves due to upregulated inhibitory pathways that oppose the sensitized excitatory pathways that cause OIH [7]. Due to this, termination of OIH occurs when a new balance of excitatory and inhibitory neuronal activity is reached – levels of activity that are much higher than the state before OIH occurred [7]. This new equilibrium of high neuronal activity is at risk for derangements which can indicate higher pain susceptibility [7]. In summary, OIH can be reversed, but it is thought that once a patient undergoes OIH, they will be at increased risk for redeveloping it especially if they are exposed to opioid agonists or antagonists in the future.

Discussion

Prevalence

There has not been a reported prevalence of OIH. In one longitudinal study of 197 chronic pain patients on chronic opioid therapy, 27.6% of them needed increasing doses of opioids that were not related to disease progression or increase in activity [27]. Most authors believe it is not a rare observance and that it is likely under diagnosed. In either case, OIH is an issue that has lasting and devastating consequences unless it is recognized and dealt with.

Differential Diagnosis

1. Opioid-induced tolerance
2. Opioid withdrawal
3. Allodynia

Opioid-induced hyperalgesia and opioid tolerance are at the top of the differential for this case. These two entities are often confused in clinical practice [28]. If a patient has OIH, the look for the following clinical features during ongoing opioid administration: increased pain intensity over time, diffuse pain or new pain in new locations, and increased pain sensation to mechanical pressure, heat, and tactile stimuli [1, 28]. Increased opioid doses will worsen OIH [1]. Furthermore to diagnose OIH, other entities such as disease progression, opioid tolerance, or opioid withdrawal must be ruled out [1]. These other entities will have improved pain with an increase of opioid while the opposite is true of OIH [1]. Tolerance will have a reappearance of pain of the same intensity as prior to treatment [1]. Opioid withdrawal will have accompanying symptoms such as lacrimation, rhinorrhea, dilated pupils, hydrosis, diarrhea, dysphoric mood, insomnia, and yawning [1].

OIH is largely a clinical diagnosis and is reliant on history and physical exam. A patient who states that his or her pain is worsening despite an increase in the opioid dose, the pain has become diffuse or spread to new areas, and/or is becoming increasingly sensitive to mildy painful stimuli, is very likley has developed opioid induced hyperalgesia. On exam they will appear in distress and will have pain out of proportion to any stimuli or even pain with non-painful stimuli. At this time, there are no lab tests or imaging studies that can diagnose OIH, but studies are ongoing in finding new receptor systems, genes, and biomarkers that are associated with OIH. If an appropriate biomarker is found and validated, it could revolutionize and simplify the diagnosis of OIH leading to improved outcomes.

Unfortunately, there is no one agreed-upon treatment for OIH. Most experts will agree that reducing or completely discounting opioid therapy is necessary [12, 22]. Multimodal techniques have also been shown to be helpful [19]. There are several drugs that have been proposed to help with this situation. Ketamine is perhaps the most widely accepted and has the strongest evidence [7, 12, 19]. Other treatment modalities are not widely accepted or are still in experimental stages. Furthermore, the fact that no guidelines on the treatment of OIH exists further complicates the situation. Until research on the subject progresses, treatment will be largely practitioner dependent.

Future Directions and Clinical Trials

Research has shown that targeting NMDA receptors and using multimodal analgesia does not always fix the problem of OIH [12]. Due to this, further research needs to be done to study other receptor systems to find a better response to OIH. The link seen with microglia in OIH might mean glial inhibitors may help fight OIH but more work in this area is needed [29]. The glial inhibitor ibudilast is being currently studied and has shown reduction of neuropathic pain in the animal model and a threefold increase in morphine analgesic potency [1]. It is still in the preclinical stages but has completed safety testing in humans [1]. Neurosteroids (e.g., progesterone, pregnanolone) are steroids that are made in the brain and have inhibitory effects through GABA receptors, glycine receptors, and calcium channels [1]. These neurosteroids have been shown to reduce pain sensation in rat models and promote analgesia [1]. These steroids are another possible treatment for OIH because of their effects; however, they tend to have low bioavailability and rapid metabolism which can make clinical use difficult [1]. Cannabinoid targets have not been evaluated in treating OIH, but this should be done in the future as these receptors are located in areas that are involved in pain processing (periaquaductal gray, rostroventral medulla [3, 16], microglia, and the dorsal spinal cord) [1]. Logistically speaking it would make sense for these receptors to have a potential role in OIH, and further work is needed to determine if this is true. Another recent study in mice has suggested that 5-HT3 antagonists such as ondansetron either systemically or intrathecally can prevent and reverse OIH [14]. Chronic morphine use induces gene expression in the dorsal root ganglion including CGRP, NMDA receptor, and the B adrenergic receptor all of which are involved in OIH and tolerance [9]. This study showed ondansetron prevents this morphine-enhanced gene expression and therefore giving it a possible role in the treatment of OIH [11, 14]. This still needs to be tested in clinical models of OIH, but ondansetron is a safe medication (major side effect of

QTc prolongation) and is already widely used making it a potential future agent against OIH. N-acetyl-cysteine has been shown to decrease remifentanil-induced hyperalgesia by suppressing matrix metalloproteinase 9 in the dorsal root ganglia in rodents [29]. This is yet another potential future target. Most of the few controlled experiments on OIH that exist are done in patients who have surgical procedures and are given remifentanil infusions followed by opioids after the procedure and then are found to have a state of hyperalgesia [30]. While these studies are useful, future studies must focus on OIH in patients on long-acting opioid therapy for chronic pain as this use of opioids has surpassed the original intent of treating acute surgical pain in today's world. OIH must be better recognized as a clinical issue by practitioners, and improved information is needed regarding prevalence, differences in acute versus chronic opioid exposure, effect of type of opioid used [9], and clear guidelines on diagnosis and treatment. In addition, further research needs to be done on new potential treatments in the human model so they can be implemented into practice.

Conclusion

Opioid-induced hyperalgesia is real but difficult to diagnose entity. This is because objective methods to diagnose it are difficult and usually rely on subjective measurements such as postoperative opioid use and patient supplied pain scores. Guidelines and diagnostic criteria of OIH need to be developed so this becomes less of an issue. Only when the condition is realized can it be appropriately treated; otherwise, the reflex treatment of giving more opioids will only exacerbate it. The amount or duration of opioid intake that is enough to cause OIH still needs to be elucidated along with information on whether certain types of opioids are more likely to cause it. This will certainly prove difficult as many factors play into this, and it is probably unique to each patient. Until this information is determined, it would be prudent to limit opioid dosages and duration of therapy to the minimum amount needed [31]. While there are several proposed treatments of OIH, there is no consensus on what is best or what has the strongest evidence. There are many ways to go about treating it, but as of now it should likely involve some combination of reducing or stopping opioid therapy, initialing multimodal analgesia [19], and using drugs such as the NMDA receptor antagonist ketamine [7, 19]. Several involved receptor systems and drugs that interact with them have been proposed to fight OIH; however, most of them are in early experimental stages and have not been tested in the human model. A tremendous amount remains to be known about OIH, and the more research is accomplished and we discover about it, the better we will be able to avoid, recognize, and treat it.

References

1. Arout CA, Edens E, Petrakis IL, Sofuoglu M. Targeting opioid-induced hyperalgesia in clinical treatment: neurobiological considerations. CNS Drugs. 2015;29(6):465–86.
2. Tompkins DA, Campbell CM. Opioid-induced hyperalgesia: clinically relevant or extraneous research phenomenon? Current Pain Headache Rep. 2011;15(2):129–36.
3. Raffa RB, Pergolizzi JV. Opioid-induced hyperalgesia: is it clinically relevant for the treatment of pain patients? Pain Manage Nursing. 2013;14(3):e67.
4. Mao J. Opioid-induced abnormal pain sensitivity. Curr Pain Headache Rep. 2006;10(1):67–70.
5. Matthias MS, Johnson NL, Shields CG, Bair MJ, Mackie P, Huffman M, et al. "Im not gonna pull the rug out from under you": patient-provider communication about opioid tapering. J Pain. 2017;18(11):1365–73.
6. Krumova EK, Bennemann P, Kindler D, Schwarzer A, Zenz M, Maier C. Low pain intensity after opioid withdrawal as a first step of a comprehensive pain rehabilitation program predicts long-term nonuse of opioids in chronic noncancer pain. Clin J Pain. 2013;29(9):760–9.
7. Angst M, Clark J. Opioid-induced hyperalgesia: a qualitative systematic review. Acute Pain. 2006;8(4):191.
8. Vera-Portocarrero LP, Zhang E-T, King T, Ossipov MH, Vanderah TW, Lai J, et al. Spinal NK-1 receptor expressing neurons mediate opioid-induced hyperalgesia and antinociceptive toler-

ance via activation of descending pathways. Pain. 2007;129(1):35–45.
9. Pud D, Cohen D, Lawental E, Eisenberg E. Opioids and abnormal pain perception: new evidence from a study of chronic opioid addicts and healthy subjects. Drug Alcohol Depend. 2006;82(3):218–23.
10. Gong K, Bhargava A, Jasmin L. GluN2B N-methyl-D-aspartate receptor and excitatory amino acid transporter 3 are upregulated in primary sensory neurons after 7 days of morphine administration in rats. Pain. 2016;157(1):147–58.
11. Liang D-Y, Li X, Clark JD. 5-Hydroxytryptamine type 3 receptor modulates opioid-induced hyperalgesia and tolerance in mice. Anesthesiology. 2011;114(5):1180–9.
12. Leal PDC, Clivatti J, Garcia JBS, Sakata RK. Opioid-induced hyperalgesia (OIH). Brazilian J Anesthesiol. 2010;60(6):639–47.
13. King T, Gardell LR, Wang R, Vardanyan A, Ossipov MH, Malan PT, et al. Role of NK-1 neurotransmission in opioid-induced hyperalgesia. Pain. 2005;116(3):276–88.
14. Roeckel L-A, Coz G-ML, Gavériaux-Ruff C, Simonin F. Opioid-induced hyperalgesia: cellular and molecular mechanisms. Neuroscience. 2016;338:160–82.
15. Vardanyan A, Wang R, Vanderah TW, Ossipov MH, Lai J, Porreca F, et al. TRPV1 receptor in expression of opioid-induced hyperalgesia. J Pain. 2009;10(3):243–52.
16. Vanderah TW, Suenaga NMH, Ossipov MH, Malan TP, Lai J, Porreca F. Tonic descending facilitation from the rostral ventromedial medulla mediates opioid-induced abnormal pain and antinociceptive tolerance. J Neurosci. 2001;21(1):279–86.
17. Mao J, Sung B, Ji R-R, Lim G. Chronic morphine induces downregulation of spinal glutamate transporters: implications in morphine tolerance and abnormal pain sensitivity. J Neurosci. 2002;22(18):8312–23.
18. Ramasubbu C, Gupta A. Pharmacological treatment of opioid-induced hyperalgesia: a review of the evidence. J Pain Palliative Care Pharmacother. 2011;25(3):219–30.
19. Chou R, Gordon DB, Leon-Casasola OAD, Rosenberg JM, Bickler S, Brennan T, et al. Management of postoperative pain: a clinical practice guideline from the American Pain Society, the American Society of Regional Anesthesia and Pain Medicine, and the American Society of Anesthesiologists Committee on Regional Anesthesia, Executive Committee, and Administrative Council. J Pain. 2016;17(2):131–57.
20. Hayhurst CJ, Durieux ME. Differential opioid tolerance and opioid-induced hyperalgesia. Anesthesiology. 2016;124(2):483–8.
21. Singler B, Troster A, Manering N, Schuttler J, Koppert W. Modulation of remifentanil-induced postinfusion hyperalgesia by propofol. Anesth Analg. 2007;104(6):1397–403.
22. Savage SR. Long-term opioid therapy: assessment of consequences and risks. J Pain Symptom Manag. 1996;11(5):274–86.
23. Chu L, Clark D, Angst M. Opioid tolerance and hyperalgesia in chronic pain patients after one month of oral morphine therapy: a preliminary prospective study. J Pain. 2006;7(1):43–8.
24. Hay JL, White JM, Bochner F, Somogyi AA, Semple TJ, Rounsefell B. Hyperalgesia in opioid-managed chronic pain and opioid-dependent patients. J Pain. 2009;10(3):316–22.
25. Kidner CL, Mayer TG, Gatchel RJ. Higher opioid doses predict poorer functional outcome in patients with chronic disabling occupational musculoskeletal disorders. J Bone Joint Surg-Am Vol. 2009;91(4):919–27.
26. Townsend CO, Kerkvliet JL, Bruce BK, Rome JD, Hooten MW, Luedtke CA, et al. A longitudinal study of the efficacy of a comprehensive pain rehabilitation program with opioid withdrawal: comparison of treatment outcomes based on opioid use status at admission. Pain. 2008;140(1):177–89.
27. Low Y, Clarke CF, Huh BK. Opioid-induced hyperalgesia: a review of epidemiology, mechanisms and management. Singap Med J. 2012;53(5):357–60.
28. Veevaete L, Lavand'homme P. Opioid-induced hyperalgesia: new insights in to the chronicization of pain. Tech Region Anesth Pain Manage. 2014;18:100–4.
29. Weber L, Yeomans DC, Tzabazis A. Opioid-induced hyperalgesia in clinical anesthesia practice. Curr Opin Anaesthesiol. 2017;30(4):458–65.
30. Fishbain DA, Cole B, Lewis JE, Gao J, Rosomoff RS. Do opioids induce hyperalgesia in humans? An evidence-based structured review. Pain Med. 2009;10(5):829–39.
31. Bannister K, Dickenson AH. Opioid hyperalgesia. Curr Opin Supp Palliative Care. 2010;4(1):1–5.

A 65-Year-Old Man with Poor Cancer Pain Control Despite Intrathecal Pump

43

Tariq Malik

Case Presentation

A 64 year-old man who had refractory cancer pain secondary to squamous cell carcinoma of the lung with metastasis to the thoracic and lumbar spine. He is status post multiple extensive medical and surgical interventions. After failing a variety of conservative treatment modalities to control his back pain, an ITP was discussed and was successfully trialed. A programmable Medtronic SynchroMed II system was implanted with patient therapy management (PTM). Patient is receiving intrathecal morphine 10-mg/cc concentration at a rate of 75 mcg/h or a dose of 1.8 mg/day. He reported significant and continued pain relief with the ITP at the 3 months pump refill visit with no noted neurological or respiratory side effects. He did well for 1 year. One year after implantation, patient presents with significant increase in his pain which is no longer covered by his current ITP morphine dose despite cancer being in remission as seen on his recent positron emission tomography (PET) scan. He claims he gets some benefit from the extra dose using the PTM device, but he has noticed that the extent of pain relief is decreasing and lately, he gets no relief when he gives himself extra dose using the PTM device. His intrathecal dose is increased by 10%, and he is asked to return to the clinic in a week for further pain management.

T. Malik (✉)
Department of Anesthesia and Critical Care
University of Chicago, Chicago, IL, USA
e-mail: TMuslim@dacc.uchicago.edu

What Is Your Provisional Diagnosis?

In this case, the patient seems to be the analgesic benefit from the intrathecal device a year after it was implanted. This issue could be either due to change in the patient status or device (catheter or pump). It's important to find the exact cause to solve the problem. Patient-related factors involve progression of underlying disease, or some other disease process namely psychosocial issues. This requires detailed history and consultation with the oncologist or family members. In the absence of disease progression, the most common cause for worsening pain is from drug tolerance.

How Do You Rule Out Drug Tolerance as Cause of Increased Pain?

After proper evaluation and consultation, if the patient-related factors are excluded, next step is to increase the dose by 10–15%. It's known that after IT pump implantation, patient often need dose adjustment with time especially in the first year. This is attributed to development of tolerance. A lack of response to such dose escalation, especially when even the higher dose of PTM-based extra dose is not helping, should lead to

T. Malik (ed.), *Practical Chronic Pain Management*, https://doi.org/10.1007/978-3-030-46675-6_43

work up to exclude device (pump and catheter) dysfunction.

How Do You Evaluate Device Dysfunction?

It's important to confirm the integrity of the system from the pump to the catheter tip. Structural integrity of the system can be evaluated using imaging (X-ray, CT). The patency of the catheter can be checked using the accessory port of the pump and aspirating CSF; free-flowing CSF confirms a patent catheter. At times radiopaque dye or radioactive dye is used to rule out any leak from the catheter system. Granuloma can develop at the tip of the intrathecal catheter that can present as failure of therapy or as a mass causing nerve root or spinal cord compression. This is diagnosed by maintaining high level of clinical suspicion, and confirming it with MRI with gadolinium imaging or CT with myelogram. The granuloma presenting with compressive symptoms need urgent or emergent decompressive surgery; otherwise, cessation of intrathecal therapy can resolve the granulomatous mass over months.

How Is the Problem Managed?

Failure of intrathecal therapy should always prompt systematic trouble shooting. Device and catheter malfunction is not uncommon. Apart from patient-related factors which are diagnosed clinically, device and catheter malfunction always require some sort of testing or imaging. If the loss of pain relief is from disease progression, then intrathecal dose of medication should be increased or adjuvant medications are added to the pain pump. The micro-leaks from the catheter can be hard to diagnose, necessitating 2–3 days of daily imaging using Tc-99 or In-111 dye. Intermittent kinking of the catheter with intermittent underdoing or overdosing has also been described. In a case scenario where catheter patency or integrity cannot be confirmed, it's advisable to replace the intrathecal catheter (Fig. 43.1).

Discussion

Uncontrolled pain in patients with advanced cancer is one of the most feared symptoms by cancer patients [1–4] and is sometimes feared more than death. It was estimated that 1.7 million cancer cases occur in the United States each year [5] of which 60% will experience pain at some point while more than 20% of cancer patients will die in pain. Cancer pain can be due to the tumor effect itself, metastasis with involvement of other painful structures such as nerves, or different treatment side effects as such chemotherapeutics. Pain can occur due to soft tissue and bone destruction or nerve injury and may involve inflammatory and/or neuropathic mechanisms. The majority of cancer pain is managed by oral opioids; however, when pain is intractable or patient experiences oral opioids side effects such as respiratory depression or constipation, other modalities should be considered. Intrathecal opioid therapy provides more superior pain control as compared to systemic opioids. The advantages come from more direct medication supply to the Mu, Kappa, Delta, sodium and calcium channel, GABA, alpha 2, and NMDA receptors in substantia gelatinosa of the spinal cord dorsal horn. Thus modulating pain transition at different levels of the spinal cord with much lower doses allowing more effective pain control without crossing the blood brain barrier [6]. ITP has been shown to be superior to conventional medical management in cancer pain, with lower medication toxicity effect as measured by the National Cancer Institute Common Toxicity Criteria and improved survival in a large randomized controlled clinical trial [7] with lower medical expenses and healthcare utilization [8]. Other retrospective analysis studies have shown low rate of complications with long-term follow-up [9]; however, randomized controlled clinical trials are scarce.

The majority of patient's whom experience relief via IT therapy will require some dose adjustments during the first 6 months. Once optimal dose for pain control is achieved, ITP dose may require minimal adjustments on follow-up visits. Any sudden increase in pain that does not respond to pump adjustment should be highly

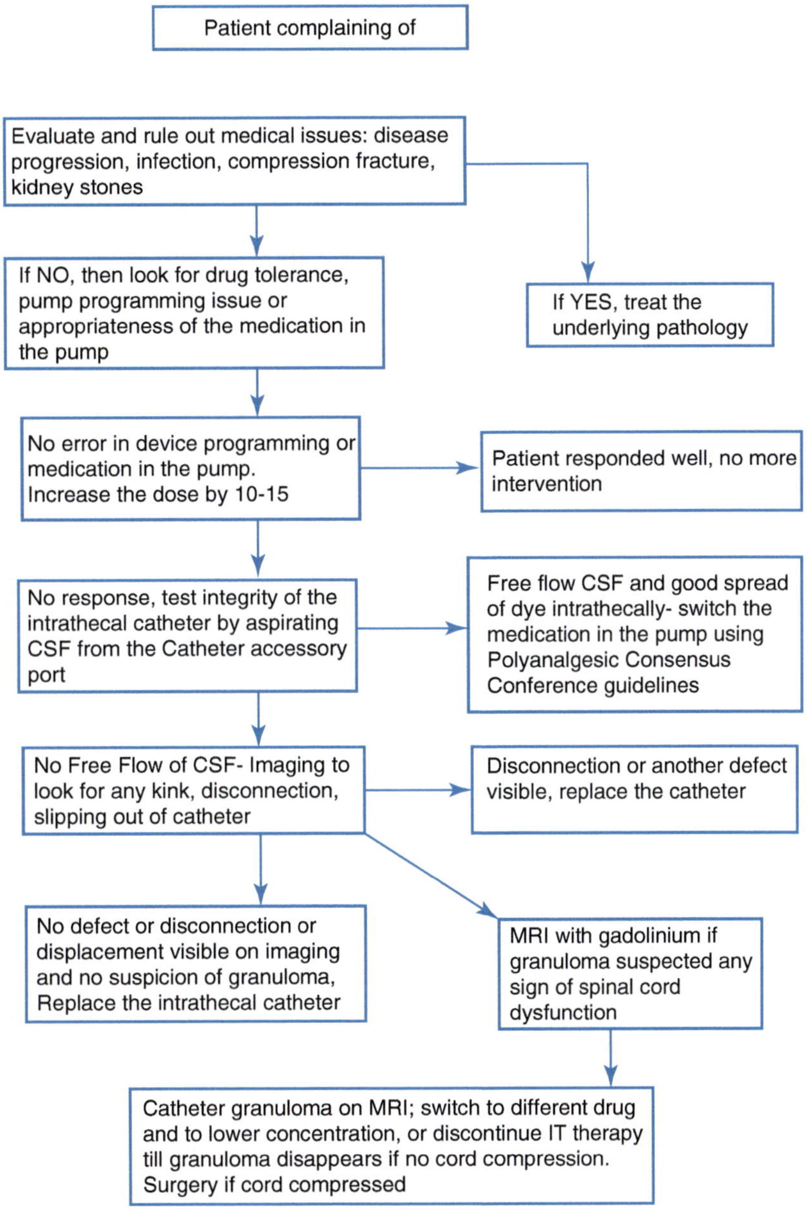

Fig. 43.1 Algorithm for management of failure of intrathecal therapy

suspicious of either pump/catheter failure/malfunction or disease progression. In both instances, imaging studies and immediate investigation are prudent to avoid withdrawal and allow proper management in a timely fashion. Potential reasons for ITP failure can be categorized into (1) device failure reasons which can be further divided into pump failure reasons or catheter failure reasons, (2) procedure-related reasons, and (3) patient-related reasons.

Pump Failure Reasons

Pump motor failure, battery depletion, and catheter access port failure. Other reasons for pump failure include hypermobility, which may lead to pump inversion. Majority of pump-related failure reasons is believed to be related to surgical implantation technique, so careful technique is highly recommended to minimize rate of complications.

Catheter-Related Failure Reasons

Catheter failure rates are three times more common than pump failure rates with a rate of 20% [10]. Catheter-related failure reasons range from dislocation or disconnection which usually occurs either at the pump site or at distal end. CSF leak from the implanted catheter is always due to the hole or holes in the catheter that most likely happens due to inadvertent catheter damage during implantation [11]. Catheter kinks, breakage, and migration have also been reported. Granuloma formation around the catheter tip is a relatively uncommon but serious complication with incidence of 0.5–3% [12]. Risk factors associated with granuloma are high intrathecal opioid concentrations [13], long duration of infusion, rapid dose escalation, spine surgery, and low flow rates of infusion. Diagnosis is made after clinical suspicion by T1-weighted MRI or CT myelogram accessing pump side port assessing catheter patency. Treatment varies according to severity of symptoms and can range from substitution of intrathecal medication with saline to urgent neurosurgical intervention in more severe cases with serious neurological deficits. If granuloma is suspected, early intervention is crucial to prevent serious complications such as spinal cord compression, paraparesis, or paraplegia [14].

Procedure-Related Reasons

Seromas and hygromas can occur; a more serious complication is pump site infection and bacterial meningitis. Surgical technique and hypervigillance are crucial as cancer patients are frequently malnourished and immunocompromised [15].

Patient-Related Reasons

Mostly occur due to medication side effects. Despite lower overall systemic doses required to achieve analgesia, patients with intrathecal opioids may develop side effects similar to systemic opioids such as constipation, nausea, pruritus, urinary retention, and respiratory depression. Such side effects are commonly ruled out during trial period where the need for a different medication or effective dose is investigated and a safe transition from systemic opioids to intrathecal opioids is achieved.

Other side effects that occur due to medications include opioid induced hyperalgesia, hypotension, immunological compromise, and hypogonadotropic hypogonadism [16].

Appropriate patient management can reduce long-term sequela for patients with possible ITP malfunction. Pump interrogation and assessment of end volume to computer-predicated volume of pump during follow-up and pump refill visits may lead to diagnosis prior to patient developing withdrawal symptoms. Diagnostic workup should include careful patient history and examination; pump interrogation, verification of pump contents, settings, and residual volume in the pump. Plain X-ray posterior, anterior, and lateral views can assist in visualization of the catheter. Fluoroscopy to confirm pump rotors are moving at the expected rate. Catheter dye study after side port aspiration can assist in the assessment of catheter patency and function. Immediate MRI or CT myelogram should be performed if patient demonstrates any neurological deficits. A careful evaluation of bowel and bladder function is very important as well as actively looking for the presence of any neurodeficit is important whenever there is any suspicion for the presence of catheter grauloma. Treatment of ITP failure should focus on avoiding patient experiencing withdrawal while workup and testing is complete.

Conclusion

ITP therapy has significantly advanced over the past 35 years and has emerged as an important effective treatment modality in intractable cancer pain. Meticulous surgical technique is key to avoiding complications; however, if complications do arise, early assessment and investigations are prudent to avoiding more critical potentially fatal complications if not properly managed.

References

1. Bao YJ, et al. Hydromorphone for cancer pain. Cochrane Database Syst Rev. 2016;10:CD011108.
2. Onofrio BM, Yaksh TL, Arnold PG. Continuous low-dose intrathecal morphine administration in the treatment of chronic pain of malignant origin. Mayo Clin Proc. 1981;56(8):516–20.
3. Wang JK, Nauss LA, Thomas JE. Pain relief by intrathecally applied morphine in man. Anesthesiology. 1979;50(2):149–51.
4. Neufeld NJ, Elnahal SM, Alvarez RH. Cancer pain: a review of epidemiology, clinical quality and value impact. Future Oncol. 2017;13(9):833–41.
5. Siegel RL, Miller KD, Jemal A. Cancer statistics, 2017. CA Cancer J Clin. 2017;67(1):7–30.
6. Yaksh TL, Rudy TA. Analgesia mediated by a direct spinal action of narcotics. Science. 1976;192(4246):1357–8.
7. Smith TJ, et al. Randomized clinical trial of an implantable drug delivery system compared with comprehensive medical management for refractory cancer pain: impact on pain, drug-related toxicity, and survival. J Clin Oncol. 2002;20(19):4040–9.
8. Stearns LJ, et al. Health services utilization and payments in patients with cancer pain: a comparison of intrathecal drug delivery vs conventional medical management. Neuromodulation. 2016;19(2):196–205.
9. Onofrio BM, Yaksh TL. Long-term pain relief produced by intrathecal morphine infusion in 53 patients. J Neurosurg. 1990;72(2):200–9.
10. Winkelmuller M, Winkelmuller W. Long-term effects of continuous intrathecal opioid treatment in chronic pain of nonmalignant etiology. J Neurosurg. 1996;85(3):458–67.
11. Pucks-Faes E, et al. Eleven years' experience with intrathecal baclofen – complications, risk factors. Brain Behav. 2018;8(5):e00965.
12. Deer TR. A prospective analysis of intrathecal granuloma in chronic pain patients: a review of the literature and report of a surveillance study. Pain Physician. 2004;7(2):225–8.
13. Duarte RV, et al. Intrathecal granuloma formation as result of opioid delivery: systematic literature review of case reports and analysis against a control group. Clin Neurol Neurosurg. 2012;114(6):577–84.
14. Shields DC, et al. Extramedullary intrathecal catheter granuloma adherent to the conus medullaris presenting as cauda equina syndrome. Anesthesiology. 2005;102(5):1059–61.
15. Motta F, Antonello CE. Analysis of complications in 430 consecutive pediatric patients treated with intrathecal baclofen therapy: 14-year experience. J Neurosurg Pediatr. 2014;13(3):301–6.
16. Kleinmann B, Wolter T. Intrathecal opioid therapy for non-malignant chronic pain: a long-term perspective. Neuromodulation. 2017;20(7):719–26.

A 38-Year-Old Woman with Baclofen Withdrawal

44

Lynn R. Kohan and Xiaoying Zhu

Case Description

A 38-year-old woman with history of MS and spasticity with an indwelling Medtronic 40 ml IDDS implanted presents to the pain management center for a baclofen IDDS refill and complaints of mildly increased spasticity for the past month. She was last in the office 5.5 months ago at which time she underwent an IDDS refill. Her IDDS contains a solution of baclofen 500mcg/ml and is programmed to run at 125 mcg/day. Her IDDS was implanted 5 years ago and she has been on a stable dose of intrathecal baclofen (ITB) for the past 3 years. She does not take any other medications. She does have oral baclofen as a precaution provided to all clinic patients with baclofen IDDSs. Interrogation of the IDDS showed no errors, and her expected residual volume was 2 ml greater than her calculated expected residual volume. On physical examination, she was noted to have mildly increased stiffness and spasticity (Modified Ashworth Scale 2). No clonus was noted. Since there were no unusual findings with her IDDS during interrogation and refill and her reported history and physical examination were consistent with gradual increased spasticity, it was determined that she was likely having progression of her MS disease. Her IDDS was increased to 150mcq/day to try to better alleviate her symptoms. She was instructed to call the clinic for another possible IDDS adjustment if she continued to have issues. Three days after her refill, the patient called the emergency pager at 10 pm. She stated that for the past several hours her IDDS had been beeping and she reported feeling irritable and itchy. The patient was told to immediately come into the emergency room and to take 20 mg of her oral baclofen. In the emergency room, she was found to be mildly tachycardic with an oral temperature of 100.8. All other vital signs were stable. She was noted to have a Modified Ashworth Scale of 4. She typically has a Modified Ashworth Scale of 1 at baseline. Complete metabolic panel, complete blood count, sedimentation rate, and c reactive protein were all within normal limits.

Upon interrogation of her IDDS, it was noted that a dual tone critical alarm was occurring. She was treated with intravenous diazepam and additional 20 mg of oral baclofen. She was taken to the Operating Room where a rotor IDDS study was performed. A bolus of 0.01 ml was programmed to be administered over 1 minute. This was administered after first determining that with her concentration of 500 mcq/ml a 0.01 ml bolus would only represent a 5-mcg bolus and thus there was not a risk of overdose. It was noted that the rotor did not move and thus it was determined that there was a rotor pump failure. She then underwent surgery to replace her IDDS. The

L. R. Kohan (✉) · X. Zhu
Department of Anesthesiology, University of Virginia Health System, Charlottesville, VA, USA
e-mail: lrk9g@virginia.edu; xz6b@virginia.edu

T. Malik (ed.), *Practical Chronic Pain Management*, https://doi.org/10.1007/978-3-030-46675-6_44

patient's symptoms improved following the IDDS replacement. The patient was monitored for 24 hours and was subsequently discharged in stable condition.

What Is Your Preliminary Diagnosis?

Preliminary Diagnosis in Clinic

The preliminary diagnosis at her initial presentation was increased spasticity secondary to progression of her multiple sclerosis. At the clinic visit, causes of increased spasticity were assessed. Many issues such as disease progression, acute infection, medication changes, and stress can contribute to worsening spasticity in a patient with multiple sclerosis [1]. The patient did not report any signs or symptoms of acute infection, denied recent medication changes, and denied any symptoms of acute distress. This patient reported increasing spasticity and stiffness over the past month. These symptoms are consistent with possible progression of her underlying MS disease; however, her IDDS was also interrogated to make sure there were no discrepancies. Since interrogation of her IDDS did not reveal any abnormalities, it was determined that she had progression or a flare of her MS.

Preliminary Diagnosis in Hospital

The preliminary diagnosis was increased spasticity secondary to baclofen withdrawal. The patient called reporting symptoms of acute and substantial worsening of her spasticity, itching, and irritability. Upon arrival to the emergency room she was found to be tachycardic and mildly febrile. An audible critical alarm was also audible from her IDDS. These are signs and symptoms of potential baclofen withdrawal from potential IDDS malfunction and thus treatment was promptly initiated.

How Is the Diagnosis Confirmed?

When investigating the cause of decreased or loss of effectiveness with intrathecal baclofen, a systematic approach should be taken. Saulino et al. recently published an article on best practices when troubleshooting baclofen therapy. In addition, Medtronic has published an algorithm for evaluating loss of efficacy with baclofen.

Easily detectable issues should be ruled out first. A thorough history and physical examination as well as an IDDS interrogation should be obtained. The patient's medications should be reviewed as some medications may have the potential to exacerbate or obscure symptoms. Selective serotonin reuptake inhibitors, interferons, dextroamphetamine, and theophylline have been found to increase hypertonicity [2].

Physical examination should be thorough and comprise of a targeted neuromuscular examination including evaluation of strength, range of motion, reflexes, clonus, and spontaneous or elicited spasms. Spasticity can be assessed based on the modified Ashworth Scale (Table 44.1).

Vital signs should be evaluated and a mental status examination performed. Laboratory work up should include an assessment for infection or other noxious stimuli. A complete blood count, comprehensive metabolic panel (including hepatic function), and coagulation status is advised [2]; however, the presence of abnormalities does not "diagnose" withdrawal.

Causes of acute infection or noxious stimuli also need to be investigated. Infections are thought to be involved in the pathogenesis of MS and may impact disease susceptibility and clini-

Table 44.1 Modified Ashworth Scale scores

Grade	Description
0	No increase in muscle tone
1	Slight increase in muscle tone, manifested by a catch and release or by minimal resistance at the end of the range of motion when the affected part(s) is moved in flexion or extension
1+	Slight increase in muscle tone, manifested by a catch, followed by minimal resistance throughout the remainder (less than half) of the ROM (range of movement)
2	More marked increase in muscle tone through most of the ROM, but affect part(s) easily moved
3	Considerable increase in muscle tone passive, movement difficult
4	Affected part(s) rigid in flexion or extension

From Smith and Bohannon [3], with permission

cal course [3]. A study by Correale et al. demonstrated an increased risk of relapse correlating with increased MRI activity during a systemic infection [4].

One should also rule out any programmable or refilling errors. This should be done by first interrogating the IDDS and reviewing the dosing parameters. Make sure that the IDDS's dosing parameters match the prescribed dosing. If there is any suspicion of wrong concentration, the IDDS solution should be withdrawn and the IDDS should be refilled with new solution. The IDDS's extracted reservoir volume needs to be compared to the expected volume. A large or growing discrepancy in residual volume could indicate an IDDS-related malfunction. This type of malfunction may be secondary to a pump rotor malfunction. If there is concern for a rotor failure or malfunction, the rotors in the IDDS should be imaged. As long as a bolus of approximately 10 microliters could not cause an overdose, a 0.01 ml bolus over 1 minute can be administered. Next one should wait 2 minutes to allow bolus to finish and then x-ray or use fluoroscopy to determine the new position of the pumps rotors. The pump's rotors should have moved 60 degrees. If the rotors do not move the expected amount, then a rotor failure may be present [5]. If a rotor issue is detected, the patient will need to have urgent replacement of their IDDS (Fig. 44.1).

Audible alarms will also indicate if there is a problem with the IDDS. Alarms will sound for low battery, low reservoir situations, or critical alarms. If a low reservoir alarm is detected, the patient should present immediately for a refill. If a low battery alarm is present, the patient will need to have urgent replacement of their IDDS [6]. Any critical alarm should be investigated immediately as it indicates that medication flow has ceased or is about to cease.

Once mechanical IDDS abnormalities, programming abnormalities, and solution issues have been ruled out, one should investigate for issues related to the catheter. The first step when investigating for a catheter malfunction is to obtain imaging [7]. Plain anterior/posterior (AP) and lateral radiographs of the thoracic and lumbar regions should be obtained. One should use this imaging to evaluate all the catheter tubing from site of connection to the IDDS, entry into the intrathecal space, to the catheter tip. Any connectors along this path should also be visualized. If all appears normal, a catheter study under fluoroscopic guidance should be performed. A catheter study entails accessing the catheter access port (CAP) with a 24-gauge Huber needle provided in a catheter assess kit. Cerebral spinal fluid (CSF) should be easily aspirated from the catheter access port if the catheter tip is within the intrathecal space. And the catheter is patent. As the catheter volume is usually <0.25 ml, >0.25 ml (typically at least 2 ml) should be aspirated from the catheter access port to ensure adequate aspiration of CSF and drug. If one is able to freely aspirate 2–3 ml, contrast dye should be injected under fluoroscopy. The catheter should be evaluated from its insertion point into the IDDS around the flank, into the spine, to its tip. One should pay special attention to any pooling of contrast behind the IDDS and at any connection sites. Extravasation of any dye outside of the catheter can indicate loss of catheter integrity secondary to a break in the catheter, disconnection, migration outside of the intrathecal space, or loculation [8]. If limited dye is seen in the study, the catheter may be occluded. Occlusion may due to kinking of the catheter along its course or occlusion at the tip. Although rare, a granuloma may occur at the tip of the catheter. MRI imaging with gadolinium is the diagnostic test of choice for granuloma detection [9]. A priming bolus should be performed after completion of the catheter study after a successful aspiration of the CAP in order to refill the catheter to its tip with baclofen in order to prevent withdrawal.

If one is unable to aspirate from the catheter access port, an occluded catheter or kink may be present. Contrast should not be injected if one cannot easily aspirate 2–3 ml from the catheter access port as doing so could result in ITB overdose from infusion of drug remaining in the catheter into the CSF [10]. If there is either loss of integrity noted or failure to be able to aspirate appropriate volume of CSF, the patient should be scheduled for urgent catheter revision to avoid baclofen withdrawal.

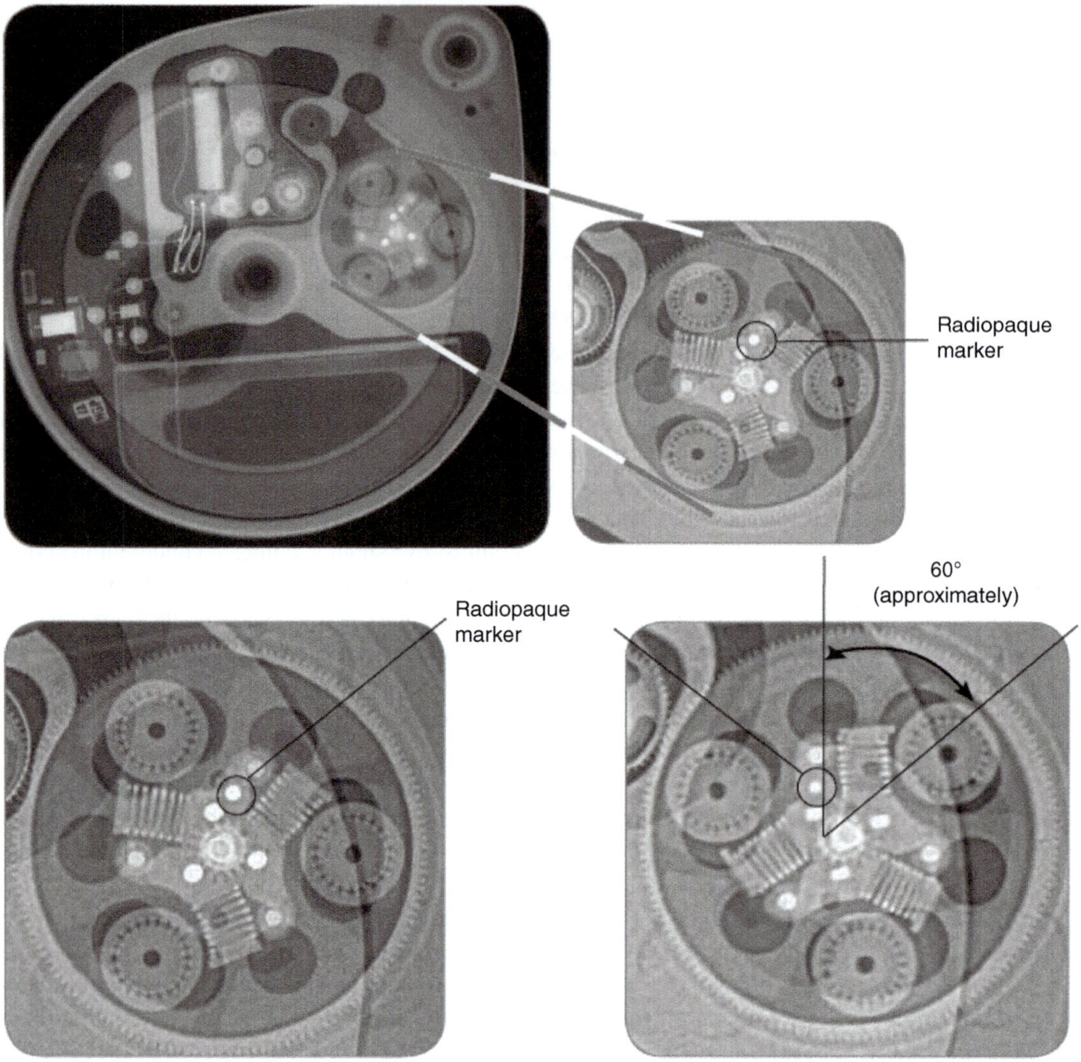

Fig. 44.1 Pump rotor study. (**a**) Pump roller of SynchroMed II pump. (**b**) Pump roller rotation of SynchroMed II pump. (Reprinted with the permission of Medtronic, Inc. (C))

What Is the Pathophysiology of This Condition?

The exact mechanism of action of baclofen as a muscle relaxant and anti-spastic agent is not fully elucidated. Baclofen inhibits both mono- and polysynaptic reflexes at the spinal cord level possibly by its actions at supraspinal sites as well as by decreasing excitatory neurotransmitter release from primary afferent terminals [11]. Baclofen also enhances vagal tone and causes inhibition of mesolimbic and nigrostriatal dopamine neurons [12]. Baclofen is a structural analog of gamma-aminobutyric acid (GABA) and may exert its effects by stimulating $GABA_B$ receptors to cause muscle relaxation. Overall baclofen decreases increased muscle tone, tendon reflexes, and ankle clonus [13] by causing increased inhibitory tone in the central nervous system and spinal cord [14]. Therefore, sudden withdrawal of baclofen results in predominantly excitatory effects such as CNS hyper-excitability and severe spasticity. Sudden cessation of ITB can result in mild symptoms such as pruritus, anxiety, and tremors or more severe symptoms such as hyperthermia, myoclonus, seizures, rhabdomyolysis, disseminated intravascular coagulation, multisystem organ failure, cardiac arrest, coma, and death [15–17].

How Is This Problem Managed?

Management of Baclofen Withdrawal

Adequate identification of the cause of loss of efficacy of ITB is essential as baclofen withdrawal can be fatal. Common signs of baclofen withdrawal include itching, twitching, and mental status changes [18, 19].

Symptoms can occur within a few hours to 48 hours with various signs and symptoms of different degrees [18, 20]. The severity of the symptoms does not always correlate with dosing levels. The clinical presentation of baclofen withdrawal can mimic sepsis, meningitis, neuroepileptic malignant syndrome, and malignant hyperthermia [18, 20, 21]. Symptoms of ITB withdrawal may include increased spasticity, stiffness, hypotension or labile blood pressure, hyperthermia, myoclonus, and mental status changes. Symptoms may progress and ultimately present as rhabdomyolysis, multiple system organ failure, coagulopathy, seizures, coma, and death [22]. Patients presenting with symptoms of withdrawal should be placed in a monitored setting since withdrawal symptoms can lead to serious morbidity. If acute signs and symptoms of baclofen withdrawal are noted, the acute withdrawal algorithm should be followed (Fig. 44.2).

Baclofen withdrawal is definitively treated with resumption of baclofen therapy. First-line treatment in severe withdrawal is to perform a lumbar puncture and administer a bolus of intrathecal baclofen. A consensus panel agreed to use the dose and how often to administer depending on many factors including the severity of withdrawal, the patients dosing prior to cessation, the time since symptoms first occurred, and the response to previous boluses [2]. It is reasonable to administer a similar or higher bolus than was given during the initial trial. If the implanted IDDS is not working, a continuous intrathecal catheter can be used with baclofen delivered through an external pump. This system would allow the patient to remain stable until a new intrathecal IDDS could be implanted. In this scenario the malfunctioning intrathecal IDDS should be set to minimum rate and the external pump could be set to run continuously or deliver boluses at the physician's discretion [18, 20]. In these cases, the patient should be monitored.

If resumption of intrathecal delivery cannot be achieved, then oral medications should be used. Oral baclofen and oral benzodiazepines can be used; however, it should be noted that oral baclofen will not stop the progression on ITB withdrawal [21]. Oral baclofen has variable absorption, a slow onset and short duration of action, and variable renal elimination thus limiting its ability as a good treatment for baclofen withdrawal [23]. In addition, there is no uniform conversion from oral to intrathecal baclofen; thus, it is hard to know a proper dose. A reasonable regimen would be to start at 10–20 mg every 6 hours but realize that a large degree of variability will exist in terms of effectiveness and tolerability [2].

Other medications that can be used are benzodiazepines and cryoheptadine. Benzodiazepines are advantageous since they have intravenous formulations and can be delivered via continuous infusions. They also activate GABA-A receptors, which circumvent the issue of resistance to oral baclofen because of the downregulation of GABA-B receptors that occurs with long-standing baclofen use [2]. For these reasons, benzodiazepines can lessen withdrawal symptoms thus improving spasticity, rigidity, and hyperthermia. Diazepam is the most commonly used followed by lorazepam and midazolam [2]. Benzodiazepines are also helpful in preventing seizures. Patients receiving benzodiazepine treatment should be monitored.

Cyproheptadine is a serotonin agonist that can be used as an adjunctive treatment in baclofen withdrawal as an off-label use. Typical dosing is 2–4 mg every 6 hours but may be increased in dose of frequency depending on the patient response. Administering cyproheptadine has been shown to decrease spastic hypertonia,

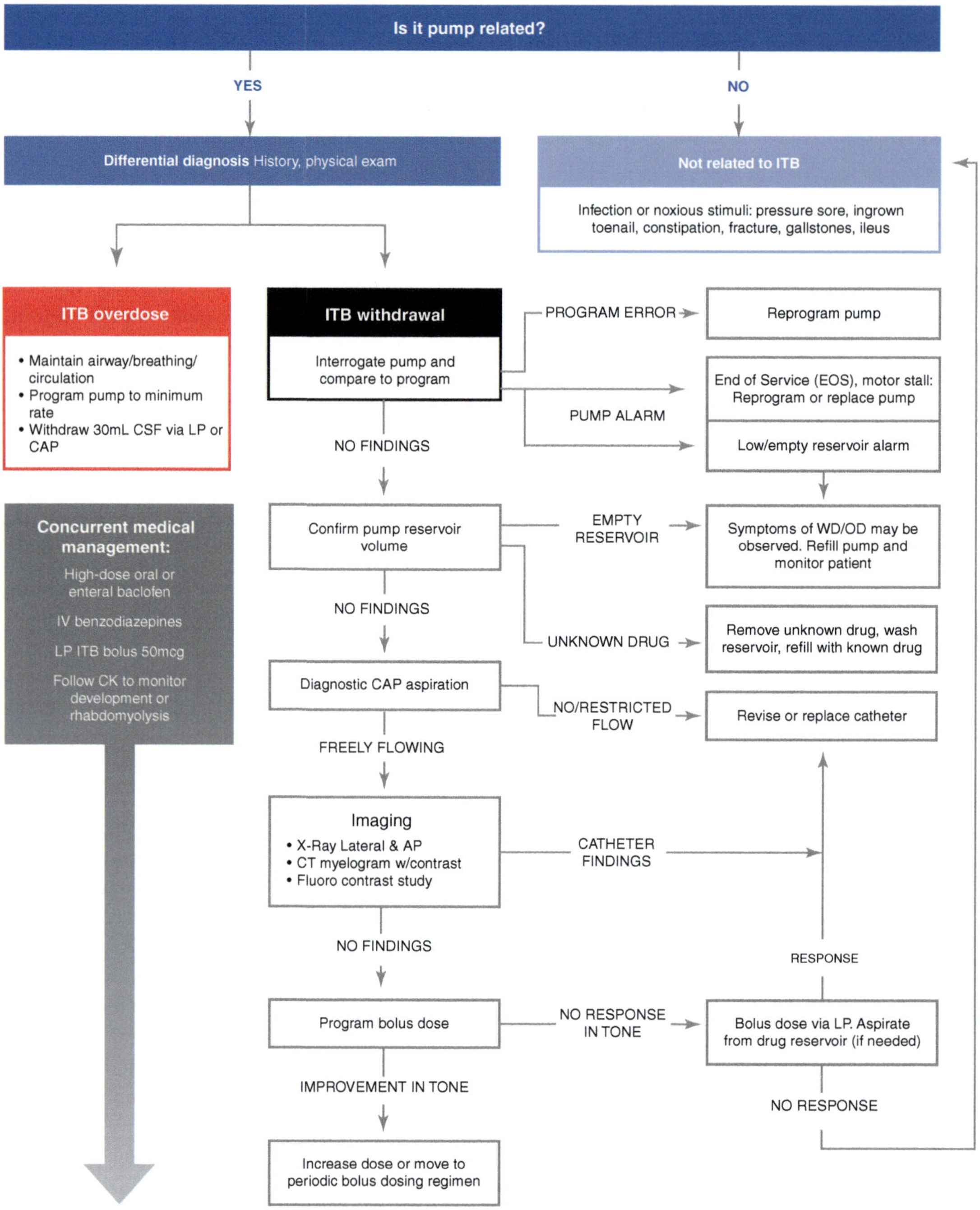

Fig. 44.2 Acute troubleshooting algorithm. (Reprinted with the permission of Medtronic, Inc. (C))

fever, and pruritus [24, 25]. There are no formal studies evaluating the effectiveness of one medication over the other; however, the panel in Saulino's study recommended benzodiazepines and cyproheptadine as first-line adjunctive medications in the treatment of ITB withdrawal [2]. The patient should undergo IDDS revision as soon as possible in order to resume intrathecal therapy. It is advised that the patient then be monitored in an in-patient setting for at least 24 hours to ensure there are no problems with over- or under-dosing [2].

What Is the Prognosis of This Condition?

Baclofen withdrawal must be recognized early as it can progress and eventually become fatal. If treated appropriately with resumption of therapy, patients will have a good prognosis. If baclofen withdrawal fails to be recognized or if appropriate treatment is not initiated, prognosis may be poor.

Discussion

Prevalence

MS affects approximately 400,000 people in the United States and has an estimated prevalence of 90 per 100,000 population [26]. Primary progressive MS is diagnosed in about 10% of patients at onset [27]. MS is caused by CNS inflammation that damages the myelin sheath as well as axons themselves. MS can cause various neurological symptoms because it can affect the brain, optic nerve, and spinal cord. Sensory and motor changes often occur resulting in leg weakness, ataxia, or spasticity.

Spasticity is a frequent symptom of MS that can affect quality of life as disease progresses. Treatment includes oral medications, but these can have limited efficacy and are often associated with significant side effects such as drowsiness [28]. ITB was approved by the US Food and Drug Administration (FDA) for treatment of severe spasticity in 1992. In select patients, ITB can ameliorate symptoms of spasticity, improve functionality, and decrease side effects associated with oral medications [29, 30]. ITB is administered through an implanted IDDS with a reservoir with an attached catheter that delivers medication directly into the intrathecal space. Baclofen decreases spasticity by binding to (GABA-B) receptors and inhibiting the release of excitatory neurotransmitters, thereby inhibiting monosynaptic and polysynaptic spinal reflexes [31]. The doses needed for effective treatment of spasticity are much lower than oral doses, thus decreasing systemic side effects.

While complications are rare, providers should be prepared to recognize them and treat them promptly. Complications can result in baclofen overdose, under-dose, or insufficient intrathecal delivery. A thorough investigation needs to be taken when a patient reports symptoms related to baclofen overdose or under-dose. In April 2002, the FDA issued a drug warning label for baclofen withdrawal syndrome. There have been 27 cases reported to the FDA of which 6 have been fatal [32].

Differential Diagnosis

Differential Diagnosis of Increased Spasticity

The differential diagnosis of increased spasticity in a patient with a baclofen IDDS include patient-related causes as well as loss of baclofen efficacy secondary to IDDS-related issues.

Patient-Related Issues

Certain conditions such as infections or increased physiological stressors can contribute to increased spasticity in patients with MS. Urinary infections, bladder distension, and urolithiasis can all increase spasticity [1]. Increased body temperatures can also contribute to increased spasticity. Increased spasticity may also be secondary to disease progression or a flare in their underlying disease. Disease progression or a flare can be investigated by MRI imaging to evaluate for increased lesions within the central nervous system. Tolerance to baclofen has also been reported [33] and can be included in the differential diagnosis but only after all other causes have been ruled out.

IDDS-Related Issues

Loss of baclofen effectiveness as previously described can be secondary to programming errors (wrong concentration or wrong dose of medication being delivered) or mechanical problems with the IDDS or catheter. Programmable errors are typically easily identified by reviewing the IDDS settings and doses carefully. Specialized pharmacies can also compound different concentrations of baclofen. There can be variations in accuracy when baclofen is compounded resulting in under-dosing.

The catheter and pump are subject to complications throughout the life of the system [34]. A study by Fluckiger et al. identified the annual rate of complications requiring surgical intervention was 10.5%. Thirty-five percent of the complications were pump related, while the remainder were catheter related [35]. IDDS-related complications can include motor stall and battery exhaustion. In June 2013, Medtronic issued a class I recall for Medtronic Synchromed II and Synchromed EL Implantable Drug Infusion Pumps [36]. The recall stated that there was potential that an electrical shorting within the IDDS could cause a motor stall thus contributing to loss of or reduction in therapy. Medtronic, Inc. was able to revise their device with FDA approval to fix this issue.

Combinations of medications can also contribute to IDDS malfunction. Medtronic published information stating that corrosive agents originating from drug formulations may be contributing factors [37]. Spontaneous IDDS stalls are rare due to the high integrity and reliability of the system. The most common time for an IDDS to stall is after an MRI and thus all IDDSs should be interrogated in some form approximately 20 minutes after an MRI to assure motor function has resumed. This assessment can be performed by interrogating the IDDS logs [38]. If the IDDS has not resumed, a second interrogation should be performed in 20 minutes to assess for any delayed resumption of function. If the IDDS still has not resumed function, the IDDS manufacturer should be called and appropriate care taken to prevent withdrawal.

Other potential causes of loss of efficacy of ITB therapy can include granuloma formation at the tip of the catheter resulting in inadequate delivery of ITB or is severe spinal cord compression [39]. Granulomas are inflammatory masses that develop at the tip of the catheter. While granulomas are more often associated with opioid intrathecal medications, there have been cases reported in the literature of granulomas occurring in patients receiving intrathecal baclofen [40]. MRI is the preferred imaging modality to diagnose a catheter tip granuloma [41].

Differential Diagnosis of Baclofen Withdrawal

Other medical conditions can also mimic baclofen withdrawal including sepsis, meningitis, neuroleptic malignant syndrome, autonomic dysreflexia, serotonin syndrome, and malignant hyperthermia [18, 20] as they may present with similar mental status changes, hypo- or hyperthermia, changes in respiratory rate and blood pressure, as well as muscle rigidity. Typically, the mental status changes that occur with intrathecal baclofen withdrawal include anxiety, agitation, and/or hallucinations [2]. Pruritus without a rash is highly associated with intrathecal baclofen withdrawal [18, 20].

Predictive Value of Different Clinical Features

There are no specific predictive values regarding the clinical features of baclofen withdrawal syndrome; however, it is thought to advance on a spectrum. Mild baclofen withdrawal is often associated with increase in tone, pruritus without a rash, and irritability. As the syndrome progresses, patients may experience return of their underlying baseline tone, altered mental status, mild dysphoria, increased creatine phosphokinase levels, decreased blood pressure, paresthesias, and become febrile. Severe baclofen withdrawal is often associated with substantial increase in tone, coma, signs of rhabdomyolysis, and seizures [2].

Strength of Evidence

Evidence for best course for identification and treatment of loss of efficacy of baclofen and baclofen withdrawal is based currently on expert consensus panels.

Future Directions

Current treatment of intrathecal baclofen withdrawal remains inadequate. Definitive treatment remains resumption of intrathecal baclofen. Current research is investigating the creation of an IV formulation of baclofen. A recent study by Schmitz et al. showed that an IV formulation of baclofen was well tolerated clinically. The drug showed a bioavailability of 80% which suggests that a dose reduction of 20% in IV dose would be advised compared to oral [42]. Therefore, IV baclofen might prove beneficial in preventing baclofen withdrawal at least in cases where there has been cessation of oral baclofen. It is unclear how effective it will be in cases of intrathecal baclofen withdrawal. More studies are needed to develop better easier treatments.

Summary/Conclusions

In summary, treatment of spasticity with ITB can be very effective and safe. Patients with ITB therapy may present with increased spasticity. The increased spasticity may be secondary to many different causes including patient-related issues as well as issues secondary to malfunctions of the catheter or pump itself. A systematic approach should be utilized when identifying the causes of increased spasticity and should be treated appropriately. One should carefully assess for any signs or symptoms of baclofen withdrawal since it can lead to significant morbidity and mortality and thus must be promptly recognized.

References

1. Vaidyanathan S, Soni BM, Oo T, et al. Delayed complications of discontinuation of intrathecal baclofen therapy: resurgence of dyssynergic voiding, which triggered off autonomic dysreflexia and hydronephrosis. Spinal Cord. 2004;42(10):598–602.
2. Saulino M, et al. Best practices for intrathecal baclofen therapy: trouble shooting. Neuromodulation. 2016;19:632–41.
3. Smith MB, Bohannon RW. Interrater reliability of a modified Ashworth scale of muscle spasticity. Am Phys Ther Assoc. 1987;67(2):206–7.
4. Ascherio A, Munger KL. Environmental risk factors for multiple sclerosis. Part I: the role of infection. Ann Neurol. 2007;61(4):288–99.
5. Correale J, Fiol M, Gilmore W. The risk of relapses in multiple sclerosis during systemic infections. Neurology. 2006;67:652–9.
6. SynchroMed IsoMed indications, drug stability, and emergency procedures. Minneapolis: Medtronic; 2017.
7. Sgouros S, Charalambides C, Matsota P, et al. Malfunction of Synchromed II baclofen pump delivers a near-lethal baclofen overdose. Pediatr Neurosurg. 2010;46(1):62–5.
8. Dvorak EM, McGuire JR, Nelson ME. Incidence and identification of intrathecal baclofen catheter malfunction. PMR. 2010;2(8):751–6.
9. Turner MS. Assessing syndromes of catheter malufunction with SynchroMed infusion systems: the value of spiral computed tomography with contrast injection. PMR. 2010;2(8):757–66.
10. Deer T, Raso L, Coffey J, Allen J. Intrathecal baclofen and catheter tip inflammatory mass lesions (granulomas): a reevaluation of case reports and imaging findings in light of experimental, clinicopathological, and radiological evidence. Pain Med. 2008;9(4):391–5.
11. Lew SM, Psaty EL, Abbott R. An unusual cause of overdose after baclofen pump implantation: case report. Neurosurgery. 2005;56:E624. Discussion E624.
12. Allerton CA, Boden PR, Hill RG. Actions of the GABAB agonist, (−)-baclofen, on neurones in deep dorsal horn of the rat spinal cord in vitro. Br J Pharmacol. 1989;96:29–38.
13. Peng CT, Ger J, Yang CC, Tsai WJ, Deng JF, Bullard MJ. Prolonged severe withdrawal symptoms after acute-on-chronic baclofen overdose. J Toxicol Clin Toxicol. 1998;36:359–63.
14. Mohammed I, Hussain A. Intrathecal baclofen withdrawal syndrome-a life-threatening complication of baclofen pump: a case report. BMC Clin Pharmacol. 2004;4:6.
15. Kroin JS, Bianchi GD, Penn RD. Intrathecal baclofen down-regulates GABAB receptors in the rat substantia gelatinosa. J Neurosurg. 1993;79:544–9.
16. Green LB, Nelson VS. Death after acute withdrawal of intrathecal baclofen: case report and literature review. Arch Phys Med Rehabil. 1999;80:1600–4. https://doi.org/10.1016/S0003-9993(99)90337-4.
17. Sampathkumar P, Scanlon PD, Plevak DJ. Baclofen withdrawal presenting as multiorgan system failure. Anesth Analg. 1998;87:562–3.
18. Meinck HM, Tronnier V, Rieke K, Wirtz CR, Flugel D, Schwab S. Intrathecal baclofen treatment for stiff-man syndrome: pump failure may be fatal. Neurology. 1994;44:2209–10.
19. Coffey RJ, Edgar TS, Francisco GE, et al. Abrupt withdrawal from intrathecal baclofen: recognition and management of a potentially life-threatening syndrome. Arch Phys Med Rehabil. 2002;83:735–41.

20. Ben Smail D, Hugeron C, Denys P, Bussel B. Pruritus after intrathecal baclofen withdrawal: a retrospective study. Arch Phys Med Rehabil. 2005;86:494–7.
21. Ross JC, Cook AM, Stewart GL, Fahy BG. Acute intrathecal baclofen withdrawal: a brief review of treatment options. Neurocrit Care. 2011;14:103–8.
22. Medtronic. Lioresal Intrathecal (baclofen injection) Full Prescribing Information. http://professional.medtronic.com/pt/neuro/itb/fpi/index.htm. 2013.
23. Berweck S, Lutjen S, Voss W, et al. Use of intrathecal baclofen in children and adolescents: interdisciplinary consensus table 2013. Neuropediatrics. 2014;45:294–308.
24. Agarwal SK, Kriel RL, Cloyd JC, et al. A pilot study assessing pharmacokinetics andtolerability of oral and intravenous baclofen in healthy adult volunteers. J Child Neurol. 2015;30:37–41.
25. Saveika JA, Shelton JE. Cyproheptadine for pediatric intrathecal baclofen withdrawal: a case report. Am J Physical Med Rehabil. 2007;86:994–7.
26. Meythaler JM, Roper JF, Brunner RC. Cyproheptadine for intrathecal baclofen withdrawal. Arch Phys Med Rehabil. 2003;84:638–42.
27. Hersh C, Fox R. Multiple sclerosis. The Cleveland clinic foundation center for continuing education June 2014, Lyndhurst, Ohio.
28. The Mutliple Sclerosis Foundation.
29. Haselkorn JK, Loomis S. Multiple sclerosis and spasticity. Phys Med Rehabil Clin N Am. 2005;16:467–81.
30. Dario A, Tomei G. Management of spasticity in multiple sclerosis by intrathecal baclofen. Acta Neurochir Suppl. 2007;97:189–92.
31. Anderson W, Jallo G. Intrathecal baclofen therapy and the treatment of spasticity. Neurosurg Q. 2007;17:185–92.
32. Penn RD. Intrathecal baclofen for severe spasticity. Ann N Y Acad Sci. 1988;531:157–66.
33. http://www.fda.gov/medwatch/safety/2002/baclofen.htm.
34. Heetla HW, Staal ML, Kliphuis C, van Laar T. Tolerance to continuous intrathecal baclofen infusion can be reversed by pulsatile bolus infusion. Spinal Cord. 2010;48(6):483–6.
35. Follet KA, Naumann CP. A prospective study of intrathecal catheter-related complications of intrathecal drug delivery systems. J Pain Symptom Manag. 2000;19(3):209–15.
36. Flückiger B, Knecht H, Grossmann S, Felleiter P. Device-related complications of long-term intrathecal drug therapy via implanted pumps. Spinal Cord. 2008;46:639–43.
37. FDA. FDA—Medtronic SynchroMed II and SynchroMed EL implantable drug infusion pumps—feed through failure. 2016;1–3.
38. Medtronic Inc. Increased risk of motor stall and loss of or change in therapy with unapproved drug formulations. 2012;1–2.
39. Kosturakis A, Gebhardt R. SynchroMed II intrathecal pump memory errors due to repeated magnetic resonance imaging. Pain Physician. 2012;15:475–7.
40. Arnold P, Viraat H, Oliphant S. Spinal cord compression secondary to intrathecal-induced granuloma: a report of four cases. Evid Based Spine Care J. 2011;2(1):57–62.
41. Deer T, Krames ES, Hassenbusch S, et al. Management of intrathecal catheter-tip inflammatory masses: an updated 2007 consensus statement from an expert panel. Neuromodulation. 2008;11(2):77–91.
42. Schmitz N, Krach L, Coles L, Mishra U, Agarwal S, Cloyd J, Kriel R. A randomized dose escalation study of intravenous baclofen in healthy volunteers: clinical tolerance and pharmacokinetics. Am Acad Phys Med Rehabilitat. 2017;9:743–50.

Chemotherapy-Induced Peripheral Neuropathy

45

Dan Fischer and Tariq Malik

Case Description

A 62-year-old women presents to the pain clinic with long-standing symptoms of numbness, tingling, and occasionally needle-like pain in her feet and hands. She first noticed these symptoms 2 weeks ago, and she has found little to no relief with over-the-counter NSAIDS and acetaminophen. She reports that she has a history of right breast cancer for which she underwent a right mastectomy 6 months ago and initiated subsequent chemotherapy with placitaxel and cisplatin 6 weeks ago. She was warned about the possibility of neuropathy but was told it is unlikely and, even if happens, it is not that bad and would go away. Now she has developed these symptoms and nothing she has taken has worked so far, and she has been sent by the oncology service for further management. Physical examination shows decreased sensation to touch in vibration in the distal extremities bilaterally, and there is a concurrent diminished Achilles reflexes bilaterally.

D. Fischer
Department of Anesthesiology and Critical Care, University of Chicago, Chicago, IL, USA
e-mail: dfischer2@dacc.uchicago.edu

T. Malik (✉)
Department of Anesthesia and Critical Care, University of Chicago, Chicago, IL, USA
e-mail: TMuslim@dacc.uchicago.edu; tmalik@dacc.uchicago.edu

What Is Your Preliminary Diagnosis?

The patient is reporting numbness and tingling that started few months after she was started on chemotherapeutic agents. Her symptoms are distributed in a glove and stocking fashion and are affecting the distal parts of the limbs much more prominently. These are telltale sign of chemo-induced nerve damage. But since she has history of cancer which can metastasize especially to bone and can cause nerve compression, imaging study is warranted especially if the symptoms are progressively getting worse.

How Is Diagnosis Confirmed?

Chemotherapy-induced neuropathy (CIPN) is often a clinical diagnosis largely dependent on history and physical exam; however, other more objective modalities have been explored. It often presents as a sensory neuropathy characterized by tingling, numbness, and pain that typically starts in the toes and fingers before spreading proximally in a "stocking-glove" distribution [1]; however, symptoms can also include hypersensitivity to cold or touch, loss of proprioception, decreased perception of vibration and pinprick, and decrease or loss of deep tendon ankle reflexes [2]. To assess clinical parameters, such as history of chemotherapy treatment and distribution of sensory pathology, several scales have been used to evaluate patients for CIPN. The most common tools used are the Total Neuropathy Score (TNS), the Common Toxicity Criteria of the National Cancer Institute (NCI-CTC), the National Cancer Institute Common

T. Malik (ed.), *Practical Chronic Pain Management*, https://doi.org/10.1007/978-3-030-46675-6_45

Terminology Criteria for Adverse Event (NIC-CTCAE), World Health Organization criteria, Eastern Cooperative Oncology Group criteria, and Ajani criteria for assessing therapy-induced toxicity [3, 4].

Measurement of sensory and motor nerve conduction velocities (NCV), sensory nerve action potentials (SNAP), and compound muscle action potential (CMAP) together with needle electromyography (EMG) are the standard neurophysiological tests used to aid in diagnosis. Axonal loss from sensory nerves is thought to be represented by diminished amplitude of SNAP and sensory NCV, but changes in NCV have weaker correlation of CIPN from drugs affecting dorsal root ganglia (DRG), such as platinum derivatives, and weaker correlation when small sensory fibers are involved [5]. Sural and other whole nerve biopsies have been used in the past but are now seen as rarely indicated when evaluating CIPN, but a joint task force report of the European Federation of Neurological Societies and the Peripheral Nerve Society indicates that the role of skin biopsy is evolving in the evaluation of neuropathies and possibly CIPN [5, 6].

It is important to note, however, that EMG and nerve conduction studies are regarded as having limited utility in clinical diagnosis. One study comparing nerve conduction studies to clinical examination in patients treated with cisplatin showed no diagnostic advantage [3].

Distinguishing CIPN from other potential neuropathies in patients with cancer requires evaluation of the patients' symptom presentation and therapy course. Analysis of the administered drug, whether or not it is associated with CIPN, cumulative dosage, and the characteristics and associated timeline of symptom development are required to aid in the diagnosis of CIPN, which emphasizes the importance of a detailed history in conjunction with physical exam and other diagnostic tools [7].

What Is the Pathophysiology of This Condition?

The pathophysiology of CIPN is not entirely known, but several theories have been derived from animal models and postmortem studies for various chemotherapeutic agents. A unifying theory that the cytotoxic mechanisms of these agents used to trigger cancer cell death also acts on various cells of the nervous system. Sometimes the side effects of these therapies can be so severe that they lead to dose reduction or discontinuation, ultimately inhibiting patients to receive effective therapy.

Platinum derivatives are able to alter the structure of DNA by forming intra-strand adducts and inter-strand crosslinks. Formation of platinum-DNA adducts is the mechanism of action for triggering cancer cell death [8], but this disruption of the tertiary structure of DNA is also a proposed method of neural apoptosis. Other proposed mechanisms triggered by platinum agents include oxidative stress, mitochondrial dysfunction, and increased activity of regulatory genes such as p53, p38, and ERK ½ [4].

Dorsal root ganglia (DRG) have been implicated as susceptible to the deposition of platinum compounds like cisplatin and oxaliplatin, ultimately leading to DRG neuron apoptosis and contributing to the sensory dysfunction consistent with CIPN. Postmortem studies have showed retention of cisplatin in the dorsal root ganglion cells with associated reduction in nuclear size [3]. Dorsal root ganglia lack the protection of a blood-brain barrier, and since they are vascularized by fenestrated capillaries that permit exposure to circulating compounds, DRG are particularly vulnerable to chemotherapeutic agents like platinum derivatives.

Cisplatin is additionally able to disrupt mitochondria DNA synthesis through the formation of adducts [4], and in cultured rat embryo dorsal root ganglion models, cisplatin was found to consistently inhibit axonal growth in a dose-dependent manner at similar concentrations believed to be neurotoxic in humans [3].

Oxaliplatin is unique in that it can induce both acute and chronic neuropathy. The acute neuropathy is believed to be caused by transient activation of voltage-gated sodium channels of peripheral nerves due to chelation of calcium by oxaliplatin. This triggers a hyperexcitability of peripheral nerve membranes, but as the activation is acute and transient, it is also believed to be reversible [3].

Chronic exposure of oxaliplatin can lead to an accumulation in DRG cells to produce gradual morphological and functional changes, but the proposed mechanisms are still hypothetical.

Some experimental studies theorize that the accumulation of oxaliplatin in cell bodies decreases cellular metabolism and axoplasmic transport [3].

Carboplatin has been found to be less neurotoxic than other platinum derivatives, but it is often dose-limited by hematologic toxicity [3].

Vincristine, a common vinca-alkaloid used since the 1960s for its antineoplastic properties, has been known to have both motor and sensory side effects, including peripheral neuropathy and chronic neuropathic pain. Other vinca-alkaloids, such as vinblastine, vinflunine, and vinorelbine, have been found to be less neurotoxic [5]. The mechanism of action of vincristine is primarily due to its high binding affinity to β-tubulin and prevents the formation of microtubules necessary for cellular structure and intracellular transport. Vincristine's ability to disrupt microtubule polymerization leads to the development of inflammation, swelling, and damage in myelinated and unmyelinated neuronal axons. With respect to pain, vincristine has been found in rat models to enhance the responsiveness of C-fiber nociceptors to both nociceptive and non-nociceptive stimuli, thus contributing to a state of chronic neuropathic pain [8].

The taxanes, specifically paclitaxel as it is more neurotoxic than docetaxel and abraxane [5], inhibit tubulin depolymerization and therefore disrupt intracellular structure as well as cell division. This disturbance of the cellular environment ultimately contributes to mitochondrial abnormalities and calcium release within the cell. A study in 2006 observed that rats treated with paclitaxel developed painful peripheral neuropathy-associated swollen and vacuolated mitochondria in the axons of peripheral nerves [8]. Paclitaxel is able to trigger the opening of the mitochondrial permeability transition pore (mPTP), a pore that spans the outer membrane of mitochondria, contains β-tubulin, and contains a voltage-dependent anion channel. Opening of these pores leads to the release of calcium from mitochondria, which can also lead to calcium triggered calcium release from the endoplasmic reticulum. This organelle dysfunction then leads to the disruption of membrane ion potentials and creates reactive oxygen species that cause cellular injury. Paclitaxel has been associated with injury of sensory neurons, alterations in dorsal root ganglion cells, hyperplasia of macrophages in the peripheral nervous system, and increased microglial and astrocyte activation within the spinal cord. It is through this diverse series of downstream targets that paclitaxel is thought to contribute to a state of sensory dysfunction and pain consistent with CIPN [4].

Bortezomib is a generally well-tolerated and effective drug used primarily to treat multiple myeloma and some types of solid tumors, but its use is often limited by the onset of severely painful peripheral neuropathy characterize by paresthesias, burning sensations, numbness, sensory loss, and reduced sensation of vibration and proprioception. Bortezomib's mechanism of action involves the inhibition of protein degradation through binding specifically and reversibly to the 26S proteasome subunit, and in doing so, causes an inhibition of the cell cycle which leads to an increase in apoptosis.

Several studies, however, have revealed a variety of ways bortezomib can disrupt neural cellular function and/or cause cell death. Both in vivo and in vitro studies have showed that bortezomib can induce tubulin polymerization and stabilization, specifically with α-tubulin. The ability of microtubules to remain dynamic is essential for their function in cellular architecture, and it is thought that bortezomib's alteration of tubulin dynamics contributes to the onset of peripheral neuropathy. Furthermore, studies of animals treated with bortezomib have observed intracytoplasmic vacuolation of dorsal root ganglia attributed to mitochondrial and endoplasmic reticulum enlargement that ultimately disrupts intracellular calcium homeostasis and triggers apoptosis in those cells. Schwann cells have also been found to have vacuoles in the cytoplasm as well as perinuclear inclusion bodies after treatment with bortezomib; it is believed that stress to the endoplasmic reticulum caused by bortezomib causes macro-autophagy and results in cell death. Bortezomib is also a potent inducer of excessive reactive oxygen species production which makes it a potent inducer of mitochondrial damage, and a recent study demonstrated that bortezomib was associated with an increase in reactive oxygen species in dorsal root ganglia. Reactive oxygen species are known to play a crucial role in bortezomib-induced apoptosis [8].

How Is This Problem Managed?

In a review article published in *Supportive Care in Cancer*, the most strongly supported pharmacologic intervention for CIPN is Duloxetine, a serotonin-norepinephrine reuptake inhibitor (SNRI), with a "B" level of evidence [1]. A multi-institutional, double-blind crossover trial involving 231 patients with CIPN secondary to treatment with taxanes or oxaliplatin chemotherapy experienced a significantly larger average decrease in mean pain score and greater degree of improvement in functional and quality of life scores after taking Duloxetine with a target dose of 60 mg PO Daily for 5 weeks when compared to placebo [1]. Duloxetine initial dosing is recommended to be 60 mg once daily; however, lower initial doses may be considered in patients when tolerability is a concern. In the Pachman study, participants started with 30 mg daily for 1 week before achieving target dose of 60 mg daily for 4 weeks. Use of duloxetine should be avoided in patients with severe renal impairment (creatinine clearance <30 mL/minute) and end-stage renal disease (ESRD). Duloxetine should also be avoided in hepatic impairment, and its use is contraindicated if patients are also using monoamine oxidase (MAO) inhibitors due to risk of serotonin syndrome. Common side effects (~10% of users) include headache, drowsiness, fatigue, nausea, xerostomia, abdominal pain, muscle weakness, and weight loss [9]. In the 2014 study involving duloxetine therapy for CIPN, the most common side effects were fatigue (7%), insomnia (5%), and nausea (5%) [10].

Other pharmacologic interventions have been studied due to their use in successfully treating neuropathic pain not caused by chemotherapeutic agents, but there is limited evidence to support efficacy of several treatments specifically for CIPN. The discomfort associated with CIPN leads clinicians and patients to attempt therapies that could provide some relief, even in the absence of studies proving efficacy. Tricyclic antidepressants (TCAs) such as nortriptyline and amitriptyline have been studied with mixed results. A randomized control trial (RCT) involving 51 patients with cisplatin-induced neuropathy had patients start taking 25 mg nortriptyline daily with increasing doses 25 mg weekly to a maximum target dose of 100 mg daily in two 4-week phases separated by a 1-week washout period; nortriptyline appeared to have a modest benefit in the second treatment period, but there was no significant difference between groups. No significant differences in paresthesias between groups were observed in the first treatment period. Meanwhile, an RCT of amitriptyline of 44 patients with daily doses between 10 mg and 50 mg failed to improve sensory neuropathic symptoms in patients suffering from CIPN from a variety of chemotherapeutic agents. Both studies lacked statistical power to be able to definitively evaluate TCAs for the treatment of CIPN, and as such, nortriptyline and amitriptyline have garnered a Class C recommendation for CIPN therapy. If utilized, recommended dosing entails starting at 10–25 mg at bedtime and doubling doses every 3–7 days until a target dose of 150 mg daily has been reached. The trial period should be 6–8 weeks with at least 2 weeks at the maximum tolerated dosage. Side effects include sedation, dry mouth, weight gain, blurry vision, urinary retention, memory impairment, confusion, thrombocytopenia, and orthostatism; caution should be used in patients with cardiac disease as doses greater than 100 mg daily have been associated with cardiac death. Other precautions to consider include glaucoma, seizure disorder, serotonin syndrome, and the risk of suicidal behavior associated nortriptyline and amitriptyline [1].

Gabapentoids such as gabapentin and pregabalin are antiepileptics that have been studied and also have been found to have limited supporting evidence in the treatment of CIPN. In a study, 75 patients with CIPN secondary to taxane- and/or platinum-based chemotherapy were treated with 800 mg Gabapentin and compared with 35 controls. Among patients with moderate neuropathic pain, 72% of patients in the gabapentin intervention group reported to have experienced either complete or partial relief when compared to 4% in the control group. However, a phase III randomized, double-blind crossover trial of gabapentin with a median maximal dose of 2700 mg daily involving 115 CIPN patients secondary to a variety of chemotherapeutic agents failed to demonstrate any benefit of gabapentin therapy. Recommended starting doses for gabapentin include 100–300 mg at bedtime or 100–300 mg three times a day followed by increasing daily dosage by 300 mg every 4–7 days as tolerated until reaching a target dose of 3600 mg per day divided by three doses. Trial of therapy should be over the course of 3–8 weeks for titration and 2 weeks at maximum dose to observe therapeutic benefits; side effects include sedation, dizziness, headaches, and peripheral edema. Precautions include renal insufficiency due to suboptimal drug clearance and withdrawal syndromes associated with abrupt discontinuation. Other benefits of gabapentin include improvement of sleep disturbance, hot flashes, and anxiety symptoms as well as the lack of clinically significant interactions with other drugs. Despite the many benefits of gabapentin therapy, the lack of evidence supporting efficacy in patients with CIPN has only garnered a Class C recommendation [1].

Pregabalin therapy for CIPN has been investigated in a single-arm study that included 23 gastrointestinal cancer patients with oxaliplatin-induced neuropathy. Patients were treated with pregabalin by starting at 50 mg three times a day followed by a dose increase in 50 mg increments until symptoms improved or the maximum dose of 150 mg three times daily was achieved. The patients who reported the best overall benefit were the 5 of 23 (22%) who achieved the maximum dose of 150 mg three times daily; however, a total of 48% of study participants reported an improvement in their neuropathy within 2–6 weeks of initiating therapy. As there is a lack of additional supportive evidence other than this small study, pregabalin only has a Class C recommendation for the treatment of CIPN. Dosing recommendations involve starting at 50 mg three times daily or 75 mg twice daily as tolerated followed by increasing dosage to a total of 300 mg daily after 4–7 days of therapy. After this trial, daily dosage can be increased by 150 mg a day every 4 to 7 days as tolerated until a target dose of 600 mg per day has been achieved. Similar to gabapentin, side effects include sedation, dizziness, and peripheral edema; unique to pregabalin is the possible side effect of euphoria. Precautions include concomitant psychiatric disease to the risk of euphoria, withdrawal syndromes with abrupt discontinuation, and renal insufficiency. Much like gabapentin, associated benefits include improvement with sleep disturbances and anxiety symptoms as well as having a lack of clinically significant drug interactions [1].

A randomized control trial of topical amitriptyline, baclofen, and ketamine was performed in 208 patients with CIPN secondary to a variety of chemotherapeutic agents. A pluronic lecithin organogel (PLO) compounded with baclofen 10 mg, amitriptyline HCL 40 mg (3%), and ketamine 20 mg (1.5%), abbreviated as BAK-PLO, was topically applied to areas affected by neuropathic pain twice daily and compared to a placebo gel. The intervention group had significantly greater improvement in both sensory and motor neuropathy compared to the placebo group, and there were no associated toxicities with BAK-PLO therapy. As such, topical gel with compounded baclofen, amitriptyline, and ketamine at these doses currently earns a Class B recommendation; however, it is not as strongly supported by ASCO due the need for additional supportive evidence other than this single RCT. Recommended dosage is application of affected areas 2 to 4 times daily over a trial period of 4 weeks. Currently there is no evidence of local or systemic toxicities, which gives therapy a favorable risk-benefit profile [1].

As for nonpharmacologic interventions, there is promising evidence regarding the use of neuromodulation in the treatment of CIPN. A pilot trial from 2014 investigated the effect of Scrambler therapy, a device which treats pain via noninvasive cutaneous electrostimulation, on patients with established CIPN. Among 37 enrolled patients, 25 patients were treated primarily on lower extremities while 12 were treated primarily upper extremities. All subjects reported at least 1 month or more duration of tingling and/or pain described as 4 or greater on a scale of 10 the week prior to Scrambler therapy. Patients were then treated in affected areas for up to 10 daily 30-minute sessions, and symptoms were monitored using a neuropathy questionnaire consisting of numerical scales from 0 to 10 both daily before therapy and weekly for the 10 week follow-up period after therapy. The study observed a 53% reduction in pain score from baseline to day 10, a 44% reduction in tingling, and a 37% reduction in numbness. These benefits appeared to last throughout 10 weeks of follow-up, and no significant adverse effects from therapy were observed [11].

The basis of Scrambler therapy is an attempt to substitute "pain" information with "nonpain" information by using 16 different electrical currents that simulate normal nerve action potentials in various algorithms surrounding the area(s) of pain [11]. The success of Scrambler therapy in CIPN is still being explored, and the next step will likely involve randomized controlled trials [12].

Another intervention that utilizes neuromodulation is neurofeedback. Neurofeedback acts as a form of operant conditioning designed to reinforce positive consequences of preferred behavior. In the cases of CIPN, patients have the potential to train their brains to experience decreased symptom severity. A randomized controlled trial was conducted among cancer survivors with CIPN. Participants were randomized to a neurofeedback (NFB) group, in which they received 20 sessions of NFB over a maximum of 10 weeks, or a wait-list control (WLC) group. Participants in the NFB group were instructed to watch a computer monitor with quantitative electroencephalogram (qEEG) monitoring. Participants were required to keep the amplitude of a desired EEG waveform above a certain threshold while inhibiting the amplitude of other, less desired waveforms during episodes of neuropathic pain. Visual and auditory rewards were given for voluntary changes in EEGs to more desired waveforms. Subjects in the NFB group demonstrated greater improvement (−2.43 [95% Confidence Interval, −3.58 to −1.28]) than controls (0.09 [95% Confidence Interval, −0.72 to −0.90]) on the Brief Pain Inventory (BPI) worst-pain item, a validated, self-administered questionnaire used to assess pain severity and impact of pain on daily functioning [12, 13].

As effectiveness of treatments available for CIPN is limited and variable, many patients opt for complementary therapies such as herbal medicine, acupuncture, nutrients, sensorimotor training, or mind-body therapy such as imagery and relaxation, yoga, meditation, and qigong. Success of these therapies is also quite variable and but not well studied. The *Journal of Oncology Practice*, an American Society of Clinical Oncology (ASCO) Journal, only recommends the use of Duloxetine based on the current available evidence in their most recent practice guidelines [14]. The ASCO Guidelines also list other therapies that the society does not officially recommend but presents as options for clinicians. They admit it is reasonable to try TCAs, such as nortriptyline or despiramine, for patients with CIPN; however, they encourage clinicians to discuss the paucity of scientific evidence for their efficacy in CIPN treatment as well as the potential harms, benefits, cost, and patient preferences. Although data is limited supporting gabapentin and pregabalin, the ASCO panel also believes a trial of gabapentoids is reasonable provided patients are informed about the limited scientific evidence for CIPN, potential harms, costs, and benefits from their use. Topical therapy with compounded ketamine 20 mg, baclofen 10 mg, and amitriptyline HCL 40 mg is currently not an official recommendation by the ASCO; however, due to the potential benefit exhibited by a single RCT, it is still considered reasonable to try this topical therapy so long as patients are informed of the limited scientific evidence for CIPN treatment, potential harms, benefits, and costs [14].

What Is the Prognosis of This Condition?

The long-term prognosis of CIPN is difficult to determine given the variability of chemotherapeutic agents, dosages, age of exposure, and total exposure time in different patient populations. However, a recent meta-analysis including 31 studies with data from 4179 patients suggests a high overall prevalence of CIPN, which maximizes within the first month after chemotherapeutic treatment and is less likely over time. However, meta-analysis estimated that approximately one-third of patients undergoing chemotherapy can expect to have chronic CIPN 6 months or more after the end of chemotherapy [15].

Some studies of specific chemotherapeutics have found potential improvement and in some cases reversibility with discontinuation of treatment.

Neuropathy associated with vincristine therapy is frequently found to be dose limiting, although reportedly it can worsen for a few months after discontinuation in a phenomenon known as "coasting." The process of recovery itself can last for many months; however, vincristine neuropathy has a fairly good prognosis overall as it is usually reversible [3].

Peripheral neuropathy caused by bortezomib is found to usually improve or completely resolve approximately 3 to 4 months after therapy discontinuation. One study showed that 64% of patients with at least grade 2 peripheral neuropathy secondary to bortezomib treatment experienced symptomatic improvement or resolution when compared to baseline at a median of 110 days [5].

Long-term follow-up examination of patients treated with taxanes, however, describes a prolonged effect of CIPN in some individuals often associated with a negative effect on quality of life. Similar findings have been found in patients treating with platinum compounds across multiple studies looking at neuropathy and neuropathic pain years after discontinuation of treatment [5].

There are insufficient long-term studies to determine if CIPN is curable, and at present, only treatment of symptoms is available. With regard to prevention, only avoidance, dose adjustments, or discontinuation of chemotherapy has been shown to prevent the pain associated with CIPN. However, one study showed that exercise through a moderate-intensity progressive walking and resistance exercise program over the course of 6 weeks while receiving chemotherapy experienced a reduction in some CIPN symptoms including numbness, tingling, and hot/coldness in hands/feet [16]. Although this study does show that exercise can help prevent some CIPN symptoms, it does not provide data regarding the effect of exercise on pain secondary to CIPN.

Discussion

Prevalence

The occurrence of CIPN has been studied for decades, and research has shown that therapies most likely to induce CIPN include cisplatin, oxaliplatin, vincristine, paclitaxel, and bortezomib but with varying rates. However, the occurrence of CIPN is generally related to agent dosing, both with respect to amount of drug administered and in the number of drug administrations [17].

The epidemiology of CIPN is unclear due to the variable methods of assessment and underreporting. A recent meta-analysis including 31 studies with data from 4179 patients estimated CIPN prevalence was approximately 68.1% (95% CI 57.7–78.4) among patients after the first month of chemotherapy, 60.0% (36.4–81.6) at 3 months, and 30.0% (6.4–53.5) at 6 months or more. It was noted, however, that there is significant heterogeneity in the estimates of different studies due to variable times of assessment, variance in cumulative chemotherapy dose, and different types of chemotherapy being used [15].

Differential Diagnosis

Symptoms of CIPN are not necessarily specific and can often be found in other forms of peripheral nerve disease. Before making the diagnosis of CIPN, other etiologies of peripheral neuropathy should be considered. Patients with diabetes mellitus can present with a peripheral neuropathy symptomatically similar to CIPN, which is why establishing symptom onset and progression as compared to the chemotherapeutic regimen is important to help distinguish CIPN from diabetic neuropathy. It is theorized that patients with diabetes mellitus may be at greater risk of developing CIPN due to the increased risk of underlying neuronal demyelination [7].

With regard to cancer patients, clinicians must take into account the onset and progression of neuropathic symptoms in conjunction with the timing of chemotherapy administration. In rare instances, cancer can be associated with the development of paraneoplastic neuropathy, which is theorized to be caused by onconeural antibodies which can target the peripheral nervous system and produce neurological syndromes that can present similarly to CIPN. As such, paraneoplastic neuropathies can occur in patients already undergoing chemotherapeutic treatment, making it difficult to distinguish paraneoplastic neuropathy from CIPN, or it can occur prior to the initiation of chemotherapy, which can aid in diagnosis. Anti-hu antibodies have been associated with patients with small cell lung cancer experiencing subacute sensory neuropathy, and anti-CV2 antibodies have implicated in causing sensorimotor peripheral neuropathy in patients with small cell lung cancer or thymoma [18].

Hematologic malignancies can also be associated with paraneoplastic neuropathies. Patients with multiple myeloma can experience paraneoplastic neuropathy at reported rates of 20% of patients prior to treatment, and more than 50% of patients may have objective evidence of small- or large-fiber nerve dysfunction [18]. Amyloid deposition in peripheral nerves can also be linked in paraproteinemic neuropathies such as Waldenstrom's disease [7]. Demyelinating paraneoplastic neuropathy is also associated with patients who have lymphoma [18]. The possibility of a paraneoplastic neuropathy being the etiology of patients' systems indicates the importance of a detailed history in order to establish a diagnosis of CIPN according to type of cancer, symptom onset, and timeline of therapeutic intervention.

Patients with cancer presenting with neuropathic pain can also be experiencing malignant infiltration of peripheral nerves by tumor cells. Lymphomas are commonly implicated as cancers that can infiltrate nerves or nerve roots, but they often present with prominent pain and an asymmetrical distribution, whereas CIPN more commonly presents in a symmetrical manner. Examination of cerebrospinal fluid can be helpful as cell count and protein levels are typically increased when there is malignant infiltration of nerve roots [19].

Autoimmune neuropathies should also be considered as bone marrow transplantation resulting in graft versus host disease can be associated with Guillain-Barre syndrome (GBS) and chronic inflammatory demyelinating polyradiculopathy (CIDP) [7].

Predictive Value of Different Clinical Features (Both on History and Physical Exam), and Lab Testing/Imaging

There is insufficient data to elaborate on the predictive value of different clinical features, but a systematic review and meta-analysis in 2014 examined 31 different studies that utilized several diverse methods to assess the presence or grade of CIPN. A post hoc sensitivity analysis revealed that 17 of those studies, which in all were composed of 449 patients, used neurophysiological examination (NPS: quantitative sensory testing and/or nerve conduction studies) to assess for CIPN. Sixteen of those 17 studies used NPS in conjunction with another assess method, but in these 17 studies, CIPN prevalence was higher within 1 month of chemotherapy cessation (73.3%, 58.6–87.3%), at 3 months (70.1%, 41.8–98.4%), and at 6 months or more (39.9%, 3.9–76.0%) [15]. As discussed previously, measurement of sensory and motor nerve conduction velocities (NCV), sensory nerve action potentials (SNAP), and compound muscle action potential (CMAP) together with needle electromyography (EMG) are the standard neurophysiological tests used for diagnosis.

Strength of Evidence for Different Treatment Modalities

The evidence on the effectiveness is not very strong for the available therapies that are currently being used to treat or prevent CIPN. The National Cancer Institute sponsored 15 clinical trials that studied chemo-induced neuropathy prevention (alpha lipoic acid, intravenous calcium/magnesium, vitamin E, acetyl-L-carnitine, or glutathione) or its treatment (nortriptyline, gabapentin, lamotrigine, amifostine, topical amitriptyline/ketamine, topical baclofen/amitriptyline/ketamine, or duloxetine). Of these studies, only duloxetine was shown to help neuropathic pain in established CIPN. Most medications (gabapentin, topical preparations, etc.) are used in an off-label fashion. The neuromodulation techniques have shown effectiveness in case reports and observational studies, but benefits have not been confirmed in a true large randomized clinical trial.

Future Directions or Clinical Trials in Progress

There are currently two clinical trials listed in the European Union Registry investigating ways to prevent chemotherapy-induced neuropathy. A phase II randomized study by UNICANCER is studying the effectiveness of riluzole in the prevention of oxaliplatin-induced peripheral neuropathy in patients with colorectal cancer (stage II/III) with adjuvant oxaliplatin-based chemotherapy. There is also a study by PledPharma of their product PledOx, also known as calmangafodipir, which is marketed as a chemoprotectant acetate. The current study is a phase III, double-blind, multicenter, placebo-controlled study of PledOx use on top of modified FOLFOX6 (5-fluorouracil, folinic acid, and oxaliplatin) to prevent CIPN patients with metastatic colorectal cancer [20].

A therapeutic study utilizing cryotherapy for the prevention of CIPN is currently underway at the University of Texas Health Science Center at San Antonio. Recruited patients will wear an Elasto-Gel cold glove and sock on one hand and one foot (same side) 15 minutes prior to and 15 minutes following each infusion of taxane chemotherapy. The study is designed to see if cryotherapy can alter the rate and severity of CIPN in treated extremities [21].

A randomized interventional clinical trial investigating the possible benefit of intraneural facilitation (INF), a physical therapy technique used with the aim of restoring blood flow to damaged nerves and treat neuropathic pain, is currently underway at Loma Linda University. In this study, the patients with newly diagnosed breast cancer stages I to III without preexisting peripheral neuropathy planning to received platinum-based and/or taxane-based chemotherapy will either be randomized into a treatment arm with INF or standardized muscle stretching and strength exercises in order to see if INF can help prevent or reduce the degree of chemotherapy-induced neuropathy [21].

Neuromodulation also continues to show promise for the future of CIPN treatment. The use of repetitive transcranial magnetic stimulation (rTMS) to treat CIPN is currently underway at MD Anderson Cancer Center. The study aims to see if small magnetic impulses from a magnetic coil placed against the scalp can change brain activity in a manner that will reduce the symptoms of CIPN when compared to controls who do not receive rTMS. Study participants will be composed of colorectal cancer patients with oxaliplatin-induced neuropathy, and the intervention group will complete total of 10 one-hour long rTMS sessions [12, 21].

Conclusion/Summary

Chemotherapy-induced neuropathy is a common cause of neuropathic pain. Its pathogenesis is poorly understood, is poorly evaluated by treating physicians, and often poorly managed. With ever-increasing success in treating cancer, it is more likely that cancer will become more of a chronic medical condition that is a life threatening condition. The current state of managing this painful condition is far from satisfactory, and the available medications or interventions being used to treat the problems are based on empirical evidence. Not all chemotherapeutic agents–induced neuropathy pain are the same; so what is required is a more targeted approach to investigate the mechanism of pain from each chemo agent and treat it. What it basically means is more basic science and bench research is needed before the puzzle of chemo-induced neuropathic pain will be solved. Till then we are stuck in reactionary mode of treating damaged nerves instead of a proactive approach of saving nerves from getting damaged.

References

1. Pachman DR, Watson JC, Lustberg MB, Wagner-Johnston ND, Chan A, Broadfield L, Cheung YT, Steer C, Storey DJ, Chandwani KD, Paice J. Management options for established chemotherapy-induced peripheral neuropathy. Support Care Cancer. 2014;22(8):2281–95.
2. Fehrenbacher JC. Chemotherapy-induced peripheral neuropathy. InProgress in molecular biology and translational science, vol. 131: Academic Press; 2015. p. 471–508.
3. Miltenburg NC, Boogerd W. Chemotherapy-induced neuropathy: a comprehensive survey. Cancer Treat Rev. 2014;40(7):872–82.
4. Brewer JR, Morrison G, Dolan ME, Fleming GF. Chemotherapy-induced peripheral neuropathy: current status and progress. Gynecol Oncol. 2016;140(1):176–83.
5. Grisold W, Cavaletti G, Windebank AJ. Peripheral neuropathies from chemotherapeutics and targeted agents: diagnosis, treatment, and prevention. Neuro-Oncology. 2012;14(suppl_4):iv45–54.
6. Lauria G, Hsieh ST, Johansson O, Kennedy WR, Leger JM, Mellgren SI, Nolano M, Merkies IS, Polydefkis M, Smith AG, Sommer C. European Federation of Neurological Societies/peripheral nerve society guideline on the use of skin biopsy in the diagnosis of small fiber neuropathy. Report of a joint task force of the European Federation of Neurological Societies and the peripheral nerve society. Eur J Neurol. 2010;17(7):903–e49.
7. Staff NP, Grisold A, Grisold W, Windebank AJ. Chemotherapy-induced peripheral neuropathy: a current review. Ann Neurol. 2017;81(6):772–81.
8. Carozzi VA, Canta A, Chiorazzi A. Chemotherapy-induced peripheral neuropathy: what do we know about mechanisms? Neurosci Lett. 2015;596:90–107.
9. https://online.lexi.com/lco/action/login
10. Smith EM, Pang H, Cirrincione C, Fleishman S, et al. Effect of duloxetine on pain, function, and quality of life among patients with chemotherapy-induced painful peripheral neuropathy: a ramdomized clinical trial. JAMA. 2013;309(13):1359–67.
11. Pachman DR, Weisbrod BL, Seisler DK, Barton DL, Fee-Schroeder KC, Smith TJ, Lachance DH, Liu H, Shelerud RA, Cheville AL, Loprinzi CL. Pilot evaluation of scrambler therapy for the treatment of chemotherapy-induced peripheral neuropathy. Support Care Cancer. 2015;23(4):943–51.
12. Munch J. Managing chemotherapy-induced neuropathy. MD Anderson Cancer Center. Available from: https://www.mdanderson.org/publications/oncolog/november-december-2017/manging-chemotherapy-induced-neuropathy.html.
13. Prinsloo S, Novy D, Driver L, Lyle R, Ramondetta L, Eng C, McQuade J, Lopez G, Cohen L. Randomized controlled trial of neurofeedback on chemotherapy-induced peripheral neuropathy: a pilot study. Cancer. 2017;123(11):1989–97.
14. Hershman DL, Lacchetti C, Dworkin RH, Lavoie Smith EM, Bleeker J, Cavaletti G, et al. Prevention and management of chemotherapy-induced peripheral neuropathy in survivors of adult cancers: American Society of Clinical Oncology clinical practice guideline. J Clin Oncol. 2014;32(818):1941–67.
15. Seretny M, Currie GL, Sena ES, Ramnarine S, Grant R, MacLeod MR, Colvin LA, Fallon M. Incidence, prevalence, and predictors of chemotherapy-induced peripheral neuropathy: a systematic review and meta-analysis, PAIN®. 2014;155(12):2461–70.
16. Kleckner IR, Kamen C, Gewandter JS, Mohile NA, Heckler CE, Culakova E, Fung C, Janelsins MC, Asare M, Lin PJ, Reddy PS. Effects of exercise during chemotherapy on chemotherapy-induced peripheral neuropathy: a multicenter, randomized controlled trial. Support Care Cancer. 2018;26(4):1019–28.
17. Boyette-Davis JA, Walters ET, Dougherty PM. Mechanisms involved in the development of chemotherapy-induced neuropathy. Pain Manag. 2015;5(4):285–96.
18. Park SB, Goldstein D, Krishnan AV, Lin CS, Friedlander ML, Cassidy J, Koltzenburg M, Kiernan MC. Chemotherapy-induced peripheral neurotoxicity: a critical analysis. CA Cancer J Clin. 2013;63(6):419–37.
19. Windebank AJ, Grisold W. Chemotherapy-induced neuropathy. J Peripher Nerv Syst. 2008;13(1):27–46.
20. www.clinicaltrialsregister.eu
21. https://clinicaltrials.gov

A 35-Year-Old Opioid-Tolerant Patient with Uncontrolled Pain After Surgery

46

Darshan Patel and Dalia H. Elmofty

Case Description

A 35-year-old man with a history of depression and low back pain after a fall at work 3 years earlier is scheduled for ventral hernia repair. He has chronic back pain with baseline pain scores averaging 7–8/10. His pain regimen includes oxycodone extended release 20 mg PO TID, gabapentin 600 mg PO TID, and Cymbalta 60 mg PO QHS. He has had a L4-L5 and L5-S1 laminectomy. During his visit to the anesthesia perioperative medicine clinic, the patient expresses concern regarding management of his postoperative pain. He states that, historically, even very high doses of opioid medications have failed to alleviate his pain.

On the day of surgery, the patient is visibly anxious in the preoperative holding area and refusing regional anesthesia. Intraoperatively, the patient develops tachycardia and hypertension that persists despite administering hydromorphone in divided doses. A total of 250 mcg of fentanyl and 2 mg of hydromorphone are administered. In the post-anesthesia care unit, the patient complains of significant pain, which he rates at 9/10. He is given another milligram of hydromorphone in divided doses without significant pain relief. Ultimately, the patient is started on a hydromorphone PCA along with methadone 5 mg IV every 8 hours and a ketamine infusion with improvement in his pain.

D. Patel
Department of Anesthesiology, St. Francis Medical Center, Evanston, IL, USA
e-mail: dpatel1@dacc.uchicago.edu

D. H. Elmofty (✉)
Department of Anesthesia, University of Chicago, Chicago, IL, USA
e-mail: delmofty@dacc.uchicago.edu

What Is Your Preliminary Diagnosis?

The preliminary diagnosis is opioid tolerance. Opioid tolerance is defined by the United States Food and Drug Administration (FDA) as the use of greater than or equal to 60 mg of oral morphine equivalents per day for a period of 7 days or longer [1–3]. Clinically, opioid tolerance is a state of adaptation in which exposure to a drug induces changes that result in a diminution of one or more of the drug's effects over time. However, development of opioid tolerance is not necessarily a sign of addiction [4]. Often, a higher dose of the opioid is necessary to achieve pain relief [5].

How Is the Diagnosis Confirmed?

Diagnosis of opioid tolerance is a clinical one that can be suspected in patients with minimal pain relief despite being treated with opioid pain medications. These patients have been on opioid

T. Malik (ed.), *Practical Chronic Pain Management*, https://doi.org/10.1007/978-3-030-46675-6_46

therapy for longer than two weeks while requiring escalating doses.

What Is the Pathophysiology of This Condition?

Opioid tolerance is thought to occur secondary to a combination of pharmacokinetic and pharmacodynamic changes. The pharmacokinetic changes include upregulation of the metabolic process responsible for elimination of the drug; the pharmacodynamic changes include downregulation of the opioid receptor or desensitization. Downregulation, or a decrease in the number of active receptor sites, occurs from chronic agonist exposure. Concomitantly, it is postulated that there is decreased action or desensitization via an uncoupling of the opioid receptor from the GTP binding subunit [6]. The opioid receptor is linked to a G-protein, which, when activated, leads to a decrease in cyclic adenosine 3, 5-monophosphate (cAMP) that subsequently inhibits sodium and calcium influx. Over time, changes in G-protein function can lead to desensitization and development of opioid tolerance.

How Is This Problem Managed?

Managing opioid tolerance requires first dispelling several misconceptions regarding its development, including the following: (1) It takes time for opioid tolerance to develop and the perioperative period is too short of a timeframe for its manifestation; (2) Even if opioid tolerance occurs, the problem can be overcome by simply giving more opioids, which are not that costly; (3) With increased opioid analgesic tolerance comes increased tolerance to side effects; (4) Increasing opioid doses does not increase the risk to the patient.

However, studies show that opioid tolerance can develop quickly—within a matter of hours—in a phenomenon known as tachyphylaxis. Patients may already be tolerant to opioids before they present to the perioperative setting, often from presurgical opioid use. There is a difference in tolerance rate and degree among the various opioid receptors. Opioid tolerance is quickest for analgesia, less for respiratory depressant effects, and least for the slowing of gastrointestinal (GI) motility. The decrease in GI motility is especially significant in the perioperative setting where faster return of GI transit and earlier oral intake are associated with earlier hospital discharge and subsequent cost savings. Adequately treating the opioid-tolerant patient's pain may require higher doses of opioids compared to treating the opioid-naive patient's pain; this puts the opioid-tolerant patient at higher risk for respiratory depression [7].

When a patient develops tolerance to an opioid, opioid rotation should be considered. Opioid rotation involves switching from one opioid to another as there is incomplete cross-tolerance. The rationale is that the rotated opioid will act on another receptor subtype. It is recommended to calculate opioid equivalent dosing when switching from one drug to another and then starting the patient on the new drug with at least a 25–50% reduction in equivalent dosing [4, 8].

Managing patient expectations plays a key role in the perioperative management of the opioid-tolerant patient. Complex-pain patients require special consideration in each phase of the perioperative process: preoperative, intraoperative, and postoperative.

Phase 1: Preoperative Management

Surgeons should refer patients with preexisting pain syndromes to anesthesia preoperative clinics or pain clinics to establish their baseline pain disorders, manage expectations, and implement preemptive analgesic measures. This visit allows the anesthesiologist to review the patient's current pain regimen and ascertain what has and has not worked in the past [8]. Moreover, listening to the patient's concerns and validating the complexity of the patient's pain may relieve some of his or her anxiety and allow the physician to set realistic expectations of postoperative pain [8]. Pain scoring systems can be used to identify patients at risk for developing severe postoperative pain [9].

Patients should be educated about multimodal analgesia, including discussing regional techniques such as epidurals or peripheral nerve blocks and/or catheters. Gulur et al. found that opioid-tolerant patients have a significantly longer length of stay and higher rates of 30-day readmissions when compared to a control group [1]. A study by Duncan et al. demonstrated the cost-saving effects of multimodal analgesia, even in non-opioid-tolerant patients. Given the cost savings afforded by multimodal analgesia, and the added benefit of decreased risk for opioid-related adverse events, a multimodal approach should be an essential part of the patient's perioperative care plan.

On the day of surgery, non-steroidal anti-inflammatory drugs (NSAIDs), non-aspirin pain relievers (acetaminophen), and membrane stabilizers such as gabapentin can be given preoperatively to reduce the requirement of postoperative opioids [4]. These modalities also form an integral part of many enhanced recovery after surgery (ERAS) pathways that have been created to achieve early recuperation [10]. ERAS a paradigm shift in perioperative care that began in colorectal surgery has since spread to almost all major surgical specialties because of significant improvements in clinical outcomes and cost savings. ERAS is an evidence-based, multimodal, multidisciplinary approach to the surgical patient that involves surgeons, anesthesiologists, unit staff members/nurses, and often an ERAS coordinator working together to implement a care protocol. The care protocols published by the ERAS Society are evidence-based guidelines for several surgical procedures, including the following: shift from "NPO after midnight" to carbohydrate loading via clear liquids up to 2 hours prior to surgery; shift from a large, open procedure to a minimally invasive procedure; shift to approach that includes early mobilization, early removal of drains and tubes, and earlier resumption of PO intake (even the same day as the operation). The benefits of ERAS protocols include a 30% to 50% reduction in hospital stays, fewer complications and readmissions, and lower costs [11].

Phase 2: Intraoperative Pain Management

Anesthetic technique can influence the development of opioid tolerance. For patients with a history of chronic pain requiring opioid therapy, an intraoperative multimodal therapy can facilitate postoperative pain control and reduce the risk of developing opioid tolerance in the postoperative timeframe (see Tables 46.1, 46.2, and 46.3). One benefit of multimodal therapy is a reduction in the overall use of opioid medications, which is especially vital during these times of national drug shortages and the growing problem of the opioid epidemic.

Intraoperative multimodal therapy consists mainly of IV adjunct therapy and IV infusion therapy; regional anesthesia should also be considered.

- *IV adjunct therapy* (Table 46.1). IV adjunct therapy includes methadone, buprenorphine, acetaminophen, and ketorolac.

  Methadone has become the mainstay for treating chronic pain, especially for cancer and neuropathic pain. Yet, in the perioperative setting, its utilization for treating acute pain has been minimal, largely because of many misconceptions regarding the onset, duration, and metabolism of methadone. These misconceptions, which have been debunked, include widely variable clearance, longer time to peak analgesia, short duration of analgesia relative to its elimination half-life, and cross reactions with other medications. Methadone's potential benefits include its duration of action and incomplete cross-tolerance with opioid rotation. It may, however, be associated with respiratory depression, sedation, and prolongation of QT.

  For treating acute pain, methadone can provide many advantages over the conventional acute pain regimen of opioids. Methadone is both a μ receptor agonist and has properties of NMDA antagonism. This antagonism is thought to counteract the development of opioid-induced tolerance and hyperalgesia [12–14]. Methadone also provides analgesia

Table 46.1 Intraoperative multimodal therapy: intravenous adjunct therapy

Medication	Dose	Mechanism of action	Possible side effects
IV methadone	2.5–5 mg q 8-12 hr	μ receptor agonist, N-methyl-D-aspartate (NMDA) receptor antagonist	Respiratory depression, sedation, prolonged QT
IV buprenorphine	300 mcg q 6-8 h	Partial μ receptor agonist, ORL-1 agonist, kappa receptor antagonist	Respiratory depression, sedation
IV ketorolac	400–800 mg q 6 hr	Inhibits cyclooxygenase	Renal insufficiency, platelet inhibition, GI upset
IV acetaminophen	1 g q 6 hr	Unknown	Hepatic toxicity
IV ketamine	0.5 mg/kg bolus prior to incision 0.5 mg/kg/hr infusion	NMDA receptor antagonist	Psychomimetic

Adapted from Elmofty [21]

Table 46.2 Intraoperative multimodal therapy: infusion therapy

Medication	Dose	Mechanism of action	Possible side effects
IV ketamine	0.5 mg/kg bolus prior to incision 0.5 mg/kg/hr infusion	NMDA receptor antagonist	Psychomimetic
IV magnesium	30–50 mg/kg bolus prior to incision 10-15 mg /kg/hr infusion	NMDA receptor antagonist	Respiratory depression, hypotension, cardiac depression
IV lidocaine	1.5 mg/kg bolus prior to incision 1.5 mg/kg/hr infusion	Na + channel blocker	Nausea, vomiting, dizziness, dysrhythmia, methemoglobin
IV dexmedetomidine	0.5–2 mcg/kg bolus prior to incision 0.2–0.7mcg/kg/hr infusion	Alpha 2 agonist	Hypotension, bradycardia, sedation

**IV* intravenous, *GI* gastrointestinal
Adapted from Elmofty [21]

by inhibiting the reuptake of serotonin and norepinephrine (SNRI).

Buprenorphine is a kappa antagonist, partial μ receptor agonist, and an opioid receptor like-1 (ORL-1) agonist. As a kappa antagonist, it may prevent opioid-induced tolerance and hyperalgesia [14].

Acetaminophen is an analgesic and antipyretic medication. The exact mechanism through which acetaminophen exerts these effects has yet to be fully elucidated. However, it is postulated that acetaminophen may raise the pain threshold by inhibiting the nitric oxide (NO) pathway, which is mediated by a variety of neurotransmitter receptors, including substance P and NMDA. The antipyretic effects are likely secondary to inhibition of prostaglandin synthesis and release in the central nervous system and its effects on the anterior hypothalamic heat-regulating center [15].

Ketorolac, a member of the NSAID family of drugs, is unique in its availability as an IV formulation. NSAIDs have properties of anti-inflammation, antipyresis, and analgesia. NSAIDs work by inhibiting cyclooxygenase enzymes, which inhibit production of prostaglandins, which are implicated in peripheral and central sensitization by facilitating the release of excitatory neurotransmitters [16].

- *IV infusion therapy* (Table 46.2). IV infusion therapy includes ketamine, magnesium, lidocaine, and dexmedetomidine.

Ketamine and *magnesium* are used intraoperatively to prevent opioid-induced tolerance

Table 46.3 Regional techniques for abdominal surgery

Analgesia desired	Regional block(s)
Somatic and visceral organs	Epidural Paravertebral block
Skin and muscles of the anterior abdominal wall in upper abdomen	Subcostal block
Skin and muscles of the anterior abdominal wall in lower abdomen	Transversus abdominis plane block (TAP)

Adapted from Elmofty [21]

and hyperalgesia [4, 8, 17, 18]. Both are antagonists of the NMDA receptor.

Lidocaine is a local anesthetic with antiarrhythmic properties. Its use as an analgesic is derived from its property of stabilizing neuronal cell membranes by binding and inhibiting voltage-gated sodium channels. This inhibition relieves pain by blocking the initiation and conduction of neuronal impulses [19].

Dexmedetomidine is an alpha-2 receptor agonist that provides analgesia along with sedation without respiratory depression by binding to receptors in the spinal cord and locus ceruleus. In this manner, it may also help prevent opioid tolerance. When dexmedetomidine is used in addition to morphine PCA, Lin et al. demonstrated a 29% decrease in opioid consumption and an overall reduction in morphine-related side effects when compared to conventional morphine PCA alone [20].

- *Regional anesthesia* (Table 46.3). Regional anesthesia such as neuraxial anesthesia and peripheral nerve blocks as well as paravertebral blocks should also be considered [21].

  Neuraxial anesthesia for abdominal surgery. Thoracic neuraxial anesthesia is a cornerstone for perioperative pain management after major abdominal surgery. In addition to the desired analgesia, thoracic neuraxial anesthesia provides the added benefit of improved intestinal motility and reduced perioperative cardiovascular events [22].

  Contraindications to neuraxial analgesia include coagulopathy, infection of the skin overlying the point of needle entry, and patient refusal. For the purposes of standardization and patient safety, the American Society of Regional Anesthesia (ASRA) published guidelines for the placement and removal of indwelling catheters or single shot injections.

  Peripheral nerve blocks for abdominal surgery. The cutaneous innervations of the anterior abdominal wall arise from the anterior rami of the T7-T11, T12 subcostal, and L1 (iliohypogastric and ilioinguinal) nerves. The intercostal nerves course between the internal oblique and the transversus abdominis muscle. The transversus abdominis plane block (TAP) is one peripheral nerve block that can be performed for postoperative abdominal pain control. The TAP block was initially introduced in 2000 as a blind technique involving the injection of local anesthetic into the lumbar triangle of petit. It has since evolved to include surgical and ultrasound guided approaches. The fascial layer between the internal oblique muscles and the transversus abdominis muscles forms the transversus abdominis plane. The spinal nerves mentioned above pass between these layers [23]. Although not a technically challenging procedure, liver lacerations and other complications have been reported. Using ultrasound guidance helps to reduce these risks. The TAP blocks should be performed bilaterally to provide analgesia for a midline incision. Although studies vary in the coverage level that can be achieved with a single shot administration of local anesthetics, generally at least a T10 level can be attained. Subcostal blocks can help supplement coverage and provide reliable analgesia from T7-T10.

  Paravertebral blocks have been described for thoracic and breast surgery but are less frequently used for abdominal surgery. A paravertebral block is a unilateral block of the spinal nerve, including the dorsal and ventral rami, and the sympathetic chain ganglion. It provides somatic and sympathetic coverage, but no visceral coverage unless there is spread into the epidural space. Postoperative abdominal pain can be effectively controlled with a multimodal approach that incorporates the use of regional anesthesia [24].

Phase 3: Postoperative Pain Management

Multimodal analgesia should be continued postoperatively. Epidural catheters can remain in place for continuous infusions and/or intermittent boluses. Infusion therapy can also be continued in the postoperative time frame. IV lidocaine infusion therapy has been shown to reduce morphine consumption up to 24 hours after abdominal surgery [25].

It is vital to remember that when employing regional techniques, baseline opioids should only be decreased up to 50% as the patient taking chronic opioids can go into opioid withdrawal perioperatively [4, 8]. Because opioid dosing regimens vary greatly for the opioid-naive patient versus the opioid-tolerant patient, standard dosing for all patients is not an effective treatment strategy [5].

Postoperative pain assessment should include the conventional visual analogue scale (VAS), but more emphasis should be placed on recovery of function, early ambulation, and recovery of bowel and bladder functions, which is in line with many ERAS guidelines [10].

When working with opioid-tolerant patients, it is necessary to also be sensitive to the psychological aspect of their care. Patients will often exhibit pain catastrophizing or the tendency to magnify the threat value of pain and to feel helpless within the context of pain. Patients with chronic pain tend to be more sensitive to painful conditions and are more likely to be deconditioned due to their underlying chronic pain disorder. These patients often are frustrated with the healthcare system secondary to incomplete coverage of their pain from providers' hesitation to prescribe the higher doses required by opioid-tolerant patients. These patients are also more likely to be irritable from dysfunction in their personal lives and from chronic sleep deprivation secondary to pain [8, 26]. Pain scores for these patients are higher and take longer to decrease [25].

What Is the Prognosis of This Condition?

Opioid-induced tolerance seems to be a chronic and persistent problem that is associated with a significantly longer length of stay and a greater 30-day-all-cause readmission rate when compared to the control group ($P < 0.01$) [1]. This is due to one of three possibilities: (1) inadequate control of perioperative pain, (2) chronic opioid users are prone to androgen deficiencies, leading to decreased muscle mass and fatigue and ultimately to a prolonged recovery after an acute event, and (3) chronic opioid use leads to immunosuppression that makes the patient more prone to infections [1].

Discussion

Prevalence

In 2011, the Institute of Medicine estimated that 100 million individuals in the United States were in pain. However, the incidence has been difficult to analyze because the calculations and definitions vary from source to source. In 2001, JCAHO advocated for pain to be the "fifth vital sign" and ever since the use of opioids for pain management has increased exponentially each year [1].

Opioids are mistakenly thought of as the first line of treatment for pain. The United States appears to be the main consumer of opioids, accounting for 56% of morphine and 81% of oxycodone usage globally [2]. It is estimated that 35 million Americans, or about 14% of the US population, have misused prescription opioids during their lifetimes [6]. And there is growing evidence that opioids may have a negative impact on postoperative pain.

Differential Diagnosis

Chronic opioid exposure can lead to opioid-induced tolerance or opioid-induced hyperalgesia (OIH). Clinical differentiation between the two can be challenging. Both opioid-induced tolerance and OIH are included in the differential of postoperative pain that is difficult to control. For many practitioners the initial response is to prescribe more medications, often escalating the opioid dose. If no response is observed with this

Table 46.4 OIH mechanism of action and treatment options

Mechanism of action	Inactivation of μ-receptor Genetic polymorphisms of COMT Enhanced response to nociceptive neurotransmitters Spinal dynorphin release Activation of dorsal horn NMDA receptors
Treatment options	Decrease/discontinue opioid Employ opioid rotation Add NMDA receptor antagonists

Table 46.5 Opioid tolerance mechanism of action and treatment options

Mechanism of action	Possible down-regulation of opioid receptors Right-shift of the opioid dose-response curve
Treatment options	Increase opioid dosage

**NMDA* N-methyl-D aspartate, *COMT* Catechol-O-methyltransferase, *OIH* opioid-induced hyperalgesia
Adapted from Elmofty [21]

empiric method, the practitioner should consider the development of opioid-induced tolerance or OIH. Tables 46.4 and 46.5 summarize the causes of opioid non-responsiveness and the mechanisms of action and treatment options for both opioid-induced tolerance and OIH.

Opioid-induced hyperalgesia is a paradoxical response to opioids. Patients experience a worsening of pain with administration of opioids [4, 8]. OIH differs from opioid tolerance in that an increase in dose worsens pain and a reduction in dose alleviates pain. Quantitative sensory testing (QST) can be utilized before initiating opioid therapy and at routine intervals after initiating therapy to detect the development of OIH [27].

The reasons why OIH affects some, but not all, patients are not completely understood. Some animal models indicate that sex may play a role. For instance, in modeling male and female rats, females were found to develop OIH earlier and for a longer duration of time than males [28]. Genetic predisposition may also be a factor. It has been postulated that catechol-O methyltransferase (COMT) polymorphisms may play a role in predisposing certain patients to OIH [29]. Psychosomatic factors such as increased preoperative anxiety regarding pain may also play a role in patient susceptibility to developing OIH [30].

Opioid tolerance is a physiological process in which there is a progressive lack of response to opioids. It often requires an escalation in dosing to elicit the same effect. A right-shift of the dose-response curve is seen in opioid tolerance.

Summary

- Opioid tolerance is a state of adaptation in which exposure to a drug induces changes that result in a reduction of one or more of the drug's effects over time.
- Opioid tolerance is defined as the use of greater than or equal to 60 mg of oral morphine equivalents per day for a period of 7 days or longer.
- Opioid tolerance is thought to occur from a combination of pharmacokinetic and pharmacodynamic changes.
- Diagnosis of opioid tolerance is a clinical one, which can be suspected in a patient with minimal pain relief despite escalating doses of opioid pain medications.
- When a patient develops tolerance to an opioid, the problem is managed by opioid rotation and the use of adjunct therapy.
- For patients with a history of chronic pain requiring opioid therapy, a multimodal approach and introduction of adjunct therapy perioperatively may improve postoperative pain control and reduce the risk of developing OIH and opioid tolerance.
- It is crucial for surgeons to refer patients with preexisting pain problems to anesthesia preoperative clinics or pain clinics. During these visits patients must be educated about multimodal analgesia, which decreases opioid-related adverse events, length of hospital stays, and overall costs.
- When working with opioid-tolerant patients, it is also necessary to be sensitive to the psychological aspect of their care.

References

1. Gulur P, Williams L, Chaudhary S, Koury K, Jaff M. Opioid tolerance—a predictor of increased length of stay and higher readmission rates. Pain Physician. 2014;17(4):E503–7.
2. International Narcotics Control Board. Narcotic drugs technical reports. Estimated world requirements for 2011. https://www.incb.org. Accessed 24 May 2018.
3. Food and Drug Administration. Extended-release (ER) and long-acting (LA) opioid analgesics risk evaluation and mitigation strategy (REMS). FDA REMS modification. 2015;10.
4. Hadi I, Morley-Forster PK, Dain S, Horrill K, Moulin DE. Brief review: perioperative management of the patient with chronic non-cancer pain. Can J Anesth. 2006;53(12):1190–9.
5. Lewis NL, Williams JE. Acute pain management in patients receiving opioids for chronic and cancer pain. Continuing Education in Anaesthesia, Critical Care & Pain. 2005;5(4):127–9.
6. Mahathanaruk M, Hitt J, de LeonCasasola OA. Perioperative management of the opioid tolerant patient for orthopedic surgery. Anesthesiol Clin. 2014;32(4):923–32.
7. Hayhurst CJ, Durieux ME. Differential opioid tolerance and opioid-induced hyperalgesia: a clinical reality. Anesthesiology. 2016;124(2):483–8.
8. Tumber PS. Optimizing perioperative analgesia for the complex pain patient: medical and interventional strategies. Canadian J Anesth. 2014;61(2):131–40.
9. Janssen KJ, Kalkman CJ, Grobbee DE, Bonsel GJ, Moons KG, Vergouwe Y. The risk of severe postoperative pain: modification and validation of a clinical prediction rule. Anesth Analg. 2008;107(4):1330–9.
10. Melnyk M, Casey RG, Black P, Koupparis AJ. Enhanced recovery after surgery (ERAS) protocols: time to change practice? Can Urol Assoc J. 2011;5:342.
11. Ljungqvist O, Scott M, Fearon KC. Enhanced recovery after surgery: a review. JAMA Surg. 2017;152(3):292–8.
12. Manfredi PL, Houde RW. Prescribing methadone, a unique analgesic. J Support Oncol. 2003;1(3):216.
13. Toombs JD, Kral LA. Methadone treatment for pain states. Am Fam Physician. 2005;71(7):1353–8.
14. Lee M, Silverman S, Hansen H, Vikram P. A comprehensive review of opioid-induced hyperalgesia. Pain Physician. 2011;14:145–61.
15. NCI Thesaurus [Internet]. Ncit.nci.nih.gov. 2018 [cited 24 May 2018]. Available from: https://ncit.nci.nih.gov/ncitbrowser/ConceptReport.jsp?dictionary=NCI_Thesaurus&ns=NCI_Thesaurus&code=C198.
16. Tröster A, Sittl R, Singler B, Schmelz M, Schüttler J, Koppert W. Modulation of remifentanil-induced analgesia and postinfusion hyperalgesia by parecoxib in humans. Anesthesiology. 2006;105(5):1016–23.
17. Koppert W, Sittl R, Scheuber K, Alsheimer M, Schmelz M, Schüttler J. Differential modulation of remifentanil-induced analgesia and postinfusion hyperalgesia by S-ketamine and clonidine in humans. Anesthesiology. 2003;99(1):152–9.
18. De Oliveira GS, Castro-Alves LJ, Khan JH, McCarthy RJ. Perioperative systemic magnesium to minimize postoperative pain: a meta-analysis of randomized controlled trials. Anesthesiology. 2013;119(1):178–90.
19. NCI Thesaurus [Internet]. Ncit.nci.nih.gov. 2018 [cited 24 May 2018]. Available from: https://ncit.nci.nih.gov/ncitbrowser/ConceptReport.jsp?dictionary=NCI_Thesaurus&version=18.03d&ns=ncit&code=C614&key=517506826&b=1&n=null.
20. Lin TF, Yeh YC, Lin FS, Wang YP, Lin CJ, Sun WZ, Fan SZ. Effect of combining dexmedetomidine and morphine for intravenous patient-controlled analgesia. Br J Anaesth. 2008;102(1):117–22.
21. Elmofty D. Opioid-induced hyperalgesia, tolerance and chronic postsurgical pain; a dilemma complicating postoperative pain management. In: Anitescu A, editor. Pain management review: a problem-based learning approach. New York, NY, USA: Oxford University Press. p. 303–9.
22. Freise H, Van Aken HK. Risks and benefits of thoracic epidural anaesthesia. Br J Anaesth. 2011;107(6):859–68.
23. Siddiqui MR, Sajid MS, Uncles DR, Cheek L, Baig MK. A meta-analysis on the clinical effectiveness of transversus abdominis plane block. J Clin Anesth. 2011;23(1):7–14.
24. Finnerty O, Carney J, McDonnell JG. Trunk blocks for abdominal surgery. Anaesthesia. 2010;65(s1):76–83.
25. Dunn LK, Durieux ME. Perioperative use of intravenous lidocaine. Anesthesiology. 2017;126(4):729–37.
26. Shah S, Kapoor S, Durkin B. Analgesic management of acute pain in the opioid-tolerant patient. Curr Opin Anesthesiol. 2015;28(4):398–402.
27. Silverman SM. Opioid induced hyperalgesia: clinical implications for the pain practitioner. Pain Physician. 2009;12(3):679–84.
28. Juni A, Cai M, Stankova M, Waxman AR, Arout C, Klein G, Dahan A, Hruby VJ, Mogil JS, Kest B. Sex-specific mediation of opioid-induced hyperalgesia by the melanocortin-1 receptor. Anesthesiology. 2010;112(1):181–8.
29. Jensen KB, Lonsdorf TB, Schalling M, Kosek E, Ingvar M. Increased sensitivity to thermal pain following a single opiate dose is influenced by the COMT val158met polymorphism. PLoS One. 2009;4(6):e6016.
30. Edwards R, Wasan A, Jamison R. Hyperalgesia in pain patients at elevated risk for opioid misuse. J Pain. 2010;11(4):S45.

Correction to: 45-Year-Old Man with Leg Pain and Numbness

Robert Fuino and Waqar Waheed

Correction to: Chapter 32 in T. Malik (ed.), *Practical Chronic Pain Management*, https://doi.org/10.1007/978-3-030-46675-6_32

The content of the chapter 32 has been changed. In the originally published version, chapters 32 and 40 were duplicates of the same chapter. The former chapter 32 has now been replaced with a new chapter entitled "45-Year-Old Man with Leg Pain and Numbness."

The updated version of this chapter can be found at https://doi.org/10.1007/978-3-030-46675-6_32

T. Malik (ed.), *Practical Chronic Pain Management*, https://doi.org/10.1007/978-3-030-46675-6_47

Index

T. Malik (ed.), *Practical Chronic Pain Management*, https://doi.org/10.1007/978-3-030-46675-6

P

GPSR Compliance

The European Union's (EU) General Product Safety Regulation (GPSR) is a set of rules that requires consumer products to be safe and our obligations to ensure this.

If you have any concerns about our products, you can contact us on ProductSafety@springernature.com

In case Publisher is established outside the EU, the EU authorized representative is:

Springer Nature Customer Service Center GmbH
Europaplatz 3
69115 Heidelberg, Germany

Batch number: 10732807

Printed by Printforce, the Netherlands